MW01493001

COMBAT
Orthopedic Surgery

Lessons Learned in Iraq and Afghanistan

STRYKER QUALITY
STRYKER EXPERIENCE
STRYKER TRAUMA AND EXTREMITIES

COMBAT
Orthopedic Surgery

Lessons Learned in Iraq and Afghanistan

Edited by

LTC Brett D. Owens, MD, MC USA
Chief, Orthopaedic Surgery Service
Keller Army Hospital
West Point, New York

LTC Philip J. Belmont Jr, MD, MC USA
Program Director
Orthopaedic Surgery Residency Program
William Beaumont Army Medical Center/
Texas Tech University Health Sciences Center
El Paso, Texas

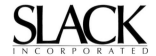
SLACK
INCORPORATED

www.slackbooks.com

ISBN: 978-1-55642-965-1

Copyright © 2011 by SLACK Incorporated

Cover/section opener illustration by LTC Anthony A. Beardmore, MD, MC USA, *San Antonio Military Medical Center, San Antonio, Texas.*

All rights reserved. No part of this book may be reproduced, stored in a retrieval system or transmitted in any form or by any means, electronic, mechanical, photocopying, recording or otherwise, without written permission from the publisher, except for brief quotations embodied in critical articles and reviews.

The procedures and practices described in this book should be implemented in a manner consistent with the professional standards set for the circumstances that apply in each specific situation. Every effort has been made to confirm the accuracy of the information presented and to correctly relate generally accepted practices. The authors, editor, and publisher cannot accept responsibility for errors or exclusions or for the outcome of the material presented herein. There is no expressed or implied warranty of this book or information imparted by it. Care has been taken to ensure that drug selection and dosages are in accordance with currently accepted/recommended practice. Due to continuing research, changes in government policy and regulations, and various effects of drug reactions and interactions, it is recommended that the reader carefully review all materials and literature provided for each drug, especially those that are new or not frequently used. Any review or mention of specific companies or products is not intended as an endorsement by the author or publisher.

SLACK Incorporated uses a review process to evaluate submitted material. Prior to publication, educators or clinicians provide important feedback on the content that we publish. We welcome feedback on this work.

Published by: SLACK Incorporated
                   6900 Grove Road
                   Thorofare, NJ 08086 USA
                   Telephone: 856-848-1000
                   Fax: 856-848-6091
                   www.slackbooks.com

Contact SLACK Incorporated for more information about other books in this field or about the availability of our books from distributors outside the United States.

Library of Congress Cataloging-in-Publication Data
    Combat orthopedic surgery : lessons learned in Iraq and Afghanistan / [edited by] Brett D. Owens, Philip J. Belmont Jr.
        p. ; cm.
    Includes bibliographical references and index.
    ISBN 978-1-55642-965-1 (alk. paper)
    1. Surgery, Military. 2. Orthopedic surgery. 3. Afghan War, 2001---Medical care. 4. Iraq War, 2003---Medical care. I. Owens, Brett D., 1972- II. Belmont, Philip J., 1969-
    [DNLM: 1. Orthopedic Procedures--methods. 2. Afghan Campaign 2001-. 3. Evidence-Based Medicine. 4. Iraq War, 2003 -. 5. Military Medicine. 6. Musculoskeletal System--injuries. WE 190]
    RD153.C66 2011
    617.9'9--dc22
                                    2010050086

For permission to reprint material in another publication, contact SLACK Incorporated. Authorization to photocopy items for internal, personal, or academic use is granted by SLACK Incorporated provided that the appropriate fee is paid directly to Copyright Clearance Center. Prior to photocopying items, please contact the Copyright Clearance Center at 222 Rosewood Drive, Danvers, MA 01923 USA; phone: 978-750-8400; web site: www.copyright.com; email: info@copyright.com.

Printed in the United States of America

Last digit is print number: 10 9 8 7 6 5 4 3 2 1

Dedication

I would like to thank my wife, Julie, without whom none of this would have been possible, and my children—Cassidy, Ryan, Jocelyn, and Bennett—who inspire me every day. I also thank my partner and friend, Philip—the perfect person to join me on this endeavor.

—*LTC Brett D. Owens, MD*

I would like to thank my wife, Madra, for her love, support, and never-ending friendship as well as my loving children, Alanna and Ava. The family we have created has brought more joy and meaning to my life than I could have ever imagined.

—*LTC Philip J. Belmont Jr, MD*

Contents

Acknowledgments

The authors would like to express their gratitude for the patriotism, fidelity, and honor exhibited by the US military force during the Iraq and Afghanistan Wars. These brave soldiers, sailors, marines, and airmen should always be recognized and remembered for their daily sacrifices, as each individual made a personal choice to meet the call to arms when the United States needed their service. The all-volunteer force's exceptional performance coupled with the sacrifice of its human treasure upon the battlefields of Iraq and Afghanistan should continually remind us all that service in the defense of the country is a fundamental responsibility of citizenship.

War is an ugly thing, but not the ugliest of things. The decayed and degraded state of moral and patriotic feeling which thinks that nothing is worth war is much worse. The person who has nothing for which he is willing to fight, nothing which is more important than his own personal safety, is a miserable creature and has no chance of being free unless made and kept so by the exertions of better men than himself.
—John Stuart Mill, English economist and philosopher (1806-1873)

The editors would like to thank SLACK Incorporated for their support, namely John Bond, April Billick, Jennifer Cahill, Debra Toulson, Michelle Gatt, and Carrie Kotlar. Carrie, we could not have done it without you!

The views presented in the book are those of the individual authors and do not necessarily represent the views of the Department of Defense, its Components, or the US Government.

About the Editors

LTC Brett D. Owens, MD is a Distinguished Graduate of the United States Military Academy in West Point, New York. He graduated from the Georgetown University School of Medicine in Washington, DC and completed his internship at Walter Reed Army Medical Center. He completed his orthopaedic surgery residency at the University of Massachusetts and the John A. Feagin Jr Sports Medicine Fellowship at West Point. He is currently an Associate Professor of Surgery (Orthopaedics) at the Uniformed Services University of the Health Sciences in Bethesda, Maryland. He served as an orthopaedic surgeon with the 86th Combat Support Hospital in Iraq and is currently Chief of Orthopaedic Surgery Service, Keller Army Hospital, West Point, New York.

LTC Philip J. Belmont Jr, MD is a Distinguished Graduate of the United States Military Academy in West Point, New York. He graduated from the Duke University School of Medicine in Durham, North Carolina and completed his internship and orthopaedic surgery residency at Walter Reed Army Medical Center in Washington, DC. He is currently an Associate Professor of Surgery (Orthopaedics) at the Uniformed Services University of the Health Sciences in Bethesda, Maryland. He served as an orthopaedic surgeon with the 228th Combat Support Hospital in Iraq and is currently the Chief of Adult Reconstruction and Program Director of the William Beaumont Army Medical Center/Texas Tech University Health Sciences Center Orthopaedic Surgery Residency Program at William Beaumont Army Medical Center, El Paso, Texas.

Contributing Authors

LTC(P) Romney C. Andersen, MD, MC USA
(Chapters 21, 27)
Chairman, Department of
Orthopaedics and Rehabilitation
Walter Reed National Military Medical Center
Washington, DC
Uniformed Services University of the Health Sciences
Bethesda, Maryland

LTC(P) Martin F. Baechler, MD, MC USA (Chapter 19)
Hand Surgeon
Department of Orthopaedics and Rehabilitation
Walter Reed National Military Medical Center
Bethesda, Maryland

CPT Michael J. Beltran, MD, MC USA (Chapter 21)
Department of Orthopaedics and Rehabilitation
San Antonio Military Medical Center
San Antonio, Texas

James P. Bradley, MD (Chapters 18, 25)
Department of Surgery
Division of Plastic and Reconstructive Surgery
University of California
Los Angeles, California

Trevor S. Brown, PhD (Chapter 9)
Scientist
The Regenerative Medicine Department
Operational and Undersea Medicine
Naval Medical Research Center
Silver Spring, Maryland

COL Chester C. Buckenmaier III, MD, MC USA
(Chapter 19)
Chief, Defense and Veterans
Pain Management Initiative
Walter Reed Army Medical Center
Associate Professor of Anesthesiology
Uniformed Services University of the Health Sciences
Bethesda, Maryland

MAJ Travis C. Burns, MD, MC USA (Chapter 24)
Orthopaedic Surgery Service
Keller Army Community Hospital
West Point, New York

LCDR Joseph Carney, MD, MC USN (Chapter 15)
Orthopaedic Surgery Residency Director
Department of Orthopaedic Surgery
Naval Medical Center San Diego
San Diego, California

CAPT D.C. Covey, MD, MC USN (Chapter 15)
Chairman, Department of Orthopaedic Surgery
Naval Medical Center San Diego
San Diego, California

CPT Jonathan F. Dickens, MD, MC USA (Chapter 26)
Department of Orthopaedics and Rehabilitation
Walter Reed National Military Medical Center
Washington, DC

MAJ Matthew L. Drake, MD, MC USA (Chapter 19)
Hand Surgeon
Orthopaedic Surgery Service
Tripler Army Medical Center
Honolulu, Hawaii

COL Gerald L. Farber, MD, MC USA (Chapter 17)
Orthopaedic Surgery Service
Tripler Army Medical Center
Honolulu, Hawaii
Department of Surgery
Uniformed Services University of the Health Sciences
Bethesda, Maryland

COL James R. Ficke, MD, MC USA (Chapter 5)
Chairman, Department of
Orthopaedics and Rehabilitation
Orthopaedic Consultant, US Army Surgeon General
San Antonio Military Medical Center
San Antonio, Texas

CDR Mark E. Fleming, DO, MC USN (Chapter 11)
Director, Orthopedic Trauma Service
Walter Reed National Military Medical Center
Assistant Professor, Department of Surgery
Uniformed Services University of the Health Sciences
Bethesda, Maryland

LCDR Jonathan Agner Forsberg, MD, MC USN
(Chapters 9, 10, 22)
Director of Orthopaedic Research
Operational and Undersea Medicine Directorate
Naval Medical Research Center
Silver Spring, Maryland
Integrated Department of Orthopaedic Surgery
Walter Reed National Military Medical Center
Assistant Professor, Department of Surgery
Uniformed Services University of the Health Sciences
Bethesda, Maryland

MAJ Brett A. Freedman, MD, MC USA (Chapter 8)
Chief, Spine and Neurosurgery Service
Landstuhl Regional Medical Center
Landstuhl, Germany

COL Tad Gerlinger, MD, MC USA (Chapter 3)
Chief, Adult Reconstruction
Program Director
San Antonio Uniformed Services
Health Education Consortium
Orthopaedic Surgery Residency
San Antonio Military Medical Center
San Antonio, Texas

CPT Gens P. Goodman, DO, MC USA (Chapter 2)
Department of Orthopaedics and Rehabilitation
William Beaumont Army Medical Center/
Texas Tech University Health Sciences Center
El Paso, Texas

LtCol Wade Gordon, MD, MC USAF (Chapter 27)
Director, Integrated Orthopaedic Trauma Services
Walter Reed National Military Medical Center
Washington, DC and Bethesda, MD
Uniformed Services University of the Health Sciences
Bethesda, Maryland

CDR David E. Gwinn, MD, MC USN (Chapter 29)
Department of Orthopaedics and Rehabilitation
Walter Reed National Military Medical Center
Washington, DC

LT Kathryn H. Hanna, MD, MC USN (Chapter 16)
Orthopaedic Surgeon
Department of Orthopaedic Surgery
Naval Medical Center San Diego
San Diego, California

Zach Harvey, BS, CPO (Chapter 23)
Walter Reed Army Medical Center
Washington, DC

COL (Ret) Roman Hayda, MD, MC USA (Chapter 7)
Associate Professor
Orthopaedic Surgery
Brown University
Warren Alpert School of Medicine
Providence, Rhode Island

CAPT Eric P. Hofmeister, MD, MC USN (Chapter 16)
Chairman, Department of Orthopaedic Surgery
Naval Medical Center San Diego
San Diego, California
Assistant Professor, Department of Surgery
Uniformed Services University of the Health Sciences
Bethesda, Maryland

LTC Joseph R. Hsu, MD, MC USA (Chapters 21, 24)
Orthopedic Surgeon
US Army Institute of Surgical Research
Chief, Orthopaedic Trauma Service
San Antonio Military Medical Center
San Antonio, Texas

Wesley Jackson, PhD (Chapter 12)
Walter Reed National Military Medical Center
Washington, DC
Clinical and Experimental Orthopaedics Group
National Institute of Arthritis and
Musculoskeletal and Skin Diseases
National Institutes of Health
Bethesda, Maryland
Orthopaedic Surgery Service
McDonald Army Health Center
Ft. Eustis, Virginia

CPT Daniel G. Kang, MD, MC USA (Chapter 28)
Department of Orthopaedics and Rehabilitation
Walter Reed National Military Medical Center
Washington, DC

CPT Kelly G. Kilcoyne, MD, MC USA (Chapter 26)
Department of Orthopaedics and Rehabilitation
Walter Reed National Military Medical Center
Washington, DC

CPT Matthew Kluk, MD, MC USA (Chapter 27)
Department of Orthopaedics and Rehabilitation
Walter Reed National Military Medical Center
Washington, DC

COL John F. Kragh Jr, MD, MC USA (Chapter 14)
Orthopedic Surgeon
Damage Control Resuscitation
US Army Institute of Surgical Research
Fort Sam Houston, Texas

LCDR Leo T. Kroonen, MD, MC USN (Chapter 16)
Director, Hand and Microvascular Surgery
Department of Orthopaedic Surgery
Naval Medical Center San Diego
San Diego, California
Assistant Professor, Department of Surgery
Uniformed Services University of the Health Sciences
Bethesda, Maryland

*CDR (Ret) Anand R. Kumar, MD, MC USN
(Chapters 18, 25)*
Department of Plastic and Reconstructive Surgery
Walter Reed National Military Medical Center
Bethesda, Maryland

LTC Ronald A. Lehman Jr, MD, MC USA (Chapter 28)
Chief, Pediatric and Adult Spine
Integrated Department of
Orthopaedics and Rehabilitation
Associate Professor, Department of Surgery
Assistant Professor of Neurology
Uniformed Services University of the Health Sciences
Bethesda, Maryland

CAPT Alan A. Lim, MD, MC USN (Chapters 18, 25)
Plastic and Reconstructive Surgery
Naval Medical Center Portsmouth
Portsmouth, Virginia
Assistant Professor, Department of Surgery
Uniformed Services University of the Health Sciences
Bethesda, Maryland

Capt Robert McGill, MD, MC USAF (Chapter 20)
Department of Orthopaedics and Rehabilitation
San Antonio Military Medical Center
San Antonio, Texas

LTC Clinton K. Murray, MD, MC USA (Chapter 13)
San Antonio Uniformed Services
Health Education Consortium
Infectious Disease Fellowship Program Director
Associate Professor, Department of Medicine
Uniformed Services University of the Health Sciences
Bethesda, Maryland

MAJ Leon J. Nesti, MD, PhD, MC USA (Chapters 8, 12)
Hand and Upper Extremity Reconstructive Surgeon
McDonald Army Health Clinic
Ft. Eustis, Virginia
Chief, Clinical and Experimental Orthopaedics
National Institute of Arthritis and
Musculoskeletal and Skin Diseases
National Institutes of Health
Bethesda, Maryland

LTC Mark Pallis, DO, MC USA (Chapter 3)
Chief, Department of Surgery
Blanchfield Army Community Hospital
Fort Campbell, Kentucky

*MAJ Benjamin K. Potter, MD, MC USA
(Chapters 9, 10, 22, 23, 26)*
Director, Musculoskeletal Oncology
Orthopaedic Surgery Liaison
Amputee Patient Care Program
Integrated Department of Orthopaedics and Rehabilitation
Walter Reed National Military Medical Center
Washington, DC
Assistant Professor, Department of Surgery
Uniformed Services University of the Health Sciences
Bethesda, Maryland

Col Damian Rispoli, MD, MC USAF (Chapter 20)
Chief of Shoulder and Elbow Surgery
Vice Chairman, Department of
Orthopaedics and Rehabilitation
San Antonio Military Medical Center
San Antonio, Texas

LTC Michael K. Rosner, MD, MC USA (Chapter 29)
Chief of Neurosurgery
Walter Reed National Military Medical Center
Washington, DC
Associate Professor, Department of Surgery
Uniformed Services University of the Health Sciences
Bethesda, Maryland

MAJ Andrew J. Schoenfeld, MD, MC USA (Chapters 1, 4)
Department of Orthopaedic Surgery
William Beaumont Army Medical Center/
Texas Tech University Health Sciences Center
El Paso, Texas
Assistant Professor, Department of Surgery
Uniformed Services University of the Health Sciences
Bethesda, Maryland

LTC Scott B. Shawen, MD, MC USA (Chapter 26)
Program Director, Orthopaedic Surgery Residency
Director, Orthopaedic Foot and Ankle Surgery
Walter Reed National Military Medical Center
Washington, DC

MAJ Dirk L. Slade, MD, MC USA (Chapter 4)
Department of Orthopaedic Surgery
William Beaumont Army Medical Center/
Texas Tech University Health Sciences Center
El Paso, Texas

CPT Daniel J. Stinner, MD, MC USA (Chapter 24)
Department of Orthopaedics and Rehabilitation
San Antonio Military Medical Center
San Antonio, Texas

CDR Joseph E. Strauss, DO, MC USN (Chapter 27)
Department of Orthopaedics and Rehabilitation
Walter Reed National Military Medical Center
Washington, DC
Uniformed Services University of the Health Sciences
Bethesda, Maryland

LTC(P) Kenneth F. Taylor, MD, MC USA (Chapter 17)
Orthopaedic Surgery Service
Tripler Army Medical Center
Honolulu, Hawaii
Assistant Professor, Department of Surgery
Uniformed Services University of the Health Sciences
Bethesda, Maryland

COL Joachim Jude Tenuta, MD, MC USA (Chapter 6)
Orthopaedic Surgery Service
United States Military Academy
West Point, New York

LT Scott Tintle, MD, MC USN
(Chapters 18, 19, 22, 25)
Department of Orthopaedics and Rehabilitation
Walter Reed National Military Medical Center
Washington, DC

LCDR Jared A. Vogler, DO, MC USN (Chapter 12)
Walter Reed National Military Medical Center
Washington, DC
Clinical and Experimental Orthopaedics Group
National Institute of Arthritis and
Musculoskeletal and Skin Diseases
National Institutes of Health
Bethesda, Maryland

MAJ Scott Waterman, MD, MC USA (Chapter 11)
Department of Orthopaedics and Rehabilitation
Walter Reed National Military Medical Center
Washington, DC

Preface

The need for a comprehensive text detailing evidence-based medicine and clinical best practices concerning orthopedic combat-related injuries sustained by US military servicemembers has been widely recognized by military orthopedic surgeons. Musculoskeletal wounds have comprised a majority of combat wounds experienced by US military personnel in conflicts from World War II through Vietnam. As of October 1, 2010, more than 40,000 US military servicemembers have been wounded in action in the Iraq and Afghanistan Wars, of which nearly 12,000 have required medical evacuation from theater. Prior reports on the spectrum of orthopedic injuries in the Iraq and Afghanistan Wars estimate that over half of all combat-wounded soldiers sustained a musculoskeletal injury to the extremity.

The combat medical experience of US military personnel in the irregular warfare of the Iraq and Afghanistan Wars presents unique challenges and paradigms that have not been previously encountered. The widespread use of individual and vehicular body armor, evolution of enemy tactics to include its reliance on improvised explosive devices, and the effectiveness of treatment rendered at military treatment facilities has resulted in a large burden of complex orthopedic injuries.

During the course of the Iraq and Afghanistan Wars, military orthopedic surgeons have made significant technical and philosophic changes in the treatment of musculoskeletal combat casualties. This book aspires to be the essential guide to providing optimal care for combat casualties both initially in theater as well as definitively at tertiary care facilities within the United States. Military surgeons fully understand not only their role in providing optimal treatment to musculoskeletal combat casualties in order to conserve the fighting strength of the military, but also the solemn covenant of providing the best possible musculoskeletal surgical care to those brave US military servicemembers who defend our nation.

He who wishes to be a surgeon should go to war.
—Hippocrates

Foreword

It is with humbling pride on many levels that I write this Foreword to *Combat Orthopedic Surgery: Lessons Learned in Iraq and Afghanistan*. Humbling because I deployed the first time in October 2001, long before this text was available, and I think back to the mistakes I made and the real costs of these lessons learned. Humbling, too, as I have had the honor of serving closely with many of the authors, knowing what sacrifices they and their families have borne, in order to care for our nation's wounded. But I also write with a fierce pride to have witnessed what we in military orthopedics have become as a result of this war.

In the early years we boarded planes for Afghanistan and Iraq with a copy of Rockwood and Green and Hoppenfeld's *Surgical Exposures*, only to find that none of the improvised explosive device blasts we were seeing resembled those hallowed texts. There is a loneliness one feels when faced with such cases where there is so little to guide one's hand. But one learns. From Balad and Bagram and a dozen unnamed places to Landstuhl and Walter Reed grew a cadre of surgeons and a culture of cooperation that truly embodies Duty, Honor, Country. This cadre returned to share their lessons in courses like the Combat Extremity Surgical Course, the SOMOS (Society of Military Orthopaedic Surgeons) Disaster Toolbox, and at the annual meeting of SOMOS where those who have been teach those who will go, allowing combat surgery to constantly evolve based on the best science and experience available from the field.

This text represents the culmination of 10 years of scientific application in combat orthopedic surgery. It represents the work of hundreds of warrior physicians who have had the courage to take a hard line at what works—and what doesn't—in caring for the combat casualty. I have no doubt that it will become a most trusted companion, and the first thing packed in the bags of those orthopedic surgeons deploying and redeploying to serve our nation's wounded.

It is with this humble but fierce pride that on behalf of SOMOS and the countless patients that this work will impact, I express my gratitude to the contributors to this project, especially its editors, who recognized the need for this text, and saw it through to its fruition. No effort has contributed greater to the mission of those who serve the wounded warrior.

—LtCol John M. Tokish, MD, MC USAF
President, Society of Military Orthopaedic Surgeons

Foreword

Writing this Foreword to *Combat Orthopedic Surgery: Lessons Learned in Iraq and Afghanistan* is truly an honor. Our discipline of orthopedic surgery as well as the discipline of surgery itself was founded and advanced on the field of battle and with the subsequent care of the wounded warrior. The term *practice of medicine* is no better illustrated than during times of combat. Lieutenant Colonels Brett D. Owens and Philip J. Belmont Jr have captured the essence of "the practice of orthopedics" during these first 10 years of the conflicts in Iraq and Afghanistan.

Owens and Belmont have assembled a cadre of authors who have experienced and participated in the evolution of change in combat care that has resulted from the Iraq and Afghanistan conflicts. Many of these orthopedic surgeons were educated at our finest military academies and at the Uniform Services University of the Health Sciences. This training prepared them for combat, but as this book so markedly illustrates, no training or education could adequately prepare them for the mission they faced.

This book is extremely well organized into 3 parts. The first part outlines the triage system and the operation of that system that has evolved through the 10-year experience in the Iraq and Afghanistan theaters. The second part demonstrates the advances in the discipline of orthopedics used to care for our soldiers inflicted with injuries, many of which have never been encountered by the treating orthopedic surgeon or the orthopedic community in general. The comprehensive final part is sectioned into the upper extremity, lower extremity, and spine and pelvic sections which will provide a field manual as well as a definitive reference for all orthopedic surgeons who care for modern day soldiers and their injuries, or who have an interest in this important field of orthopedics. A testament to the broader audience that this book should and will reach are those civilian orthopedic surgeons who provide care in areas afflicted with natural disasters such as the recent earthquake in Haiti.

I speak for all those who have previously served in the armed forces, hats off to the editors and authors of *Combat Orthopedic Surgery: Lessons Learned in Iraq and Afghanistan*. You have enhanced the legacy that military medicine has provided to advance the field of orthopedic surgery, and more importantly to help all of us provide better outcomes for our patients, especially those who have honorably served our nation in combat.

—John Callaghan, MD
President, American Academy of Orthopaedic Surgeons
Lawrence and Marilyn Dorr Chair
Professor, Department of Orthopaedics and Rehabilitation
University of Iowa Health Care
Iowa City, Iowa

Introduction

When we set out to produce a written account of the combat orthopedic surgery experience over the past decade during the Iraq and Afghanistan Wars, we began by examining the peer-reviewed literature. We selected those individuals who had been most active academically in documenting their surgical, medical, and rehabilitative experience of treating the complex musculoskeletal combat injuries sustained by US military servicemembers. When significant gaps existed within the peer-reviewed literature, we called upon the subject matter experts who were most involved in treating these combat musculoskeletal injuries. Our authors span multiple locations, specialty areas, and service connections. Overall, we relied on relationships—some old, some new—to produce a definitive text of the recent US military combat orthopedic experience. Nearly all of the experts who were solicited to participate enthusiastically did so, and their tireless efforts have produced an exceptionally thorough and in-depth account of their experiences in caring for US combat casualties.

The text is divided into sections, with the first being devoted to an overview of general topics. The second section covers scientific topics and their clinical application to musculoskeletal combat casualties. The final 3 sections are devoted to the anatomic regions of focus with the chapters being mostly clinical in nature. All of these chapters are authored by expert military surgeons who shoulder the burden of care for our injured military servicemembers and illustrative case examples are often utilized.

We hope that the reader will find this text informative and complete. The past decade has seen advances that are a direct result of these military conflicts, and we are hopeful for the dissemination of the knowledge gained to the orthopedic community at large. However, after nearly a decade of combat, our greatest desire is that a second edition of this text is unnecessary.

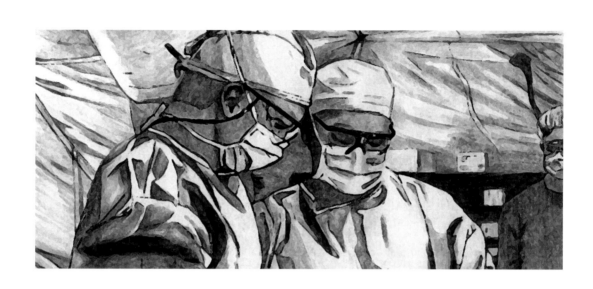

Section I
Principles

Chapter **1**

THE HISTORY OF COMBAT ORTHOPEDIC SURGERY

MAJ Andrew J. Schoenfeld, MD

"He who wishes to be a surgeon should go to war," said Hippocrates Ascelpiades, the most storied physician in the Western world.[1] While the sentiment is true for surgery as a whole, it applies most readily to the field of orthopedics. Although recognized as an independent discipline only in the late 19th century, orthopedics emerged from the field of surgery fully formed, having developed over the course of millennia, with all principal developments engendered during times of war.

Prior to the technological advances of the late 19th century, it is possible to argue that the majority of survivable combat surgery was orthopedic in nature: extremity amputations, setting of fractured limbs, and removal of bullets and/or other projectiles. Military surgeons were the world's first orthopedic surgeons. Long before Nicholas Andry coined the term *orthopedics*, Persian surgeons had performed the first battlefield amputations, Egyptian military physicians had reduced cervical spine fractures, and the Byzantine Paul of Aegina had successfully executed a laminectomy to relieve impending paraplegia.[2-4] Indeed, from the time of Homer, when the first soldier-surgeons developed concepts of battlefield wound care, to the American Civil War, when the unique experience of military surgeons led to the recognition of orthopedics as an independent discipline, combat surgery has been a driving force in the development of orthopedic surgery. Additionally, advancements in the arena of combat orthopedics, particularly during World War II, made significant contributions to and even changed the face of civilian orthopedic surgery. The goal of this chapter is to provide a brief synopsis of significant war-related orthopedic developments and experiences from the Ancient Era to the end of the 20th century.

The Ancient Period (1700 BCE to 7th Century CE)

The development of medicine is shrouded in the prehistory of early man. From the time when pioneering Cro-Magnon developed tools capable of trephening the skulls of injured cave-dwellers, there have been individuals practicing the physical art of health care. Although the Western tradition is generally traced to Ancient Greece and the works of the Hippocratic school (5th century BCE), by the time of Hippocrates, medicine and combat surgery had already been practiced for centuries in the Mediterranean littoral and the Fertile Crescent.[3-5] The Edwin Smith Papyrus (c. 1700 BCE) speaks of Egyptian military surgeons attempting to treat soldiers with combat wounds to the cervical spine,[4] and the Papyrus of Ani refers to the successful reduction of a cervical dislocation sustained during combat.[3,4]

The first surgeons to function as soldier-physicians, traveling with and fighting alongside other soldiers in addition to treating the wounded, emerged in the armies of Mycenaean Greece (1500-1100 BCE). *The Iliad* mentions Podalirius and Machaon, who not only served as physicians but actively fought against the Trojans.[6] In this epic, the more well-known Patroclus and Achilles (Figure 1-1) are also depicted as combat surgeons, although it is clear that these warriors were not physicians by training.

Owens BD, Belmont PJ Jr, eds. *Combat Orthopedic Surgery: Lessons Learned in Iraq and Afghanistan (pp 3-12)*
© 2011 SLACK Incorporated

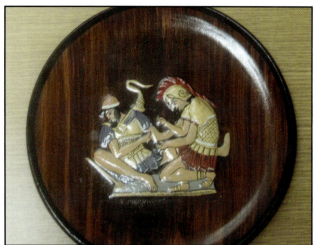

Figure 1-1. Reproduction plate of a pictograph from an Ancient Greek drinking goblet representing Achilles (right) tending to the arm wound of his friend, Patroclus. (Author's private collection.)

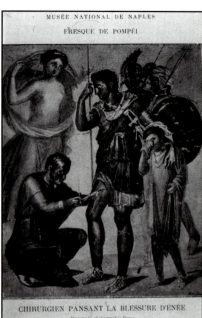

Figure 1-2. Fresco from Pompeii (1st century CE) depicting a surgeon (left), guided by the goddess Isis, excising an arrow head from the leg of Aeneas. (Reprinted from the National Library of Medicine.)

During this Greek period, armored warriors fought in close quarters, either in linear formation or in small groups. Armor generally covered the head and torso, with the extremities, face, and neck largely exposed. As would be the case with most modes of combat until the advent of musketry, significant combat wounds to the head, neck, chest, and abdomen were usually fatal.[5,7] Survivable injuries often occurred in the extremities and were only treated at the end of the conflict once the wounded were collected and physicians were no longer needed to participate in the fighting. The majority of penetrating wounds in this period, however, resulted in the death of the soldier. In their historical review of wounds sustained in the wars of Ancient Greece, Pikoulis and colleagues calculated that stabbing sword wounds carried 100% mortality, while spear wounds resulted in 80% mortality.[7] Slingshots and arrows were somewhat less lethal, but wounds from these ballistic missiles still resulted in significant mortality, ranging from 42% to 67%.[7]

Extremity wounds were treated with irrigation using water and wine. Debridement of devitalized tissue was performed, and foreign bodies, including wood, metal fragments, and arrow heads, were removed. In the case of fractures, reductions were performed using traction/countertraction, and correction was maintained with the use of splints.[8] If the extremity wound or fracture was extensive or if an open fracture was present, amputations were performed, and a wooden prosthesis fashioned.[2,9] The proficiency of Greek physicians in manufacturing prostheses allowed some warriors to continue in the profession of arms despite their amputation.

According to Herodotus, one of the first physicians to perform an amputation was Hegesistratus the Persian.[10] This soldier-surgeon amputated his own foot in order to escape from a Spartan stockade and then devised a wooden prosthesis that allowed him to return to battle. Unfortunately, this surgical innovator was recaptured by the Spartan forces and, in light of his evasive ingenuity, was sentenced to death.

The advent of Imperial Rome (44 BCE-476 CE) witnessed the rise of the military surgeon who did not actively participate in battle. Moreover, it was during this period that physicians became a regular institution within the organization of the military. More numerous than their soldier-physician forbears, Roman army surgeons included military physicians, civilian camp followers, and slaves who may have been free physicians captured during periods of Roman conquest. Roman surgeons were posted on the frontiers and traveled with their assigned units, although most treatment was rendered at the conclusion of battle. The Romans also developed the concept of the field hospital, established close enough to the conflict that wounded soldiers could be transported with relative ease and expedience.[8] Roman medicine differed little from its classical Greek antecedent, however, and no significant advancements in the treatment of musculoskeletal injuries occurred during this period. Simple wound debridement and removal of foreign bodies (Figure 1-2), combined with the reduction and splinting of closed fractures, were the main interventions, and amputations were the only major surgical procedure performed with any regularity.[8,11,12]

The famous physician Galen of Pergamum (129-200 CE) garnered much of his early medical experience working among both gladiators and soldiers. He refined a technique for the management of arrow and sword wounds and developed an apparatus capable of reducing significantly displaced long-bone fractures.[11] The late Roman physician, Paul of Aegina, may have been one of the first practitioners to employ casting in the treatment of extremity fractures[11] and was also the first to successfully perform surgical decompression in the event of spine laminar fractures.[4]

The Medieval Period (7th Through 16th Centuries)

The collapse of the Roman Empire combined with the onset of religious absolutism in Europe and the Middle East led to a general stagnation in the practice of medicine for nearly a millennium. Rather than develop new ideas in the areas of surgical science, Christian and Islamic scholars held the works of Galen and Hippocrates as incontrovertible codices. Experimentation, scientific investigation, and dissent from the accepted teachings of these ancient scholars were heavily discouraged throughout this period. It is unknown whether skilled physicians were considered regular additions to the Crusading armies as they had been in Roman times, although medical experiences during the Crusades led to the re-establishment of the hospital in Europe.[12] Certainly, in this age of armor, there was little treatment that could be afforded by physicians for injuries resulting from the blows of broad swords, battle axes, and spiked maces. Additionally, in the feudal period, the hierarchy of medicine dictated that surgical intervention was beneath the standing of aristocratic physicians, who were trained at universities. Surgical treatments, and consequently the care of wounded soldiers, fell to uneducated barber-surgeons who derived from the lower strata of medieval society.[2,11]

The mainstays of treatment in this era included wound debridement, splinting or casting of fractures, and surgical amputations. Most procedures were performed in a less elegant fashion than they were in Ancient Greece or Rome. For example, hot irons were used to cauterize wounds, and boiling oil was used in the treatment of open injuries.[2,11,13,14]

In Western Europe, at least, the surgical innovators who appeared sprang from the ranks of military physicians.[4,13,14] The 13th century French surgeons Lanfranchi of Milan and Henri de Mondeville developed improved techniques for the suturing of wounds, and de Mondeville also fabricated surgical devices for the extraction of missiles.[4] At the same time, the German Heinrich von Pfolspeundt sought to develop a systematic approach to the treatment of war wounds, particularly the more severe injuries caused by the introduction of gunpowder.[13] Guy de Chauliac, a 14th century surgeon who served as Chief Physician to the Avignon Papacy, developed a doctrine on wound care that would inform wound management in the Western world for more than 2 centuries. De Chauliac's principles included removal of foreign bodies, tissue preservation, and primary closure wherever possible.[14] In 1517, the German military surgeon Hans von Gersdorff published a treatise on the treatment of extremity wounds, which included a description of his screw-traction device for the reduction of fractures and dislocations. This portable contraption, which applied a controlled force at the physician-operator's discretion, represented one of the most significant advances in fracture management since Ancient times.[13]

The Age of Gunpowder (16th Through 18th Centuries)

The introduction of gunpowder and artillery to European warfare marked the end of the feudal traditions of knightly combat and heavily armored cavalry. Whereas warfare previously occurred in chaotic close confrontations between groups of skilled soldiers, the introduction of musketry permitted the creation of large-scale forces capable of inflicting considerable damage on opponents from greater distances. Musketry still proved lethal, especially in the event of gunshot wounds to the chest and abdomen, but an increased survivability relative to the sword and spear injuries of medieval warfare challenged military practitioners of the time and stimulated significant developments in the field of medicine.

Chief among the military physicians of the 16th century was Ambrose Paré, Court Surgeon to the French King Henry II. Paré, who in his youth had garnered significant battlefield experience in the humble role of barber-surgeon, served in the French army during the Italian Wars of the 16th century and the Wars of Religion.[2,5,12] He successfully railed against the use of hot oil and cautery irons in the treatment of gunshot wounds and developed a suture technique that enabled the successful performance of thigh amputations.[5,8,13] Paré also employed the royal armorers in the creation of spinal orthoses and the first prosthetic limbs with functional joints.[2]

It was in this period that the essential role that military surgeons played in the conservation of the fighting force was recognized. For the first time since the days of Rome, European armies were regularly supplied with their own physicians and surgeons, recognized as integral components to the combat force.[5,12] At the end of the 16th century, the Spanish Army founded the first permanent military medical hospital.[8]

During this time, battlefield surgeons were most effective in their management of soft tissue wounds, effecting primary muscle and tendon repairs, and reducing fractures and dislocations. Gunshot wounds were explored, and enlarged if necessary, in order to eliminate debris, remove projectiles, and debride devitalized tissue. The fear of sepsis, however, led to an increased reliance on amputations, especially in the case of open fractures or shattered bones.[8] Such an approach was enabled by the work of the French army surgeon Jean Louis Petit (1674-1750), who developed the 2-stage circular amputation technique and introduced the screw tourniquet to manage bleeding during the procedure.[5,11] Similar to von Gersdorff's traction device, the screw tourniquet enabled the surgeon to apply variable amounts of pressure to compress the vessels of the upper or lower extremities. Petit reported that the application of his tourniquet device reduced mortality rates following lower limb amputations by 50%.[11]

At the start of the American Revolution (1775-1783), the Continental Congress authorized one military surgeon for each American regiment. As there were few professionally trained practitioners in the colonies at the time, most Revolutionary War surgeons had been educated in the apprentice system that was a holdover from the European barber tradition.[15] Almost none of the American Revolutionary War surgeons had any prior combat experience, including the first Surgeon General of the Army, Dr. Benjamin Church. A notable exception was Dr. John Jones, who had been trained by the famous John Hunter (Surgeon General of the English Army during the Revolutionary War) and had served as a military surgeon during the French and Indian War (1755-1763).[5,8,16]

In response to the pressing need for a text capable of directing inexperienced practitioners with no prior combat experience, Jones authored *On the Treatment of Wounds and Fractures: Designed for the Use of Young Military Surgeons in North America*.[8,16,17] Jones advocated the use of opium for pain and emollients made from bark to cauterize small vessels. Pistol or musket balls were to be removed as atraumatically as possible, and primary closure was avoided. If primary closure was deemed necessary, an onion was placed in the wound, and secondary exploration was performed within a few days.[5] Amputations were often delayed until surgeons were able to appreciate how soldiers were responding to their initial injury. During the Battle of Harlem, Continental surgeon Charles Gillman made the serendipitous discovery of the ameliorative effect of alcohol on infection.[15,16] Despite the fact that Gillman's use of rum to clean wounds echoed the Ancient Greek application of wine as an irrigant, this unique battlefield treatment was not adopted by the medical department of the Continental Army.[16]

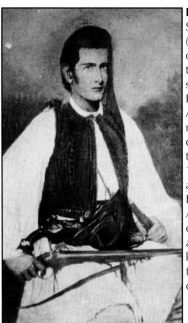

Figure 1-3. Portrait of Samuel G. Howe, MD (1801-1876) in the service dress of a Greek revolutionary. A Harvard-trained surgeon from Boston, Howe would introduce American surgical techniques to the Balkans during his participation in the Greek Revolution of 1821. Besides working as a physician and surgeon, Howe returned to the Ancient Greek tradition of soldier-physicians and also participated in combat operations. (Reprinted from the National Library of Medicine.)

The Early 19th Century

Western warfare in the 19th century differed little from the line techniques developed by military practitioners in the 17th and 18th centuries, although the introduction of rifled muskets, the minie ball, and grapeshot made combat more lethal and injuries substantially more severe. The minie ball traveled at a higher velocity (950 ft/sec) than musket bullets and struck the body with greater kinetic energy, resulting in more complex fractures and greater soft tissue damage.[5,17] During this period in the United States, military surgeons A. B. Boyer and William Gibson explored the use of emergent fasciotomies during the War of 1812 and the Black Hawk War, respectively.[16] Samuel G. Howe, a Harvard-trained surgeon, would export American amputation and surgical techniques to the Balkans during his service in the Greek Revolution (1821-1829) (Figure 1-3).

Developments in America were overshadowed, however, by the Napoleonic wars and one of the greatest military medical innovators of all time, Baron Dominique Jean Larrey (Figure 1-4).[5,8,18] Often referred to as the father of modern military surgery, Baron Larrey rose from the modest role of apprentice-surgeon to become the Surgeon-Major of the French Rhine Army and then Physician-General of Napoleon's Grande Armée.[18] Larrey devised the modern concept of a triage system, developed the first military ambulances to expeditiously evacuate wounded soldiers during battle (the famed flying ambulance corps), and invented novel techniques for successful hip and shoulder amputations.[5,8,18] A skilled surgeon, Larrey performed more than 400 amputations during

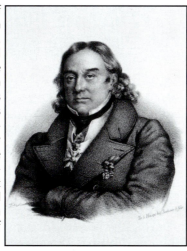

Figure 1-4. Portrait of Baron Dominique Jean Larrey (1766-1842). From humble Provencal origins, Larrey would rise to become the Surgeon in Chief of Napoleon's Grande Armée. He is credited with the foundation of modern military medicine, including the development of the triage system and emergent evacuation for wounded soldiers. (Reprinted from the National Library of Medicine.)

the French retreat from Russia[8,18] and was lauded by Napoleon as "…[one of] the most virtuous [men] I have ever known."[18] The French Emperor also recognized Larrey's surgical prowess as playing a vital role in the remarkable success of his army.

The European experience in the Crimean War (1853-1856) foreshadowed the gruesome trauma of the American Civil War. This conflict was the first to experience the widespread use of the destructive minie ball, whose proclivity for soft tissue destruction and severe long-bone fractures led to extraordinarily high mortality rates following gunshot wounds.[5] Although amputations were performed fairly quickly following injury, postoperative sepsis and mortality were shockingly high: 23% for below-the-knee amputations, 50% for above-the-knee amputations, and 100% for hip disarticulations.[19] During this war, the regular use of plaster of Paris for casting was instituted, and the British medical corps became the first service to use chloroform as a general anesthetic.[5,8]

The American Civil War (1861 to 1865)

Neither the Union Army nor the Confederate States could have prepared for the enormous number of combat casualties that would result from the most destructive war in American history. The American armed forces of 1860 contained fewer than 100 physicians, many of whom had no formal medical education.[17,19] Some of these military surgeons resigned their commissions to enlist in the Confederate Army, and both sides had to make a concerted effort to marshal enough physicians to treat the immense casualties that appeared with the commencement of hostilities. More than 3 million soldiers would serve on both sides over the course of the 4-year conflict,

with more than 600,000 servicemembers dying in action.[17,19-23] Approximately 500,000 soldiers survived the conflict with permanent disabilities, providing significant experience for surgeons, particularly in the area of operative orthopedics. Gunshot wounds were the most common mode of injury during the war, and, while head, neck, chest, and abdominal wounds were often fatal, 86% to 94% of soldiers with extremity wounds survived.[17] Furthermore, 65% to 71% of all wounds in the Civil War involved the extremities, providing invaluable orthopedic operative experience to military surgeons.[5,20,21]

As most formal medical schools were located in the North, the Confederacy found itself bereft of experienced medical personnel. A prominent Confederate surgeon, Julian J. Chisholm, who had trained at the University of South Carolina before the war, composed an instructional manual to assist Confederate physicians in the performance of their duties. This text, *A Manual of Military Surgery for the Use of Surgeons in the Confederate Army*, outlined principles of wound management and provided a decision algorithm for performing amputations.[19] According to Chisholm, indications for primary amputation included devitalized limbs, damage to major blood vessels or nerves, extensive soft tissue destruction, and open fractures.[19]

Given the profound fear of sepsis or gangrene, most Civil War surgeons would perform a primary amputation for any fracture caused by a gunshot wound. An experienced surgeon could perform a major amputation in less than 15 minutes,[19] and more than 60,000 of these procedures would be performed on Union soldiers over the course of the war.[5] Popular perceptions notwithstanding, the majority of these procedures were performed with the benefit of anesthesia.

Many Civil War surgeons rigidly followed the doctrines outlined by Chisholm or Samuel Gross in their approaches to wound and fracture management. Others, however, were true surgical pioneers and experimented with techniques that would not be seen again for 100 years. In 1863, Middleton Goldsmith, a Union surgeon, reported on his experience with the use of bromine spray in the treatment of hospital-acquired gangrene.[5,17] This novel intervention reduced mortality from 60% to 3% in patients with this condition.[5] J. F. Zacharias, a surgeon with the Confederacy, employed maggots in the treatment of osteomyelitis and for debridement of gangrenous wounds. S. Weir Mitchell from Philadelphia experimented with direct suture repair of nerve lacerations caused by gunshot.[24]

George Otis, who later edited the *Medical and Surgical History of the War of the Rebellion*, initiated attempts at limb salvage, performing resection arthroplasties of damaged shoulder or hip joints in lieu of amputations (Figure 1-5).[17,23] Hip resections were performed using

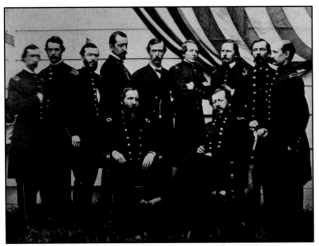

Figure 1-5. Photograph of Surgeon General Joseph K. Barnes (seated right) and his staff during the Civil War. Standing, second from right, is George Otis, assistant surgeon in the Union Army. Under the direction of General Barnes, Otis would later play an integral role in compiling the *Medical and Surgical History of the War of the Rebellion*. (Reprinted from the National Library of Medicine.)

a lateral incision based off of the greater trochanter, and patients who survived the procedure were usually able to ambulate with the use of a cane and shoe lift.[17] In a series of 1086 patients who received resection arthroplasty of the shoulder, only 14 individuals subsequently required an amputation.[20]

The Civil War also witnessed the first serious attempts at open reduction and internal fixation of fractures.[17] Several of these procedures were performed by Benjamin Howard, a federal surgeon from New York. Howard, who believed that the advantage of internal fixation solely lay in the resultant ease of patient transport, resected the ends of fractured fragments and then approximated the freshened ends with wire. Other surgeons attempted to fix femur fractures with metal wires and pinned radial fractures with brass.[17] In 1864, James Bolton, a Confederate physician, published his experience with external fixation for long-bone fractures in the *Confederate States Medical and Surgical Journal*.[25]

By 1865, the meager workforce of 100 physicians with limited combat experience that existed before the war had been transformed into more than 15,000 professional military surgeons.[17] The Civil War provided the surgical experience and training that directly led to the recognition of orthopedic surgery as an independent specialty in the United States.[17] Most American orthopedic pioneers of the later 19th century were influenced by experiences resulting from the Civil War, including 2 of the first 6 presidents of the American Orthopaedic Association, Newton Shaffer and Benjamin Lee, who were themselves veterans of the conflict.[17]

The Late 19th Century (1865 to 1914)

Great advances were made in the arena of combat orthopedic surgery from the end of the Civil War until the start of the next great conflict in American history, World War I. In the United States, Assistant Surgeon General A. C. Girard mandated the use of antiseptic surgical techniques according to Listerian principles in 1877.[16] This development was closely followed by Colonel Robert Murray's use of antiseptic surgery for elective procedures in military personnel.[16]

During the Franco-Prussian campaign (1870-1871), Prussian Surgeon General Johann Friedrich von Esmarch popularized the use of his compression bandage and developed new techniques to expedite battlefield wound management and surgery.[5] More effective wound management was achieved via the use of sublimate solutions and the application of iodoform powder to open wounds.[16] von Esmarch also expanded on Larrey's triage system, adding the necessity to not only treat the most serious survivable injuries, but to do so in light of maximizing military medical resources. Shortly after the cessation of European hostilities, von Esmarch's battlefield innovations were widely adopted by the medical departments of France, England, Russia, and the United States (Figure 1-6).

Possibly the most significant addition to the performance of combat orthopedic surgery in this period was the introduction of x-ray equipment to theaters of combat. An Italian physician, Lieutenant Colonel Giuseppe Alvaro, first used radiographs to locate bullet fragments in wounded soldiers during the Abyssinian War (1895), but the practice was quickly implemented by the British, German, and American medical corps.[5,22] The British brought radiographic equipment into combat hospitals during the Greco-Turkish War (1897)[26] and the 2nd Boer War (1899-1902).[22] Although rudimentary compared to modern imaging, late 19th century radiographs were capable of depicting fractures as well as locating bullet fragments and shrapnel. This allowed surgeons to target fragments atraumatically and eliminated the need for probing, a factor that had contributed significantly to wound contamination.[5]

At the start of the Spanish-American War (1898), the US Army established 3 hospital barges in the Cuban theater, all equipped with x-ray machines.[5] The Spanish-American War was the first major American military operation since the introduction of aseptic surgical techniques and antisepsis to the medical department. Despite the fact that the metal-jacketed high-velocity bullets used during this conflict caused

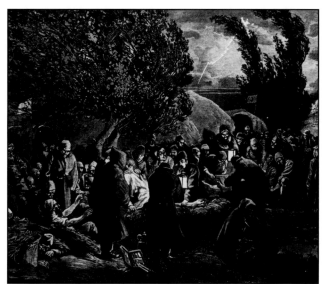

Figure 1-6. Amputation scene in a Turkish field hospital during the Russo-Turkish War (1877-1878). Although the medical departments of the Great Powers had adopted modern surgical techniques and Listerian principles of antiseptic surgery, many medical departments of the Balkan nations operated in conditions unchanged since the Napoleonic wars. (Reprinted from the National Library of Medicine.)

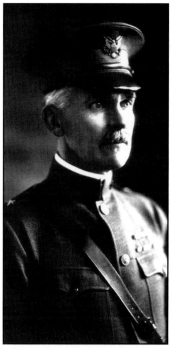

Figure 1-7. Colonel Joel E. Goldthwait (1867-1961), Director of the Division of Orthopaedic Surgery in the American Expeditionary Force during World War I. As Chairman of the Department of Orthopaedic Surgery at Massachusetts General Hospital, Goldthwait played a leading role in ensuring state-of-the-art orthopedic services were available to injured servicemembers on the Western Front. The Division of Orthopaedic Surgery consisted of 42 orthopedic surgeons, hand-picked by Goldthwait, to participate in the war effort. (Reprinted from the National Library of Medicine.)

greater wound cavitation and soft tissue damage than the minie ball, advances in medical and surgical care significantly reduced mortality and amputation rates for American soldiers. Among the 1,990 American combat casualties, the mortality rate was 7.4%, and only 29 gunshot wounds were treated with amputations.[5,27]

World War I (1914 to 1918)

The start of the Great War witnessed the devastating introduction of modern military armaments to 19th century warfare. Horse cavalry and line infantry ran up against high-explosive shells, machine guns, and mechanized artillery for the first, and last, time in history. American military and medical observers had 3 years of neutrality to formulate a war plan for the US Army medical department in light of the tremendous casualties and horrendous injuries that would result from this new mode of warfare.

In 1916, the American Orthopaedic Association was asked by the War Department to develop a committee on orthopedic preparedness for anticipated entry into the conflict.[28] A Department of Military Orthopaedic Surgery was formed within the Office of the Surgeon General under the command of Major E. G. Brackett.[29] An orthopedic section was also established at Walter Reed General Hospital, and orthopedic training schools were created at a number of military posts in order to train Army and Navy physicians.[8,28,29]

The core of military orthopedic surgeons in 1917 was principally derived from civilian departments at Harvard and Johns Hopkins.[28,29] Colonel Joel E. Goldthwait (Figure 1-7), Chairman of Orthopedic Surgery at Massachusetts General Hospital, was appointed director of the Division of Orthopaedic Surgery within the American Expeditionary Force (AEF). The division consisted of 42 orthopedic surgeons and 12 orthopedic nurses dispersed throughout the Western Front. Members of the division were present at all echelons of care, from the front lines where they supervised corpsmen in splint application to the major military hospitals in the rear where surgical interventions were performed.[5,8,12,22,28,29] The skill of American orthopedic surgeons can be attested by the 15.6% mortality rate following open femur fracture for American personnel in the Great War, compared to an 80% mortality rate for British soldiers with similar injuries.[28]

Important developments during World War I also occurred in the medical services of other nations. Antoine Depage, a Belgian surgeon, expounded on his positive experiences with radical debridement for contaminated open injuries and delayed wound closure.[5] The French surgeon Alexis Carrel invented a technique of antiseptic wound irrigation using Dakin's solution.[30] Open wounds were treated with this solution and then left open for 1 to 2 days, following which they were re-examined and debrided if necessary.[8,28-30] Delayed closure, facilitated by the work of Depage and Carrel, also allowed surgeons to experiment with the retention of fracture fragments and virtually eliminated the use of primary amputation for injuries caused by gunshot.[5,8] The Austrian Otto Marburg and the French 5th Army Surgeons Georges Guillain and J. A. Barre independently advocated for emergent surgery on all soldiers with spinal cord injuries.[22] Colonel Henry Gray of the British 3rd Army even composed a list of emergent indications for spinal cord decompression in the combat theater, including severe radicular pain, progressive neurologic deficit, or large open spinal wounds.[22]

World War II and Korea (1941 to 1953)

Many of the young physicians who had trained as orthopedic surgeons during World War I or served in the AEF re-enlisted to form the core of the Orthopaedic Surgery Division at the start of World War II. The period from 1941 to 1953 would represent a time of remarkable advancements in the orthopedic field, many of which were spurred by American military experiences in World War II.[5,8,29,31] The introduction of antibiotics and blood replacement enabled more advanced surgical techniques, including reconstructive surgery and aggressive attempts at internal fixation.[8] Orthopedic achievements were also directly inspired by the Surgeon General, Major General Norman T. Kirk (Figure 1-8), the first orthopedic surgeon to serve in the role of Army Surgeon General.[31]

Major General Kirk, who had treated 33% of all American amputees during World War I, spearheaded the development of orthopedic specialty hospitals and amputee centers. He also tapped Dr. Sterling Bunnell to establish a series of specialty hand centers throughout the country and to train a cadre of surgeons in reconstructive techniques relative to the hand. These important developments directly contributed to the establishment and recognition of hand surgery as a subspecialty within the discipline of orthopedics.

American orthopedic surgeons experimented with limb salvage procedures during the Second World War and developed established principles for the use of external fixation.[5,8,32] The Bankart, Putti-Platt, and Magnuson-Stack procedures were described in servicemembers with persistent shoulder dislocations due to war injuries.[29] During World War II, radical debridements and skin grafting were used for the first time in the treatment of lower extremity osteomyelitis.[33,34] Bone grafting was also developed for the treatment of massive intercalary bone defects.[31] On the German side, Dr. Gerhard Kuntscher pioneered the technique of intramedullary nailing of long-bone fractures, a procedure that was quickly adopted by American surgeons once they saw the benefits in

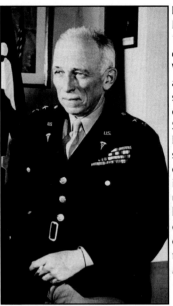

Figure 1-8. Major General Norman T. Kirk (1888-1960), Surgeon General of the Army during World War II. Under Kirk's guidance, the Army instituted several orthopedic specialty centers across the United States during World War II, including facilities that specialized in amputee care and hand surgery. His initiatives directly contributed to the recognition of hand surgery as a subspecialty within the discipline of orthopedics. (Reprinted from the National Library of Medicine.)

Allied prisoners of war who had been treated by the Germans.[5,8,11,31,35] Numerous orthopedic surgeons who had witnessed Kuntscher's successful treatment in Allied airmen during World War II would widely apply intramedullary fixation for long-bone fractures in the Korean War.[5,8,29,31]

The introduction of helicopter evacuation systems during the Korean War also enabled the construction of fixed army hospitals, capable of accommodating up to 200 patients, close to the forward edge of battle.[5] These institutions, with modern medical equipment and sterile surgical facilities, allowed surgeons in theater to provide care similar to that administered to patients in the United States.[5,8] The culmination of 40 years of advancements in combat orthopedics is reflected in the fact that gas gangrene, which had a high prevalence and significant mortality rate among wounded servicemembers in World War I, was rarely encountered during the Korean War.[5]

Similar to the Civil War, which galvanized the development of orthopedic surgery as an independent field, and World War I, which prepared the way for the development of the American Academy of Orthopaedic Surgeons and the American Board of Orthopaedic Surgery, World War II and Korea played a vital role in the future of orthopedic surgery. Besides the well-recognized impact that World War II had on hand surgery, the fact that 33% of all Academy fellows were on active duty during the conflict had an immeasurable effect on the profession, especially in regard to its academic development.[31] For example, in 1945, 37% of all orthopedic articles were published by surgeons on active duty, and in the year following the end of the war, that number increased to 44%.[31]

Vietnam to the First Gulf War (1965 to 1991)

The use of helicopters was refined and continued on a larger scale during the Vietnam War (1965-1973).[27] Fixed hospitals in Vietnam were capable of providing definitive orthopedic care to most patients, although the echelon system still in use today was also devised during this period.[5,8,27,36-38] During Vietnam, the use of pulsatile lavage for the irrigation of contaminated wounds was applied for the first time,[27,39] and techniques of limb salvage were further refined by military surgeons such as Norman Rich at the Second Surgical Hospital in An Khe.[5,40]

One of the most significant innovations in the modern period was the reintroduction of armored helmets and individual body armor to warfare at the start of the Persian Gulf War.[41,42] The armored warriors who had disappeared from the battlefield with the advent of gunpowder at the start of the 15th century returned to the deserts of Kuwait at the end of the 20th. The use of armor in Desert Storm significantly mitigated what would otherwise have been life-threatening injuries, including a significant reduction in chest wounds. However, the use of such body armor had little impact on orthopedic injuries, which were significant despite the low casualties of the First Gulf War.[41,42]

Operation Desert Storm also witnessed the demise of the mobile army surgical hospital (MASH) units that had been the mainstay of care during Korea and Vietnam.[5] The nature of desert warfare, including the amount of terrain covered by combat units, made the cumbersome MASH unit obsolete. At the end of the Gulf War, a process was initiated to trim down the facilities capable of providing combat support. Due to developments in air travel and emergent medical care, it became possible to transfer wounded soldiers to state-of-the-art medical facilities in Europe or the United States. Definitive orthopedic care no longer needed to be provided in theater, and emergent treatment and provisional stabilization could be effectively administered by smaller medical units, such as the forward surgical teams and combat support hospitals that would appear during the Global War on Terror.[38,43]

Conclusion

The military orthopedic surgeon is a member of a proud tradition that extends back as long as military history itself. Rather than representing a relatively new addition to the field of combat surgery, the discipline of orthopedics has always been integral to, if not the sole mainstay of, military medicine. As the face of warfare has changed, so too has the nature of combat orthopedics. In every conflict, the field of orthopedic surgery has risen to meet the needs of the fighting force, and, in most instances, developments on the battlefield and combat hospitals eventually made positive contributions to the care of civilians as well. As the nature of war and combat injury is drastically different in the Global War on Terror from its antecedents in Europe and Southeast Asia, the advancements and contributions of the present conflict to the field of orthopedic surgery remain to be seen, although they will be, no doubt, momentous.

Standing on the shoulders of the giants who preceded us, we surgeons form a proud heritage of human links...from generation to generation.... A thousand years from now our current accomplishments as surgeons will not be ridiculed. Rather, like explorers to the New World, we will be admired for the courage and skill during a time when people were cut open to be healed. (TR Thompson, personal communication)

References

1. Schein M. *Aphorisms and Quotations for the Surgeon.* Shrewsbury, Shropshire, UK: Tfm Publishing; 2003:143.
2. Banta JV. Armorers and barber surgeons: a remarkable legacy. Graduation address for the Newington Orthotics and Prosthetics School. May 20, 1996. *Conn Med.* 1997;6(17):423-425.
3. Filler AG. A historical hypothesis of the first recorded neurosurgical operation: Isis, Osiris, Thoth, and the origin of the djed cross. *Neurosurg Focus.* 2007;23(1):E6.
4. Goodrich JT. History of spine surgery in the ancient and medieval worlds. *Neurosurg Focus.* 2004;16(1):Article 2.
5. Manring MM, Hawk A, Calhoun JH, Andersen RC. Treatment of war wounds: a historical review. *Clin Orthop Relat Res.* 2009;467(8):2168-2191.
6. Homer. *The Iliad.* Lombardo S (trans). Indianapolis, IN: Hackett Publishing Co; 1997.
7. Pikoulis EA, Petropoulos JC, Tsigris C, et al. Trauma management in ancient Greece: value of surgical principles through the years. *World J Surg.* 2004;28(4):425-430.
8. Noe A. Extremity injury in war: a brief history. *J Am Acad Orthop Surg.* 2006;14(10):S1-S6.
9. Helling TS, McNabney WK. The role of amputation in the management of battlefield casualties: a history of two millennia. *J Trauma.* 2000;49:930-939.
10. Strassler RB, Purvis A. Herodotus. *The Landmark Herodotus: The Histories.* New York, NY: Pantheon; 2007.
11. Colton CL. The history of fracture treatment. In: Browner BD, Jupiter JB, Levine AM, Trafton PG, eds. *Skeletal Trauma.* 3rd ed. Philadelphia, PA: WB Saunders; 2003:3-28.
12. Gabriel RA, Metz KS. *Contributions in Military Studies: A History of Military Medicine.* New York, NY: Greenwood Press; 1992.
13. Beasley AW. Orthopaedic aspects of medieval medicine. *J R Soc Med.* 1982;75(12):970-975.
14. Riesman D. *The Story of Medicine in the Middle Ages.* New York, NY: PB Hoeber; 1936.

15. Pruitt BA Jr. Combat casualty care and surgical progress. *Ann Surg.* 2006;243:715-729.

16. Cozen LN. Military orthopaedic surgery. *Clin Orthop Relat Res.* 1985;200:50-53.

17. Kuz JE. The ABJS Presidential Lecture, June 2004. Our orthopaedic heritage: the American Civil War. *Clin Orthop Relat Res.* 2004;429:306-315.

18. Skandalakis PN, Lainas P, Zoras O, Skandalakis JE, Mirilas P. To afford the wounded speedy assistance: Dominique Jean Larrey and Napoleon. *World J Surg.* 2006;30(8):1392-1399.

19. Franchetti MA. Trauma surgery during the Civil War. *South Med J.* 1993;86(5):553-556.

20. Barnes JK. *Medical and Surgical History of the War of the Rebellion.* Washington, DC: Surgeon General's Office; 1875-1888.

21. Bengtson BP, Kuz JE. *Photographic Atlas of Civil War Injuries: Photographs of Surgical Cases and Specimens—Otis Historical Archives.* Grand Rapids, MI: Medical Staff Press; 1996.

22. Hanigan WC, Sloffer C. Nelson's wound: treatment of spinal cord injury in 19th and early 20th century military conflicts. *Neurosurg Focus.* 2004;16(1):Article 4.

23. Otis GA. *The Medical and Surgical History of the War of the Rebellion (1861-65). Surgical History, Volume II.* Washington, DC: GPO; 1870.

24. Mitchell SW, Morehouse GR, Keen WW. *Gunshot Wounds and Other Injuries of Nerves.* Philadelphia, PA: JB Lippincott; 1864.

25. Bolton J. New method of treating ununited fracture of long bones. *Confederate States Medical and Surgical Journal.* 1864;1:55-56.

26. Abbott FC. Surgery in the Graeco-Turkish war. *Lancet.* 1899;21:151-156.

27. Burkhalter WE. *Orthopaedic Surgery in Vietnam.* Washington, DC: Office of the Surgeon General and Center of Military History; 1994.

28. Peltier LF. The division of orthopaedic surgery in the AEF a.k.a. the Goldthwait Unit. *Clin Orthop Relat Res.* 1985;200:45-49.

29. Brav EA. Military contributions to the development of orthopaedic surgery by the Armed Forces, USA since World War I. *Clin Orthop Relat Res.* 1966;44:115-126.

30. Dunlop J. The Carell-Dakin treatment at Oxford: an observation of the Carrel-Dakin method of treating chronic wounds in an orthopaedic centre in England. *Am J Orthop Surg.* 1918;16:495-498.

31. Dougherty PJ, Carter PR, Seligson D, Benson DR, Purvis JM. Orthopaedic surgery advances resulting from World War II. *J Bone Joint Surg Am.* 2004;86(1):176-181.

32. Coates JB Jr, Cleveland M, McFetridge EM, eds. *Orthopaedic Surgery in the Mediterranean Theater of Operations.* Washington, DC: Office of the Surgeon General, Department of the Army; 1957.

33. Kelly RP. Skin grafting in the treatment of osteomyelitic war wounds. *J Bone Joint Surg Am.* 1946;28:681-691.

34. Knight MP, Wood GO. Surgical obliteration of bone cavities following traumatic osteomyelitis. *J Bone Joint Surg Am.* 1945;27:547-556.

35. Fischer S. Obituary: Gerhard Kuntscher. *J Bone Joint Surg Am.* 1974;56(1):208-209.

36. Hardway RM. 200 years of military surgery. *Injury.* 1999;30: 387-397.

37. Hardaway RM. Viet Nam wound analysis. *J Trauma.* 1978;18: 635-643.

38. Bagg MR, Covey DC, Powell ET IV. Levels of medical care in the Global War on Terrorism. *J Am Acad Orthop Surg.* 2006; 14:S7-S9.

39. Keblish DJ, DeMaio M. Early pulsatile lavage for the decontamination of combat wounds: historical review and point proposal. *Mil Med.* 1998;163(12):844-846.

40. Rich NM, Rhee P. An historical tour of vascular injury management: from its inception the new millennium. *Surg Clin North Am.* 2001;81:1199-1215.

41. Uhorchak JM, Rodkey WG, Hunt MM, Hoxie SW. *Institute Report #469: Casualty Data Assessment Team Operation Desert Storm.* San Francisco, CA: Letterman Army Institute of Research; 1992.

42. Belmont PJ Jr, Schoenfeld AJ, Goodman G. Epidemiology of combat wounds in Operation Iraqi Freedom and Operation Enduring Freedom: orthopaedic burden of disease. *J Surg Orthop Adv.* 2010;19(1):2-7.

43. Rush RM Jr, Stockmaster NR, Stinger HK, et al. Supporting the Global War on Terror: a tale of two campaigns featuring the 250th Forward Surgical Team (Airborne). *Am J Surg.* 2005;189:564-570.

Chapter 2

THE COMBAT ENVIRONMENT AND EPIDEMIOLOGY OF MUSCULOSKELETAL COMBAT CASUALTIES

LTC Philip J. Belmont Jr, MD and CPT Gens P. Goodman, DO

Overview of the Iraq and Afghanistan Wars' Tactical and Operational Environment

The majority of US armed conflicts prior to the 21st century, with the exception of portions of the Vietnam War, took place along the lines of traditional general warfare in which forces conduct major combat operations against an organized, uniformed enemy. The US military over the past 2 centuries has successfully employed a military strategy based upon the principle foundations of advanced technology, discipline, aggressive military action, ability to change and conserve military practices as the needs arise, and power to finance wars.[1] This "Western Way of War" has become the dominant mode of warfare throughout the world. Countries employing its principles have consistently fielded armies with greater fighting potential than their enemies.

The conflicts in Iraq and Afghanistan markedly differ from previous US military engagements in that these are irregular wars in which there is a violent struggle among state and nonstate actors for legitimacy and influence over the civilian population. Additionally, there is neither a uniformed enemy nor defined front lines, and alliances can easily shift.[2] Enemies of the coalition forces in Iraq and Afghanistan are unable to successfully challenge the US military in traditional general warfare. Therefore, they have principally used unconventional tactics of terrorism, insurgency, and guerrilla warfare to counteract the traditional US military advantages of superb military discipline and advanced technology.

As a result, most combat casualties in Iraq and Afghanistan occur due to ambush or, increasingly, from the use of improvised explosive devices (IEDs).[3,4] IEDs are destructive weapons deployed in unconventional methods that are designed to hinder and defeat the opposing force's superior military assets in the field. IEDs are constructed from homemade, commercial, or military explosive material and are most often tactically used in the form of buried artillery rounds, antipersonnel mines, and car bombs.[5,6] The rampant use of IEDs and other terrorist tactics by al-Qaeda and the Sunni insurgents against US and coalition forces in Iraq has been directed at thwarting US military efforts and damaging the Iraqi civilian population's perception that the sovereign representative Iraqi government could provide stability and order. The ultimate goal of these attacks by IEDs and related vehicular-borne IEDs, commonly referred to as "suicide car bombs," has been to sway public opinion enough to effectively delegitimize the Iraqi government or to pressure the democratically elected civilian leadership to capitulate to the enemies' demands. To this end, the US and coalition forces' most important and yet difficult task has been to protect the "soft target" of the general Iraqi population.

At the onset of the Iraq War, the US military's overall operational strategy was predicated upon the total defeat and destruction of the enemy in accordance with the principle of aggressive military action

Owens BD, Belmont PJ Jr, eds. *Combat Orthopedic Surgery: Lessons Learned in Iraq and Afghanistan (pp 13-22)*
© 2011 SLACK Incorporated

espoused by the Western Way of War. There is little debate that the US military's initial success in the overthrow of Saddam Hussein and the Ba'ath Party was directly attributable to the principles of military discipline and the power to finance a highly trained and technologically advanced army. Conversely, the emphasis on offensive operations directed toward the total defeat and destruction of the enemy came at the expense of defensive operations and of stability and reconstruction during the initial years of the Iraq War. These facts only served to fuel the Sunni insurgency.

The US military's unique ability to adapt to and overcome the changing conditions on the battlefield and to implement a comprehensive counterinsurgency strategy has been pivotal in achieving greater success in the Iraq War. During "The Surge" of 2007-2008, General Petraeus employed the "clear, build, and hold" counterinsurgency strategy developed by Colonel H. R. McMaster. This resulted in an overall dramatic increase in security and a decrease in overall violence against US and coalition forces, as well as the Iraqi civilian population.[7,8] The indelible success of The Surge was to stem the rising tide of the Sunni-Shiite sectarian conflict within Iraq and to provide physical security to the population. The US military then was able to conduct stability and reconstruction operations and place the country under the control of the Iraqi government. Similar counterinsurgency operational concepts are only now in 2010 being applied on a large scale in the Afghanistan War against the Taliban.

The current counterinsurgency strategy used by US military forces in Iraq and Afghanistan, coupled with the enemies' increasing reliance on explosive ordinance such as IEDs, have resulted in combat injury patterns that substantially differ from prior US conflicts. US troops are routinely exposed to a nonuniformed enemy as they actively provide security to the civilian populace while simultaneously denying safe haven to the enemy. The combat medical experience of US military personnel in this irregular warfare presents unique challenges that have not been encountered to such a degree in the history of American military medicine.

Combat Casualty Definitions and Statistics

A casualty in customary military usage refers to an active-duty soldier lost to the theater of operations for any medical reason, including illness and nonbattle injury.[9] Combat (battle) injury is defined as "any casualty incurred as the direct result of hostile action sustained in combat or sustained going to or from

a combat mission."[10] The treatment of combat injuries begins at Echelon I (which includes intravenous fluid resuscitation, hemorrhage control, and fracture immobilization), is provided by military combat medics at the point of injury, and ends upon arrival at the unit's battalion aid station staffed by a trained military physician or physician's assistant. A more intensive level of care, Echelon II, as compared to a battalion aid station, is provided by forward surgical teams where general and orthopedic surgeons and anesthetists employ advanced trauma life support protocols and provide surgical stabilization. The Echelon III level of care is provided at a combat support hospital where combat casualties receive care from surgical subspecialists, and there is intensive care capability and further advanced treatment. After medical stabilization, combat casualties are then medically evacuated for further treatment if necessary through Landstuhl Regional Medical Center in Germany (Echelon IV) and eventually reach a military treatment facility (Echelon V) within the United States.

It is important to correctly categorize casualties and their final disposition in order to maintain consistency when comparing casualty statistics between wars (Figure 2-1). Soldiers who die from combat injuries before reaching an Echelon II level of care are defined as killed in action (KIA), whereas soldiers who survive until arrival at an Echelon II level of care are defined as wounded in action (WIA).[11] The WIA group is further divided into soldiers who died of wounds (DOW) as a result of combat injuries, those treated and medically evacuated (MEDEVAC), and those treated and returned to duty (RTD) within 72 hours.[11] It is imperative to consistently apply exact definitions for combat casualty classifications in order to obtain valid comparisons between conflicts, as well as between studies, when analyzing combat casualty statistics.

Additionally, clearly identifying the casualty population (denominator) is necessary to perform valid comparisons between wars and reach meaningful conclusions. Most casualty reports previous to the Iraq and Afghanistan Wars have not had clearly defined casualty populations from which the denominator being studied is known.[12] As a result, the reporting of musculoskeletal combat casualty statistics from previous wars is potentially biased toward more severe injuries, with less significant wounds being disregarded. The inclusion of soldiers KIA, soldiers RTD, and nonbattle injuries in any cohort examined will affect the distribution of wounds and mechanism of injury. Combat casualties who were RTD and excluded from casualty statistical analysis will bias the reported results toward more severe injuries. Additionally, including only the primary or dominant wound without taking into account secondary wounds can also lead to inaccurate data analysis.

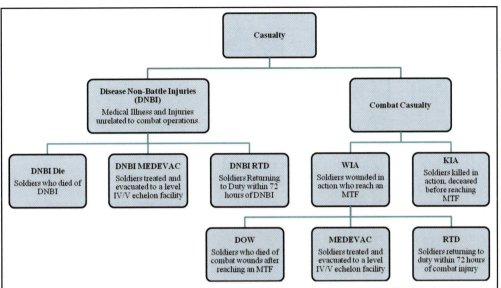

Figure 2-1. Schematic of military casualty definitions and classifications. Wounded in action (WIA), killed in action (KIA), military treatment facility (MTF), died of wounds (DOW), medically evacuated (MEDEVAC), returned to duty (RTD), disease non-battle injury (DNBI).

Most existing reports published on combat casualties prior to, and during, the initial years of the Iraq and Afghanistan Wars have been from either forward surgical teams,[13-17] combat support hospitals,[18-20] or individual military medical centers.[21-24] The combat casualty statistics calculated from individual military treatment facilities underestimate the scale and scope of combat injuries because the denominator consists only of those reaching these facilities.[25] Reports from the Department of Defense administrative health databases focus only on hospital admission rates for combat and nonbattle casualties and fail to account for those soldiers treated in an ambulatory setting and RTD.[26,27] Thorough and correct combat casualty statistical analysis is dependent upon incorporating data from ambulatory casualties who are RTD together with hospitalization and mortality data.

Recent advances in electronic casualty data collection have resulted in the ability to report more detailed and accurate combat casualty care statistics. The Joint Theater Trauma Registry (JTTR) is a prospective database of all Department of Defense combat and other trauma-related casualties beginning at Echelon II and continuing through US military medical treatment facilities. The JTTR is used to document and provide timely information on care and outcomes of military and civilian trauma patients through the echelons of care. Additionally, in December 2007, the Army's Medical Communication for Combat Casualty Care organized a method to electronically capture and transmit trauma data to the US Army Institute of Surgical Research at Fort Sam Houston, Texas, where the JTTR data resides, in order to improve the quality of reported data.[28] There have been more than 40,000 trauma cases entered within the JTTR database, and data collection now occurs over a period of days

instead of months. The JTTR has been used to assess the epidemiology of combat injuries[3,29,30] and musculoskeletal combat injuries to the extremities[31,32] as well as to evaluate the effectiveness of treatment modalities on combat casualty outcomes. Similar to other casualty collection methods, however, the JTTR only records data on soldiers severely injured, including those who DOW and MEDEVAC, and often excludes soldiers KIA and RTD. The US Army also employs a comprehensive electronic medical records system (AHLTA), which has been used to capture additional casualty data on all soldiers WIA.[3]

Historical Comparison of Combat Casualties to Disease and Nonbattle Injury Casualties

Historical comparisons between major conflicts are difficult because data prior to World War I (WWI) are based upon incomplete records in many cases.[33] Additionally, when analyzing the primary data sources for combat casualties and for disease and nonbattle injury (DNBI) casualties, comparisons are challenging because the methods for defining a combat casualty differed between conflicts. Reports from World War II (WWII),[34] the Korean War,[35] the Vietnam War,[36] and the early stages of the Iraq War[26] have relied upon hospital admission rates, while reports from WWI[34] and the later stages of the Iraq War[3,32,37] used ambulatory casualty data along with hospitalization data. Nevertheless, reports from major US conflicts dating back to WWII have consistently found that DNBI has resulted in significantly more hospitalizations and

Table 2-1

Historical Comparison of Casualty Mortality Data for Disease Nonbattle Injury Versus Combat (Battle) Injury

Casualty Classification	WWI	WWII	Korea	Vietnam[33]	Iraq/Afghanistan[33]
Combat deaths	53,402[33]	291,557[33]	33,739[33]	47,434	4,171
DNBI deaths	63,114[33]	113,842[33]	2,835[33]	10,786	1,167
Ratio deaths DNBI:combat casualty	1.1[33,34a]	0.33[33,34b]	0.08-0.1[33,35]	0.23	0.28

[33]Department of Defense: Data available on all combat and DNBI deaths in the principal wars in which US military personnel participated. Data from Iraq and Afghanistan includes March 19, 2003 to February 6, 2010.

[34a]Reister (1975): Data available on all combat and DNBI deaths in the European theater only from April 1, 1917 to December 31, 1918.

[34b]Reister (1975): Data available on all combat and DNBI deaths in the European theater only from December 7, 1941 to December 3, 1945.

[35]Reister (1973): Data available on all combat and DNBI deaths in Korea from July 1950 to July 1953.

time lost than combat injuries.[25,34-36,38,39] The ratio of DNBI to combat casualties was 4.6 to 4.8 in the European theater in both WWI and WWII,[34] 2.4 in the Vietnam War,[36] and has been reported to be as low as between 2.2 and 3.0 in the current conflicts.[3,26,37] Despite the significant decrease in the ratio of DNBI to combat casualties, DNBI casualties continue to represent a significant loss of military personnel within the theater of operations. Since the beginning of the Iraq and Afghanistan Wars in 2001 through February 6, 2010, 47,365 military servicemembers have required medical air transports for DNBI, compared to 10,813 requiring medical air transports as a result of being WIA.[33]

A historical comparison of casualty mortality data, which is more consistently defined among US conflicts, finds a substantial decrease in the ratio of deaths attributable to DNBI compared with those from combat injury (Table 2-1). In WWI, the ratio of DNBI deaths to combat deaths was 1.1 and then subsequently decreased greater than 3-fold in WWII to 0.33.[34] This significant decrease can be largely attributed to the widespread use of antibiotics. Acute respiratory illnesses and infectious diseases were the most prominent causes of hospitalization of US military servicemembers in both conflicts, but the peak incidence was nearly 50% less for acute respiratory illnesses in WWII when compared to WWI.[38] The ratio of DNBI deaths to combat deaths has leveled off to 0.23 to 0.28 since the Vietnam War.[3,36,37]

The loss of troops in the combat zone caused by musculoskeletal nonbattle injuries and the resulting impact on the fighting force has received markedly less attention than the loss caused by musculoskeletal combat casualties; however, it is of significant scope and magnitude to warrant further research. The findings of 2 longitudinal cohort studies of a US Army Brigade Combat Team participating in the counterinsurgency operation "The Iraq War Troop Surge" from 2006-2007 found that there were more than 3 times as many nonbattle musculoskeletal casualties compared to combat (battle) musculoskeletal casualties.[32,37]

Additionally, these studies found that 48% of all musculoskeletal casualties MEDEVAC were a result of nonbattle injuries. The incidence of anterior cruciate ligament rupture and first-time shoulder dislocation as a result of nonbattle injuries during deployment have been found to occur at rates nearly 5 times that of the civilian population.[37] DNBI casualty care statistics are dependent on many factors, including the intensity of combat, type of unit, branch of military service, climate, environment, and duration of deployment.[27,40-42] Higher overall DNBI casualty rates have been reported during periods of increased combat intensity,[26,27,40-42] but this has yet to be determined for the subset of musculoskeletal nonbattle injuries.

The relative increase in the percentage of combat casualties and combat casualty deaths, measured by a decrease in both the ratio of DNBI to combat casualties and the ratio of DNBI deaths to combat deaths, has raised the importance of providing optimal treatment to combat casualties in order to conserve the fighting strength. Additionally, musculoskeletal nonbattle injuries have been reported to account for more than 50% of all DNBI casualties in the current conflicts, warranting significant attention to minimize their effect on the attrition of US military personnel.[37]

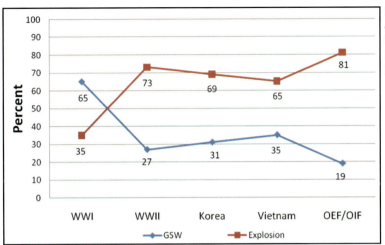

Figure 2-2. Comparison of percentage of combat casualties from gunshot wounds versus explosion injuries.[30,35,43,44] World War I (WWI), World War II (WWII), Operation Enduring Freedom/Operation Iraqi Freedom (OEF/OIF), gunshot wound (GSW).

Mechanism of Injury

During the past 100 years, the United States has been involved in 5 major conflicts: WWI, WWII, the Korean War, the Vietnam War, and the Iraq and Afghanistan Wars. There has been a consistent upward trend in the number of combat casualties resulting from explosive mechanisms of injury, including mortars, rocket-propelled grenades, landmines, and IEDs, when compared to gunshot wounds (Figure 2-2). Explosive mechanisms of injury accounted for 35% of all recorded combat casualties in WWI,[43] 65% in Vietnam,[44] and comprise as much as 84% in the current conflicts.[3,29]

The irregular warfare tactics employed by the enemy coupled with the application of the US' counterinsurgency "clear, build, and hold" doctrine, where large numbers of soldiers actively provide physical security to the civilian population, has caused a growing number of US combat casualties to occur from ambush and explosive mechanisms of injury, particularly IEDs. IEDs are estimated to be responsible for more than 62%[4] of all coalition deaths and more than 80% of all combat casualties during the Iraq War.[3,29] The lethality of IEDs can be measured by the recently reported 26.5% KIA rate,[3] which is calculated by the following equation[11]:

$$\%KIA = KIA/[KIA + (WIA - RTD)] \times 100$$

The %KIA provides a measure of the initial lethality of weapons and is dependent upon the critical body regions injured, the effectiveness of immediate care by medics, and the overall efficiency of battlefield evacuation.[11]

Explosion injuries are classified as primary, secondary, or tertiary with the corresponding etiology of each being the blast wave, projectiles from the munitions, and the victim being thrown against the ground

or an object, respectively.[45] The effects of the primary blast wave decrease exponentially as distance from the explosion increases.[46] Effects of the primary blast wave also depend upon whether the blast occurs within a closed space, increasing both mortality and severity of injury.[45,47,48] Miscellaneous blast injuries, often referred to as quaternary blast injury, include exposure to dust, thermal burns from an explosion, and burns from a fire or blast.[49]

Distribution, Pattern, and Types of Musculoskeletal Combat Wounds and the Effects of Individual Body Armor

Explosive ordinances generally injure multiple body regions simultaneously in contrast to gunshot wounds, which most commonly involve a single body region.[50] Owens and colleagues[31] reviewed the spectrum of orthopedic injuries to the extremities during Operation Iraqi Freedom/Operation Enduring Freedom (OIF/OEF) from October 2001 through January 2005. This study found that explosions were responsible for 75% of extremity combat wounds, representing the highest proportion attributable to explosions in US military history, while gunshot wounds accounted for only 16% of extremity combat wounds. A subsequent report detailing injuries sustained during the The Surge found that the percentage of explosive injuries increased to 81% of all musculoskeletal combat casualties, and the subset of IED-related casualties accounted for 70% as enemy tactics evolved during the course of the Iraq War.[32] In this latter study, when analyzing the mechanism of musculoskeletal combat injury by the combat casualty classification, explosion injuries resulted in a higher RTD rate compared to a gunshot wound (66.9% versus 41.7%) because many combat casualties who survive the initial blast are outside the effective primary blast radius; sustain less severe secondary, tertiary, or quaternary blast injuries; and can be expeditiously treated.[51] This also explains why gunshot wounds have resulted in a moderately increased risk for being MEDEVAC when compared to explosion injuries (58.3% compared to 31.7%).

The overall percentage of soldiers KIA by IEDs has been reported to range from 22% to 26%,[3,52] demonstrating the enemies' tactical success in the use of these weapons. Despite advancements in the US military's individual and vehicular body armor, these figures are still comparable to prior US conflicts.[9,11,25,53,54] Explosive mechanisms with primary blast wave pressures above 80 psi are associated with greater than 50% mortality.[55] Fragments from the explosive munitions have been reported to reach initial velocities of 6000 m/sec, which are capable of causing secondary blast injuries far beyond the primary blast zone, resulting in significant mortality and morbidity.[56,57] Although the percentage of those KIA remains high, the use of individual body armor has reduced the proportion of thoracic injuries among all combat casualties,[58] and most likely has kept the KIA percentage for explosions lower by allowing more soldiers to survive outside the primary blast radius. More quantifiably, individual body armor has reduced the lethality of gunshot wounds, estimated to be 33% prior to the Iraq and Afghanistan Wars[59] but now reported to be 4.6%.[3]

Belmont and colleagues[3] reported that soldiers who survived until arrival at a military treatment facility had a 3.2% DOW rate for all mechanisms of injury, which is the lowest reported for US ground troops in WWII, Korea, Vietnam, and the initial stages of OIF/OEF.[11,53] Despite the enemies' increased use of IEDs and tactical improvements in their deployment, the uniform use of individual body armor and the effectiveness of treatment provided to soldiers, including the rapid use of prehospital tourniquets,[60,61] has increased battlefield survivability of combat injuries. As a result, soldiers are surviving more complex wounding patterns, creating unique challenges to the orthopedic surgeon in the management of combat orthopedic injuries.

The musculoskeletal combat casualty wound incidence rates during OIF are provided in Table 2-2.[31,32,62] Members of a brigade combat team were found to have a major amputation incidence of 2.1 per 1000 soldier combat-years during combat deployment.[32] The aforementioned study and a review of the US JTTR and Military Amputee Research Program databases from 2001 through 2006 have reported major extremity amputation rates from 7.4% to 9.4%

Table 2-2

Musculoskeletal Fractures in the Current Conflict

	Owens[31]	Belmont[32]
Upper extremity	50.4% (461)	41.1% (30)
Lower extremity	49.6% (454)	42.5% (31)
Axial skeleton	N/A	16.4% (12)[62]

Rates are reported as percentage (N).
Upper extremity includes clavicles, scapula, and distal upper extremity. Lower extremity starts at proximal femur. Axial skeleton includes cervical spine, thoracic spine, lumbosacral spine, and pelvis.

among all combat casualties with extremity injuries who were unable to return to duty within 72 hours of injury.[32,63] Five of 6 (83%) amputees in the US Army brigade combat team[3] had more than one major limb amputation compared to the study by Stansbury and colleagues,[63] which reported a figure of 18%. The increased rate of major extremity amputation and the prevalence of multiple major limb amputations within the brigade combat team studied by Belmont and colleagues[32] are likely attributable to the evolution of tactics and improvement in the enemy's weaponry over the 4 years of combat prior to The Surge operation. Valid comparisons of the major extremity amputation rate with reports from previous conflicts are precluded by lack of consistently applied definitions.[35,64-66] Many studies report on the individual amputee, not the number of major extremity amputations, and thus underreport the overall incidence of extremity amputations and how the denominator is calculated.

Previous studies of the Iraq and Afghanistan Wars have found that soft tissue wounds are the most common musculoskeletal combat wound and comprise 36% to 53% of total wounds.[31,32] Fractures have been reported to account for between 24% and 26% of musculoskeletal combat wounds, and a staggering 44% to 82% are open fractures.[31,32] Additionally, the subset of spine, pelvis, and long-bone fractures have accounted for more than half of all fractures sustained in combat in Iraq and Afghanistan.[32] In soldiers wounded in action, which excludes KIA, gunshot wounds (46%) when compared to explosive mechanism of injury (11%) resulted in a greater percentage of open fracture.[32] It is understandable that nearly half of all soldiers sustaining high-velocity gunshot wounds had open fractures. Most military small arms have a 3- to 10-fold greater muzzle kinetic energy than bullets fired by civilian handguns,[25,67] often resulting in severely comminuted fracture patterns with large associated soft tissue defects. Combat fractures caused by high-velocity gunshot wounds with soft tissue defects are often accompanied by significant morbidity. The complications of wound infection (77%), recurrent infection (37%), and delayed union/nonunion (37%) and subsequent amputation (14%) were reported in a recent study of combat-associated type III open tibial fractures.[68]

These changes in wounding patterns can be largely attributed to the enemy's increasing use of IEDs. Soldiers in close proximity to an explosive mechanism may sustain significant primary and secondary blast injuries, which can cause a direct limb amputation in up to 95% of cases. Blasts may also precipitate a significant musculoskeletal combat wound that may necessitate a later surgical amputation.[69-71] Explosive mechanisms in the current conflict have been reported to account for long-bone amputation rates of 7.7%, as compared to a 0% rate for gunshot wounds.[32] Cadaveric tests demonstrate that traumatic amputations occurring as a result of explosive mechanism are primarily caused by shock wave coupling that directly causes extremity fracture and massive soft tissue destruction.[70,72] Thus, the advanced orthopedic surgical care provided to deployed US forces in Iraq and Afghanistan means that the likelihood of an amputation is largely dependent upon the initial tissue destruction rather than infection or isolated neurologic or vascular injury as in previous US conflicts. Additionally, during the initial stage of OIF, long-bone amputations were more often caused by gunshot wounds,[65] but this was supplanted by explosive mechanisms in 88% of amputees as the enemy's tactics evolved.[63]

All US soldiers use advanced individual body armor including protective vests and Kevlar (DuPont, Wilmington, DE) helmets. Some of the currently used outer tactical vests consist of fine Kevlar weaves capable of providing protection from 9-mm pistol rounds. Additionally, Small Arms Protective Inserts (SAPI), which are made of boron carbide ceramic with a spectra shield backing, can resist munitions fragments up to a 7.62-mm round with muzzle velocities of 2750 feet per second (Figure 2-3).[73] The current body armor provides initial protection for the head, thorax, and abdomen, reducing the impact of what might otherwise be life-threatening injuries. This is reflected in the reduction in thoracic injuries, from 13% in Vietnam to 5% in the current conflicts.[3,44] Meanwhile, there has been a relative increase in the number of injuries in the unprotected regions of the body, including the head/neck and extremities, sustained by troops in Iraq and Afghanistan.

Furthermore, improvements in care provided at the Echelons I and II levels of care, coupled with the rapidity of medical evacuation, have resulted in casualties surviving injuries that often leave them with increas-

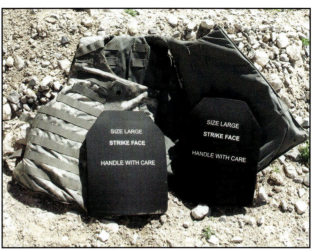

Figure 2-3. SAPI, made of boron carbide ceramic with a spectra shield backing, can resist munitions fragments up to a 7.62-mm round with muzzle velocities of 2750 feet per second.[73]

ingly morbid conditions. The medical and casualty evacuation system routinely employs ground and helicopter transport to forward surgical teams or combat support hospitals within 1 hour. The overall percentage of soldiers who die of wounds after reaching medical treatment facilities in OIF has been found to be 3.2%,[3] which is nearly 7-fold less than the %KIA. This compares favorably to the 8.8% DOW rate reported by the Israeli Defense Forces, who used a similar personal armor system during the Second Palestinian Uprising.[74] The current %DOW also represents a significant reduction compared to reports for US ground troops in WWII, Korea, Vietnam, and the initial stages of OIF/OEF (%DOW range 3.2% to 6.7%).[1,11,74] The %DOW provides a measure of the appropriateness of field triage and the effectiveness of treatment rendered at the forward surgical team and combat support hospital, which are staffed by medical providers, including general and orthopedic surgeons.

Evolution of Enemy Tactics and the Development and Fielding of the Mine-Resistant Ambush-Protected Vehicle

The asymmetric tactical use of IEDs against US military forces in Iraq and Afghanistan has continued to evolve, with both total use and sophistication increasing as the wars have progressed. The US military's global data concerning explosive ordinance, including IEDs, remain classified to prevent extremists from gaining information the United States has obtained. The most reliable known data from a private company

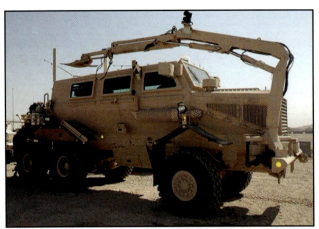

Figure 2-4. MRAP vehicles more effectively counter the threat of IEDs, largely in part due to the development of the "V"-shaped hulls, which has helped reduce US military fatalities.

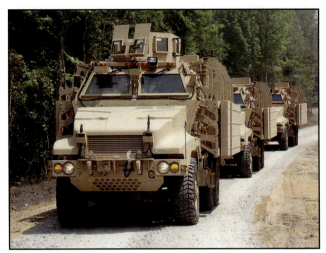

Figure 2-5. Convoy of MRAP vehicles.

that analyzes the use of IEDs estimate that, by 2009, the annual number of IED attacks in Afghanistan had grown nearly 2-fold from 515 in 2006.[75] The increase in IED attacks along with the doubling of American troop levels in 2009 has led overall coalition fatalities in Afghanistan to rise from 295 in 2008 to 520 in 2009.[76] In February 2007, faced with increasing IED attacks and resultant deaths, the Department of Defense addressed the urgent operational need to improve armored tactical vehicles and thereby increase crew protection by initiating the mine-resistant ambush-protected (MRAP) vehicle program (Figures 2-4 and 2-5). Shortly thereafter, in May 2007, the Department of Defense declared the acquisition of MRAP vehicles its highest priority.[77] The MRAP program relied only on proven technologies and commercially available products; established minimal operational requirements; and undertook a concurrent approach to producing, testing, and fielding the vehicles.

The MRAP program demonstrated 3 of the principal foundations of the Western Way of War. First, US combatant commanders changed military practices as the needs arose by identifying the need to better protect US troops in hazardous fire areas against IEDS, rocket-propelled grenades, and small arms fire. Second, the US Department of Defense had the power to finance the production of 16,203 MRAP vehicles as of July 2009 at a cost of $22.7 billion.[77] Third, US research and industry were able to develop and produce the technologically advanced MRAP vehicles to more effectively counter the threat of IEDs. Casualty figures suggest that the quick pace of the development of MRAP vehicles with "V"-shaped hulls has helped to reduce US military fatalities from IED attacks. Figures compiled on the Web site www.icasualties.org reveal that, in 2009, the percentage of US military servicemembers who were killed in IED attacks decreased to 40% compared to 50% in 2008.[76] Additionally,

the MRAP vehicle has never lost an entire crew to a single IED explosion. The increased personnel protection afforded by the MRAP will result in fewer battle deaths but will undoubtedly result in more complex combat casualty wounds that might have otherwise proved fatal.

Conclusion

More than two-thirds of all soldiers medically evacuated from theater have sustained injuries to the musculoskeletal system. US servicemembers MEDEVAC from Iraq and Afghanistan receive continued care at Echelon V facilities within the United States. The musculoskeletal combat casualty care statistics, distribution of wounds, and mechanisms of injury are dependent on many factors, including the intensity and type of combat, type of unit, branch of service, and duration of deployment. The estimated initial hospitalization and projected disability benefits for soldiers sustaining combat extremity wounds in Iraq and Afghanistan between October 2001 and December 2005 is $1.66 billion.[29] The complex orthopedic injury patterns found in the Iraq and Afghanistan Wars, including the high incidence rates of major amputations and open fractures, have important implications for the treatment of soldiers at Echelons IV and V. Additionally, the fiscal cost and responsibility for ongoing care of combat-injured soldiers must be borne by the federal government, military treatment facilities, and the Veterans' Administration.[29] Despite the willingness, experience, and expert care provided by military orthopedic surgeons, the elimination of morbidity and preservation of life has proven to be difficult. Advancement in individual and vehicular body armor in conjunction with evolving enemy tactics and weaponry have afforded the enemy a greater capacity for impairing and incapacitating soldiers deployed to the theater of operations.

References

1. Parker G. Introduction: the Western way of war. In: Parker G, ed. *The Cambridge Illustrated History of Warfare*. Cambridge, UK: Cambridge University Press; 1995:2-9.

2. Covey DC. From the frontlines to the home front: the crucial role of military orthopaedic surgeons. *J Bone Joint Surg Am.* 2009;91:998-1006.

3. Belmont PJ Jr, Goodman GP, Zacchilli M, Posner M, Evans C, Owens BD. Incidence and epidemiology of combat injuries sustained during "The Surge" portion of Operation Iraqi Freedom by a US Army Brigade Combat Team. *J Trauma.* 2010;68:204-210.

4. Bird SM, Fairweather CB. Military fatality rates (by cause) in Afghanistan and Iraq: a measure of hostilities. *Int J Epidemiol.* 2007;36(4):841-846.

5. Covey DC. Blast and fragment injuries of the musculoskeletal system. *J Bone Joint Surg Am.* 2002;84:1221-1234.

6. Mazurek MT, Ficke JR. The scope of wounds encountered in casualties from the global war on terrorism: from the battlefield to the tertiary treatment facility. *J Am Acad Orthop Surg.* 2006;14:S18-S23.

7. Packer G. The lesson of Tal Afar. *The New Yorker.* (10 Apr 2006):48-65. http://www.newyorker.com/archive/2006/04/10/060410fa_fact2?currentPage=all. Accessed April 3, 2010.

8. McMaster HR. Colonel H.R. McMaster (USA) holds a Defense Department news briefing via teleconference from Iraq on operations in Tal Afar. *FDCH Political Transcripts.* September 13, 2005.

9. Bellamy RF. Combat trauma overview. In: Zajtchuk R, Grande CM, eds. *Textbook of Military Medicine, Anesthesia and Perioperative Care of the Combat Casualty.* Falls Church, VA: Office of the Surgeon General, United States Army; 1995:1-42.

10. Atlas of injuries in the United States Armed Forces. *Mil Med.* 1999;164(8 Suppl):S1-S89.

11. Holcomb JB, Stansbury LG, Champion HR, et al. Understanding combat casualty care statistics. *J Trauma.* 2006;60(2):397-401.

12. Holcomb JB. The 2004 Fitts Lecture: current perspective on combat casualty care. *J Trauma.* 2005;59:990-1002.

13. Beekley AC, Watts DM. Combat trauma experience with the United States Army 102nd Forward Surgical Team in Afghanistan. *Am J Surg.* 2004;187(5):652-654.

14. Chambers LW, Rhee P, Baker BC, et al. Initial experience of US Marine Corps Forward Resuscitative Surgical System during Operation Iraqi Freedom. *Arch Surg.* 2005;140(1):26-32.

15. Patel TH, Wenner KA, Price SA, et al. A U.S. Army Forward Surgical Team's experience in Operation Iraqi Freedom. *J Trauma.* 2004;57(2):201-207.

16. Peoples GE, Gerlinger T, Craig R, et al. Combat casualties in Afghanistan cared for by a single forward surgical team during the initial phases of Operation Enduring Freedom. *Mil Med.* 2005;170(6):462-468.

17. Rush RM, Stockmaster NR, Stinger HK, et al. Supporting the Global War on Terror: a tale of two campaigns featuring the 250th Forward Surgical Team (Airborne). *Am J Surg.* 2005;189(5):564-570.

18. Acosta JA, Hatzigeorgiou C, Smith LS. Developing a trauma registry of a forward deployed military hospital: a preliminary report. *J Trauma.* 2006;61(2):256-260.

19. Murdock AD. Experience at the 332d Air Force Theater Hospital: evacuation hub for Iraq. *J Trauma.* 2007;62(6 Suppl):S19.

20. Cho JM, Jatoi I, Alarcon AS, et al. Operation Iraqi Freedom: surgical experience of the 212th Mobile Army Surgical Hospital. *Mil Med.* 2005;170(4):268-272.

21. Johnson BA, Carmack D, Neary M, et al. Operation Iraqi Freedom: the Landstuhl Regional Medical Center experience. *J Foot Ankle Surg.* 2005;44(3):177-183.

22. Lin DL, Kirk KL, Murphy KP, et al. Evaluation of orthopaedic injuries in Operation Enduring Freedom. *J Orthop Trauma.* 2004;18(5):300-305.

23. Montgomery SP, Swiecki CW, Shriver CD. The evaluation of casualties from Operation Iraqi Freedom on return to the continental United States from March to June 2003. *J Am Coll Surg.* 2005;201(1):7-13.

24. Wolf SE, Kauvar DS, Wade CE, et al. Comparison between civilian burns and combat burns from Operation Iraqi Freedom and Operation Enduring Freedom. *Ann Surg.* 2006;243(6):786-795.

25. Champion HR, Bellamy RF, Roberts P, et al. A profile of combat injury. *J Trauma.* 2003;54:S13-S19.

26. Zouris JM, Wade AL, Magno CP. Injury and illness casualty distributions among U.S. Army and Marine Corps personnel during Operation Iraqi Freedom. *Mil Med.* 2008;173:247-252.

27. Wojcik BE, Humphrey RJ, Czejdo B, Hassell H. U.S. Army disease and nonbattle injury model, refined in Afghanistan and Iraq. *Mil Med.* 2008;173:825-835.

28. Simmons L. Trauma registry system crunches data mining time, improves battlefield care and equipment. The Gateway. 2009;4(6). http://www.mc4.army.mil/mc4newsletter/2009_6/feature_story.asp. Accessed March 1, 2010.

29. Masini BD, Waterman SM, Wenke JC, et al. Resource utilization and disability outcome assessment of combat casualties from Operation Iraqi Freedom and Operation Enduring Freedom. *J Orthop Trauma.* 2009;23(4):261-266.

30. Owens BD, Kragh JF Jr, Wenke JC, Macaitis J, Wade CE, Holcomb JB. Combat wounds in Operation Iraqi Freedom and Operation Enduring Freedom. *J Trauma.* 2008;64:295-299.

31. Owens BD, Kragh JF Jr, Macaitis J, Svoboda SJ, Wenke JC. Characterization of extremity wounds in Operation Iraqi Freedom and Operation Enduring Freedom. *J Orthop Trauma.* 2007;21:254-257.

32. Belmont PJ Jr, Thomas D, Goodman GP, Schoenfeld AJ, Zacchilli M, Burks R. Combat musculoskeletal wounds in a U.S. Army Brigade combat team during Operation Iraqi Freedom. *J Trauma.* (In press).

33. Directorate for Information Operations and Reports, Department of Defense. Military casualty information http://siadapp.dmdc.osd.mil/personnel/CASUALTY/castop.htm. Accessed February 23, 2010.

34. Reister FA. *Medical Statistics in World War II.* Washington, DC: The Surgeon General, Department of the Army; 1975:3-75.

35. Reister FA. *Battle Casualties and Medical Statistics: U.S. Army Experience in the Korean War.* Washington, DC: The Surgeon General, Department of the Army; 1973:1-45.

36. Palinkas LA, Coben P. Disease and non-battle injuries among U.S. Marines in Vietnam. *Mil Med.* 1988;153(3):150-155.

37. Belmont PJ Jr, Goodman GP, Waterman B, DeZee K, Burks R, Owens BD. Disease and nonbattle injuries sustained by a U.S. Army Brigade combat team during Operation Iraqi Freedom. *Mil Med.* 2010;175(7):469-476.

38. Hoeffler DF, Melton LJ. Changes in the distribution of Navy and Marine Corps casualties from World War I through the Vietnam Conflict. *Mil Med.* 1981;146:776-779.

39. Holland BD, Long AP. Cost of non-battle injuries and diseases compared to battle casualties. *Mil Med.* 1955;117(1):46-50.

40. Blood CG, Anderson ME. The battle for Hue: casualty and disease rates during urban warfare. *Mil Med.* 1994;159:590-595.

41. Blood CG, Gauker C. The relationship between battle intensity and disease rates among Marine Corps infantry units. *Mil Med.* 1993;158:340-344.

42. Blood CG, Jolly R. Comparisons of disease and non-battle injury incidence across various military operations. *Mil Med.* 1995;160:258-263.

43. Beebe GW, DeBakey ME. *Battle Casualties: Incidence, Morality, and Logistic Considerations.* Springfield, IL: Charles C. Thomas; 1952:74-147.

44. Hardaway RM. Viet Nam wound analysis. *J Trauma.* 1978;18(9): 635-643.

45. Cooper GJ, Maynard RL, Cross NL, et al. Casualties from terrorist bombings. *J Trauma.* 1983;23(11):955-967.

46. Leibovici D, Gofrit ON, Stein M, et al. Blast injuries: bus versus open-air bombings—a comparative study of injuries in survivors of open-air versus confined-space explosions. *J Trauma.* 1996;41(6):1030-1035.

47. Cullis IG. Blast waves and how they interact with structures. *J R Army Med Corps.* 2001;147(1):16-26.

48. Arnold JL, Halpern P, Tsai MC, et al. Mass casualty terrorist bombings: a comparison of outcomes by bombing type. *Ann Emerg Med.* 2004;43(2):263-273.

49. DePalma RG, Burris DG, Champion HR, et al. Blast injuries. *N Engl J Med.* 2005;352(13):1335-1342.

50. Peleg K, Aharonson-Daniel L, Stein M, et al. Gunshot and explosion injuries: characteristics, outcomes, and implications for care of terror-related injuries in Israel. *Ann Surg.* 2004;239(3):311-318.

51. Ramasamy A, Harrisson SE, Clasper JC, Stewart MPM. Injuries from roadside improvised explosive devices. *J Trauma.* 2008;65(4):910-914.

52. Nelson TJ, Clark T, Stedje-Larsen ET, et al. Close proximity blast injury patterns from improvised explosive devices in Iraq; a report of 18 cases. *J Trauma.* 2008;65(1):212-217.

53. Bellamy RF, Maningas PA, Vayer JS. Epidemiology of trauma: military experience. *Ann Emerg Med.* 1986;15(12):1384-1388.

54. Gawande A. Casualties of war—military care for the wounded from Iraq and Afghanistan. *N Engl J Med.* 2004;351(24):2471-2475.

55. Mellor SG, Cooper GJ. Analysis of 828 servicemen killed or injured by explosion in Northern Ireland 1970-84: the Hostile Action Casualty System. *Br J Surg.* 1989;76(10):1006-1010.

56. Clark MA. The pathology of terrorism: acts of violence directed against citizens of the United States while abroad. *Clin Lab Med.* 1998;18(1):99-114.

57. Bellamy RF, Zajtchuk R. The physics and biophysics of wound ballistics. In: Zajtchuk R, ed. *Textbook of Military Medicine, Part I: Warfare, Weaponry, and the Casualty, Vol. 5, Conventional Warfare: Ballistic, Blast, and Burn Injuries.* Washington, DC: Office of the Surgeon General, Department of the Army, United States of America; 1991:107 162.

58. Uhorchak JM, Rodkey WG, Hunt MM, Hoxie SW. *Institute Report #469: Casualty Data Assessment Team Operation Desert Storm.* San Francisco, CA: Letterman Army Institute of Research; 1992.

59. Bellamy RF, Zajtchuk R. Assessing the effectiveness of conventional weapons. In: Zajtchuk R, ed. *Textbook of Military Medicine, Part I: Warfare, Weaponry, and the Casualty, Vol. 5, Conventional Warfare: Ballistic, Blast, and Burn Injuries.* Washington, DC: Office of the Surgeon General, Department of the Army, United States of America; 1991:53-82.

60. Beekly AC, Sebesta JA, Blackbourne LH, et al. Prehospital tourniquet use in Operation Iraqi Freedom: effect on hemorrhage control and outcomes. *J Trauma.* 2008;64:S28-S37.

61. Kragh JF, Walters TJ, Baer DG, et al. Practical use of emergency tourniquets to stop bleeding in major limb trauma. *J Trauma.* 2008;64(2 Suppl):S38-S50.

62. Schoenfeld AJ, Goodman GP, Belmont PJ Jr. Characterization of combat-related spinal injuries sustained by a US Army Brigade combat team during Operation Iraqi Freedom. *Spine J.* 2010 Jun 10. [Epub ahead of print]

63. Stansbury LG, Lallis SJ, Branstetter JG, Bagg MR, Holcomb JB. Amputations in U.S. military personnel in the current conflicts in Afghanistan and Iraq. *J Orthop Trauma.* 2008;22(10):43-46.

64. Dougherty PJ. Wartime amputations. *Mil Med.* 1993;158(12):755-763.

65. Ramalingam T, Pathak G, Barker P. A method for determining the rate of major limb amputations in battle casualties: experiences of a British field hospital in Iraq, 2003. *Ann R Coll Sug Engl.* 2005;87(2):113-116.

66. Islinger RB, Kuklo TR, McHale KA. A review of orthopaedic injuries in three recent U.S. military conflicts. *Mil Med.* 2000;165(6):463-465.

67. Bartlett CS, Helfet DL, Hausman MR, Strauss E. Ballistics and gunshot wounds: effects on musculoskeletal tissues. *J Am Acad Orthop Surg.* 2000;8(1):21-36.

68. Johnson EN, Burns TC, Hayda RA, et al. Infectious complications of open type III tibial fractures among combat casualties. *Clin Infect Dis.* 2007;45(4):409-415.

69. Frykberg ER, Tepas JJ 3rd. Terrorist bombings. Lessons learned from Belfast to Beirut. *Ann Surg.* 1988;208(5):569-576.

70. Hull JB, Cooper GJ. Pattern and mechanism of traumatic amputation by explosive blast. *J Trauma.* 1996;40(3 Suppl):S198-S205.

71. Hull JB. Traumatic amputation by explosive blast: pattern of injury in survivors. *Br J Surg.* 1992;79(12):1303-1306.

72. Hayda R, Harris RM, Bass CD. Blast injury research: modeling injury effects of landmines, bullets, and bombs. *Clin Orthop Relat Res.* 2004;422:97-108.

73. Interceptor Body Armor System. http://www.olive-drab.com/od_soldiers_gear_body_armor_interceptor.php. Accessed April 3, 2010.

74. Lakstein D, Blumenfeld A. Israeli Army casualties in the second Palestinian uprising. *Mil Med.* 2005;170(5):427-430.

75. Shanker T. Makshift bombs spread beyond Afghanistan, Iraq. *The New York Times.* October 29, 2009. http://www.nytimes.com/2009/10/29/world/29military.html. Accessed March 1, 2010.

76. Operation Enduring Freedom: coalition fatalities. http://www.icasualties.org/oef/Afghanistan.aspx. Accessed March 1, 2010.

77. The Library of Congress. *Defense Acquisitions: Rapid Acquisition of MRAP Vehicles.* Washington, DC: US Government Accountability Office; October 2009: GAO-10-155T.

Chapter 3

ECHELONS OF CARE

LTC Mark Pallis, DO and COL Tad Gerlinger, MD

Throughout the history of warfare, the principal task of military medical personnel has been to preserve combat power through medical treatment. While a considerable amount of effort has been directed toward reducing the incidence of disease and nonbattle injury, the timely evacuation, treatment, and ultimate return to duty of wounded servicemembers continues to be a high priority for modern militaries. The US military has developed a complex, integrated trauma treatment system that is arguably the largest and best in the world.

There are 5 levels or echelons of care for wounded servicemembers (Figure 3-1). Each echelon is progressively further from the forward edge of the battle area and has more advanced capabilities than the previous one. Each succeeding echelon possesses the same treatment capabilities as those echelons forward and adds a new treatment capability.[1,2] The ultimate goal of the system is to coordinate all available medical resources to provide injured personnel with the most timely and effective treatment possible given the potential geographic, security, and logistical constraints. Relatively minor injuries can be treated at a forward level and servicemembers can return to duty. More significant wounds or those requiring longer periods of rehabilitation are evacuated to higher levels of care. The system is based on the principles of basic first aid at the point of wounding, rapid evacuation, early surgical stabilization, critical care transport, and definitive care provided at hospitals located in the continental United States.

Movement of casualties generally progresses from one echelon to the next. However, depending on the severity of the injury or the tactical situation, the evacuation of the wounded may skip a level.[3] For example, a severely injured Soldier may be evacuated by helicopter from the point of wounding directly to an Echelon III facility. In the current conflict, medical regulating officers (MRO) coordinate available evacuation assets with medical treatment facilities to ensure rapid evacuation of casualties; match the severity of injury with the required surgical capabilities; and distribute the load, where possible, to prevent overwhelming the resources of a single facility.

By Joint Doctrine, tactical patient evacuation in the combat zone from Echelon I to Echelon II, from Echelon II to Echelon III, and within Echelon III is normally the responsibility of the component commands and is coordinated by a Theater Patient Movement Requirements Center (TPRMC). These movements can be by surface (land or water), rotary-wing aircraft, or tactical aeromedical aircraft. Strategic aeromedical evacuation from the combat zone (Echelon III) to the communications zone (Echelon IV) is normally the responsibility of the Air Force. Patient evacuation from theater to the continental United States is executed by the Air Force Air Mobility Command.[2] In the current conflict, the goal for casualty evacuation (Echelon I to II) is 60 minutes, for tactical evacuation (Echelon II to III) is 24 hours, and for strategic evacuation (Echelon III to IV) is 48 to 72 hours.

Because rapid evacuation of the wounded from the combat zone is now possible, care in theater is limited to the treatment necessary to save life, limb, and/or eyesight. For extremity trauma, the principles of damage control orthopedics[4] are applied in an effort to

Owens BD, Belmont PJ Jr, eds. *Combat Orthopedic Surgery: Lessons Learned in Iraq and Afghanistan (pp 23-30)*
© 2011 SLACK Incorporated

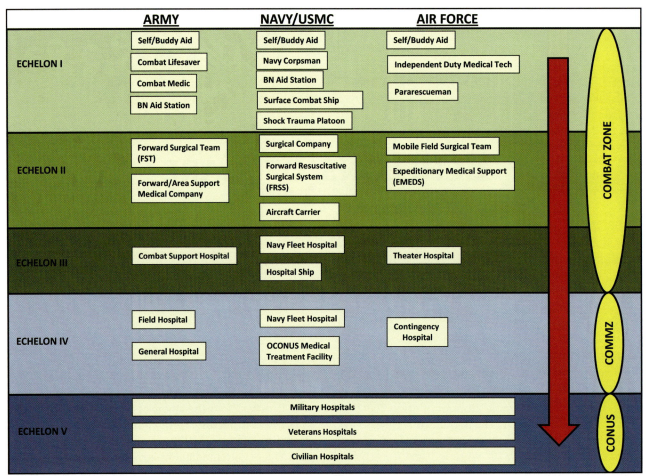

Figure 3-1. Joint Echelons of Care in the Military Health System.[13] COMMZ = communications zone, CONUS = continental United States.

control hemorrhage, prevent infection, and preserve function. Antibiotics and tetanus prophylaxis are administered. Open wounds are debrided, left open, and dressed with an absorbent dressing or wound vacuum dressing. Fractures are stabilized with either splints or external fixators. If required, immediate amputation is performed, but every attempt is made to preserve the limb when it is perfused or can be revascularized. Compartment releases are performed liberally to prevent the development of compartment syndrome during transport. Definitive treatment of extremity injuries, as well as the decision regarding reconstruction or amputation of severe injuries, is generally done after the wounded servicemember reaches the continental United States Echelon V hospital. All wounds are re-evaluated at each level of care, often in the operating room (OR), as the patient is moved through the evacuation chain.[3]

To demonstrate the scope of care provided by the military trauma system, from October 2001 through March 2010, there were 4052 combat deaths and an additional 1175 noncombat deaths in Operation Iraqi Freedom (OIF) and Operation Enduring Freedom

(OEF) combined. Of these, 942 died of wounds. There were a total of 36,906 wounded in action in OIF/OEF, and of these, 10,890 required medical air transport. An additional 47,890 servicemembers required medical air transport for nonhostile injury or illness.[5,6] These numbers, of course, do not include the tremendous workload resulting from care provided for coalition and host-nation civilian casualties.

Echelon I

Care is rendered at the unit level and includes self aid and buddy aid, examination, and emergency lifesaving measures such as maintenance of airway, control of bleeding, prevention and control of shock, and prevention of further injury by trained personnel.[7]

Combat casualty care begins at the point of injury. First responders include fellow servicemembers and service-specific medics or corpsman. Self and buddy aid is typically the first medical intervention for the wounded. First aid training is included in the various basic training courses offered by the services and focuses on the ABCs: airway, breathing, and circulation. In addition to basic CPR skills, prevention of shock, intravenous infusion, splinting of fractures, initial care of wounds to include burns, and transport of the wounded are also outlined in the *Soldier's Manual of Common Tasks, Level 1.*[8] These skills are trained and tested at the unit level for all Soldiers. Nonmedical personnel may also receive advanced basic trauma skills training through the Combat Lifesaver program[9] (Figure 3-2). A Combat Lifesaver performs lifesaving measures as a secondary duty, such as initiating intravenous access, as the tactical situation allows. Training includes advanced first aid and lifesaving procedures beyond basic first aid and may be conducted at the unit level by the unit's medical personnel, in conjunction with materials available by correspondence or online. Combat Lifesavers are a force multiplier for the combat medic.

Combat medics and corpsman are intrinsic to military units. They serve as the medical expert at the company level and lower. Their duties include conducting first aid sustainment training for the members of their unit as well as serving as the medical experts at that level. They also maintain tactical proficiency, as they are integral to the fighting unit. The medic/corpsman's focus is on basic first aid, hemorrhage control, initial treatment of wounds, and evacuation of those requiring more advanced care. After initial entry training, they attend Advanced Individual Training (MOS 68W) in the Army, "A" school in the Navy (NEC HM-0000), and Tech School in the Air Force (4N0X1) that focuses on the skills of a battlefield medical provider. Skills are equivalent to an emergency medical technician-basic (EMT-B), and many seek advance qualification.

Medical support of special operations units is characterized by an austere structure and a limited number of medical personnel. The nature of special operations forces (SOF) missions requires that SOF medical personnel possess a variety of enhanced medical skills that enable them to operate under a multiplicity of circumstances.[7]

SOF have additional requirements of their medical personnel. Due to limited access to the next higher echelon of care, SOF medical personnel are given additional medical training. Army Special Forces' medics (18D) attend year-long training and are required to maintain emergency medical technician-paramedic (EMT-P) credentials. Ranger and Special Operation Aviation medics obtain additional medical skills through the Special Operations Combat Medic Course (SOCM), which includes BLS, ACLS, EMT-B, and the opportunity to test for EMT-P. Navy, Marine Corps, and Air Force Special Operation medical personnel are also expected to maintain a higher level of proficiency than a basic corpsman and medic. They

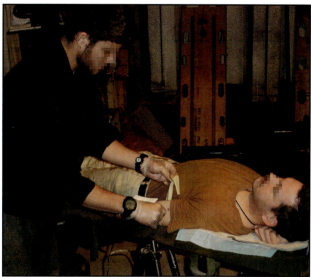

Figure 3-2. Medic intravenous access training.

attend SOCM, may earn EMT-P credentials, and Navy personnel may become qualified as Independent Duty Corpsman with additional training.

This echelon may include an aid station that has physicians or physician assistants. Treatment at the aid station includes restoration of the airway by surgical procedure; use of intravenous fluids, including Ringer's Lactate and Human Albumin; antibiotics; and application of splints and bandages. These elements of medical management prepare patients for RTD or for transportation to a higher echelon of care.[7]

A physician or physician assistant staff the Army Battalion Aid Station (BAS). The BAS is the most far-forward treatment location with basic lab, moderate pharmacy, blood products, and the possibility of a patient-holding capability.[10] Initial resuscitative treatment is conducted at this level and may include emergency procedures including surgical airway, chest tube placement, and surgical venous access. The providers hold additional qualification in Advanced Trauma Life Support (ATLS), and most undergo pre-deployment training focused on combat casualty care. The Navy/Marine Corps equivalent of the BAS is the Shock Trauma Platoon, which is staffed by 2 physicians.

Evacuation of casualties is at the discretion of the provider. If the patient cannot be rapidly returned to duty, evacuation to the next echelon is coordinated by TPRMC and is generally performed by assets located at the next echelon. This evacuation may be to the supporting Echelon II facility or may be to the Echelon III facility as required by the patient's medical condition and as allowed by the available evacuation assets and tactical situation.

Echelon II

Care is administered at an HSS [health service support] organization by a team of physicians or physician assistants, supported by appropriate medical, technical, or nursing staff. As a minimum, this echelon of care includes basic resuscitation and stabilization and may include surgical capability, basic laboratory, limited x-ray, pharmacy, and temporary holding ward facilities. At this echelon, examinations and observations are accomplished more deliberately than at Echelon I. This phase of treatment applies emergency procedures, such as resuscitation, to prevent death, loss of limb, or body functions. For those patients who require more comprehensive treatment, surface or air evacuation is available to a facility possessing the required treatment capability. This is the first echelon at which Group O liquid packed red blood cells will be available for transfusion.[7]

Echelon II is the first echelon at which surgical capability exists. The Army fields Forward Surgical Teams (FST), the Air Force has the Mobile Field Surgical Team (MFST), and the Navy uses the Forward Resuscitative Surgical System (FRSS). These can be co-located with a Medical Company (Army), Expeditionary Medical Support (Air Force EMEDS), Surgical Company (Navy), or a ship with ORs. These additional assets may add patient hold, dental, lab, x-ray, mental health, preventive medicine, and optometry capabilities.

The forward surgical team (FST) is a 20-man team which provides far forward surgical intervention to render nontransportable patients sufficiently stable to allow for medical evacuation to a Level III hospital (combat support hospital [CSH]).[11]

The mission of the Army FST is to be a rapidly deployable initial surgical asset deployed forward in the Division Area of Operations. They are employed in the combat zone and may be assigned one per maneuver brigade. The unit is composed of an ATLS section, OR section, and intensive care unit (ICU) section (Figures 3-3 through 3-5). It is staffed by 2 or 3 general surgeons, 1 or 2 orthopedic surgeons, 2 CRNAs, an executive officer, and an officer in charge for each of the ATLS, OR, and ICU sections. The staff of 20 is completed with ATLS medics, OR technicians, and ICU LPNs. Doctrine states that an FST is capable of providing emergency treatment, necessary surgery, and continuous postoperative care for 30 patients in 72 hours before receiving resupply. Postoperative nursing care is limited to 8 patients for 6 hours. Capabilities include airborne and air assault insertion and the ability to maneuver with the fighting force in intrinsic vehicles. Equipment includes tentage for ATLS, OR, and ICU

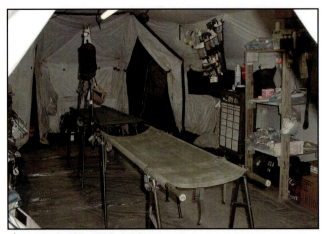

Figure 3-3. FST ATLS section.

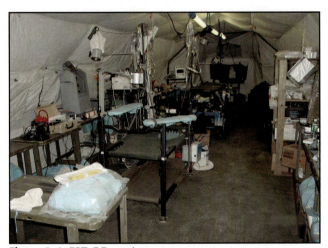

Figure 3-4. FST OR section.

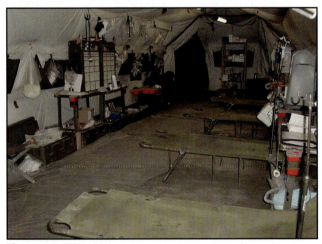

Figure 3-5. FST ICU section.

sections and the necessary equipment to resuscitate casualties, perform surgery, and recover postoperative patients who may require ventilator support. There is no patient holding capability.

FSTs may be co-located with a medical company, to which they may be assigned, which provides for additional health service capabilities. Depending on the unit to which medical companies are assigned, they may be referred to as a forward support medical company (FSMC), main support medical company (MSMC), brigade support medical company (BSMC), and division support medical company (DSMC). Tactical capabilities may also differ according to the unit to which they are assigned: armored, light infantry, airborne, and air assault. The medical companies are composed of a headquarters section, treatment platoon, ambulance platoon, mental health section, preventive medicine section, and optometry section. The treatment platoon may have up to 4 treatment squads led by a field surgeon or physician assistant, as well as lab, dental, and x-ray assets. The treatment platoon also contains a patient holding squad, led by a medical-surgical nurse, that can provide care for up to 40 patients for up to 72 hours.

The Air Force MFST may be employed as a portion of the Small Portable Expeditionary Aeromedical Rapid Response (SPEARR) team. It is a 5-member team that consists of a general surgeon, orthopedic surgeon, emergency medicine physician, anesthetist, and OR nurse or technician. It is designed to provide care for 10 trauma patients in 48 hours, and their equipment is man-portable. The complete SPEARR team adds a 3-person Critical Care Air Transport (CCAT) team and a 2-man Preventive Medicine (PM) team. The CCAT is composed of an intensive care physician (critical care, anesthesiology, or emergency medicine), and the PM team is staffed by a flight surgeon and public health officer. The complete SPEARR team is capable of 7-day operations; can provide basic primary care, postoperative care, and preventive medicine; and its equipment can be contained on a pallet-sized trailer.

The addition of an EMEDS Basic increases capabilities, providing for 24-hour sick call, dental care, limited laboratory, and x-ray. Staff is 25 members, and 4 holding beds, an OR table, and 3 tents are also added to the SPEARR footprint. An EMEDS+10 adds 6 additional beds to the EMEDS Basic, consists of a 56-member staff, and has 6 tents.

The Navy deploys the FRSS in support of the Marine Corps. It provides 1 OR and 2 surgeons and is designed to perform resuscitative surgery for 18 patients in 48 hours before resupply. It is capable of standing alone, but has no holding capability.

The FRSS is frequently employed with a surgical company, which is designed to provide surgical support for a Marine Expeditionary Force (MEF). They are normally assigned one per regiment and have a 60-bed capacity, 3 ORs, and can hold patients for up to 72 hours.

The Navy also has ship-based Echelon II capabilities. The Casualty Receiving and Treatment Ships (CRTS) are intrinsic to the Amphibious Ready Group (ARG) and contain 47 or 48 patient beds, 4 to 6 ORs, and 17 ICU beds. Troop quarters may provide up to 300 additional beds. Care is provided by FSTs, staffed by 3 or 4 physicians, 1 surgeon, 1 anesthesia provider, and additional support staff. Additional surgeons, to include orthopedic and oral maxillofacial surgeons, may be assigned. Lab and x-ray are available, and patient holding is generally limited to 3 days.

Patients who cannot be returned to duty within 72 hours are generally evacuated to Echelon III. Direct transport to Echelon IV is possible if the patient's condition is unlikely to allow return to duty within the Echelon III evacuation policy or if the medical capabilities required by the patient's condition are not available at Echelon III.

Echelon III

Care administered requires clinical capabilities normally found in a MTF that is typically located in a lower-level enemy threat environment. The MTF is staffed and equipped to provide resuscitation, initial wound surgery, and postoperative treatment. This echelon's care may be the first step toward restoration of functional health, as compared to procedures that stabilize a condition or prolong life. It does not have the crises aspects of initial resuscitative care and can proceed with greater preparation and deliberation. Blood products available include fresh frozen plasma, platelets, frozen Group O red cells, and Groups A, B, and O liquid cells.[7]

Echelon III facilities offer the most advanced level of medical and surgical care within the combat zone. These large hospitals are comparable to civilian trauma centers, providing triage, resuscitation, and surgical stabilization for combat casualties. Although each service configures its Echelon III facilities slightly differently, they all are comparably equipped and have similar capabilities. They have an emergency room and a large patient holding capability—including postoperative care wards, inpatient wards, and ICUs. Ancillary support services include laboratory, blood bank, x-ray, computed tomography scan, pharmacy, physical therapy, and occupational therapy. Patients are either treated and returned to duty or are stabilized for further evacuation.

The professional complement in these facilities is quite robust. All include general surgeons, orthopedic surgeons, vascular surgeons, thoracic surgeons, obstetrician/gynecologists, ophthalmologists, urologists, oral surgeons, anesthesiologists, nurse anesthetists, radiologists, emergency physicians, internists, and psychiatrists. The hospitals can be further augmented with additional specialists in fields such as neurosurgery, otolaryngology, intensive care, infectious disease, dermatology, and cardiology.

By doctrine, Echelon III facilities are generally located in rear areas of the combat zone or near major lines of communication (harbor, airfield, large highway). This provides security for the hospital but also facilitates evacuation of casualties and resupply. They are modular by design, allowing the medical commander to tailor the medical support to a given operation or tactical situation.[3] These facilities are also designed to be mobile; however, their large size requires several weeks to move, set up, and become operational.

The Army Echelon III facility is the Combat Support Hospital (CSH), a 248-bed unit that is divided into a 164-bed and an 84-bed hospital company capable of operating independently in split-based operations.[12] The hospital facility is the Deployable Medical System (DEPMEDS), which consists of temper tents and ISO shelters (Figure 3-6). The 84-bed hospital company has a total of 168 personnel and is composed of an emergency medical treatment section with a dispensary, 1 OR (2 tables), 2 ICUs each composed of 12 beds, 3 intermediate care wards (ICW) each composed of 20 beds, and a central material services section. The 164-bed hospital company has 253 personnel, 2 ORs (4 tables), 2 ICUs (24 beds), and 7 ICWs (140 beds). When fully deployed, the 248-bed hospital covers 5.7 acres.[3]

The Navy Fleet Hospital is a 500-bed hospital composed of 970 personnel, 3 ORs (6 tables), 80 ICU beds, and 420 acute-care beds. It requires 28 acres and 2 weeks to be fully set up. The Navy Expeditionary Medical Support System (NEMSS) is a smaller, scalable Echelon III facility. It is composed of 260 personnel, 1 OR (2 tables), 5 to 20 ICU beds, and up to 96 acute care beds. It requires 2 acres and 2 days to be fully set up. The Navy also has 2 hospital ships (USNS Mercy and USNS Comfort) that can operate as an Echelon III or IV facility. Each has 1200 personnel, 12 ORs, 100 ICU beds, 400 intermediate care beds, and 500 minimal care beds. Patient holding capability for these ships is limited to 5 days.[3]

The Air Force Air Transportable Hospital has 3 packages that can be deployed in increments or as an entire entity. The first increment is composed of 37 personnel, 1 OR, 1 ICU bed, 2 ICW beds, and 7 minimal care beds. The second increment is composed of 51 personnel, 2 ORs, 2 ICU beds, 3 ICW beds, and 20 minimal care beds. The third increment is composed of 68 personnel, 4 ORs, 4 ICU beds, 6 ICW beds, and 20 minimal care beds. Each increment can be operational within 24 hours and requires 26,000 to 50,000 square feet to be fully operational. The hospital can also be augmented with a Patient Retrieval Team (4 ambulances and 14 medical technicians) and/or a Patient Decontamination Team (19 medical technicians).

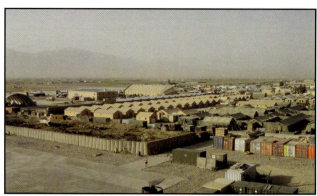

Figure 3-6. Combat support hospital in Afghanistan.

Within each theater of operations, the Air Force also operates Aeromedical Staging Facilities. For strategic aeromedical evacuation, these are fixed facilities located on or near an enplaning or deplaning airbase or airstrip. They have 50 to 250 beds, are staffed by physicians and nurses, and can hold patients for up to 24 hours. They provide reception, administrative processing, ground transportation, feeding, and limited medical care for patients entering, en route to, or departing the aeromedical evacuation system. The Air Force also has smaller Mobile Aeromedical Staging Facilities staffed by flight nurses and medical technicians to support tactical aeromedical evacuation within the combat zone. These are located near runways/taxiways of forward airfields or operating bases.[13]

Prior to movement from Echelon III to Echelon IV, all patients are evaluated by an Air Force Flight Surgeon to determine stability for flight and to confirm that appropriate medications and treatment plan have been provided. Although electronic medical records have been developed to allow all providers within the continuum of care to access and document medical/surgical treatment provided to patients, it has been standard practice to write the surgical plan on the patient's dressing as a precautionary measure (Figure 3-7).

Severely injured patients who have been stabilized are transported by critical care air transport teams (CCATTs). These are flying ICUs staffed by a critical care physician, a critical care nurse, and a respiratory therapist. They can transport critically ill casualties on ventilators, as well as continue critical care resuscitation and treatment en route to the next level of care.

Echelon IV

This echelon of care will provide not only a surgical capability as provided in Echelon III, but also further definitive therapy for patients in the recovery phase who can return to duty within the theater evacuation policy. Definitive care is normally provided

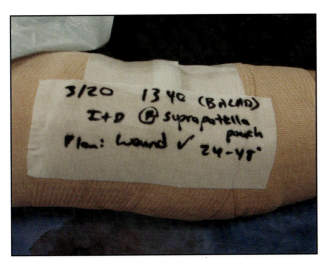

Figure 3-7. Treatment plan written on dressing prior to evacuation out of theater.

by a communications zone fleet hospital, general hospital, or overseas MTF. If rehabilitation cannot be accomplished within a predetermined holding period, the casualties/patients are evacuated to the zone of Interior, Echelon V.[7]

Echelon IV is the first level at which definitive surgical management can be provided outside the combat zone.[3] Definitive care is normally provided by a communications zone fleet hospital, CSH, or overseas medical treatment facility. If rehabilitation and return to duty cannot be accomplished within a predetermined period of time, casualties are evacuated to an Echelon V facility.

In the current conflict, the 2 Echelon IV facilities are Landstuhl Regional Medical Center (LRMC) and the US Military Hospital Kuwait (Navy Fleet Hospital). Virtually all of the combat-wounded casualties and severe nonhostile action injured patients are evacuated to LRMC. At this level, all wounds are reassessed on arrival, most commonly in the OR. Wounds undergo repeat irrigation and debridement approximately 48 hours from the time of injury, and augmentation or alteration of skeletal fixation is performed as indicated. Because wounded patients are generally held at LRMC for no more than 3 to 5 days, definitive surgical stabilization is generally only performed for simple closed injuries when it facilitates transport.[14]

Because more than 80% of the medical air transports in the current conflict were for noncombat-related illness or injury, most patients evacuated to LRMC or Kuwait did not suffer combat trauma. Many of these patients were sent to an Echelon IV facility for further evaluation, treatment, or rehabilitation. Generally, if the patient could be safely returned to the combat zone within 14 days, he or she would remain at LRMC for care and not be evacuated back to

the continental United States. Patients with meniscal tears, for example, would be treated with arthroscopy and returned to theater.

Echelon V

Care is convalescent, restorative, and rehabilitative and is normally provided by military, Department of Veterans Affairs, or civilian hospitals in CONUS. This phase may include a period of minimal care and increasing physical activity necessary to restore patients to functional health and allow their RTD or useful life.[11]

If the wounded cannot be returned to duty within the period of time allowed by the theater evacuation plan, they are transported to the continental United States for Echelon V care. This care is primarily provided at military and veterans' hospitals, but may also be provided at civilian hospitals, as described by the National Disaster Medical System. Injured servicemembers undergo definitive, restorative care and rehabilitation with the goal of return to duty. If the patient's medical conditions render him or her unfit for duty, care is designed to optimize function and return him or her to a productive civilian life.

Although any of the 59 hospitals in the Military Health System may serve as Echelon V facilities, injuries may dictate more specialized care. Care dedicated to wounded warriors and the treatment of injuries related to combat is provided at the following facilities:

- Walter Reed Army Medical Center Amputee Care Center and Gait Laboratory
- National Naval Medical Center's Traumatic Stress and Brain Injury Program
- Center for the Intrepid state-of-the-art rehabilitation facility and San Antonio Military Medical Complex Army Medical Center Burn Center at Fort Sam Houston
- Naval Medical Center San Diego Comprehensive Combat Casualty Care Center
- The multisite Defense and Veterans Brain Injury Center (DVBIC) for patient care, education, and clinical research[15]

The Walter Reed National Military Medical Complex (WRNMMC) is composed of the facilities at Walter Reed Army Medical Center and the National Naval Medical Center, as directed under the Base Realignment and Closure. The facility will consist of a 345-bed hospital, Traumatic Brain Injury/Post-Traumatic Stress Disorder Intrepid Center of Excellence, and an Amputee Care Center and Gait

Laboratory. WRNMMC provides the full spectrum of medical, surgical, and pediatric subspecialty care as well as mental health services. The Amputee Care Center and Gait Laboratory is a 31,000-square foot, $10 million center that contains a gait lab, indoor track, and computer-assisted rehabilitation environment (CAREN). It is a state-of-the-art facility designed to maximize functional outcomes in the care of the wounded.[16]

The San Antonio Military Medical Complex is made up of the former Brooke Army Medical Center and Wilford Hall Air Force Medical Center, which now serve as north and south campuses. The Burn Center at the Institute of Surgical Research and the Center for the Intrepid (CFI) state-of-the-art rehabilitation facility are additional resources available for the treatment of the wounded. The 450-bed north campus is undergoing an extensive $700 million expansion that will give it 425 beds (116 ICU and 309 ward) and 32 ORs. Capabilities will include medical, surgical, and pediatric subspecialty care, burn care, bone marrow and organ transplant, and a center for excellence for battlefield health and trauma. The south campus will host a proposed ambulatory surgical center; medical, surgical, and pediatric subspecialty clinics; and a center for excellence for eye care.[17] The CFI is a $50 million facility that opened in 2007 to provide state-of-the-art rehabilitation services to wounded warriors. The 4-story, 60,000-square foot center is equipped with an indoor running track, firing range, pool, 2-story climbing wall, prosthetic center, and a CAREN.[18]

Naval Medical Center San Diego uses a Comprehensive Combat and Complex Casualty Care (C5) program. Medical, surgical, and pediatric subspecialty care is available as well as programs and facilities that focus on mental health, traumatic brain injury, and amputee care. The C5 facility is a 30,000-square foot center that offers a climbing wall, multiterrain obstacle course, and simulated living areas to assist in rehabilitative care. It functions as the military's primary west coast center for the wounded warrior.

The multisite DVBIC focuses on care of traumatic brain injury. It is a collaboration between the Department of Defense, Veterans Affairs, and 2 civilian centers that is funded by the DoD and includes research, education, and treatment. Defense Centers of Excellence for Psychological Health and Traumatic Brain Injury, within DVBIC, provides traumatic brain injury care to wounded warriors at 19 sites.[19]

References

1. Levels of medical care. In: Szul AC, Davis LB, Walter Reed Army Medical Center Borden Institute, eds. *Emergency War Surgery.* 3rd US rev. Washington, DC: Walter Reed Army Medical Center Borden Institute; 2004:2.1-2.10.
2. The Health Service Support System in Joint Publication 4-02. P. I-1. www.dtic.mil/doctrine.
3. Bagg MR, Covey DC, Powell ET. Levels of medical care in the global war on terrorism. *J Am Acad Orthop Surg.* 2006;14: S7-S9.
4. Hildebrand F, Giannoudis P, Krettek C, Pape HC. Damage control: extremities. *Injury.* 2004;35:678-689.
5. Department of Defense. Global War on Terrorism—Operation Iraqi Freedom: by casualty category within service. March 19, 2003 through October 4, 2010. http://siadapp.dmdc.osd.mil/ personnel/CASUALTY/oif-total.pdf. Accessed October 11, 2010.
6. Department of Defense. Global War on Terrorism—Operation Enduring Freedom: by casualty category within service. October 7, 2001 through October 4, 2010. http://siadapp.dmdc.osd. mil/personnel/CASUALTY/wotsum.pdf. Accessed October 11, 2010.
7. Doctrine for Health Services Support in Joint Operations JP 4-02(95). www.dtic.mil/doctrine.
8. STP 21-1-SMCT. *Soldier's Manual of Common Tasks, Warrior Skills, Level 1.* Washington, DC: Department of the Army; June 18, 2009.
9. Army FM 4-02.4. *Medical Platoon Leader's Handbook Tactics, Techniques, and Procedures.* Washington, DC: Department of the Army: Appendix C.
10. Army FM 8-55. *Planning for Health Service Support.* Washington, DC: Department of the Army; February 15, 1985.
11. Army FM 4-02.25(03)(FM 8-10-25). *Employment of Forward Surgical Teams Tactics, Techniques, and Procedures.* Washington, DC: Department of the Army.
12. Aeromedical evacuation. In: Szul AC, Davis LB, Walter Reed Army Medical Center Borden Institute, eds. *Emergency War Surgery.* 3rd US rev. Washington, DC: Walter Reed Army Medical Center Borden Institute; 2004:4.1-4.9.
13. Smith MW. *Medical Operations Handbook.* www.cs.amedd. army.mil/simcenter/Library/Medical%20Operations%20Book/ medopsbk.pps. Accessed December 3, 2010.
14. Tenuta JJ. From the battlefields to the states: the road to recovery. The role of Landstuhl Regional Medical Center in US military casualty care. *J Am Acad Orthop Surg.* 2006;14:S45-S47.
15. Military Health System. Wounded warrior care. http://www. health.mil/About_MHS/Health_Care_in_the_MHS/Wounded_ Warrior_Care.aspx. Accessed October 11, 2010.
16. Baker FW III. New amputee care center opens at Walter Reed. http://www.defense.gov/news/newsarticle.aspx?id=47432. Accessed October 11, 2010.
17. San Antonio Military Medical Center. San Antonio Medical BRAC. http://www.sammc.amedd.army.mil/sa_medical_brac. asp. Updated March 20, 2009. Accessed October 11, 2010.
18. Wilson E. $50 million rehabilitation center opens on Fort Sam Houston. Jan 30, 2007. www.army.mil/-news/2007/01/30/1570-50-million-rehabilitation-center-opens-on-fort-sam-houston/.
19. Defense and Veterans Brain Injury Center. Home page. http:// www.dvbic.org. Accessed October 11, 2010.

Chapter 4

THE FORWARD SURGICAL TEAM

MAJ Andrew J. Schoenfeld, MD; MAJ Dirk L. Slade, MD; and
LTC Philip J. Belmont Jr, MD

The forward surgical team (FST) represents the US military's second level of care in the 5-tiered echelon of care system.[1,2] In the Navy, the services provided by an Army FST may be replicated in a surgical company or a forward resuscitative surgical system (FRSS) paired with a shock trauma platoon.[1] The Air Force gives Echelon II care to wounded servicemembers through mobile field surgical teams (MFST) or expeditionary medical support (EMEDS) units.[1] Regardless of the branch of service, the Echelon II site is often the first location where wounded soldiers are evaluated and treated by physicians and surgeons.[1-5] In addition, the Echelon II facility is the setting where initial surgical resuscitation can be performed. The conflicts in Iraq and Afghanistan were the first to witness the use of FSTs and other Echelon II units on a large scale.[3-8] The doctrine regarding deployment and use of these units is still evolving and will likely change with the nature of armed conflict (ie, conventional warfare versus insurgency), tactical considerations, and the likelihood for combat unit mobility.

Historical Development of the Forward Surgical Team

The concept of the FST was developed by the British Royal Army Medical Corps during World War II (1939-1945).[3] Charles Rob, surgical consultant to the British 1st Airborne Division, devised the FST as a means to provide immediate medical care to wounded paratroopers during the North Africa Campaign.[3] The FSTs were intended to be rapidly mobile, with physicians and equipment parachuted into combat zones. The FSTs were also designed to operate under austere conditions with very limited resources.

Despite the British success with these mobile surgical units during World War II, the concept was not readily adopted by the US military. Up until after the first Gulf War (1990-1991), operating rooms (ORs) were only located in American mobile army surgical hospitals (MASH) or combat support hospitals (CSH).[2,3] The military's experience in the invasion of Grenada (1983), where the first MASH did not arrive until 4 days after the start of hostilities, highlighted the need for highly mobile surgical units that could maneuver quickly and effectively treat casualties close to the front lines.[3] In response to Grenada, the Army began to train small airborne surgical squads, similar to the British FSTs of World War II. These airborne surgical squads made combat jumps during the airborne invasion of Panama (1989), and, within the next 5 years, the Army created 2 fully equipped airborne FSTs: the 274th Medical Detachment (Airborne) and the 250th Medical Detachment Surgical (Airborne).[3]

At the start of Operation Enduring Freedom (OEF), the 274th and the 250th were both reflagged as FSTs and were deployed in support of Special Forces Operations in Afghanistan.[7,8] The 274th FST was initially located in Uzbekistan and then moved to Bagram.[7] The 250th deployed first to Oman and was then moved to Kandahar after the fall of the Taliban government.[8] There, the unit supported Task Force K-Bar, the 26th Marine Expeditionary Unit, and the

Owens BD, Belmont PJ Jr, eds. *Combat Orthopedic Surgery:
Lessons Learned in Iraq and Afghanistan (pp 31-38)*
© 2011 SLACK Incorporated

3/101 Airborne Brigade Combat Team (BCT). In 2003, the 250th FST also made a combat jump into Northern Iraq with the 173rd Airborne Brigade, establishing the second front in Operation Iraqi Freedom (OIF).[4] The 555th FST and 745th FST supported BCTs of the 3rd Infantry Division, spearheading the initial invasion of Iraq from Kuwait.[5]

Since the initial phases of OIF and OEF, numerous FSTs have deployed to Iraq and Afghanistan. At the present time, FSTs are engaged in surgical and civil-affair missions, working in outposts amidst the rugged terrain of Afghanistan, augmenting the medical staff of CSHs in Iraq, and supporting Special Forces Operations in Southeast Asia.[1,3-9] In most instances, the current use of FSTs does not strictly adhere to the doctrine regarding their use according to *Field Manual 8-10-25: Employment of Forward Surgical Teams.*[10]

Doctrinal Composition and Mission of the Forward Surgical Team

According to Army doctrine, an FST consists of 20 uniformed personnel: 10 officers and 10 enlisted.[3,4,9,10] The surgical cadre is composed of 3 general/trauma surgeons and 1 orthopedic surgeon. One of the 4 surgeons will usually serve as the FST commander, assisted in this duty by an administrative medical service corps officer who functions as executive officer.[3,10] The other officers of the FST are critical care nurse/head nurse (1), emergency room nurse (1), nurse anesthetist (2), and OR nurse (1). Enlisted personnel assigned to the FST are team sergeant (1), intensive care licensed practical nurse (3), OR technician (3), and emergency medical technician/combat medic (3).

For standard land-based operations, the FST is supplied with 6 high-mobility multipurpose wheeled vehicles that are capable of transporting the entire unit and all equipment.[5] The high-mobility multipurpose wheeled vehicles are designed to support chemical/biological protected shelter system tents and lightweight multipurpose shelters, which form the triage area, OR, and recovery room once the FST is operational.[3,5,6] The high-mobility multipurpose wheeled vehicle engines, or a tactical generator, are used to provide power and to support heating, cooling, ventilation, and air filtration.

The FST doctrinally supports 2 OR tables in a single tent, with procedures performed by a team of 2 general surgeons, or 1 general surgeon and 1 orthopedic surgeon.[3-5,9] Surgical procedures may be performed simultaneously, side by side, with 1 OR technician supporting each procedure and 1 OR nurse facilitat-

ing both cases at the same time. The FST is capable of providing basic bedside laboratory studies and has 20 units of packed red blood cells available for transfusion. According to doctrine, the FST does not have access to x-ray equipment or fluoroscopic machinery.[9,10]

The Naval FRSS consists of 9 to 10 servicemembers capable of providing surgical treatment.[1] The FRSS cannot hold patients and does not have intrinsic evacuation capabilities. The EMEDS team of the Air Force is composed of 25 individuals, while the augmented EMEDS+10 has 56 members and can accommodate up to 15 patients.[1]

The FST is designed to support brigade/regiment-sized units and is attached to these formations. The FST mobilizes with the parent line unit and deploys forward, remaining 3 to 5 km behind the front line.[4] The FST will often be located with the combat unit's medical company and forward support battalion, and these organizations can be used to augment the FST's human or material resources.[1,3-5] The forward support battalion will also provide logistical support to the FST and will assist in arranging for medical evacuation of the wounded.

The FST is constructed in 4 sections: 3 shelter systems attached to high-mobility multipurpose wheeled vehicles and an administrative section operated by the medical service corps officer.[3,5] The administrative section is responsible for record keeping and coordinating medical evacuation. The 3 shelter systems serve as triage/Advanced Trauma Life Support (ATLS) section, OR section, and recovery room section (Figures 4-1 through 4-4).[3-5,9] If necessary, wounded soldiers can enter through the triage tent, proceed to the OR, and leave the FST via the recovery room (see Figure 4-1). One emergency room nurse and combat medics operate the triage tent, with one of the surgeons assisting/supervising as deemed necessary. The OR section is run by the 4 surgeons, 2 nurse anesthetists, 3 OR technicians, and 1 OR nurse. Three critical care practical nurses and 1 critical care registered nurse manage the recovery room.

The mission of the FST is to provide emergency medical care to incoming wounded; to triage, stabilize, and evacuate those individuals who will tolerate transport and require higher levels of care; to provide surgery and postoperative care to those wounded who will not survive transport to an Echelon III facility; to provide continuous postoperative critical care to ventilated or nonventilated patients for 6 to 8 hours; and to rapidly deploy via high-mobility multipurpose wheeled vehicles or fixed-wing aircraft in the wake of combat units.[3-5,9,10] Combat units operating within an hour of a CSH do not require an attached FST.[3,4,6] Additionally, if the scope of the conflict changes such that casualties are being evacuated directly to a CSH,

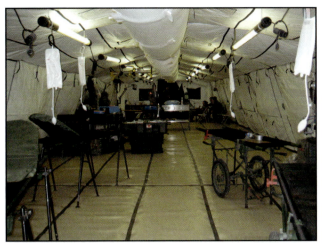

Figure 4-1. Interior of the 772nd FST, which supported the 101st Airborne Division during OEF. The 772nd FST's shelter systems were constructed without separation so that there was no division between the triage, OR, and recovery room sections. Here, the picture shows a clear view from the recovery room section (foreground) through the OR (center) to the triage section (rear).

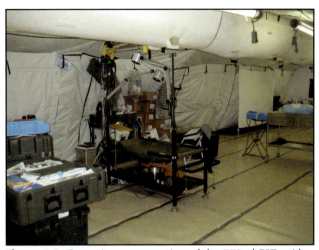

Figure 4-3. Operating room section of the 772nd FST, with a view of one of the 2 operating tables. The second operating table could be set up opposite, or adjacent, to the standard table in the picture. The OR trays and surgical scrub table are visible on the left and right sides of the image, respectively.

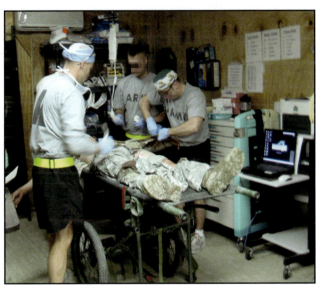

Figure 4-2. ATLS/triage section of an FST.

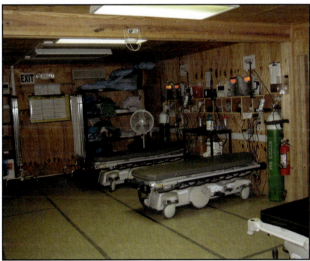

Figure 4-4. Recovery room section of an FST.

the FST doctrinally must stand down and be redeployed to another operational zone.[3,6,10]

Some FSTs may also have a designated airborne FST, a small echelon intended to provide far forward surgical support to Special Forces, Airborne, or Light Infantry units.[4] These airborne surgical echelons will parachute into drop zones and provide care for a maximum of 48 hours. Care is limited to ATLS protocol procedures, and these small units generally must rejoin the main FST after 48 hours due to personnel exhaustion and resource consumption.[4]

The FST is designed to maximally support 30 operations in 72 hours.[1,3,4] Additionally, the FST can provide critical postoperative care for 4 ventilated patients and 8 nonventilated patients up to 6 to 8 hours after surgery.[3,4] At this point, the patients should be stable enough to allow medical evacuation to a CSH. The Naval FRSS is capable of supporting 18 surgeries in 48 hours, while Air Force MFSTs can operate on 10 patients in 24 to 48 hours.[1] An Air Force EMEDS team is also capable of 10 surgeries in a 24-hour time period.[1]

All surgical procedures performed at an FST are "damage control" in nature. Wounded personnel capable of surviving their wounds until they are transported to a CSH are not treated with surgery at an FST. Furthermore, expectant soldiers receive only supportive care. The decision to operate on individuals with such life-threatening wounds that they cannot be evacuated to a CSH, but who may also not be immediately stabilized using "damage control" principles, rests with the treating surgeons. If good medical supply and low casualty flow allow, these cases may be taken to the OR. If supplies are scant or the casualty flow is heavy, such wounded servicemembers may not be deemed operable.

Typically, surgical interventions at an FST are designed to save life, limb, or eyesight and stabilize wounded servicemembers to the point where they can medically tolerate transport to a CSH.[1,3-8] Common procedures performed include chest tube thoracotomy, exploratory laparotomy, irrigation and debridement of soft tissue wounds, external fixator placement, fasciotomies, and amputations. In situations where orthopedic and general surgeons are both present at the FST, the orthopedic surgeon will function as a hand surgeon and orthopedic traumatologist.[3-5,7,8] In locations where only general surgeons are staffing an FST, they will perform all surgical procedures, including those typically conducted by orthopedic surgeons in a civilian setting.[9]

After 30 surgical procedures or 72 hours of continuous treatment of casualties, the FST becomes nonmission capable due to exhaustion of materiel as well as manpower.[1,3,4] Once an FST is identified as nonmission capable, the unit must stand down and mobilize to the division rear, where it will co-locate with a CSH or medical brigade.[3,4] Here, the unit will be resupplied, broken equipment may be repaired or replaced, surgical materials are sterilized, and personnel can recover. If no high-volume casualties are anticipated in the operational sector, the FST may remain at the CSH, augmenting the surgical capabilities of the Echelon III facility.[1,3,4]

Operational Experience of Forward Surgical Teams

Several publications have documented the operational experience of various FSTs in Iraq and Afghanistan during each phase of the spectrum of these conflicts.[4,5,7-9,11] Technically, FSTs were only employed in a doctrinally correct manner during the first portion of OIF (March through May 2003).[3-6] Prior to the start of OIF, the 274th and 250th FSTs had deployed to Afghanistan in support of special forces operations in Afghanistan.[7,8] As no Echelon III care was available in Afghanistan at the time, both the 274th and 250th FST functioned as Echelon II/III hybrid facilities. Additionally, these units were stationary once they deployed to Afghanistan and did not follow the tactical units they supported.

Peoples and colleagues reviewed the experience of the 274th FST in Afghanistan from October 2001 to May 2002.[7] During this time period, 224 combat casualties were treated by the unit. Sixty-eight percent of those treated at the FST were American soldiers while approximately 10% were enemy prisoners of war (POWs). A total of 180 procedures in 103 patients were performed by the FST, with close to 80% of the surgeries classified as trauma. The extremities were the most commonly involved body part in patients presenting to the FST, and the majority of procedures performed were orthopedic in nature.[7] These included 8 fasciotomies, 6 amputations, 5 closed reductions, and 6 placements of an external fixator. Approximately 8% of those servicemembers presenting to the 274th FST died of their injuries.[7]

Place and colleagues documented the performance of the 250th FST in Afghanistan from October 2001 through April 2002.[8] This FST treated 196 patients and performed 68 surgeries on 50 individuals. Half of these patients were US or coalition forces. Fifty-eight percent of all injuries involved the extremities, and extremity procedures represented 65% of all surgical cases. The FST's orthopedic surgeon was the primary surgeon in 51% of the operations.[8]

Patel and colleagues described the tactical and operational experience of the 555th FST during the general warfare phase of OIF, when the unit was in direct support of the 2/3 Infantry BCT.[5] The FST participated in combat-related maneuvers for a 24-day period and treated 154 wounded. The plurality of patients were American soldiers, but 30% were Iraqi POWs. Sixty-two percent of injuries among US personnel involved the extremities, while extremity trauma was present in 71% of Iraqi POWs.[5] Twenty-five surgeries were performed by the FST, including irrigation and debridement of open fractures, external fixator application, and amputations. The overall mortality rate for patients presenting to the FST was 1.9% but the surgical mortality was 12%. All those patients who died during or after surgery were Iraqi POWs.[5] Iraqi POWs generally sustained a more significant degree of combat-related trauma than Americans treated at the FST due to the technical superiority of American weaponry and the absence of personal protective equipment among Iraqi forces.[5]

Rush and colleagues examined the performance of the 250th FST during its tour in support of the 173rd Airborne Brigade in Operation Northern Delay (OIF).[4] Fifty-one percent of all injuries evaluated involved the extremities, with 94% of all procedures performed due to trauma.[4] One external fixator placement, 2 amputations, and multiple fasciotomies were performed. Injuries treated at the time of the initial combat jump into Iraq included one tibia-fibula fracture and a servicemember with bilateral shoulder dislocations.[4]

Less information is available regarding the performance of FSTs during the counterinsurgency phases of OIF and OEF. Recently, Eastridge and colleagues investigated outcomes among servicemembers initially treated at FSTs compared to those evacuated directly to CSHs.[11] The average Injury Severity Score (ISS) of soldiers initially evaluated at FSTs was 35, while those directly transported to a CSH had mean ISS of 32. The overall mortality for those servicemembers wounded in action for FSTs was 2.3% compared to a 3.1% mortality at CSHs. Among servicemembers considered severely injured (ISS >25), the mortality at FSTs and CSHs was 19.1% and 19.9%, respectively.[11] No statistically significant differences in outcome could be established for those treated at a FST versus soldiers directly evacuated to a CSH, leading the authors to conclude that FSTs were capable of achieving the same level of care provided at the more robust Echelon III facilities.[11]

Nessen and colleagues reviewed the operational viability of the 541st FST (Airborne) in OEF.[9] This unit was split, in a nondoctrinal manner, into two 10-person teams that operated in mutually exclusive and remote locations within Afghanistan. One site functioned with 2 general surgeons (one serving as the commanding officer) while the other was operated by 1 general surgeon and 1 orthopedic surgeon, with the unit executive officer serving as officer in charge. The augmented/split FST as described by these authors had additional nondoctrinal upgrades, including access to fresh frozen plasma and cryoprecipitate, some patient-holding capacity, basic x-ray equipment, and a fluoroscopic machine.

Both FST sites experienced a high volume of casualties, with 761 wounded treated over a 14-month period.[9] Forty-three percent of these received surgical intervention. In this FST, the plurality of individuals seen were local nationals, while only 23% were wounded US military servicemembers.[9] Extremity wounds again composed the largest percentage of injuries, and complex open wounds presented in 54 cases. Fractures were documented in 55 of those injured, traumatic amputations in 15, and traumatic arthrotomies in 8.

Similar to other FST reports, the largest caseload was orthopedic in nature. However, at one FST site, only 2 general surgeons were in attendance. At this location, all orthopedic procedures were performed by the general surgeons.[9] Additionally, the overall mortality for injured patients evaluated at the 541st FST was 2.4%, which is considerably lower than the previously reported mortality for counterinsurgency operations in Iraq and Afghanistan (4.5%).[9]

Challenges and Future Directions

The most substantial challenge to the effective use of FSTs at present includes the fact that the doctrine regarding their deployment is still evolving and the nature of the current counterinsurgency phases of OIF and OEF do not truly lend themselves to the employment of FSTs.[3,4,9,10] The FST was devised as a rapidly mobile medical unit that could quickly maneuver behind advancing American forces.[3-5] The FST's mission requires it to provide emergent medical care, surgical intervention that is "damage control" in nature, and evacuate casualties to an Echelon III facility within 6 to 8 hours of presentation.[1,10] An FST can also be used to support airborne operations or Special Forces strikes deep behind enemy lines.[4]

If the FST is operating in a zone without active casualties, it is doctrinally required to co-locate at an Echelon III site or to redeploy to a more active area of hostilities.[3,10] Furthermore, if combat units are able to directly evacuate casualties to a CSH within an hour of their zone of operations, the need for an attached FST is obviated. These requirements are meant to conserve military health care resources and also provide a means for the surgical staff of the FST to remain actively employed so that their cognitive and technical skills do not degrade.[3,4,6]

At the present time, however, few FSTs are being used in a doctrinally correct manner. Stinger and Rush,[3,6] along with others,[4,9] have decried the tendency for maneuver brigade commanders to request that FSTs be attached to their units, even though the nature of their tactical assignments does not doctrinally support the deployment of an FST. Additionally, the FST is not intended to be thought of as a smaller version of a CSH, and split assignments, while shown to be feasible,[9] lie outside the existing FST doctrine and could potentially degrade the unit's ability to respond to mission-appropriate tasks.

As the FST maneuvers close to the front lines, or drives deep into enemy territory with Special Forces groups, airborne teams, or light infantry, the unit may be exposed to conventional combat in a manner not typically experienced by military medical personnel. During its mission in support of the 2/3 Infantry BCT, the 555th FST was frequently responsible for its own protection and came under small arms fire, mortar fire, and assault with surface-to-surface missiles.[5] The FST actually engaged with the enemy on more than one occasion, ultimately taking 7 POWs and capturing several caches of enemy weapons and material.[5]

Although such situations did not occur during the major combat operations of OIF, due to their location close to the front lines, the potential exists for FSTs to sustain significant casualties or to be captured by the enemy.[4,5] Recognizing these facts, Patel and colleagues emphasized the need for members of an FST to be prepared to function more like a combat unit and advocated that all personnel assigned to an FST achieve proficiency in weapons training and be familiar with precepts regarding the management of POWs.[5]

Controversy also exists regarding the correct composition of an FST, as well as the manner by which such units are trained and what equipment should be available for their use. Early on in the Iraq and Afghanistan conflicts, Stinger and Rush identified that the Modified Tables of Organization and Equipment, along with the Medical Equipment Sets, assigned to FSTs were inadequate to support the mission.[3] Specifically, these authors recommended that equipment lists for FSTs be updated to include new diesel generators, deployable rapid assembly shelters, a SonoSite (Bothell, WA) portable ultrasound system, an I-Stat (Abbott Point of Care, Princeton, NJ) portable clinical analyzer, a freezer for storing blood products, access to fresh-frozen plasma and recombinant factor VIIa, an anesthesia oxygen concentrator, a Bair Hugger (Arizant Healthcare, Eden Prairie, MN) warming unit, and a substantial list of OR equipment necessary for surgical procedures.[3] While it appears that some augmented FSTs[9] may possess some of the equipment advocated by Stinger and Rush, it is unclear whether such items are now considered standard issue for these units.

Place and colleagues highlighted the fact that differences between the nature of civilian trauma and combat-related trauma render effective training of FST surgeons exceedingly difficult.[12] Some FSTs have been able to benefit from the prior experience of combat surgeons who have deployed to hostile zones on a number of occasions,[4,7-9] but most surgeons assigned to an FST will have been trained in civilian or military centers in the United States and will have little, if any, combat medical experience. Prior to the start of the current conflicts, FST surgeons and their teams were rotated through military and civilian trauma centers in an attempt to prepare them for combat life-saving requirements.[12] Place and colleagues found that the trauma training was better at military installations than civilian centers, but neither approximated the combat-related experiences in OIF or OEF.[12] Since the start of OIF/OEF, the Army has instituted a number of programs intended to increase the combat-medical acumen of deploying surgeons. To the best of our knowledge, however, the effectiveness of these initiatives has not been studied.

At present, FSTs are assigned 3 general surgeons and 1 orthopedic surgeon. In locales where split operations have been performed, one site is staffed by 2 general surgeons and another by 1 general surgeon and 1 orthopedic surgeon.[9] Nessen and colleagues recommended that since resuscitative surgery is the principal mission of the FST, if split operations are necessitated, then at least 2 general surgeons should be assigned to each 10-person team.[9] These authors were also of the opinion that any orthopedic procedures performed at an FST could capably be administered by general surgeons.[9] It should be recognized that the plurality, if not majority, of injuries documented in all prior reports regarding FSTs fall within the realm of orthopedic surgery.[4,5,7-9] During the 250th FST's participation in OEF, the unit's orthopedic surgeon performed more than half of the surgical cases.[8] With these factors in mind, the key role of the orthopedic surgeon in an FST seems incontrovertible. However, it may be possible that, in certain situations, casualty flow and mission requirements may warrant substitution of the orthopedic practitioner with an additional general surgeon. Under such circumstances, the orthopedic surgeon could be rotated back to division rear and the Echelon III facility and return to the FST as directed by the commanding officer.

Conclusion

US military FSTs were employed for the first time in military history during the prolonged conflicts in Iraq and Afghanistan. Over the course of these 2 conflicts, FSTs have been used repeatedly and in different manners. The performance of FSTs in the peer-reviewed medical literature during the wars in Iraq and Afghanistan have consistently and reliably reported that expert medical care has been provided to US, coalition, and enemy combat casualties.

FSTs during the Iraq and Afghanistan conflicts have been successfully used both within, and outside of, their prescribed doctrine through all spectrums of conflict, including general warfare, counterinsurgency operations, and unstable peace. The strategic placement of FSTs, decreased time to medical evacuation, and sophisticated resuscitative and surgical care provided by FSTs all contribute to an exceptionally low case fatality rate for soldiers injured on the battlefield in these conflicts. The orthopedic surgeon's role in the care of combat casualties at the FST has been considerable in that almost all studies have reported that between 50% and 60% of all operative cases have been for extremity injuries. The orthopedic surgeon stationed at an FST will have the capabilities to perform limb- and sometimes life-saving measures, to include sound irrigation and debridement, closed reductions, fasciotomies, amputations, and external fixator placement.

References

1. Bagg MR, Covey DC, Powell ET IV. Levels of medical care in the Global War on Terrorism. *J Am Acad Orthop Surg.* 2006;14:S7-S9.
2. Manring MM, Hawk A, Calhoun JH, Andersen RC. Treatment of war wounds: a historical review. *Clin Orthop Relat Res.* 2009;467:2168-2191.
3. Stinger H, Rush R. The Army Forward Surgical Team: update and lessons learned, 1997-2004. *Mil Med.* 2006;171:269-272.
4. Rush RM Jr, Stockmaster NR, Stinger HK, et al. Supporting the Global War on Terror: a tale of two campaigns featuring the 250th Forward Surgical Team (Airborne). *Am J Surg.* 2005;189:564-570.
5. Patel TH, Wenner KA, Price SA, Weber MA, Leveridge A, McAtee SJ. A US Army Forward Surgical Team's experience in Operation Iraqi Freedom. *J Trauma.* 2004;57:201-207.
6. Stinger HK, Rush RM. The forward surgical team: the Army's ultimate lifesaving force. *Infantry.* 2003;92:11-13.
7. Peoples GE, Gerlinger T, Craig R, Burlingame B. Combat casualties in Afghanistan cared for by a single Forward Surgical Team during the initial phases of Operation Enduring Freedom. *Mil Med.* 2005;170:462-468.
8. Place RJ, Rush RM, Arrington ED. Forward Surgical Team (FST) workload in a Special Operations Environment: the 250th FST in Operation Enduring Freedom. *Curr Surg.* 2003;60:418-422.
9. Nessen SC, Cronk DR, Edens J, et al. US Army two-surgeon teams operating in remote Afghanistan—an evaluation of split-based Forward Surgical Team operations. *J Trauma.* 2009;66:S37-S47.
10. Headquarters, Department of the Army. *Field Manual 8-10-25: Employment of Forward Surgical Teams.* Washington, DC: US Government Printing Office; 1997.
11. Eastridge BJ, Stansbury LG, Stinger H, Blackbourne L, Holcomb JB. Forward Surgical Teams provide comparable outcomes to Combat Support Hospitals during support and stabilization operations on the battlefield. *J Trauma.* 2009;66:S48-S50.
12. Place RJ, Porter CA, Azarow K, Beitler AL. Trauma experience comparisons of Army Forward Surgical Team surgeons at Ben Taub Hospital and Madigan Army Medical Center. *Curr Surg.* 2001;58:90-93.

Chapter **5**

COMBAT SUPPORT HOSPITALS

COL James R. Ficke, MD

The US Army Echelon III or NATO Role III deployed medical treatment facility is the combat support hospital (CSH). This unit is designed to be a relatively stationary facility during stability operations and is capable of functioning as a major trauma resuscitation hospital. During advancing combat operations, the CSH is capable of moving, generally at the Corps level of operations. The CSH commander has the mission to be surgically capable within 12 hours of a jump and fully capable within 36 hours. This chapter will detail the organization, capabilities, and recent literature describing performance of the CSH in current operations.

Role III treatment facilities are those that have full or at least robust surgical capability and inpatient units that admit patients. The CSH, as a Role III facility, relies upon external lift capability to move within the combat zone, but possesses all other support internally. The current configuration, the Medical Reengineering Initiative (MRI CSH), is streamlined, but maintains quite similar physician complement, with reduced administrative personnel. This unit is equipped to operate completely independent of host nation support or neighboring organizational support, relying only upon higher level logistical support. The organization consists of a command and control element, a hospital unit base or company, an augmentation element, and a forward early-entry element. The facility is based upon modules that enable flexibility in employment, as well as adaptability to any particular mission. The CSH operates successfully in desert conditions where temperatures may range from below 0°F to over 130°F, as well as colder climates or mountainous terrain. The single requirement

is enough area to establish the facilities and preserve military security (Figure 5-1).

Organization

The CSH is designed as a stand-alone facility, with capability to provide medical and surgical care within the combat zone. This hospital has organic assets to support emergency department resuscitation, a wide variety of surgical specialties, an intensive care unit (ICU), as well as outpatient services. Additionally, the CSH has laboratory, radiology, and pharmacy services to support a vast spectrum of care. Central to these elements is the headquarters section, acting as command and control, to include military personnel support, operations and logistics, laundry, and nutrition care. The hospital is organized in a modular fashion, to best support the operational requirements in a stated mission. There is an early entry unit, consisting of 44 beds and 2 operating tables. This element has been widely used in current conflicts and constitutes the basic unit of the split operations CSH. The next major element of the CSH is the 164-bed main body—comprising the intermediate care wards, outpatient clinics, and most of the ancillary services. In addition, the 40-bed augmentation unit can be used for medical contingencies or additional modules in times of surges or additional missions to include humanitarian relief operations.

The most critical elements in the CSH are the people. This team is composed of physicians, health care professionals, and support staff as well as leaders who exist to make casualty care successful. There is doctrinal allowance for standardized composition of these

Owens BD, Belmont PJ Jr, eds. *Combat Orthopedic Surgery: Lessons Learned in Iraq and Afghanistan (pp 39-44)*
© 2011 SLACK Incorporated

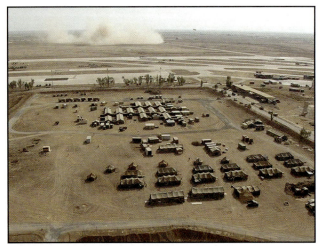

Figure 5-1. Typical CSH layout in mobility operations.

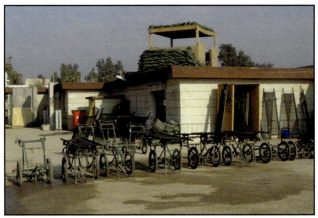

Figure 5-2. Front entrance of CSH in stability operations.

staff, but every unit mission is different, and so are the personnel required. In most situations, the physician staff will include at minimum 4 to 6 emergency physicians; 6 to 8 general surgeons; 6 to 8 anesthesia providers; 2 to 4 orthopedic surgeons; 1 urologist; 1 gynecologist; 1 oral surgeon; 1 cardiothoracic or vascular surgeon; 2 internal medicine physicians; 1 or 2 critical care intensivists; 1 psychiatrist; and several primary care physicians, physician assistants, or nurse practitioners. The fact that this extremely small staff manages the volume comparable to many major Level I civilian trauma centers is dependent upon training, teamwork, and intensity.

Headquarters

The headquarters element is similar to a battalion level command staff, with personnel, operations and planning, logistics (to include maintenance, supply, and acquisition), and communications. Security for the hospital is essential and is also within the scope of the headquarters element (Figure 5-2). Each of these sections performs functions specific to the performance of deployed military operations and is beyond the scope of this text. However, it is critical that the headquarters section remains in close communication and coordination with the medical portions of the hospital.

Early Entry Unit

The early entry unit represents the most mobile element and continues to operate at a Role III capability. This smaller hospital is designed to bring intrinsic critical care assets, including 24 intensive care beds. The unit has sections of pharmacy, radiology, and central material supply, as well as an intermediate care ward. The distinguishing feature of this element is that it retains enough resources to remain in continuous operations for several days and is independent of Role II facilities.

Main Hospital Element

By nature of size, the main hospital completes the capabilities of the modern CSH, to include outpatient services, a specialty clinic including primary care, psychiatry, urology, and obstetrics and gynecology, as well as rehabilitative services including physical therapy. This element also brings dental and oral surgery as well as a complete operating room section with at least 6 tables operating in the deployable medical sets (DEPMEDS).

Emergency Medical Treatment Section

Every deployed CSH has used emergency medical treatment in some variation of the well-known Hospital Incident Command System in place in many civilian institutions. Since the primary function of the CSH is emergency stabilization, this role has been imperative to the high levels of life-saving care afforded in recent years. This system uses trauma teams of 3 to 5 personnel focused upon a single patient, applying principles of Advanced Trauma Life Support for a rapid primary survey of airway, bleeding, breathing, circulation, and spinal injuries. The emergency medical treatment section is established in a manner to permit single-direction casualty flow, from initial triage, critical stabilization, and assessment into either the surgical suites or the ICUs. When required, blood

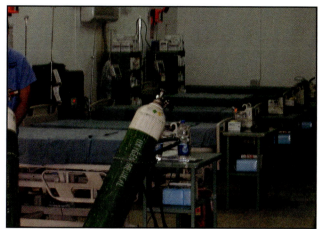

Figure 5-3. ICU 0700 rounds.

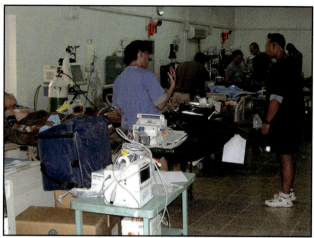

Figure 5-4. Same unit 2 hours later with mass casualty event in progress.

product support is initiated early, with most current recommendations promoting 1:1 rates of blood product to crystalloid transfusion, early application of extremity tourniquets, and rapid rewarming or prevention of hypothermia.[1,2] Additionally, the emergency medical treatment section will receive medical patients and provide basic and cardiac life support and communications with inbound evacuation vehicles.

Intermediate Care Unit

The majority of patients requiring admission sustain nonbattle injury or disease-based ailments. These patients infrequently require surgery, and less often require intensive care monitoring. Most active beds are in the intermediate care units, with routine nursing care, standard dietary requirements, and often rapid return to duty. In the event of mass casualty incidents, these patients can be discharged or transferred in order to expand the hospital's surge capacity. In this situation, surge refers to the capability of the CSH to open bed space and resources to manage the high volume and acuity of injury when faced with overwhelming or more often significantly increased care requirements over a short time.

Intensive Care Unit

Recent experience has shown improved outcomes with subspecialty-trained teams and critical care specialist direction of the ICUs.[3] Management of acute penetrating injuries most often requires surgical hemorrhage control, followed by resuscitation, rewarming, and stabilization.[4] The ICU is a focal point for severe trauma patients and is an extremely high resource consumer. Critically ill patients require extensive resources. The CSH is frequently at risk for shortage

of resources such as oxygen, electricity generation, bed space, and nearly every aspect of medical care. Depletion of these resources requires aggressive active patient management of ICU occupants—either by means of transfer to lower acuity wards or aeromedical evacuation. Figure 5-3 demonstrates an ICU early one morning; Figure 5-4 shows the same ICU a short 2 hours later in the midst of a major mass casualty incident. This surge potential is a constant risk and must be monitored in order to maintain receiving capability. Another significant factor has been the addition of a specialist trained in critical care. In fact, in a comparative study between nonintensivist management, critical care consultant, and intensivist-directed care team, the in-unit mortality was significantly reduced by the hands-on directed management by a trained intensive care specialist.[4]

Surgical Services

The operating tables within a CSH on the move in support of direct combat units may be as simple as the self-contained DEPMEDS or as elaborate as several of the fixed hardened facilities in use currently (Figure 5-5). The mainstay of all forward surgery, whether general or orthopedics, is focused upon the concepts of damage control—limited to initial life or limb salvage; rapid, timely, and essential interventions; followed by stabilization, warming, and later return to surgery for more definitive care or urgent evacuation. In the CSH, and most Role III facilities, this results in saving the most lives with limited resources in the typical austere environment.[1,5,6] One side-by-side comparison of the patient distribution and surgical procedures performed in the CSH versus a civilian Level I trauma center found comparable surgical procedures with lower Injury Severity Scores, yet a higher percentage

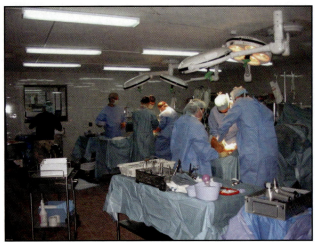

Figure 5-5. Operating room—2 tables and simultaneous damage control surgery in progress.

of penetrating injuries in the CSH.[7] Survival rates and early outcomes were comparable. One additional capability of note is the requirement for care of local nationals. Frequently, depending upon local policies (referred to as the Medical Rules of Engagement) and relationships with local medical facilities, the personnel of the CSH are required to care for locals to include host nation military, civilian, and even insurgents. This clearly increases resource requirements and must be planned for. One particularly special area of comment is that of pediatric trauma. A recent paper outlined the demographics of their busy hospital in Iraq, with approximately 3% of the 3293 patients admitted through the emergency department being children.[8] Most of these are injured as a result of blast or gunfire, and essentially none have protective armor. Most surgeons and emergency physicians only infrequently manage pediatric trauma, and these authors recommended inclusion of pediatricians with the CSH as well as additional predeployment training in physiologic management of pediatric trauma.

Ancillary Services

While the main focus during a multiple or mass casualty event is at the trauma bay or the operating room, much of the success is determined by the capabilities within pharmacy, laboratory, and radiology sections. The pharmacy of a typical CSH will dispense more than 2000 prescriptions weekly and is vital during the resuscitations in the emergency room or ICUs. With a full-time pharmacist and several technicians, the section is capable of most intravenous medications as well as parenteral nutrition management. The laboratory also functions as a blood bank, storing and processing frozen blood products, packed red cells, and

on occasion serving as the drawing service for fresh whole blood drives, a practice routinely performed in the Echelon III facilities. This source of blood, type matched and monitored, provides urgent transfusion products that retain clotting factors, another aspect of deployed trauma care well documented in recent literature.

Laboratory/Blood Bank

While the deployed laboratory services are capable of routine chemistry, urine, and hematologic analysis, the recent addition of microbiology and in some hospitals surgical pathology has greatly improved clinicians' ability to diagnose complex medical and surgical conditions. The laboratory technicians serving in the CSH are trained and credentialed through stateside hospitals and are competent to perform these tests. Most of the existing tests available are performed on automated equipment, with routine standardization testing. As a blood bank, the lab personnel work directly in the trauma bays, often facilitating massive transfusion protocols side by side with the surgeons. One of the most significant contributions has been institution of fresh whole blood drives, and then rapid transfusion. This "walking blood bank" offers more than simply red cells. The blood has active coagulating factors and platelets, and it is screened for disease by way of rapid assays and predeployment testing of US soldiers for HIV and hepatitis B.

Radiology

A deployed CSH has one assigned physician radiologist and, with recent conflicts, has also enjoyed access to modern digital imaging and teleradiology[9] as an adjunct to detailed interpretation of computerized tomographic (CT) imaging, which is routinely part of the CSH capabilities.[10] In fact, the capabilities of the CSH currently include routine use of C-arm image intensifiers, with use of contrast for advanced vascular or urologic imaging, as well as state-of-the-art CT scanners, housed in the permanent facilities. Widespread use of the focused assessment with sonography for trauma aids in the emergency department evaluation of trauma patients.

Logistics

The CSH, with 511 personnel, has a large footprint and enormous logistical requirements. Fully deployed, with 248 beds, the hospital requires 9.3 acres of space and more than 2.4 million kilowatts daily for power. Water requirements are also enormous, totaling more than 17,000 gallons daily.[11] These comprise some of the basic operational requirements, and the medical supplies are commensurate. The CSH has intrinsic oxygen collecting and concentrating capabilities as well. Most of the support staffing requirements exist for this fundamental reason and are equally as important as the physicians and health care professionals working inside the facility.

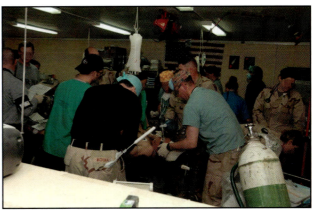

Figure 5-6. Trauma team during resuscitation.

Trauma Management Capabilities

One published account of the experience in the CSH for 6 months noted acute admission of more than 1054 patients, with 446 admitted for trauma-related conditions.[7] Most of these trauma patients arrive in groups of 3 to 5 casualties; however, frequent events involving multiple casualties create turmoil within treatment teams and strain on the available resources of the CSH. Every physician assigned to a deployed CSH should have training in principles of Advanced Trauma Life Support and should be comfortable managing a trauma team (Figure 5-6). The division of effort relies first upon a deliberate trauma response plan, a solid communication network to reach all personnel needed to respond, and rehearsals/training drills to perform best. In the CSH, trauma is frequent enough that teams have the opportunity to evaluate themselves, improve on practices as well as the policies, and perform repetitively. This author's experience during a 12-month deployment involved 19 mass casualty events—each with more than 12 patients simultaneously arriving. The strain on resources has a wide impact—from personnel in the emergency medical services, to blood product availability, to CT scanner, to OR capacity, to power. Trauma is the highest priority for the CSH and is what sets it apart from similar civilian facilities.

Conclusion

The modular CSH represents the Army's "workhorse" for combat casualty care. While the primary mission is to provide Role III combat casualty trauma care, diseases and nonbattle injuries comprise the heaviest burden of patients. The CSH has the distinction of managing heavy trauma admission volumes, similar to a major trauma center in a civilian environment. Where battle injuries are most notably penetrating in nature, the casualties managed in the CSH depend heavily upon the surgical capabilities therein. And where penetrating injuries abound, those involving the extremities are the largest area requiring surgical attention. This chapter has outlined the overall capabilities of the CSH and is intended to form a framework from where the initial stabilization of orthopedic war injuries takes place. In the austere environment of the combat zone, where everything from electricity to oxygen to damage control amidst extremes of temperatures, and injury severity must be managed on site, the CSH has that capability.

References

1. Beitler A, Wortmann GW, Hofmann LJ, Goff JM Jr. Operation Enduring Freedom: the 48th Combat Support Hospital in Afghanistan. *Mil Med.* 2006;17(3):189-193.
2. Martin M, Oh J, Currier H, et al. An analysis of in-hospital deaths at a modern combat support hospital: lessons learned from combat support hospital experience in Operation Iraqi Freedom. *J Trauma.* 2009;66(4 Suppl):S51-S60.
3. Lettieri C, Shah AA, Greenburg DL. An intensivist-directed intensive care unit improves clinical outcomes in a combat zone. *Crit Care Med.* 2009;37(4):1256-1269.
4. Grathwohl K, Venticinque SG. Organizational characteristics of the austere intensive care unit: the evolution of military trauma and critical care medicine; applications for civilian medical care systems. *Crit Care Med.* 2008;36(7 Suppl):S275-S83.
5. Blackbourne L. Combat damage control surgery. *Crit Care Med.* 2008;36(Suppl):S304-S310.
6. Holcomb JB, Jenkins D, Rhee P, et al. Damage control resuscitation: directly addressing the early coagulopathy of trauma. *J Trauma.* 2007;62(2):307-310.
7. Schreiber M, Zink K, Underwood S, Sullenberger L, Kelly M, Holcomb JB. A comparison between patients treated at a combat support hospital in Iraq and a level I trauma center in the United States. *J Trauma.* 2008;64(2 Suppl):S118-S121.
8. McGuigan R, Spinella PC, Beekley A, et al. Pediatric trauma: experience of a combat support hospital in Iraq. *J Ped Surg.* 2007;42(1):207-210.
9. McKay J, Keen EF 3rd, Bowden RA. Rapid communication and consultation in the combat support hospital. *Mil Med.* 2009;174(2):vii-x.

10. Harcke H, Statler JD, Montilla J. Radiology in a hostile environment: experience in Afghanistan. *Mil Med.* 2006;171(3):194-199.

11. US Army, Williams D, AMEDD, Organization and Personnel Systems Division, Directorate of Combat and Doctrine Development, eds. *Combat Support Hospital (CSH) (248 BED) Logistical Planning Requirements (Medical) Fact Book (Oct 16, 2009).*

Chapter **6**

LANDSTUHL REGIONAL MEDICAL CENTER

COL Joachim Jude Tenuta, MD

Combat casualty care is a dynamic process that continues to evolve with respect to types of injuries, frequency, timing of treatment, and location of care.[1-4] The transformation of the modern battlefield with respect to weaponry, modes of transportation, enemy capabilities and location, along with technologic advances have greatly altered our military's tactical approach to the mission, which includes care of our wounded warriors.[2,5] The Global War on Terror (GWOT), which includes the military operations in Afghanistan (Operation Enduring Freedom [OEF]) and in Iraq (Operation Iraqi Freedom [OIF]), has demonstrated these alterations on a large scale, and the medical response to these changes has kept pace with this 21st century conflict. The principles of managing orthopedic trauma with these combat casualties have remained clear: life/limb preservation, skeletal stabilization, aggressive wound debridement while adjusting to the new environment of armed conflict, and applying new technologies.[2-4,6,7] Landstuhl Regional Medical Center (LRMC) is a military medical facility located in Germany (Figure 6-1). It has a unique perspective in this process because it is the initial receiving facility for all casualties from the combat theaters of operations (OIF and OEF). Landstuhl is the only military medical center in that hemisphere, and any combat planning involves the use of this hospital along the evacuation chain from the hostile environment.[8]

A US military medical facility has existed in Landstuhl, Germany since the later aspects of World War II and the subsequent occupation thereafter. It has provided a utility for US forces in this region of the world since its inception (Cold War positioned

forces and subsequent engagements/deployments [eg, Lebanon, Desert Storm, Balkan Conflicts]). Prior to the onset of OIF in March 2003, planning for casualty care was conducted by the administrative and command staff of LRMC using information with regard to troop strength, enemy capabilities, and other information pertinent to casualty rates for the upcoming engagement. Of note, OEF, which commenced in Afghanistan in October 2001, was an ongoing engagement that was being supported at LRMC by only the assigned staff of that facility, without augmentation. While the recipient of casualties during the initial phases of OEF obviously created an increased workload for the clinicians at LRMC and occasionally disrupted day-to-day services, timing and numbers were inconsistent, and proper management was provided without any significant strain on assigned resources. For the anticipated invasion of Iraq, casualty estimates were difficult because there had been no recent large-scale conflict, enemy resolve was questionable, and use of chemical or biological agents on our troops needed to be considered. Along with combat casualty care, Landstuhl is also responsible for the evacuation of nonbattle injuries from theater. These range from outpatient-type injuries to multisystem injured inpatients (eg, motor vehicle accident in theater). Additionally, planning included maintaining routine patient care provided by LRMC prior to the start of GWOT (Figure 6-2). Military planners estimated/desired an evacuation time of casualties from theater medical facilities to Landstuhl to be approximately 7 days. The planned evacuation time from Landstuhl to the continental United States (CONUS) was presumed to be about 14 days. After consideration of all factors, creating

Owens BD, Belmont PJ Jr, eds. *Combat Orthopedic Surgery: Lessons Learned in Iraq and Afghanistan* (pp 45-50)
© 2011 SLACK Incorporated

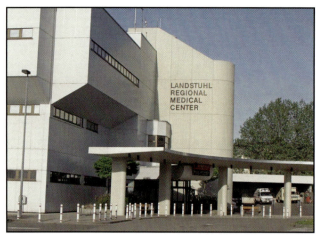

Figure 6-1. Landstuhl Regional Medical Center, Landstuhl, Germany.

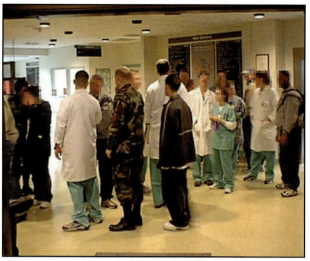

Figure 6-3. Predesignated hospital staff available for patient transport upon arrival to LRMC.

Figure 6-2. A snapshot of the typical workload provided by LRMC prior to the Global War on Terrorism.

LRMC	2001
Admissions	16
OR Cases	9
ICU Census / Acuity	1.6 / 2.7
Meals	700
Births	2.9
Ave. length of Stay	4.5
Pharmacy Products	1,059

casualty estimates with all available information, it was determined that 8 orthopedic surgeons stationed at Landstuhl would be able to provide the care required. In order to provide adequate augmentation for all services at LRMC, a Reserve General Hospital was activated and assigned to Landstuhl. The arrival of this rather large number of staff provided a logistical challenge for the hospital, but the Reserve Component orthopedic surgeons were able to assimilate quickly and provided immediate, energetic support of the mission.[9]

Pre-invasion planning within the orthopedic surgery service was focused on obtaining the appropriate number of augmented staff in order to provide the estimated services, but also required an assessment of patient flow within the hospital and the clinic area. With the often overlooked need for evaluating and managing large numbers of nonbattle injuries (predominately orthopedic injuries), the clinic staff

required a plan of management for this large number of patients. Experienced physician assistants were able to devise a plan of care that allowed for efficient flow of patients within the physical confines of the existing clinic structure with assigned clinic support staff.

This group was responsible for the assessment/ reassessment of all orthopedic injuries that arrived from theater on an outpatient basis. Determination of further care and continued evacuation was performed at that time.

Hospital planning prior to the onset of OIF provided a method for admitting critically injured and other predetermined inpatients into LRMC. The plan used available resources for transporting patients upon arrival to the medical center and allowed for a "retriage" with a more definitive determination of injury severity and proper disposition of wounded (inpatient ward versus intensive care unit [Figure 6-3]). Triage at the point of arrival was performed by a previously designated triage officer with immediate consultation support from the general surgery service, along with the orthopedic surgery service (Figure 6-4). Initial assessment was performed, along with a review of any pertinent information that arrived with the wounded servicemember, and determination was made for appropriate placement in the LRMC facility. All casualties admitted to the orthopedic surgery service were evaluated with a complete history and physical examination upon admission. Radiographic re-evaluation was performed at that time. Determination for surgical treatment/re-evaluation was also done at that time.

From the beginning of the OIF combat phase (March 2003), a majority of patients arrived to LRMC from theater approximately 12 to 48 hours from injury and initial evaluation. This evacuation time from the-

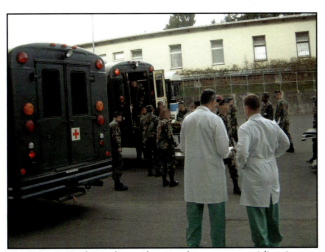

Figure 6-4. Orthopedic and general surgery providing immediate consultation upon arrival.

Daily Resources	2001	2004/5	Change
Admissions	16	28	175%
OR Cases	9	26	289%
ICU Census / Acuity	1.6 / 2.7	10.8 / 5.2	675% / 192%
Meals	700	1800	257%
Births	2.9	2.9	0%
Average LOS	4.5	4	-11%
Pharmacy Products	1,059	1,934	183%

Figure 6-5. A demonstration of the significant change in workload with OEF/OIF depicted by various averages daily.

ater has been considerably faster than any previous conflict and more rapid than predicted in preconflict planning. In general, combat and traumatic noncombat injuries are stabilized in theater through the initial 3 levels of care (combat medic/lifesaver, battalion aid station, and combat support hospital/forward surgical team).[3] Life-/limb-threatening injuries are addressed, skeletal trauma is stabilized in the field-expedient manner, and soft tissue injuries are treated with aggressive, initial debridement and irrigation.[2,4,10] Length of stay in the theater medical facilities is dependent upon stability of the patient and medical evacuation aircraft availability. Triage upon arrival to LRMC was performed by the designated representative from the surgery department. Casualties with multisystem involvement were assigned to the general surgery service. The orthopedic surgery service was the primary service for patients with isolated extremity injuries and was consulted on all other patients with orthopedic injuries. All wounds were re-evaluated. Most wounds that required an operative procedure in theater were re-evaluated in the operating room. All major procedures involving extremity injuries were performed by an orthopedic surgeon. This usually consisted of a repeat debridement within 48 hours from the time of injury, reassessment of skeletal stabilization with augmentation, or alteration of initial stabilization as indicated. Because LRMC was the first medical facility outside of a combat zone, patients could be reassessed in a safer, more stable environment. All patients had an assessment upon arrival to LRMC and, after admission, had a complete reassessment by the admitting service. Additional injuries were addressed as necessary. Due to the significant energy transmitted to the extremities with these combat injuries, findings of further tissue injury and necrosis were not uncommon, in spite of the

appropriate, outstanding care performed in theater by the orthopedic surgeons working in the combat zone in austere and often hazardous surroundings.[2]

From the onset of OIF in March 2003, the pace and workload at LRMC changed permanently (Figure 6-5). Previously for the medical center, a planeload of casualties was the exception (eg, USS Cole attack, October 2000) rather than the rule. During OIF, as the theater situation matured and aircraft availability for casualty transport was more consistent, daily evacuations were received, with patient information transmitted prior to arrival, which helped with planning of resources. Naturally, all evacuated patients required an assessment upon arrival, in order to provide optimum care upon arrival to LRMC. A representative for all surgical services continued to provide triage support in order to appropriately assign patients to respective specialties. With this systemic approach, the orthopedic surgery service was able to maintain its routine mission of outpatient clinic visits and elective surgery with minimal, and very short-term, interruption.

Another advancement and change in the management of combat injuries was the time of transport from Landstuhl to the CONUS, which averaged 4 to 5 days.[9] This is a significant difference as compared to the Vietnam era evacuation timeframe (45 days to return to CONUS).[11] Because of this relatively short time at LRMC along with the significant injury to the soft tissues, Landstuhl frequently was not the site for definitive bony stabilization with respect to the open, high-energy combat injuries to the extremities. Emphasis was upon adequate debridement of the wounds and providing adequate bony stabilization that would allow for ease of transport and not interfere with definitive care.[2,4] Because of the nature of the medical evacuation flights both from theater to LRMC and from LRMC to CONUS, traction was not used. Difficulty with unsupervised traction and/or loss of traction in flight makes this a less than desirable means. External fixation was the appropriate choice for many traumatic extremity injuries requiring bony stabilization. This provided adequate stabilization while allowing for ease of transport from each mode of transportation to the next along the evacuation route (Figure 6-6). The orthopedic surgery service at LRMC was also responsible for ensuring this continued, rapid, and efficient evacuation to CONUS. Based upon injury and military unit location, each patient was evacuated to the appropriate military medical treatment facility in the United States. The orthopedic surgery capabilities of the medical treatment facilities in the United States were the essential factors in this decision-making process. Patients with significant injuries requiring multiple and extensive procedures were generally evacuated to the regional military medical center closest to the servicemember's home duty station (eg, Walter Reed Army Medical Center, Brooke Army Medical Center, Naval Medical Center San Diego), which were able to provide more specialized care. Timing of definitive fixation and reconstructive procedures was determined by the receiving facility.[12]

With the improved time to return to the United States, the advances in all areas of prosthetics (design, fit, performance), and the advent of designated amputee facilities within the military medical system, the approach to amputations (upper and lower extremity of all levels) at Landstuhl required special attention. LRMC was not the definitive care facility for any amputation. Obviously, any amputation was performed for life- or limb-threatening reasons. Almost all of these were performed in theater because most patients were stabilized prior to their evacuation out of the combat zone. The goal at Landstuhl was adequate debridement of the limb. All viable tissue was preserved as best as possible. The determination of definitive amputation level was decided at the amputation center (Walter Reed Army Medical Center, Brooke Army Medical Center).[12] Soft tissue coverage, flaps, and prosthetic fitting are all performed at the designated amputation center; therefore, any viable tissue was spared to offer the amputation team an opportunity to decide further treatment (Figure 6-7). Because patients arrive so rapidly to Landstuhl from theater, timing of discussion of amputation or need for revising amputation level is not ideal, and these patients are informed, in general terms, of the possible scenarios regarding future treatments. Medical evacuation of amputees from LRMC to CONUS was directly to the designated amputation centers where the multispecialty approach to each injury was given.

A majority of military personnel evacuated from theater to Landstuhl did not have traumatic battle injuries.[1] The less urgent orthopedic conditions were evaluated by the LRMC Orthopedic Surgery Service

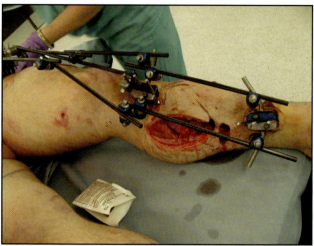

Figure 6-6. Use of external fixation for stabilization and ease of transport for multiple level extremity injury.

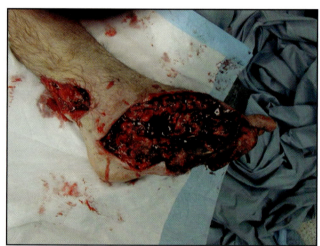

Figure 6-7. At LRMC, all viable tissue is preserved as appropriate. Determination of definitive amputation level is conducted by amputation centers in CONUS.

(Figure 6-8). Assessment upon arrival was performed, and a determination for further care was made. If a patient could be treated and returned to theater able to perform all rigorous activities of a combatant within 14 days, then that servicemember was treated and remained at LRMC until he or she could return to his or her unit in theater. In general, nearly all of those types of injuries (that allowed the warrior to return to duty within 14 days) were treated in theater and did not evacuate to Germany.[2] All other less urgent injuries were assessed for proper stabilization prior to further evacuation to the servicemember's home station in the United States. Definitive fixation was performed on nonemergent orthopedic injuries if it facilitated transport and adequate resources were available.

Because Landstuhl is the funnel for all casualties from theater, the need for reassessment of these

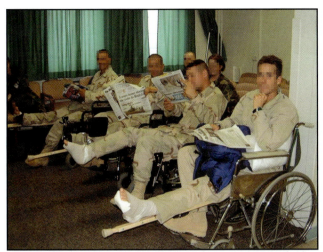

Figure 6-8. Nonurgent, nonbattle injuries awaiting further evaluation and treatment in the outpatient orthopedic clinic at LRMC.

wounded warriors applying the principles of life/limb preservation, skeletal stabilization, and aggressive wound debridement is paramount. The improvements in body armor have reduced axial trauma and have increased the overall percentage of skeletal trauma on the modern battlefield.[1] Other battlefield changes have allowed for the wounded to be evacuated from the theater to a safer location in such a rapid time that focus continues on wound management and stabilization, not definitive procedures at the medical facility in Landstuhl. The severity of the wounds and the amount of energy absorbed by the limbs with modern battlefield injuries cannot be overemphasized.[1,2] The ability to reassess these wounds in a safer, less time-constrained environment allows the orthopedic team at Landstuhl to better determine further management of these injuries. Proper coordination with receiving facilities in the United States sends these casualties to the appropriate location in order for their care to be completed in a most expeditious manner. Constant communication with all involved facilities (in the combat theaters and in CONUS) and with the aeromedical evacuation teams has helped create an efficient process, allowing for the wounded service-members to receive optimum care along all stops on the evacuation chain. The courageous and superior efforts by the combat medic/lifesaver and the orthopedic surgeons in theater have been critical on the road to recovery. LRMC continues to play a critical role in combat casualty care, ensuring these servicemembers receive timely and appropriate care throughout their evacuation.

References

1. Owens BD, Kragh JF, Macaitis J, Svoboda SJ, Wenke JC. Characterization of extremity wounds in Operation Iraqi Freedom and Operation Enduring Freedom. *J Orthop Trauma*. 2007;21:254-257.
2. Covey DC. From the frontlines to the home front. The crucial role of military orthopedic surgeons. *J Bone Joint Surg Am*. 2009;91:998-1006.
3. Bagg MR, Covey DC, Powell ET. Levels of medical care in the Global War on Terrorism. *J Am Acad Orthop Surg*. 2006;14:S7-S9.
4. Ficke JR, Pollak AN. Extremity war injuries: development of clinical treatment principles. *J Am Acad Orthop Surg*. 2007;15:590-595.
5. Holcomb JB, Stansbury LG, Champion HR, Wade C, Bellamy RF. Understanding combat casualty care statistics. *J Trauma*. 2006;60:397-401.
6. Covey DC. Combat orthopaedics: a view from the trenches. *J Am Acad Orthop Surg*. 2006;14:S10-S17.
7. Gawande A. Casualties of war—military care for the wounded from Iraq and Afghanistan. *N Engl J Med*. 2004;351:2471-2475.
8. Bellamy RF. A note on American combat mortality in Iraq. *Mil Med*. 2007;172:i,1023.
9. Tenuta JJ. From the battlefields to the States: the road to recovery. The role of Landstuhl Regional Medical Center in US Military Casualty Care. *J Am Acad Orthop Surg*. 2006;14:S45-S47.
10. Bowyer G. Debridement of extremity war wounds. *J Am Acad Orthop Surg*. 2006;14:S52-S56.
11. Bellamy RF. Why is Marine combat mortality less than that of the Army? *Mil Med*. 2000;165:362-367.
12. Hayda RA, Mazurek MT, Powell ET, et al. From Iraq back to Iraq: modern combat orthopedic care. *Instr Course Lect*. 2008;57:87-99.

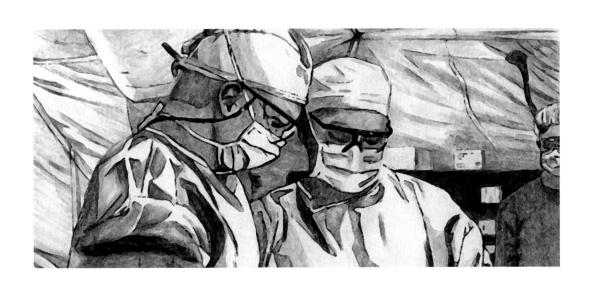

SECTION II

ADVANCEMENTS

Chapter 7

BALLISTIC, BLAST, AND BURN INJURY: SCIENCE AND CLINICAL IMPLICATIONS

COL (Ret) Roman Hayda, MD

The bombs and high-velocity firearms used in modern war create unique injuries unlike those encountered in civilian trauma. The conflicts in Iraq and Afghanistan have added a great deal of experience in dealing with bomb and ballistic injury as these weapons and our understanding of the injuries they cause continue to evolve. The wounding patterns challenge those who try to save lives and restore function of the injured whether the injured are combatants or civilians. A high degree of energy is focused by these weapons on impact, disrupting and contaminating tissues. Open injury rates in war are 90% compared to 10% in civilian trauma, transfusion needs are 3 times higher, and yet combat mortality is at a historically low rate of 10%.[1-3] These complex injuries require expert evaluation and care. Therefore, it is imperative that medical personnel have an accurate understanding of these mechanisms to correctly prioritize and provide the optimal care. Although the specific weapons and ratio of blast to gunshot injury may vary from conflict to conflict, these continue to be the overwhelming cause of injury in any war to include the present wars in Afghanistan and Iraq.

In the conflicts in Afghanistan and Iraq, the causes of casualties are blast injury in 78% of cases and ballistic injury in 18%.[4] In comparison, during World War II, 35% of casualties were generated by explosions and 65% by gunshots. In this analysis by Owens of 1566 injured warriors between 2001 and 2005, each casualty sustained an average of 4.2 wounds. Injuries involved the extremities in 55% of patients, similar to previous conflicts. However, the authors noted that there was a decrease in chest injury rate and an increase in injuries to the head and neck. These changes were attributed to the use of protective gear and increased survival rates.

Blast injuries have been caused by a variety of bombs, particularly improvised explosive devices (IEDs), in this conflict. These devices have been made from a wide variety of materials to include artillery rounds and ammonium nitrate bombs in various common containers, such as pressure cookers and soda cans. These have been triggered through sensors or remotely, inflicting a vast number of injuries. Rocket-propelled grenades and mortars were also used, while firearms included the AK-47, hunting, and sniper rifles.

Bombs and Blasts

Explosive devices have been used with great effect by traditional forces, insurgencies, and terrorists because of their ability to destroy property and to kill and injure personnel. A fundamental understanding of blast physics helps to explain the type of injuries encountered.[5] The destructiveness of blasts is related to the explosive material and quantity as well as the environment in which the detonation occurs. High-order blasts are caused by dynamite, TNT, and semtex among others, which explode at supersonic speeds up to 3000 to 8000 m/sec while low-order explosives include gas or alcohol bombs, which are subsonic.[6]

Owens BD, Belmont PJ Jr, eds. *Combat Orthopedic Surgery:*
Lessons Learned in Iraq and Afghanistan (pp 53-64)
© 2011 SLACK Incorporated

BLAST PHYSICS

In an explosion, the solid or liquid chemical components are rapidly converted into gas. This rapid expansion occurs in milliseconds, creating a blast wave that travels at supersonic speeds. The area of overpressure is followed by a rapid decline and subsequent negative pressure phase described by the Friedlander curve. This overpressure is responsible for the majority of the destructiveness in the epicenter of a blast. The impact and shattering force of an explosion is termed *brisance*. Fortunately, these forces rapidly decay in the expanding blast sphere as a function of inverse r³. Associated with the explosion is the blast wind that further disseminates debris throughout the blast field.

Projectiles are dispersed by the bomb blast, creating a great number of casualties. These may be from the bomb casing; objects deliberately packed in and around the bomb such as nails, bolts, or other hardware; or dirt and debris from the surrounding environment.[7] These projectiles create the open, highly contaminated wounds seen in blast victims. A vast number of projectiles are typically irregular, leading to inefficient flight and rapid decay in velocity, unlike gunshot injury. Nonetheless, it has been estimated that the safe stand-off distance for survivable injury from fragments is 100 times larger than survivable blast wave injury and hence the far greater number of bomb fragmentation injuries (Figure 7-1).[5]

The projectile may also be deliberately formed and directed by the device as in the case of the explosively formed projectile.[8] This novel improvised device seen on the battlefield was devised to overcome the protective armor of vehicles. In this type of bomb, the forces of the blast are directed to rapidly melt a metal that is projected in a planned direction to penetrate an armored vehicle, killing or injuring the personnel inside.

The environment of the explosion is also critical in determining its destructive nature. Walls and enclosures reflect blast waves, magnifying their effects. In contrast, in an open environment, the blast is dissipated in a spherical manner. Hence, a smaller blast will be much more destructive in an enclosed space as has been reported in the Israeli and United Kingdom experience with terrorist blasts.[9,10]

BLAST-RELATED INJURY

As a result of a blast, 4 general types or classes of injury to personnel are observed, each related to a particular physical aspect of the blast.[11] Patients may discretely manifest only one or any combination of these injury types. Understanding and recognizing these patterns leads to more effective triage and patient management.

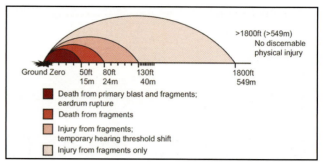

Figure 7-1. Estimated risk of death and injury relative to distance from detonation of a 155-mm shell IED. (Reprinted with permission from Champion HR, Holcomb J, Young LA. Injuries from explosions: physics, biophysics, pathology, and required research focus. *J Trauma.* 2009;66:1468-1477.)

Primary Blast Injury

Primary blast injury is caused by the blast wave and overpressure phenomena. It occurs closest to the epicenter and may cause immediate death.[6,12] As the blast wave travels through materials and tissues of different densities, its velocity changes, creating stress, shear, and shock waves. The bodily tissues are damaged macroscopically and microscopically through spalling, implosion, and shear. Spalling involves fragmentation of tissue of higher density into one of lesser density, much like boiling water. Shear occurs between tissues as they move differentially, potentially severing vascular and other attachments. Tissues with the greatest density differential are most prone to injury.

The tympanic membranes, lungs, and the gastrointestinal organs are most susceptible to primary blast injury. The tympanic membrane can be disrupted by the overpressure wave at relatively low pressures as low as 5 psi.[6] Although as many as 9% of casualties from Iraq and Afghanistan may have tympanic membrane disruption, it is not a reliable marker for other, more significant primary blast injuries with a sensitivity of only 29%.[6,13,14]

In pulmonary blast injury, the alveolar membrane is injured, resulting in edema, infiltrates, and inflammation.[15] The radiographic and clinical signs are quite similar to acute respiratory distress syndrome, often requiring a high level of respiratory support in survivors.[6,16] The gastrointestinal tract, particularly the large bowel, may also be susceptible to blast injury at the tissue interfaces, but this is much less common than pulmonary injury, being observed in 0.3% to 0.6% of blast survivors.[6] Bowel perforations may present late with acute abdominal symptoms secondary to segmental ischemia. A review of 181 patients with abdominal injury following terrorist events found that, in 94.4% of cases, blast projectiles were the predominant cause of abdominal injury and not the primary blast wave.[17]

It is increasingly recognized that the central nervous system and the cardiovascular system can also be injured by the blast wave with potentially persistent sequelae in the case of traumatic brain injury.[18] Several mechanisms have been implicated for blast-related brain injury to include air embolism, cerebrovascular spasm[19] and aneurysm,[20] and disruption of neural pathways.[21] Authors have documented electroencephalography changes in blast victims, and others have documented persistent cognitive and behavioral defects following blast injury.[22]

Nonetheless, Bell and colleagues, in a review of 408 casualties with war-related head injury evaluated at Bethesda Naval Medical Center and Walter Reed Army Medical Center, noted that penetrating brain injury was the most common form of blast injury to the nervous system in this conflict, despite high rates of protective helmet use.[23] In this cohort, 56% were injured by blast mechanism, and 71% of all penetrating injuries were caused by blast. Complications included pulmonary embolism (7%), cerebrospinal fluid leak (8.6%), meningitis (9.1%), and cerebrovascular injury (27%). They also noted a previously unreported association of head injuries with spinal cord and column injuries in 9.8% of cases. They also noted that, among severely head-injured casualties presenting with Glasgow Coma Scores of 5 or less and high Injury Severity Scores (ISS) requiring longer intensive care unit stays, mortality was only 4.4%. Meaningful recovery in patients with Glasgow Outcome Scores of 3 or higher was achieved in half of these at 1 and 2 years of follow-up.

Previous experience with terrorist blasts has found that traumatic amputation due to a primary blast wave is an ominous sign of injury associated with very high mortality.[24,25] Hull and Cooper analyzed 73 blast casualty amputations from the conflict in Northern Ireland and subsequently modeled blast activity in a computer model and then in 9 goat hind limbs. They found that a blast wave does not cause amputation by flailing of the limb. Their study demonstrated the blast shock wave causes diaphyseal fracture and subsequent amputation. However, on the battlefield, it may be hard to distinguish a primary blast amputation from one caused by blast projectiles unless other signs of primary blast injury are evident.

Primary blast injury occurs in close proximity to the blast epicenter, is associated with high mortality, and may involve multiple systems. Prompt recognition of blast lung with appropriate ventilatory support and supportive care of brain injury are critical in the recovery of the combatant.

Secondary Blast Injury

Secondary blast injury is caused by bomb fragments and from surrounding debris accelerated by the blast (Figure 7-2). These irregular fragments have very high velocity and energy initially, which are dissipated during flight. Therefore, the injury radius is much higher than primary blast injury but much less than a projectile of similar velocity and size from a firearm. Protective measures, such as vehicle armor, protective vests, and helmets, have been effective in limiting but not eliminating injury.[4] Even simple protective glasses have limited eye injury.[26]

Secondary blast injury is responsible for the high number of wounds and fractures seen in those killed or injured by the number of projectiles created.[27,28] Champion et al pointed out that, on the battlefield, secondary blast injury is the predominant cause of death.[5] Near the epicenter in the zone of primary blast injury, there is such an overwhelming number of projectiles that "total body dismemberment" by blast projectiles is observed on autopsy.[28] Ramasamy and colleagues reported on 100 consecutive casualties from the Afghanistan conflict, 78 of which were caused by blasts.[8] The explosively formed projectile caused of 91.3% injuries; 22.6% were killed or died of wounds. Primary blast injury was observed in only 3.7% blast deaths and in none of the survivors. All deaths had penetrating injuries with half sustaining amputations, 67% suffering abdominal thoracic and pelvic wounds, and 4.7 anatomic areas injured per casualty. In contrast, survivors had 2.6 anatomic areas injured with 7% amputations and no injuries to the chest or abdomen.

In survivors of secondary blast injury, the wounds are highly contaminated and contain devitalized tissue, increasing the infection risk. Indeed, high infection rates have been seen in these battlefield injuries despite early debridement and prophylactic antibiotic use.[29]

Blast projectiles most commonly cause soft tissue wounds. If the projectile carries sufficient energy and strikes bone, the bone fractures, creating a complex wound with secondary projectiles. In the series by Owens et al analyzing extremity injuries, 82% of all battlefield fractures were open.[30] These mangling injuries may involve all tissue planes to include skin, muscle, nerves, vessels, and bone with varying degrees of loss of each tissue type. There is an ongoing debate whether the severe injuries that do not result in traumatic amputation are best treated with reconstruction or amputation.

For the surgeon treating these injuries, it is important to understand that, unlike civilian open fractures and wounds, blast debris that violates the skin and injures underlying tissue can propagate widely. The contaminants travel along soft tissue planes, causing a wider zone of injury than initially suspected from a cursory evaluation or debridement. Although each fragment may not require excision, consideration of this wider zone of injury is critical in creating a

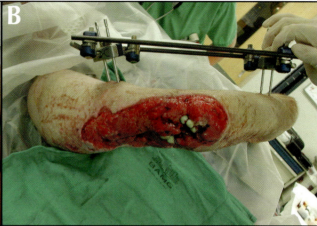

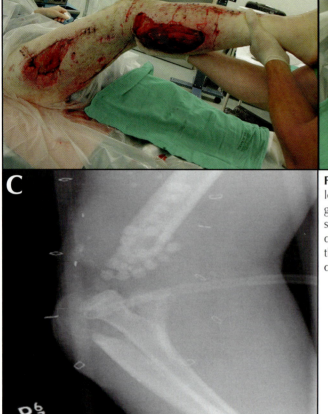

Figure 7-2. IED blast casualty with multiple injuries. (A) Right lower extremity with multiple wounds but no fracture from gravel projected by the blast. Note fasciotomy wounds and skin debridement. The smaller wounds were not explored or debrided, and debris is retained. (B) Right elbow with loss of the distal humerus and distal triceps. (C) Radiographs of right distal humerus.

treatment plan. Indeed, pursuing each fragment may cause greater soft tissue damage and threat to the patient than the initial injury. Bowyer performed a study of experimental soft tissue wounding in gelatin blocks and 28 pigs finding minimal cavity and tissue necrosis. Only 3 animals developed a soft tissue infection.[31] Subsequently, a clinical study of 83 casualties with 1200 wounds in Afghanistan was performed.[32] In 850 soft tissue only wounds, treatment was nonoperative only with dressings and antibiotics. Only 2 local infections developed, which were treated with simple debridement, confirming that a majority of wounds do not require operative debridement. Careful and sound judgment is required in treating these patients. Open fractures require thorough debridement and stabilization. External fixation usually provides initial stabilization and often provides definitive fixation, particularly in the lower extremity.

Tertiary Blast Injury

Tertiary injury is caused by gross movement of the victim into stationary objects by the forces of the blast. This mechanism results in blunt injury as is seen in motor vehicle crashes and falls from a height and may

be more familiar to medical personnel. Nonetheless, these injuries can be much more severe, as described in the USS Cole experience and seen in personnel in armored vehicles struck but not penetrated by IEDs.[33,34] In these cases, the armor plating or deck is accelerated rapidly by the blast impulse lasting only milliseconds causing blunt open and closed fractures with marked comminution (Figure 7-3).

Quaternary Blast Injury

Quaternary injury represents all other forms of injury associated with blasts. The most problematic of these are burns. The fireball associated with the explosion can burn the extremities and cause inhalation injury. The blast itself may be the cause, or flammable material in the area of the blast may ignite, causing injury to the casualty. In this conflict, approximately 5% to 10% of casualties have sustained burns, but it is not possible at this time to determine how many are associated with blasts or other mechanisms.[35,36] This rate of burn injury is similar to previous conflicts. The military surgeon must therefore be familiar with the treatment of burn casualties. Wolf and colleagues analyzed outcomes of 273 military burn casualties

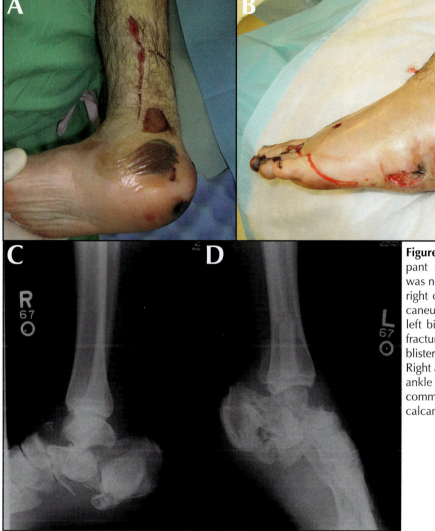

Figure 7-3. IED injury to occupant of armored vehicle that was not penetrated, resulting in right closed and left open calcaneus and talus fractures with left bimalleolar and metatarsal fractures. (A) Right ankle with blisters. (B) Left open ankle. (C) Right ankle radiograph. (D) Left ankle radiograph. (Note severe comminution of the talus and calcaneus in C and D.)

from Iraq and Afghanistan compared to a cohort of civilian burn casualties treated contemporaneously at the same institution.[37] Despite military casualties having a higher ISS (9 versus 5) and higher inhalation injury (8% versus 3%), the burned total body surface areas were similar as were the survival rates. It should be noted that the military burn casualties obtained their initial care under austere conditions and were transported across continents within days of injury. Of course, these patients also sustained other blast injury patterns.

ORTHOPEDIC MANAGEMENT OF BURN CASUALTIES

The treatment of burn casualties requires particular expertise.[36] In theater, these patients were resuscitated and stabilized. Escharatomy and fasciotomy were performed as the clinical situation dictated. Open wounds required debridement. Careful fluid replacement was performed to manage electrolyte imbalances.

Ventilatory support, particularly in those with inhalation injury, was critical. Patients with significant burns, particularly those of the face and hands, were transported by specialized teams to the Institute of Surgical Research by a burn air transport team following initial stabilization. Tangential skin excision was typically performed within days of injury, usually upon return to facilities in the continental United States. This was followed by the laborious process of skin grafting to obtain complete coverage. Depending on the area to be covered, weeks or months may be required, all the while fighting the risk of infection, contracture, and heterotopic ossification. Casualties with more than 90% burned total body surface area have survived.

Although burn surgeons and therapists are adept at management of contractures, recalcitrant contractures of the ankle, elbow, and hand have required surgical release. Some have benefited from placement of external fixators and K-wires prophylactically and also after release. In selective cases, circular frames have been used to correct deformities.

Figure 7-4. IED casualty with severe burns and multiple fractures. (A) Clinical intraoperative photograph at debridement in a facility in the continental United States. Note external fixators to right lower extremity. (B) Radiograph of open femur fracture and femoral neck fracture. (C) Radiograph of definitive fixation of femur fracture with 6-mm pin external fixator. (D) Healed femur fracture and ankylosed right hip after girdlestone debridement of the femoral neck fracture.

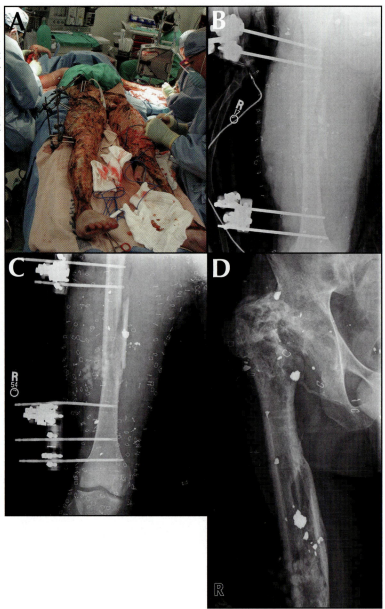

Burn victims may have open and closed fractures in the burned and nonburned extremities. When fractures occurred in the burned extremity, generally operative fracture care was required for unstable fractures that could not be splinted adequately. However, external fixation was preferred, as internal fixation risks contamination and deep infection (Figure 7-4). Internal fixation in the burned extremity was undertaken with extreme caution.

Burn casualty may also require amputation due to unreconstructible fracture patterns or severe burns with exposed vital structures. Due to their critical illness, these patients may not be candidates for complex skeletal reconstruction or free tissue transfer, therefore requiring amputation. However, due to skin loss, amputation is challenging, requiring careful rotation of available soft tissue to cover critical areas of bone and neurovascular structures (Figure 7-5). Nonetheless, prosthetic fitting and ambulation are possible.

SYSTEMIC RESPONSES TO BLASTS

In addition to discrete organs being affected by the blast wave and projectiles, systemic effects of blasts are becoming increasingly appreciated. Cernak and colleagues in the conflict in Yugoslavia sampled 65 blast victims and 62 nonblast victims with similar ISS and Red Cross Wound Classification.[22] The blast victims had higher blood thromboxane, prostacyclin, and sulfidopeptide levels. Investigators in China evaluated the relationship of blast and fragmentation injury in a dog model.[38] The highest level of thromboxane

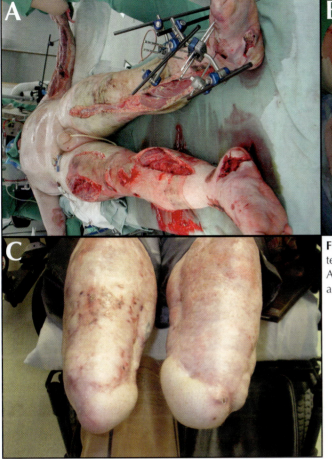

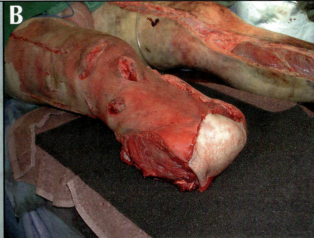

Figure 7-5. Burn casualty amputation with preserved skin strategically placed. (A) Clinical picture prior to amputation. (B) Amputation preserving unburned skin at boot top. (C) Healed amputations.

and the most severe pulmonary injury was found in the combined blast/fragmentation group, suggesting a synergistic effect between primary and secondary blast injury mediated by systemic inflammatory mediators. Other animal studies have documented bradycardia, hypotension, and apnea that are not fully explained by thoracic injury or vagal effects.[39,40] Further systemic effects of blast injury and means of their modulation remain to be elucidated.

On the horizon is the ability to modulate tissue response to blast injury through pharmacologic means. Chavko et al investigated the ability of antioxidants to alter pulmonary blast injury in a rat pulmonary blast injury model.[41] The administration of N-acetylcysteine (NACA) following blast exposure reduced neutrophil activation and chemokine markers of inflammation.[41] The clinical effectiveness of such systemic treatments for blast injury is unknown but suggests that treatment of blast effects may extend beyond surgical and supportive care.[18]

BLAST PROTECTION

Protective measures for blast mitigation have undergone an evolutionary change. New materials have been developed, such as Kevlar (DuPont, Wilmington, DE) and advanced ceramics, that prevent penetrating injury from bombs and high-velocity firearms. The modern vests and helmets made of these materials have been credited with mitigating the effects of blasts and the unprecedented survivability of combatants.[5] Several investigators have looked at the effectiveness of these protective measures. Investigators have found that some vests may actually potentiate the destructive effects of the blast wave, creating a more severe primary blast injury to the lungs.[42] However, they suggested methods of wave decoupling, which can preserve the protective benefits. Another group investigated the effectiveness of anti-mine footwear.[43] At the time, no footwear was found to be protective. In several cases, though, a severe open injury was avoided in the cadaver model, leaving a comminuted closed fracture. Designs of mine protective boots that stood on "legs" away from the blast lessened the blast impact. On a larger scale, evaluating protective measures of temporary shelters against vehicle bombs similarly found that distance from the epicenter is the best protection of personnel.

The use of protective equipment has been instrumental in protecting combatants from bombs and bullets. Undoubtedly, the technology will continue to improve survivability, but an improved understanding of concussive effects and protection from traumatic brain injury will be required. Furthermore, protection may come at the expense of mobility, impairing operational effectiveness particularly in remote and rugged terrain. Achieving this balance will challenge engineers and leaders.

Firearms and Ballistics

The wounding capacity of military and other firearms has been analyzed in significant detail well before this conflict.[44-46] Many surgeons have observed directly their destructive effects in Iraq and Afghanistan where 18% of US casualties sustained gunshot wounds.[4] Military firearms such as the US military AR-15 and the ubiquitous AK-47 are characteristically high-velocity weapons with the muzzle exit velocity of more than 700 m/sec. Sniper rifles also deliver high-velocity rounds. The high velocity confers high energy, and hence the potential injury capacity is high in these weapons. A shotgun injury at close proximity causes high-energy wounds as well. The total energy of a round is expressed as $\frac{1}{2}mv^2$ at the time of impact. The amount of energy expended by the round on impact determines the injury potential.

In addition to the velocity of the round, other characteristics of the round determine its destructiveness, specifically its flight characteristics and its deformability. Rifling of the barrel imparts spin on the bullet, lending it stable flight much like a gyroscope. The round may yaw, which is essentially wobbling along the flight path. Finally, it may also tumble, which increases the tissue directly contacted and disrupted by the round. The yaw and tumble of the round increase the amount of tissue directly impacted by the round, creating a permanent cavity.

In addition to the permanent cavity, its velocity also creates a temporary cavity, which disrupts the soft tissues. This cavitation is dependent on the thickness or depth of the traversed tissues. If the body part is of sufficient thickness, a much wider zone of injury and tissue devitalization will be observed than the entry and exit wounds suggest. Because skin is elastic and less prone to injury compared to muscle, it is an unreliable marker of internal injury (Figure 7-6). When a large cavitational wound is created, a thorough debridement is required to remove the devitalized tissue. Such a wounding pattern should be suspected when there is prolonged bleeding from a bullet wound or fluctuation suggestive of a large fluid collection or significant muscle disruption. Compartment syndrome may also be seen in these injuries.

The material composition and shape of the round determines the likely deformation of the round on contact. Military rounds are typically jacketed. When traveling through soft tissues, this jacket remains intact, and the bullet does not deform. Bullets with hollow points or material of relatively soft composition, such as lead at the point, may deform or even fragment causing secondary projectiles and further injury.[47]

The most critical element of the injury capacity of a military firearm or for that matter any weapon is its absolute energy dissipated upon contact with the casualty.[48] Although much has been written on high-velocity wounding patterns, the velocity of the round is but one component of this equation. Indeed, a high-velocity round may completely pass through an extremity, particularly if the limb is of small diameter and the bone is not struck. Very little damage occurs as the round loses little energy. Similarly, if the shot occurs at a great distance and the round has lost its velocity, little damage will occur on impact. However, a round may have a great deal of energy, either because of its weight or velocity. If most or all of the energy is dissipated by the bullet strike, a very significant injury will occur. Such an energy transfer will occur if the bullet fragments or strikes a bone, fragmenting it.

The clinician should look for signs of high-energy transfer from the round to the casualty to direct management. Clues suggestive of such energy dissipation include severe bone comminution, large cavitational or fluctuant wound, compartment syndrome, or vascular injury. The clinician must therefore carefully examine the patient's wounds and radiographs to determine the timing and extent of wound debridement.

Clinical Principles

Effective treatment of the blast casualties and high-energy firearms requires a highly knowledgeable and coordinated team effort. Certainly, the initial step is prevention. This conflict has demonstrated the effectiveness of protective equipment, which includes Kevlar vests and helmets, protective eyewear, and vehicle armor.[3-5,49] The relative decrease in injury to the thorax and abdomen in this conflict has been directly attributed to the use of personal protective armor.[4] Additional modifications of the vest over the shoulder and groin area have increased the area of protection, particularly against blast fragmentation injury at the expense of mobility. The ceramic plates are designed to withstand direct small arms fire. When the protective armor is struck but not penetrated, the combatant is still subject to the blunt force and may suffer from soft tissue injury. Severe penetrating

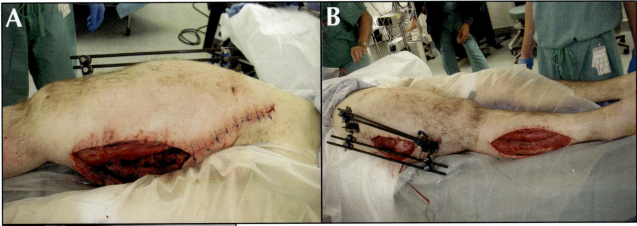

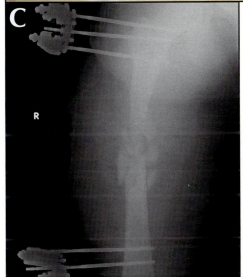

Figure 7-6. Gunshot injury to femur with compartment syndrome. (A) Medial thigh. (B) Lateral thigh, note severe swelling but little skin loss. (C) Radiograph of femur with comminution.

injury may also occur if the missile strikes the areas that cannot be covered, such as sniper shots to the shoulder.[50,51]

Upon presentation of the casualty to the medical facility, strict adherence to trauma principles must be maintained. The obvious mangling injury of the extremity distracts from other, potentially more life-threatening injuries. The whole casualty must be fully inspected to assess all injuries, as the majority of blast victims may have 3 or more injuries.[4,8] Hemorrhage is controlled with appropriate dressings and, when appropriate, tourniquet application. Wounds that are highly contaminated, are associated with fractures, are adjacent to joints, or may have significant necrotic tissue must be explored and debrided. Other clinical signs suggestive of a more severe injury are compartment syndrome and significant wound drainage. Because blast and missile debris tend to travel along tissue planes, these must be investigated to ensure thorough debridement. As Bowyer described and other clinicians have experienced, it is impossible and unnecessary to fully remove all debris from each blast

casualty. Fragmentation wounds involving only the skin and muscle may be safely treated by wound care and antibiotics.[31,32]

Fractures require appropriate stabilization with external fixation, K-wires, and splinting. At the definitive care facility, a recovery plan is made that may require multiple disciplines to include vascular surgery, plastic surgery, physical and occupational therapy, anesthesia, and social work. When amputation is a treatment consideration, involvement of the prosthetist is also important. Clinicians must stay wary of infection complicating recovery efforts. Initial wound debridement and appropriate antibiotic coverage are critical. Fracture implant choices may also influence long-term infection rates. Some authors have suggested circular frames for definitive treatment of these complex injuries.[52,53] Certain fracture patterns are more dependent on internal fixation (such as fractures of the distal humerus) for functional recovery, which may be performed in appropriately prepared cases.

The development of heterotopic ossification has clearly been associated with blast injury (Figure 7-7).

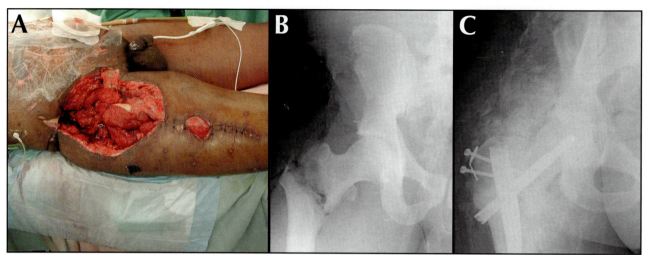

Figure 7-7. RPG causing multiple extremity and abdominal injury. (A) Right proximal thigh wound. (B) Right intertrochanteric fracture. (C) Hip ankylosis.

Potter and associates found that up to 80% of amputations performed through the zone of injury were associated with formation of heterotopic bone in blast victims while only 55% of those with amputations secondary to firearms were associated with formation of heterotopic bone.[54] In this same group of 193 amputations, the heterotopic bone was moderate (involving 25% to 50% of the diameter) or severe in 45% of blast amputations and was observed in only 25% of firearm injuries. This high rate was corroborated in a subsequent study by Forsberg and colleagues who found an association with age younger than 30 years, amputation, multiple extremity injury, ISS of 16 or higher, and head injury.[55] Neither study could find an association with the use of negative pressure wound therapy. Although the precise pathophysiology has not been elucidated, the large zone of soft tissue injury in blast victims appears to be related to the formation of heterotopic bone. At this time, no effective means of prediction or prophylaxis is available following injury. Treatment is rendered if the patient is symptomatic.

The treatment of severe extremity injury from blasts and high-velocity weapons remains challenging. Efforts are ongoing to analyze outcomes data to provide further information for optimal treatment for these severe multidimensional problems and to avoid further complications.

References

1. Perkins JG, Schreiber MA, Wade CE, Holcomb JB. Early versus late recombinant factor VIIa in combat trauma patients requiring massive transfusion. *J Trauma*. 2007;62:1095-1099.
2. Niles SE, McGlaughlin DF, Perkins JG. Increased mortality associated with the early coagulopathy of trauma in combat casualties. *J Trauma*. 2008;64:1459-1465.
3. Holcomb JB, McMullin NR, Pearse L, et al. Causes of death in U.S. Special Operations Forces in the global war on terrorism: 2001-2004. *Ann Surg*. 2007;245:986-991.
4. Owens BD, Kragh JF, Wenke JD, et al. Combat wounds in Operation Iraqi Freedom and Operation Enduring Freedom. *J Trauma*. 2008;64:295-299.
5. Champion HR, Holcomb J, Young LA. Injuries from explosions: physics, biophysics, pathology, and required research focus. *J Trauma*. 2009;66:1468-1477.
6. Ritenour AE, Baskin TW. Primary blast injury: update on diagnosis and treatment. *Crit Care Med*. 2008;36:S311-S317.
7. Stein M, Hirshberg A. Medical consequences of terrorism. *Surg Clin North Am*. 1999;79:1537-1552.
8. Ramasamy A, Harrisson SE, Clasper CC, Stewart MP. Injuries from roadside improvised explosive devices. *J Trauma*. 2008;65: 910-914.
9. Leibovici D, Gofrit ON, Stein M, et al. Blast injuries: bus versus open-air bombings—a comparative study of injuries in survivors of open-air versus confined-space explosions. *J Trauma*. 1996;41(6):1030-1035.
10. Waterworth TA, Carr MJT. An analysis of the post-mortem findings in the 21 victims of the Birmingham pub bombings. *Injury*. 1995;7(2):89-95.
11. Hull JB. Blast: injury patterns and their recording. *J Audiov Media Med*. 1992;15:121-127.
12. Nelson TJ, Clark T, Stedje-Larsen ET, et al. Close proximity blast injury patterns from improvised explosive devices in Iraq: a report of 18 cases. *J Trauma*. 2008;65:212-217.
13. Leibovici D, Gofrit ON, Shapira SC. Eardrum perforation in explosion survivors: is it a marker of pulmonary blast injury? *Ann Emerg Med*. 1991;34:168-172.
14. Harrison CD, Bebarta VS, Grant GA. Tympanic membrane perforation after combat blast exposure in Iraq: a poor biomarker of primary blast injury. *J Trauma*. 2009;67:210-211.
15. Chavko M, Prusaczyk WK, McCarron RM. Lung injury and recovery after exposure to blast overpressure. *J Trauma*. 2006;61:933-942.
16. Nguyen BT, Riley G. Thoracic manifestations of blast injury: a Walter Reed experience. *Chest*. 2005;128(4):1305-1306.
17. Bala M, Rivkind AI, Zamir G, et al. Abdominal trauma after terrorist bombing attacks exhibits a unique pattern of injury. *Ann Surg*. 2008;248(2):303-309.

18. Desmoulin GT, Dionne J-P. Blast-induced neurotrauma: surrogate use, loading mechanisms, and cellular responses. *J Trauma.* 2009;67(5):1113-1122.

19. Bell RS, Vo AH, Porter C. Wartime neurovascular injuries: review of the effectiveness of early, aggressive, endovascular management in the setting of blast-related cerebral vasospasm. *Neurosurg.* 2006;59:455.

20. Bell RS, Vo AH, Roberts R, et al. Wartime traumatic aneurysms: acute presentation, diagnosis, and multimodal treatment of 64 craniocervical arterial injuries. *Neurosurg.* 2010;66:66-79.

21. Nakagawa A, Fujimura M, Okuyama H, et al. Mechanism of primary blast injury: insight from microexplosive generated shock wave-induced brain injury animal model and engineering experiments. *Neurosurg.* 2009;65:413.

22. Cernak I, Savic J, Ignjatovic D, et al. Blast injury from explosive munitions. *J Trauma.* 1999;47:96-103.

23. Bell RS, Vo AV, Neal CJ, et al. Military traumatic brain and spinal column injury: a 5-year study of the impact blast and other military grade weaponry on the central nervous system. *J Trauma.* 2009;66:S104–S111.

24. Hull JB. Traumatic amputation by explosive blast: pattern of injury in survivors. *Br J Surg.* 1992;79:1303-1306.

25. Hull JB, Cooper GJ. Pattern and mechanism of traumatic amputation by explosive blast. *J Trauma.* 1996;40(3):S198-S205.

26. Gondusky JS, Reiter MP. Protecting military convoys in Iraq: an examination of battle injuries sustained by a mechanized battalion during Operation Iraqi Freedom. *Mil Med.* 2005;170(6):546-549.

27. Mellor SG. The relationship of blast loading to death and injury from explosion. *World J Surg.* 1992;16:893-898.

28. Kelly JF, Ritenour AE, McLaughlin DF, et al. Injury severity and causes of death from Operation Iraqi Freedom and Operation Enduring Freedom: 2003–2004 versus 2006. *J Trauma.* 2008;64(2 Suppl):S21–S27.

29. Murray C. Epidemiology of infections associated with combat-related injuries in Iraq and Afghanistan. *J Trauma.* 2008;64:S232-S238.

30. Owens B, Kragh JF, Macaitis J, Svoboda SJ, Wenke JC. Characterization of extremity wounds in Operation Iraqi Freedom and Operation Enduring Freedom. *J Orthop Trauma.* 2007;21:254-257.

31. Bowyer GW, Cooper GJ, Rice P. Small fragment wounds: biophysics and pathophysiology. *J Trauma.* 1996;40(3S):159S-164S.

32. Bowyer GW. Management of small fragment wounds: experience from the Afghan border. *J Trauma.* 1996;40(3S):170S-172S.

33. Davis TP, Alexander BA, Lambert EW, et al. Distribution and care of shipboard blast injuries (USS Cole DDG-67). *J Trauma.* 2003;55:1022-1028.

34. Langworthy MJ, Sabra J, Gould M. Terrorism and blast phenomena: lessons learned from the attack on the USS Cole (DDG67). *Clin Orthop Rel Res.* 2004;422:82-87.

35. Kauvar DS, Wolf SE, Wade CE, et al. Burns sustained in combat explosions in Operations Iraqi and Enduring Freedom (OIF/OEF explosion burns). *Burns.* 2006;32:853-857.

36. White CE, Renz EM. Advances in surgical care: management of severe burn injury. *Crit Care Med.* 2008;36:S318-S324.

37. Wolf SE, Kauvar DS, Wade C. Comparison between civilian burns and combat burns from Operation Iraqi Freedom and Operation Enduring Freedom. *Ann Surg.* 2006;243:786-795.

38. Huang JZ, Yang Z, Wang Z, Leng H. Study on characteristics of blast-fragment combined injury in dogs. *J Trauma.* 1996;40(3):S63-S67.

39. Guy RJ, Kirkman E, Watkins PE, et al. Physiologic responses to primary blast. *J Trauma.* 1998;45:983-987.

40. Ohnishi M, Kirkman E, Guy RJ, et al. Reflex nature of the cardiorespiratory response to primary thoracic blast injury in the anaesthetized rat. *Exp Physiol.* 2001;86:357-364.

41. Chavko M, Adeeb S, Ahlers ST, McCarron RM. Attenuation of pulmonary inflammation after exposure to blast overpressure by N-acetylcysteine amide. *Shock.* 2009;32(3):325-331.

42. Cooper GJ, Townsend DJ, Cater SR, Pearce BP. The role of stress waves in thoracic visceral injury from blast loading: modification of stress transmission by foams and high density materials. *J Biomech.* 1991;24:273-285.

43. Hayda R, Harris RM, Bass CD. Blast injury research: modelling injury effects of landmines, bullets, and bombs. *Clin Orthop Rel Res.* 2004;422:97-108.

44. Fackler ML, Malinowski JA, Hoxie SA, Jason A. Wounding effects of the AK-47 used by Patrick Purdy in the Stockton, California Schoolyard Shooting of January 17, 1989. *Am J Forensic Med Pathol.* 1990;11(3):185-189.

45. Ordog GJ. Wound ballistics: theory and practice. *Ann Emerg Med.* 1984;13:1113-1122.

46. Fackler ML, Surinchak JS, Malinnowski JA, Bowen RE. Wounding potential of the Russian AK-74 assault rifle. *J Trauma.* 1984;24(3):263-266.

47. Fackler ML, Surinchak JS, Malinnowski JA, Bowen RE. Bullet fragmentation: a major cause of tissue disruption. *J Trauma.* 1984;24(1):35-39.

48. Hull JB. Management of gunshot fractures of the extremities. *J Trauma.* 1996;40(3S):193S-197S.

49. Mabry RL, Holcomb JB, Baker AM. United States Army Rangers in Somalia: an analysis of combat casualties on an urban battlefield. *J Trauma.* 2000;49:515-529.

50. Kosashvili Y, Hiss J, Davidovic N. Influence of personal armor on distribution of entry wounds: lessons learned from urban-setting warfare fatalities. *J Trauma.* 2005;58:1236-1240.

51. Hofmeister EP, Mazurek M, Ingari J. Injuries sustained to the upper extremity due to modern warfare and the evolution of care. *J Hand Surg Am.* 2007;32-A(8):1141-1147.

52. Keeling JJ, Gwinn DE, Tintle S, et al. Short-term outcomes of severe open wartime tibial fractures treated with ring external fixation. *J Bone Joint Surg Am.* 2008;90:2643-2651.

53. Lerner A, Fodor L, Soudr M. Is staged external fixation a valuable strategy for war injuries to the limbs? *Clin Orthop Rel Res.* 2006;448:217-224.

54. Potter BK, Burns TC, Lacap AP, Granville RR, Gajewski DA. Heterotopic ossification following traumatic and combat-related amputations. Prevalence, risk factors, and preliminary results of excision. *J Bone Joint Surg Am.* 2007;89:476-486.

55. Forsberg JA, Pepek JM, Wagner S. Heterotopic ossification in high-energy wartime extremity injuries: prevalence and risk factors. *J Bone Joint Surg Am.* 2009;91:1084-1091.

Chapter 8

MANAGEMENT OF COMPLEX COMBAT-RELATED SOFT TISSUE WOUNDS/ NEGATIVE PRESSURE WOUND THERAPY

MAJ Brett A. Freedman, MD and MAJ Leon J. Nesti, MD, PhD

As it has been throughout time, the common denominator in the evolution of wound care is that the leaps forward have been made by military surgeons during times of war. The current conflicts in Iraq and Afghanistan, dating back to the first Gulf War, would once again fuel the progress of wound care.

Throughout modern warfare, survivable combat-related injuries have predominantly affected the extremities (60% to 75%).[1-3] More than 65% to 75% of operative cases at combat support hospitals are orthopedic in nature.[4] There has been a recent trend in pure blunt trauma mechanisms of injury yielding fractures and soft tissue injury patterns consistent with Level I civilian trauma versus mixed mechanisms with blunt and penetrating injuries that were seen prior to the up-armoring of vehicles and improvements in tactics, which reduced a soldier's exposure to fragmentation injury. Regardless of mechanism, orthopedists have come to understand that the soft tissue envelope surrounding the skeleton is the most important harbinger of successful outcome, as it directs bone healing, functional outcome, and complication potential.[5-7] This is particularly important in combat-related extremity injuries because more than 80% of fractures sustained in combat-trauma are open.[2,3]

Ritenour (a US Army general surgeon) and colleagues in 2008 provided a comprehensive epidemiological account of wound care, specifically in the setting of acute compartment syndrome (ACS), using data prospectively collected in the Joint Theater Trauma Registry developed during the Global War on Terrorism.[8] They retrospectively reviewed all admissions to Landstuhl Regional Medical Center (LRMC) between January 2005 and August 2006. During this time, 2787 patients were admitted to LRMC as evacuees from either Operation Iraqi Freedman (OIF) or Operation Enduring Freedom (OEF), for all conditions ranging from nonbattle-related medical disease to severe multitrauma. Four hundred eight of these patients (15% of all admissions) had undergone a fasciotomy in theater prior to air evacuation. To put this in context, the incidence of ACS/fasciotomy in Level I trauma centers in patients with tibial fractures, the injury pattern most at risk for ACS, is less than 10% to 20%.[9,10] Thus, this particular morbid secondary wound has become a hallmark of soft tissue management in OIF and OEF. Fitzgerald and colleagues helped reinforce the morbidity of fasciotomy wounds when they followed 60 patients long term and noted that 77% had paresthesias about the wound, approximately 33% had skin changes, ranging from scaling and pruritis to ulceration, and in 25%, the scar tethered to the underlying muscle, which alters function and cosmesis, such that 25% of patients intentionally hide their fasciotomy scars from the public.[11]

Owens BD, Belmont PJ Jr, eds. *Combat Orthopedic Surgery: Lessons Learned in Iraq and Afghanistan (pp 65-76)* © 2011 SLACK Incorporated

Management in Theater

CONTROLLING BLOOD LOSS

Wound care in theater begins on the battlefield and continues through the entire evacuation chain (Table 8-1). Medics and fellow soldiers are the first responders in the prehospital setting in combat (Echelon I). Their initial response is to stop and/or control hemorrhage, cover wounds, provisionally stabilize and/or reduce fractured extremities, remove the soldier from the hostile environment, and initiate the evacuation process. As with all previous military conflicts, hypovolemic shock secondary to hemorrhage remains the most common treatable cause of death on the battlefield.[12,13] While noncompressible internal organ hemorrhage is the most common source of exsanguination death, compressible extremity hemorrhage is the second most common source.[12] This conflict has seen an emphasis of the application of tourniquets on the battlefield. A tourniquet set has been made standard issue to all soldiers deploying to OIF/OEF. In addition, new hemorrhage controlling dressings have been tried with variable response.

HEMOSTATIC DRESSINGS WORK

Initially, hemostatic agents were granularized powders that were difficult to work with and were capable of exothermic reactions that could produce severe collateral soft tissue damage.[14] Newer dressings incorporated partially hydrated zeolite (QuickClot, Z-Medica Inc, Wallingford, CT) or chitosan (a naturally occurring polysaccharide; HemCon [HemCon Medical Technologies Inc, Portland, OR]) on specially engineered textiles to effectively obtain hemostasis without the collateral damage in challenging animal models and more importantly in clinical applications.[14] These dressings work by similar mechanisms—their constituent molecule has a very large capacity to absorb free water. In doing so, this concentrates clotting factors, which along with Ca++ ion co-factors in the dressing material and the electronic charge of the dressing promote rapid clotting at the interface between the dressing and the wound. These dressings become sticky when they contact blood, which allows the dressing to seal to the wound and stop bleeding. As a secondary benefit, this dressing acts as an antimicrobial barrier when it seals to the wound. In addition, some dressings also incorporate silver ions, which have inherent antimicrobial activity. Wedmore and colleagues recounted the use of HemCon in 64 military applications and found that 97% of the time, this dressing arrested ongoing hemorrhage.[15] In fact, 66% of the time, these dressings were successfully used after standard cotton gauze dressings and manual

Table 8-1

Steps for Preliminary Management of Complex Soft Tissue Injuries in War

1.	Hemorrhage control
2.	Temporary dressing/splint and evacuation
3.	Advanced Trauma Life Support primary survey
4.	Resuscitation and hemodynamic stabilization—Save life before limb
5.	Initiation of empiric antibiotic coverage
6.	Identification of wounds
7.	Gross decontamination
8.	Surgical debridement
9.	Irrigation
10.	Temporary stabilization of long-bone fractures (external fixation/splint)
11.	Clean moist cotton or negative pressure wound therapy dressing
12.	Evacuation to higher echelons of care for definitive management*

Steps 1 and 2 are prehospital setting tasks.
*Steps 7 through 11 should be repeated every 24 to 72 hours indefinitely until definitive soft tissue and skeletal management if possible.

pressure were unsuccessful in controlling bleeding. More recently, QuickClot Combat Gauze has been shown to be superior to HemCon in hemostasis and is the currently recommended first-line choice for hemostatic field dressing.[16]

LOW MORTALITY, BUT INCREASED WOUND SEVERITY

While these hemostatic dressings and emphasis on the importance of controlling hemorrhage (ie, liberal use of tourniquets) on the battlefield have significantly reduced preventable mortality, the concert of these efforts along with the shorter distances to medical care, enhanced capabilities of forward deployed medical units, and the efficiency of air evacuation to higher echelons of care has combined to make this conflict the most survivable in American military history.[12,13] In fact, we may be reaching a point of diminishing marginal returns in our ability to reduce mortality, as the energy and severity of combat wounds from improvised explosive devices (IEDs) create injuries that are nonsurvivable more than 75% of the time. In 2007, Holcomb and colleagues reported that 85% of the Special Forces soldiers killed in combat were deemed to have sustained nonsurvivable initial injuries and only 19% to 28% of all soldiers killed in 2003 to 2006 were deemed to have potentially survivable injuries based on autopsy.[12,13] There is an unexpected consequence to this low mortality rate, especially in the setting of high-energy traumatic mechanism of injury, which is devastating soft tissue wounds, the likes of which have not been previously encountered in war at this volume or severity.[13]

ANTIBIOTIC PROPHYLAXIS

Upon reaching the initial medical treatment facility, injured soldiers undergo a trauma survey according to the American College of Surgeons Advanced Trauma Life Support (ATLS) teachings. After controlling the airway and confirming adequate ventilation, sources of ongoing bleeding are rapidly identified and then appropriately controlled. During or immediately following completion of the trauma survey, empiric prophylactic antibiotics are started in theater and are continued for an appropriate amount of time through the evacuation process. Prophylactic antibiotics should be initiated within the first 3 hours of care and/or evacuation.[1] Hospenthal and colleagues have published a clinical practice guideline directing care of combat-related wounds, which is based on a review of the limited literature on the subject and the input from a panel of military surgeons and infectious disease specialists.[1] Patients with large, open, combat-related wounds should receive up to 72 hours of cefazolin (1 g IV every 8 hours) or a similar first-generation cephalosporin. Clindamycin (900 mg IV every 8 hours) should be used in the case of penicillin/cephalosporin drug allergy. While there is uniform agreement on this level of prophylaxis, because the most common organism to infect an open combat wound is gram-positive skin flora, there is less agreement on the use of "extended gram-negative" coverage. By convention, despite its condemnation in the Hospenthal article, currently, patients with open joints or fractures are receiving 72 hours of levofloxacin (750 mg IV/PO every day) or ciprofloxacin (400 mg IV twice daily) for extended gram-negative coverage. In patients with a penetrating abdominal injury, prophylactic coverage should be extended to a broad-spectrum antibiotic with gram-positive, gram-negative, and anaerobic coverage, like cefoxitin (1 g to 2 g IV every 6 to 8 hours) or piperacillin/tazobactam (4.5 g IV every 6 hours). This broadened coverage should be continued for 24 hours after definitive surgical cleaning of the abdomen.

With the current maturation of the battlefield, it is rare that it takes longer than 3 hours for patients to reach Echelon II/III (forward surgical teams, medi-

cal treatment facilities, or combat support hospitals). In the situation where operational tempo or weather conditions delay evacuation to Echelon II/III, it has been recommended that moxifloxacin 400 mg or levofloxacin 500 mg be given as a one-time oral dose to patients with open extremity injuries. Theater doctrine mandates that combat casualties be seen by a surgeon within 6 hours of injury, and typically this occurs in the first hour.[1,17]

Aggressive prophylactic coverage must be balanced against good practices aimed at limiting nosocomial multidrug-resistant organism (MDRO) infections.[18] At the start of these conflicts, there was no standardization regarding antibiotic prophylaxis. Antibiotics chosen were often too broad and their duration was too long, both leading to the secondary problem of MDRO generation, without an advantage in reducing infection rates. The adoption of the guidelines published by Hospenthal and colleagues and amendments to these guidelines, which have been formalized under the direction of the medical command structure in and out of theater, have gone a long way to reduce the misuse of prophylactic antibiotics.

Because the prevalence of MRDO colonization in our combat-injured patients is higher than the general population (up to 45% versus <8%), strategies have been adopted to reduce the incidence of nosocomial spread of these pathogens.[18-20] Nosocomial spread from hospital equipment or personnel is the most common mode of infection in open combat wounds. To this end, an infection control initiative started at LRMC in 2006 to 2007 and transported down-range, in which patients receive a chlorhexadine full-body wipe down on admission to the intensive care unit and then once-a-day wipe-downs with Sage (Cary, IL) antiseptic wipes, has reduced the prevalence of *Acinetobacter* on surveillance groin swab cultures from 11% to 0.6%. All patients arriving at LRMC from OIF/OEF with open wounds are treated with universal precautions, which include gown and gloves to prevent contact spread. All patients are swabbed in the bilateral groin. The groin is the most sensitive location for detecting MDRO colonization.[18] Based on the MDRO reports for the months of January and February 2010, *Escherichia coli* has become the most common MDRO micro-organism present on routine groin swabs. Since the beginning of 2010, the compliance with the groin swab surveillance protocol has been more than 95%. Only 3.5% had an MDRO organism, with *E. coli* being that organism in all but one case. Contact precautions remain in effect until these groin cultures return negative or 72 hours. Additionally, prophylactic antibiotic coverage is discontinued at 72 hours, unless there are clinical signs of active infection.

Figure 8-1. This figure demonstrates a right medial elbow and arm severe soft tissue injury sustained after an IED attack in which the soldier had his arm hanging out of the vehicle window. (A) A wound VAC has just been removed, revealing healthy pink, "beefy" granulation tissue. There is no exposed "white tissue" (bone, tendon, ligament, joint capsule, or implant). This wound is ready for definitive coverage. Delayed primary closure is not possible due to the skin loss and retraction. In this situation, split-thickness skin graft (STSG) is the ideal choice for definitive coverage. (B, C) The harvest site from the left anterior thigh and the graft that was harvested. (D) The graft in place, and (E) a Wound VAC placed over the top of the graft, left on continuous low (50 mm Hg) suction. When placing a VAC over a fresh STSG, a nonstick layer, like Adaptic (Johnson and Johnson, Inc, Arlington, TX), should be placed between the sponge and the graft. This step-wise process has led to >95% STSG take.

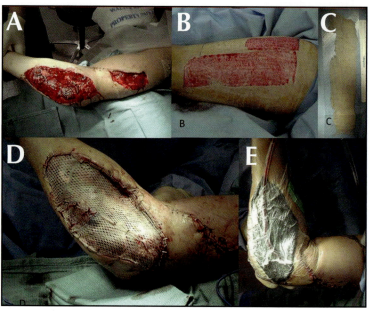

Microbiology of Combat Wound Care

The presence of bacterial colonization has not been a contraindication to wound closure or internal fixation. Unfortunately, the proper timing of closure and internal fixation has received little empiric attention in these conflicts. Anecdotally, at Walter Reed Army Medical Center (WRAMC), wounds were typically serially irrigated and debrided until the wound bed contained pink healthy-appearing muscle and granulation tissue (Figure 8-1). In addition, all "white tissue" (ie, bone, tendon, and ligament) needed to granulate over, or a reconstructive flap (local or distant) was necessary (Figure 8-2). Collagen-based artificial dermal layers (Integra, Integra LifeSciences, Plainsboro, NJ) have been used successfully in more than 93% of cases to cover exposed white tissue (bone, tendons, joint capsule) to allow a granulation layer to form capable of supporting a skin graft. This new technique, which is most commonly performed with vacuum-assisted closure (VAC), obviates the need for flap coverage. Post-wash cultures were frequently obtained at the completion of debridement procedures to provide some objective understanding of bacterial load. While it is well accepted that wound cultures obtained outside of the operating room at any point in care and those obtained at the first operation are not helpful, the evidence for the usefulness of post-washout cultures is poor and conflicting.[2] Thus, this is an Echelon V evidence recommendation (expert opinion), which is the strongest evidenced-based statement that can be made regarding the usefulness of intraoperative wound cultures.

Irrigation and Debridement

During the ATLS secondary survey, all wounds are uncovered and recorded, and the initial gross decontamination process begins. Gravel, dirt, sticks, and other large pieces of foreign material are pulled from the wounds. Varying techniques of wound irrigation may be employed from bulb syringe to special irrigation bottles to pulsed lavage (InterPulse, Stryker, Mahwah, NJ—19 psi). Irrigation and debridement is the epicenter of successful wound care in traumatic wounds because bacterial load and the failure to remove devitalized tissue are the 2 most important factors that induce deep space infection.[21] Svoboda and colleagues, in an animal model, demonstrated that pulsed lavage with 3 to 9 L of normal saline reduced bacterial load (*Pseudomonas*) by 52% to 70% versus 33% to 51% with the same volume of normal saline irrigated by bulb syringe.[22] Further, Owens and Wenke showed that the timing to the initial irrigation was also significantly related to bacterial load reduction.[23] In a goat model, if the saline pulsed lavage irrigation were started at 3 hours from time of inoculation versus 6 or 12 hours, the rate of bacterial reduction was 70% versus 52% versus 37%, respectively.[23] The specific irrigation fluid has been another source of debate over the years. In 1989, Rosenstein et al performed an experiment in dogs in which a cortical window was created in the femur and cultured methicillin-resistant *Staphylococcus aureus* (MRSA) was placed into the window for 20 minutes, and then the wound was irrigated with normal saline alone or with bacitracin and closed.[24] After 7 days, the animals were euthanized, and the dogs treated with bacitracin had significantly fewer (0% vs 50%) clinical infections, and when the femoral surgical site was

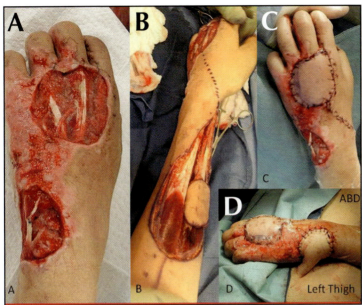

Figure 8-2. A patient after serial irrigation/debridement and wound VAC placement. The wound is now healthy for definitive coverage, but the exposed "white tissue" and the contracture risk make split-thickness skin graft (STSG) not ideal. As a result, the patient underwent a radial artery-based pedicled fasciocutaneous rotational flap to cover the dorsal full-thickness defect (B, C). Then, (D) a left groin flap was performed to cover the ulnar-sided wrist defect, which has exposed bone, joint capsule, and tendon. The left arm is left connected to the left groin area for 3 weeks. During this time, the left superficial circumflex iliac artery supplies the skin and the wound bed vascularizes the flap. The patient is then returned to the operating room, the pedicle is severed, and the edges are set neatly into the donor and harvest site. Rotational and in-set flaps such as these are the most robust, are technically simplest, and require no special equipment such as an operative microscope, as compared to the more unreliable and challenging free flaps. Rotational flaps have been the workhorse in and out of theater to cover traumatic combat wounds not amenable to STSG.

then re-exposed and cultured, cultures were positive about 2.5 times less frequently in the bacitracin-treated animals. The conclusion was that bacitracin irrigation provides an advantage over plain irrigation. More recently, Owens and colleagues in a goat model again confirmed that pulse lavage with bactericidal solutions (Castile soap > benzalkonium chloride > bacitracin) removed more of the *Pseudomonas* bacterial load acutely from an extremity wound than saline alone, but the interesting finding in this study was that when the investigators re-evaluated the wound 48 hours later, the rebound growth of *Pseudomonas* was greatest in the wounds that were treated with bactericidal solutions and pulsed lavage.[25] This suggests that there is a balance between the positive effects of bactericidal solutions and vigorous lavage and the harmful effect these agents have on local host tissue.

The basic science literature evaluating this balance is confusing and conflicting, and worsening the situation is the lack of Echelon I evidence clinical trials evaluating the best practice for irrigating contaminated wounds. In the absence of a strong evidenced-based recommendation on the best method for irrigating traumatic wounds, space, time, and logistical confinements in forward deployed military treatment facilities typically direct the method of irrigation used in theater. The most commonly used method of irrigation at Echelon IV and above has been pulsed lavage with saline or bacitracin-saline. That being said, the preference of irrigation mode, pulsed lavage versus bulb syringe, and irrigant (ie, saline with or without bacitracin) has been uniformly left to surgeon preference. Regardless, no method of irrigation can overcome the failure to clear the wound of gross debris and most importantly devitalized

tissue. A safe approach based upon the literature is employment of pulsatile lavage (on lowest power setting available) for grossly contaminated wounds and bulb syringe for mildly contaminated or clean wounds—both using normal saline without additives.

THOROUGH DEBRIDEMENT: THE MOST IMPORTANT ASPECT OF COMBAT WOUND CARE

As military surgeons have repeatedly demonstrated during the past 4 centuries, thorough debridement of foreign bodies and devitalized tissue is the single most important immediate surgical task in the treatment of combat-related open wounds.[26,27] Thus, after or in the process of surgical intervention for life-threatening conditions (ie, intra-cranial, pulmonary, solid visceral organ hemorrhage), deployed orthopedic and general surgeons need to start debriding wounds.[3] In addition to cleaning open wounds, long-bone fractures need to be stabilized. There are essentially 2 options for skeletal stabilization in theater—external fixation (Hoffmann II, Stryker) and splints. Certain hand and foot fractures may receive K-wire fixation as well. Following irrigation, debridement, and provisional skeletal stabilization, extremity wounds have been packed with saline-moistened cotton gauze, and bulky splints have been applied as needed. In particularly dirty wounds, adjuvant agents like Dakins solution (dilute bleach), an antiseptic that dates back to World War I, have been used instead of saline to provide bactericidal activity. It should be used in the lowest concentration (ie, 0.025%) to offset cytotoxic effects.[28]

Negative Pressure Wound Therapy: An Important Recent Innovation in Combat Wound Care

Until 2007, wet-to-dry dressing was the only authorized means for dressing open wounds in theater in preparation for evacuation to LRMC. This mandate stems from early attempts to evacuate patients with field-expedient vacuum dressings, which, when the vacuum failed en route, turned from infection-reducing to infection-producing dressings with catastrophic consequence in a few notable cases. In 2007, Fang and his fellow investigators recognized that a dual standard of care existed between local nationals and enemy combatants who were eligible for immediate application of negative pressure wound therapy care in theater, which was continued throughout their course of care versus injured American and NATO soldiers who were relegated to receive antiquated cotton gauze dressings.[29] Cotton gauze dressings require significantly more resources to maintain, are more painful to the patient, and require frequent exposure of large wounds to the external environment, which increases chances of nosocomial inoculation. Thus, these investigators sought to prospectively prove the safety of a specific type of negative pressure wound therapy device in air evacuation operations. Based on their research, the Freedom VAC (Kinetic Concepts Inc, San Antonio, TX) has been cleared for use on USAF air evacuation flights. Finally, American casualties in theater are able to receive immediate negative pressure wound therapy, which had long since been the standard of care for enemy combatants with open wounds who did not have to migrate through the echelons of care.

Fang and colleagues recently reported the results of their prospective observational study of combat casualties presenting to LRMC with open wounds that were treated with negative pressure wound therapy through their stay at LRMC and the air evacuation flight to the United States. They enrolled 30 patients with 41 treated wounds—20% were fasciotomy wounds and the remaining were traumatic. The average age of the patients was 26.8 years, reflecting the typical youth of combat casualties and, for that matter, civilian Level I trauma center patients. The goal of the study was to provide pilot information to substantiate the safety of negative pressure wound therapy during air evacuation flights from LRMC to the United States. Negative pressure wound therapy was successfully provided to all 30 patients—77% (23) had a completely uneventful flight, and 20% (6) required some attention (5/6 needed to have the 300-mL collection canister replaced and the other had to have a tubing piece fixed that was damaged in the

loading process). The sole significant event was the need to "milk" a clot through the tubing to restore normal suction to the wound dressing. Overall, the results of this study mirror the anecdotal successes of negative pressure wound therapy used for shorter range air evacuation missions in theater (ie, helicopter transfer between military treatment facilities/combat support hospitals). That is, uniformly, negative pressure wound therapy has been reported to be safe and effective and a substantial leap forward in the treatment of combat casualties with significant open soft tissue injuries.[29]

Definitive Management

Two Phases: Preparation and Definitive Management

Upon reaching an Echelon V medical center in the continental United States, care transitions from temporizing to definitive management. This transition occurs in 2 phases. The first is the preparation phase, and the second is definitive management. Serial irrigation and debridement remains the hallmark of complex soft tissue management in the preparation phase. Patients arriving in the continental United States undergo their first washout procedure within their first 1 to 2 days in the continental United States. The total number of washouts is dictated by the appearance of the wound, an assessment that unfortunately remains surgeon specific. While the clinical efficacy of negative pressure wound therapy is unquestioned, the process behind how it works is largely not understood. The leading concepts are that the vacuum removes exudate from the wound, which may reduce bacterial load on the wound surface. Likewise, it is supposed to accelerate the formation of granulation and wound surface area reduction. However, these 2 claims have not reliably borne out.[30,31] The vacuum effect increases local blood flow to the area, which is probably an important factor in the efficacy of the VAC, given the favorable impact on diabetic and dysvascular wounds.[31] Because the exact science of VAC therapy is poorly understood, finding the most effective modes and modifications to this class of therapy is still ongoing. Forsberg and colleagues have sought to find guidance for standardizing this decision process by measuring the composition of exudate collected from VAC dressings and patient serum.[32,33] Certain cytokine levels, like procalcitonin and metalloproteinases, seem to have some predictive value on whether a closed wound will heal uneventfully, but this evidence is early and limited. Their early findings are encouraging, but too early for practical use. As mentioned above, in addition to the gross appearance, many surgeons rely on post-wash culture results from the last washout to help dictate timing of definitive management. In the end, the current standard of care for timing of definitive surgical management is an assessment of wound health by the treating surgical team.

During the preparation phase, negative pressure wound therapy has played a vital role. Negative pressure wound therapy has been the single most important medical innovation to mature over the course of medical operations in support of OIF/OEF. It has revolutionized wound care. The KCI Wound VAC (Kinetic Concepts) has been the most frequently used negative pressure wound therapy device in this conflict. Military surgeons have stretched and then expanded the limits of negative pressure wound therapy. The potential exists for continued development of this technology for wound applications.

TIMING OF SKELETAL STABILIZATION

When unstable skeletal fractures exist in proximity to open wounds or fasciotomy sites, a decision must be made at some point regarding final definitive skeletal stabilization. This is a question that is not well answered in the civilian sector and has even less evidential support in combat casualty care. Trauma combat care doctrine dictates that these decisions and treatment be made at Echelons IV and V levels of care. Early experience in OIF/OEF with acute internal fixation at Echelons II and III resulted in unacceptable rates of infection and complications. This practice has since been discouraged. Currently, unstable long-bone fractures are provisionally stabilized with external fixation or splints. Stabilization of a fractured extremity reduces pain, improves venous return, and reduces the incidence of compartment syndrome. Since the average evacuation time from Echelon I to IV/V is 7 or more days, the timing of internal fixation must be delayed at least this long. With this delay, open wounds become colonized with potential pathogens, with an increasing frequency being MDROs.[7,18] Delays of more than 7 days in definitive fixation and coverage increase wound complication rate by 4 and delay long-bone healing time by 50%.[7,18] Mody and colleagues reported that of 58 soldiers definitively treated with intramedullary nailing for either tibia or femur fracture, 40% developed an infection.[34] Blasting mechanisms, such as following IED attack, were the primary mechanism of injury in 91% of infected cases, demonstrating that the energy imparted broadly to blast-injured tissue leads to more diffuse tissue destruction than the localized pattern following projectile or fragment wounds. This study did note that while infection was common, so were good outcomes regarding union and lack of need for subsequent surgery. Infectious complications

of combat-casualty care at the time of definitive stabilization may be unavoidable, but rapid recognition and treatment (both medical and/or surgical) has led to good outcomes.

Surgical Technique

The surgical techniques related to wound care are some of the most basic in surgery. Wound care surgery focuses on removing gross contamination and devitalized tissue, stabilizing the area of the wound, and preparing for the next stage of care. Debridement is an art and not a science. It is tedious and requires strict attention to detail. Ideally, a systematic approach is followed. One should start by debriding the skin margins to a healthy base. If and when the wound needs to be extended to access contamination that is recessed under skin flaps, this extension should be linear and longitudinal. From here, the surgeon should progress from superficial to deep, excising areas of dead and necrotic subcutaneous tissue and muscle as well as removing readily accessible foreign bodies and fully detached bone fragments. By progressing from superficial to deep, the gravity-dependant base of the wound is addressed last. The natural tendency in debridement is to underdebride. Unhealthy nonviable tissue needs to be removed. Healthy tissue should bleed, have normal color and consistency, and should contract when touched with the Bovie electrocautery. Rejection of the false belief that nonviable tissue will somehow revitalize is what separates the novice from experienced war surgeon. This separation results in fewer trips to the operating room because each trip is more effective. As stated, debridement is an art and, with increased experience, the ability to recognize what needs to occur at each operation becomes clearer.

SMALL FRAGMENTS DO NOT REQUIRE REMOVAL

There is no role for the deliberate search for penetrating small metal fragments in the deep soft tissues.[35,36] Larger fragments, which arbitrarily are defined as greater than 1 to 2 cm in largest dimension, may be retrieved. The evidence base for addressing retained metallic fragments in war wounds is limited. Baldan and colleagues reviewed the surgical database of the International Committee of the Red Cross, which contained 36,000 patients with war wounds, and concluded that the risk of bullet or metallic foreign body removal from war wounds far outweighs the benefits. Their conclusion statement sums it up best: "the metallic missile is dangerous when it is moving, not when it has come to a stop in the body."[36]

Anecdotally, metallic fragments are not common sources of delayed deep space infections, and avoiding the collateral trauma of resecting these fragments, which can often be difficult to find, outweighs the benefit of deliberately removing them. A specific caveat to this rule of thumb is, when metallic fragments are larger (a dimension defined variably by the radiologist) or near vital structures (like the orbit), the removal of these fragments may be indicated to facilitate the use of magnetic resonance imaging (MRI). A second potential indication for removal of retained metallic fragments in war wounds is to reduce lead or copper burden; however, this is such a rare event that blood levels of these ions must be confirmed to be elevated and clinical manifestation of toxicity should be present. In addition, fragments within a synovial or intrathecal space should be removed to avoid iron toxicity. Following debridement, the wound should be irrigated thoroughly. While the technique (pulsed lavage versus bulb syringe) or the solution may be debated, all agree that copious (more than 1 to 3 L) irrigation is an effective means for further reducing bacterial load in the wound.

NEGATIVE PRESSURE WOUND THERAPY

Once the wound is thoroughly irrigated and debrided, it needs to be covered. At some point in time, the wound will be healthy enough to support delayed primary closure, skin grafting, or a plastic surgical reconstructive procedure, but until this time, application of a negative pressure wound therapy dressing is the preferred mode of dressing. The benefits of negative pressure wound therapy are multiple (Table 8-2). The currently available device is the Wound VAC. This system is composed of a granular (open-cell polyurethane) foam, specialized impermeable adhesive dressing and tubing, a collection canister, and a regulated, portable vacuum source (Figure 8-3). The sponge is cut to the size of the wound. The common VAC sponge is too thick, which leads to clotting within the sponge and dead spots in the vacuum reaching the wound. A 10-blade can be used to split the thickness of the sponge in half. Next, place the sponge on the wound bed. The blood/fluid on the wound surface will create an outline on the sponge, which can be used as an outline for cutting the sponge to the margins of the wound. Next, ready the VAC machine. Place a new collection canister, and sterilely pass the tubing onto the operative field. Attach the tubing to the "lily pad" flange, which is the component of the tubing system that connects to the dressing. Completing this preparation process will allow you to immediately apply vacuum to the dressing once you have sealed it to the wound. Next, thoroughly dry the normal skin surface at the margins of the wound. Agents with a sticky

Table 8-2
Benefits of Negative Pressure Wound Therapy

1.	Reduced nursing care (dressing changes occur once every 2 to 3 days versus 3 times daily)
2.	Reduced exposure to the external environment
3.	Patient comfort
4.	Accelerated wound healing
5.	Reduced infection rate
6.	Reduced need for flap coverage

quality (benzoin or DuraPrep [3M, St. Paul, MN]) can be placed on this skin to further enhance adhesion of the cover sheets to the skin. Now, place the sponge into the wound. Use extra pieces to cover any remaining exposed portions of the wound, but do not extend the sponge onto normal skin. Doing so will lead to maceration of this skin. Immediately start placing the clear adhesive sheets over the dressing and onto the prepared skin margins. This is the key step to Wound VAC application, as failure to obtain a good seal at this step will lead to leaks and VAC failures during treatment. The sheets provided are too big; it is easiest to pre-cut the sheets into quarters prior to applying them to the wound. Once you have completely covered the sponge, make a small hole in the central portion of the dressing, and apply the "lily pad" directly over this hole. Turn on the vacuum source to 125 mm Hg continuous suction. Ensure that you have a good seal and no leak alarms.

Silver ion dressings, such as GranuFoam Silver Dressing (Kinetic Concepts), can be used to enhance bacterial load clearance under VAC dressings. Silver ions have bactericidal activity against most pathogens in open wounds, to include MRSA and vancomycin-resistant *Enterococcus*.[37,38] Care should be directed at preventing the silver dressing material from touching normal skin surface margins, as they will stain normal skin black. Intermittent instillation of irrigation fluid can also augment negative pressure wound therapy. Gabriel and colleagues have shown that a VAC dressing hooked to intermittent irrigation can halve wound healing times and wound complication rates.[39]

CONNECTING VACUUM-ASSISTED CLOSURE SPONGES IN SERIES

Soldiers injured by IED blasts often have multiple open wounds along an extremity. In this situation, a single VAC machine can be used as the vacuum source for multiple dressing sites. This is performed by follow-

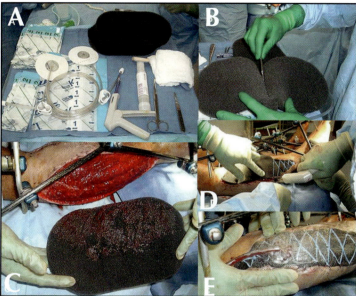

Figure 8-3. This group of images shows the pieces and steps involved in application of a Wound VAC to a lateral leg fasciotomy wound. (A) All of the pieces needed on the sterile field. Note that the occlusive "1 to 2" sheets have been cut in half to facilitate their placement. The circular pad attached to tubing is the "lily pad." The white connector end of the "lily pad" should be passed off the operative table to the nurse, who should connect it to the collection canister and the actual VAC machine. (B) The sponge being split in half to reduce the incidence of clotting in the sponge. (C) The process of placing the sponge against the wound to get an outline to cut the sponge to size. (D) Application of "Roman Sandals," which is simply large vessel loops attached to the skin margins by skin staples and then pulled to the contralateral side in a serial fashion to attempt to pull the skin margins together and reduce the area of the wound. (E) The finished product with a good seal.

ing the steps above for each wound site. Then, sponge "bridges" are created to connect each dressing site (Figure 8-4). A sponge bridge is created by first covering the skin with the adhesive sheet. Then, cut a piece of sponge about 1-inch thick to span from one dressing site to the next. Cut a hole into each dressing site and use a skin stapler to attach the sponge bridge to each dressing sponge. Next, place another adhesive sheet over this. Turn the vacuum back on, and confirm you have a good seal at each dressing site. Alternatively, a separate "lily pad" can be placed at each dressing site, and "Y"-connectors can be used to connect the tubing end of these "lily pads" to the main tubing leading back to the vacuum source.

The ideal timing for negative pressure wound therapy dressing changes has not been determined. Within the context of combat military medical care, the timing of dressing changes for most wounds is not a treatment decision point, as most wounds requiring a VAC dressing require serial debridements every 1 to 3 days. VAC changes occur as a part of the irrigation/debridement procedure, with the patient under anesthesia. The VAC sponge should not be left on for longer than 72 hours, as the open cell design of the sponge leaves dangling ends that can be entrapped by granulation tissue and left in the wound after serial dressing changes. Likewise, the sponge progressively clots over the course of therapy, which degrades the application of vacuum over this portion of the sponge. Negative pressure wound therapy should not be placed directly over injured or grafted vascular structures, as the VAC device has no means to automatically measure exudate flow rate, so an acute leak in the vessel can lead to catastrophic and even fatal hemorrhage.

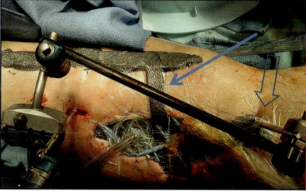

Figure 8-4. This figure shows a Wound VAC placed successfully around an external fixator. When possible, avoid pin sites, like the ones on the left side of the image. When the wound is too close to a pin site, the pin site may need to be included as well to ensure a good seal (open arrow). The solid arrow points to a "bridge" that connects 2 VAC dressings in series

Outcomes and Complications

Infection rates in combat-related orthopedic injury can be as high as more than 40%, despite careful attention to the practices outlined above.[7,34] These are large wounds caused by high energy occurring in dirty places separated by thousands of miles and levels of care from definitive surgical intervention, which often calls for the placement of internal fixation in proximity to these wounds. The current conflicts have been the most survivable to date. With this important milestone comes the acceptance that wound care in combat-injured soldiers is not a point in time activity, but a process that requires acute, intermediate, and long-term follow-up and intervention. Appropriately timed fasciotomies reduce amputation rate by half and the mortality rate by 4. It is an important tool in the tool-box of the deployed surgeon.[8] Hopefully, advances in technology may better guide and standardize the diagnosis and management of ACS, so that patients who need fasciotomy get it and those who do not need it do not get it.

ACUTE COMPARTMENT SYNDROME— LESSONS NOT YET LEARNED

The study by Ritenour and colleagues reveals that the incidence of fasciotomy in combat-injured soldiers is extraordinarily high.[8] Among patients undergoing fasciotomy in theater, 17% required revision fasci-otomy upon arrival to LRMC. In 41% of cases, this included release of a compartment that had been previously missed at the initial fasciotomy procedure. The accuracy of hastily trained surgeons, unfamiliar with the diagnosis of ACS and the techniques of fas-ciotomy, yields a rather high incidence of technically unsuccessful surgery. The author's emphasized con-clusion from this article is that missed or delayed fasciotomy for ACS doubles the rate of amputation and nearly quadruples the rate of mortality, implying more fasciotomies are needed in theater and more vigilant observation for the development of delayed ACS on the physicians higher up in the echelon chain of evacuation. In May 2007, in response to the preliminary results of this study, the Army Surgeon General issued an ALARACT explicitly stating, based on the results of the Ritenour study, "Level II and III surgeons should practice liberal use of complete fas-ciotomy." However, an important secondary observa-tion is that 35% of the fasciotomies (172 procedures) performed in theater were performed for the primary indication of prophylaxis. Thus, this article points out 2 very important lessons learned from the conflicts in Iraq and Afghanistan. First, ACS is a devastating condition that needs to be diagnosed and treated in a timely fashion. Second, the incidence of prophylactic fasciotomy is very high among soldiers treated in these conflicts. While we have seen great improve-ments in wound care technology, we still have a long way to go regarding optimal diagnosis and manage-ment of ACS.

References

1. Hospenthal DR, Murray CK, Andersen RC, et al. Guidelines for the prevention of infection after combat-related injuries. *J Trauma.* 2008;64(3 Suppl):S211-S220.

2. Owens BD, Kragh JF Jr, Macaitis J, Svoboda SJ, Wenke JC. Characterization of extremity wounds in Operation Iraqi Freedom and Operation Enduring Freedom. *J Orthop Trauma.* 2007;21(4):254-257.

3. Owens BD, Kragh JF Jr, Wenke JC, Macaitis J, Wade CE, Holcomb JB. Combat wounds in operation Iraqi Freedom and operation Enduring Freedom. *J Trauma.* 2008;64(2):295-299.

4. Murray CK, Hsu JR, Solomkin JS, et al. Prevention and manage-ment of infections associated with combat-related extremity injuries. *J Trauma.* 2008;64:S239-S251.

5. Esterhai JL Jr, Queenan J. Management of soft tissue wounds associated with type III open fractures. *Orthop Clin North Am.* 1991;22(3):427-432.

6. Utvåg SE, Grundnes O, Rindal DB, Reikerås O. Influence of extensive muscle injury on fracture healing in rat tibia. *J Orthop Trauma.* 2003;17(6):430-435.

7. Cierny G 3rd, Byrd HS, Jones RE. Primary versus delayed soft tissue coverage for severe open tibial fractures. A comparison of results. *Clin Orthop Relat Res.* 1983;178:54-63.

8. Ritenour AE, Dorlac WC, Fang R, et al. Complications after fas-ciotomy revision and delayed compartment release in combat patients. *J Trauma.* 2008;64(2 Suppl):S153-S161.

9. McQueen MM, Gaston P, Court-Brown CM. Acute compart-ment syndrome. Who is at risk? *J Bone Joint Surg Br.* 2000;82(2):200-203.

10. Shuler MS, Reisman WM, Whitesides TE Jr, et al. Near-infrared spectroscopy in lower extremity trauma. *J Bone Joint Surg Am.* 2009;91(6):1360-1368.

11. Fitzgerald AM, Gaston P, Wilson Y, Quaba A, McQueen MM. Long-term sequelae of fasciotomy wounds. *Br J Plast Surg.* 2000;53(8):690-693.

12. Holcomb JB, McMullin NR, Pearse L, et al. Causes of death in U.S. Special Operations Forces in the global war on terrorism: 2001-2004. *Ann Surg.* 2007;245(6):986-991.

13. Kelly JF, Ritenour AE, McLaughlin DF, et al. Injury severity and causes of death from Operation Iraqi Freedom and Operation Enduring Freedom: 2003-2004 versus 2006. *J Trauma.* 2008;64(2 Suppl):S21-S26; discussion S26-S27.

14. Rhee P, Brown C, Martin M, et al. QuikClot use in trauma for hemorrhage control: case series of 103 documented uses. *J Trauma.* 2008;64(4):1093-1099.

15. Wedmore I, McManus JG, Pusateri AE, Holcomb JB. A special report on the chitosan-based hemostatic dressing: experience in current combat operations. *J Trauma.* 2006;60(3):655-658.

16. Kheirabadi BS, Scherer MR, Estep JS, Dubick MA, Holcomb JB. Determination of efficacy of new hemostatic dressings in a model of extremity arterial hemorrhage in swine. *J Trauma.* 2009;67(3):450-459; discussion 459-460.

17. Bagg MR, Covey DC, Powell ET. Levels of medical care in the Global War on Terrorism. *J Am Acad Orthop Surg.* 2006;14:S7-S9.

18. Weintrob AC, Roediger MP, Barber M, et al. Natural history of colonization with gram-negative multidrug-resistant organisms among hospitalized patients. *Infect Control Hosp Epidemiol.* 2010;31(4):330-337.

19. Kaspar RL, Griffith ME, Mann PB, et al. Association of bacterial colonization at the time of presentation to a combat support hospital in a combat zone with subsequent 30-day colonization or infection. *Mil Med.* 2009;174(9):899-903.

20. Johnson EN, Marconi VC, Murray CK. Hospital-acquired device-associated infections at a deployed military hospital in Iraq. *J Trauma.* 2009;66(4 Suppl):S157-S163.

21. Evans RP, Nelson CL, Harrison BH. The effect of wound environ-ment on the incidence of acute osteomyelitis. *Clin Orthop Relat Res.* 1993;286:289-297.

22. Svoboda SJ, Owens BD, Gooden HA, Melvin ML, Baer DG, Wenke JC. Irrigation with potable water versus normal saline in a contaminated musculoskeletal wound model. *J Trauma.* 2008;64(5):1357-1359.

23. Owens BD, Wenke JC. Early wound irrigation improves the ability to remove bacteria. *J Bone Joint Surg Am.* 2007;89(8):1723-1726.

24. Rosenstein BD, Wilson FC, Funderburk CH. The use of bacitracin irrigation to prevent infection in postoperative skeletal wounds. An experimental study. *J Bone Joint Surg Am.* 1989;71(3):427-430.

25. Owens BD, White DW, Wenke JC. Comparison of irrigation solutions and devices in a contaminated musculoskeletal wound survival model. *J Bone Joint Surg Am.* 2009;91(1):92-98.

26. Noe A. Extremity injury in war: a brief history. *J Am Acad Orthop Surg.* 2006;14(10 Spec No.):S1-S6.

27. Broughton G 2nd, Janis JE, Attinger CE. A brief history of wound care. *Plast Reconstr Surg.* 2006;117(7 Suppl):6S-11S.

28. Heggers JP, Sazy JA, Stenberg BD, et al. Bactericidal and wound-healing properties of sodium hypochlorite solutions: the 1991 Lindberg Award. *J Burn Care Rehabil.* 1991;12(5):420-424.

29. Pollak AN, Powell ET, Fang R, Cooper EO, Ficke JR, Flaherty SF. Use of negative pressure wound therapy during aeromedical evacuation of patients with combat-related blast injuries. *J Surg Orthop Adv.* 2010;19(1):44-48.

30. Mouës CM, Vos MC, van den Bemd GJ, Stijnen T, Hovius SE. Bacterial load in relation to vacuum-assisted closure wound therapy: a prospective randomized trial. *Wound Repair Regen.* 2004;12(1):11-17.

31. Braakenburg A, Obdeijn MC, Feitz R, van Rooij IA, van Griethuysen AJ, Klinkenbijl JH. The clinical efficacy and cost effectiveness of the vacuum-assisted closure technique in the management of acute and chronic wounds: a randomized controlled trial. *Plast Reconstr Surg.* 2006;118(2):390-397.

32. Forsberg JA, Elster EA, Andersen RC, et al. Correlation of procalcitonin and cytokine expression with dehiscence of wartime extremity wounds. *J Bone Joint Surg Am.* 2008;90(3):580-588.

33. Utz ER, Elster EA, Tadaki DK, et al. Metalloproteinase expression is associated with traumatic wound failure. *J Surg Res.* 2010;159(2):633-639.

34. Mody RM, Zapor M, Hartzell JD, et al. Infectious complications of damage control orthopedics in war trauma. *J Trauma.* 2009;67(4):758-761.

35. Bowyer GW. Management of small fragment wounds: experience from the Afghan border. *J Trauma.* 1996;40(3 Suppl):S170-S172.

36. Baldan M, Giannou CP, Sasin V, Morino GF. The ICRC metallic foreign bodies after war injuries: should we remove them? Experience. http://www.bioline.org.br/request?js04008. Accessed February 15, 2010.

37. Cutting K, White R, Hoekstra H. Topical silver-impregnated dressings and the importance of the dressing technology. *Int Wound J.* 2009;6(5):396-402.

38. Fong J, Wood F. Nanocrystalline silver dressings in wound management: a review. *Int J Nanomedicine.* 2006;1(4):441-449.

39. Gabriel A, Shores J, Heinrich C, et al. Negative pressure wound therapy with instillation: a pilot study describing a new method for treating infected wounds. *Int Wound J.* 2008;5(3):399-413.

Chapter 9

BASIC SCIENCE OF WAR WOUNDS

LCDR Jonathan Agner Forsberg, MD; Trevor S. Brown, PhD; and
MAJ Benjamin K. Potter, MD

Throughout history, innovations in the care and treatment of wounded patients have been catalyzed by war. As discussed in Chapter 1, stepwise advances in triage and medical evacuation were documented during each major armed conflict from the American Revolution to the current conflicts in Iraq and Afghanistan.[1] These advances were driven, in part, by the cumulative understanding of the epidemiology and pathophysiology of wounding that progressed during the same intervals. In effect, more patients now survive their increasingly devastating wounds than ever before, and, as a result, patients and treating physicians alike now face new challenges over the long term. Thus, this cumulative knowledge described above is not a panacea, and research intended to benefit the wounded must continue.

Modern Clinical Challenges

Modern war wounds consist of high-energy penetrating injuries that predominately involve the extremities.[2-13] The result is distinctive patterns of injury composed of severely traumatized limbs, open fractures, disproportionately large zones of injury, and frequent bone and volumetric soft tissue loss, often in association with both gross foreign body and bacterial contamination. These devastated limbs pose unique treatment challenges at every turn.

Three of the most important problems affecting modern war injuries include wound healing, infec-

tion, and heterotopic ossification.[14-18] Though these entities are not unique to the current conflicts, they remain relatively problematic and are the foci of numerous current studies.

The Translational Approach

Clinical research requires clinician-scientists who understand both the treatment challenges as well as the basic science that drives their field of interest. The authors and other clinician-scientists interested in the treatment of high-energy penetrating injuries have adopted a translational approach to investigate important clinical problems, such as those listed above. Similar to efforts described in other disciplines,[19-23] translational research in combat trauma begins with the wounded patient. Access to patients is critical. First, clinical observations about the nature, complexity, and prevalence of particular injury patterns as well as the efficacy of various treatment modalities are assessed. Often, these assessments are retrospective, but offer valuable information regarding the epidemiology, risk factors, and basic outcomes of treatment. The results of these preliminary studies are then useful for hypothesis development and typically spawn prospective observational or preclinical (in vitro and animal) studies. The results of the preclinical work are then used in the design of clinical studies, supporting the translational paradigm of "bedside to bench and back again."

Owens BD, Belmont PJ Jr, eds. *Combat Orthopedic Surgery:
Lessons Learned in Iraq and Afghanistan (pp 77-84)*
© 2011 SLACK Incorporated

Brief Overview of Wound Healing

It is well known that wound healing follows a highly complex, interdependent sequence of events. In the simplest terms, the inflammatory phase, composed of hemostasis and inflammation, is followed by the reparative phase, made up of cell proliferation and wound maturation.[24] Platelets perform a critical initial role, not only within the coagulation pathway, but also as potent paracrine and endocrine mediators of both growth factors[25-27] and chemotaxis, luring inflammatory cells to the point of injury.[28] The fibrin clot provides an ideal matrix for cell migration, and the wound is quickly infiltrated by neutrophils and macrophages that begin removing bacteria, necrotic tissue, and foreign material. Macrophages are thought to hold the key to the progression from the inflammatory to the reparative phase of wound healing. This transition is mediated mainly by macrophage-released Interleukin (IL)-1,[29] Interferon (IFN)-γ, transforming growth factor (TGF)-β, fibroblast (FGF),[27] and other growth factors.[26] In short, these cytokines, chemokines, and growth factors are critical to the cellular and biochemical events necessary for acute wound healing (Table 9-1).[30]

Biomarkers: Cytokines and Chemokines

Because the molecular environment of the wound ultimately determines its fate,[28] it is possible to use the cytokine and chemokine profile to provide insight into the molecular pathogenesis of wound healing.[14,31,32] Biomarkers have long been used to diagnose infection and malnutrition or to predict wound healing potential in elderly or chronically debilitated patients.[33-45] Research in this area has focused traditionally on difficult-to-treat chronic wounds, predominantly in diabetics and the elderly or dysvascular. In contrast, war-time trauma victims clearly represent a different

Table 9-1

Cytokines and Chemokines: Functional Relationships and References

Protein	Description	References
Cytokines	**Unique signaling molecules produced by various cells. Can have an autocrine or paracrine effect on local cells or an endocrine effect as pyrogens.**	
IL-1	Exists in two forms: IL-1α and IL-1β. Produced by activated macrophages and monocytes in response to bacterial endotoxin or antigens. Suppressed by IL-13. Activates T-lymphocytes and upregulates production of GM-CSF. Also referred to as lymphocyte activating factor. Production of IL-1 is inhibited by IL-10.	55,57,71,72
IL-2	Produced by activated T-lymphocytes, IL-2 is a central regulator of the inflammatory response. Further stimulates T-lymphocytes (autocrine) and B-lymphocytes (paracrine) (requires IL-4). Stimulates the production of GM-CSF and IFN-γ. Also upregulates the secretion of IL-1 and TNF-α by activated macrophages. Production of IL-2 is inhibited by IL-10.	57,73,74
IL-3	Produced by activated T-lymphocytes, keratinocytes, mast cells, endothelial cells, and monocytes. Stimulates the differentiation of pluripotent hematopoietic stem cells down a myeloid lineage. Preactivates neutrophils (prerequisite for IL-8-induced chemotaxis). Stimulates hematopoesis and mast cell differentiation.	75,76
IL-4	Produced by Th2 (T-helper type-2) cells. Induces the proliferation and differentiation of B-lymphocytes. Inhibits the synthesis of IL-6 by human macrophages and blunts the expression of IL-1 and TNF-α to bacterial endotoxins or IFN-γ.	57,77-79
IL-5	Produced by Th2 cells. Responsible for differentiation of eosinophils and hematopoietic progenitor cells. Receptors for IL-5 are expressed in all hematopoietic and lymphoid cells.	78-80
IL-6	Produced by many cell types. This ubiquitous expression results in rapid increases in its concentration in response to trauma, burns, and bacterial endotoxin. Though it is commonly associated with its potent pro-inflammatory role, it does possess anti-inflammatory properties through feedback inhibition of TNF-α and IL-1 and activation of IL-1ra (receptor antagonist) and IL-10. Production of IL-6 is inhibited by IL-10.	43,57,60,81,82
IL-7	Stimulates the differentiation of pluripotent hematopoietic stem cells along a lymphoid lineage.	83

(continued)

Table 9-1 (continued)

Cytokines and Chemokines: Functional Relationships and References

Protein	Description	References
IL-10	Produced by activated Th2 cells, partially in response to IL-6. Considered anti-inflammatory, inhibits the synthesis of IFN-γ, IL-1, IL-2, IL-6, IL-12, and TNF-α and β. Co-stimulates mast cell differentiation, with IL-4.	57,84,85
IL-12	Produced by dendritic cells, macrophages, and B-lymphocytes. Stimulates the differentiation of Th1 (T-helper type-1) cells. Stimulates the production of IL-2, TNF-α, and IFN-γ (requires co-stimulation with TNF-α). Production of IL-12 is inhibited by IL-10.	86-88
IL-13	Produced by activated T-lymphocytes. Considered anti-inflammatory and regulates inflammation by inhibiting macrophage activity and in turn, decreasing production of pro-inflammatory cytokines including IL-1, IL-6, IL-12, and TNF-α. MIP-1α and certain MMPs, but also reduces IL-8 and IL-10 (anti-inflammatory chemokine and cytokine) production.	89,90
IL-15	Produced by astrocytes and glial cells in response to IL-1, IFN-γ, and TNF-α.	91,92
IFN-γ	Produced by Th1 cells, in response to IL-2. Considered pro-inflammatory, IFN-γ activates macrophages to produce TNF-α and T-cells to produce GM-CSF and the RANTES protein. Inhibits the proliferation of smooth muscle cells, endothelial cells, and myofibroblast activity through suppression of TGF-β1. Production is inhibited by IL-10.	55-57,93
Chemokines	**Chemotactic cytokines. A subset of cytokines, these molecules induce chemotaxis to sites of injury or inflammation, or play a role in the regulation thereof.**	
IL-8	Produced by monocytes, fibroblasts, and endothelial cells (but not tissue macrophages). Specifically activates neutrophils (requiring preactivation by IL-3). Considered anti-inflammatory, expression is inhibited by IL-1 and TNF-α. Necessary for angiogenesis.	57,94,95
IP-10 (interferon inducible protein-10)	Produced by lymphocytes, monocytes, and endothelial cells in response to IFN-γ in combination with TNF-α, or with bacterial endotoxin. Chemotactic for T-lymphocytes. Regulates angiogenesis. Production is inhibited by IL-4 and IL-10.	57,96,97
MCP-1 monocyte hemoattractant protein-1 (CCL-2)	Produced by monocytes, vascular endothelial cells, smooth muscle cells, and osteoblasts in respose to bacterial endotoxin, TNF-α, PDGF, IL-1 (not IL-2, TNF, or IFN-γ). Chemotactic for monocytes, basophils (not neutrophils). Regulates the expression of IL-1 and IL-6.	57,98-101
GM-CSF (granulocyte-macrophage colony-stimulating factor)	Produced by activated T-lymphocytes and macrophages in response to antigens or mitogens. Also produced by endothelial cells and fibroblasts in response to TNF-α, IL-1, IL-2, and IFN-γ. Strongly chemotactic for neutrophils, and enhances their bactericidal activity. As the name implies, stimulates the growth of granulocytes and macrophages by triggering irreversible differentiation of their progenitor cells. Synergizes with erythropoietin to stimulate the proliferation of erythrocytes and megakaryocyte progenitors.	57,102,103
MIP-1α (CCL3)	Produced by dendritic cells, and activated macrophages in response to bacterial endotoxin. Activates neutrophils to produce superoxide. Upregulates the production of other pro-inflammatory cytokines, IL-1, IL-6, and TNF-α. Inhibited by prostaglandin E2.	57,104
RANTES (CCL5)	"Regulated upon activation, normal T-cell expressed, and [presumably] secreted." Produced by T-lymphocytes (but not activated T-lymphocytes). Chemotactic for leukocytes toward sites of inflammation. Upregulated by TNF-α and IL-1, but not by IFN-γ or IL-6. Strongly suppressed by nitric oxide.	56,57
TNF-α	Produced by activated macrophages (like IL-1). Signifies a systemic inflammatory state. Upregulates production of GM-CSF in endothelial cells and fibroblasts, and the RANTES protein by T-lymphocytes. Production of TNF-α is inhibited by IL-10.	56,57

demographic, as the vast majority are young and previously healthy, if not for their acute, often severe, wounding. Wound healing, in this case, likely depends less on chronic co-morbidities and more on the degree of bacterial bioburden, adequacy of local wound perfusion, and the patient's acute nutritional and inflammatory status.

The use of serum (systemic) biomarkers is an attractive option, but it is limited by several factors. First, the wounding mechanism acutely raises the metabolic demand and primes the systemic inflammatory cascade.[46,47] Second, patients routinely undergo serial debridement procedures every 24 to 72 hours. These surgical procedures in and of themselves universally increase the concentrations of commonly referenced acute-phase reactants such as IL-6, C-reactive protein, and the erythrocyte sedimentation rate. Third, the presence of local wound and/or systemic infection further upregulates production of both acute-phase reactants and pro-inflammatory cytokines. Finally, it is the rare combat-injured patient who presents with a single wound or injured body system, precluding the use of systemic markers for local prognostication. For these reasons, nonspecific serum biomarkers such as acute-phase reactants are not commonly used in this patient population. In fact, none have accurately predicted outcome in a healthy population with acute traumatic wounds, and, as a result, means to directly measure the local wound environment have gained popularity. Nevertheless, it is probable that the systemic inflammatory response heavily influences the local wound response,[48-50] but a definitive link has yet to be made.

Wound effluent analysis of biomarkers is an attractive option for several reasons. First, wound effluent is less influenced by systemic stresses and more representative of the local wound environment than traditional systemic serum biomarkers.[51] Second, through ubiquitous mRNA expression, local wound tissues produce cytokines, chemokines, and other biomarkers and mediators of inflammation that remain extracirculatory and do not reach substantive concentrations in the serum.[14,51-54]

ENTER A COMMON CLINICAL PROBLEM IN HIGH-ENERGY WAR-TIME EXTREMITY WOUNDS

Currently, the timing of wound closure or flap coverage is a subjective clinical decision, depending predominantly on the gross appearance of the bone and soft tissues and less on routine laboratory evaluations or the patient's general condition. Yet, despite seemingly appropriate tension-free wound closure

following meticulous serial debridements and antibiotic therapy, a significant portion of wounds fail and dehisce—a devastating complication in the setting of limb salvage or when attempting to preserve residual limb length in the amputee. Conversely, some wounds with questionable appearance may possess the ability to heal, but undergo unnecessary debridements, adding treatment costs and exposing patients to additional anesthetic and surgical risks of morbidity.

Recognizing that the biomarker profiles may differ between acute and chronic wounds, one of the authors (JAF) investigated whether, by measuring them, it was possible to differentiate between the acute wounds that heal uneventfully and those that would become chronic and either become clinically infected or simply fail to heal.[14] Serum and wound fluid were collected prospectively from 50 high-energy war-time extremity wounds in 20 patients. Samples were collected at the time of wound closure, and patients were followed longitudinally for 6 weeks. Wounds requiring a return to the operating room for wound dehiscence (spontaneous opening of a previously closed wound) or impending dehiscence (a wound with persistent and increasing drainage following surgical closure or flap coverage or a wound with progressive marginal skin necrosis) and/or a clinically suspected wound infection were considered failures.

Serum and wound effluent samples were analyzed for the following biomarkers: ILs 1-8, 10, 12, 13, and 15; IFN-γ inducible protein-10 (EIP); eotaxin; IFN-γ; granulocyte-macrophage colony stimulating factor (GM-CSF); monocyte chemotactic protein (MIP)-1α, the protein regulated on activation; normal T expressed and secreted (RANTES); tumor necrosis factor (TNF)-α; and procalcitonin. This study identified notable differences in the concentrations of 3 biomarkers (RANTES, amino-procalcitonin, and IL-13) between wounds that healed uneventfully and those that went on to dehiscence. The proposed explanation for these findings was that both IL-13 and RANTES protein levels were suppressed in wounds that dehisced. IL-13, normally expressed by T-helper cells, inhibits macrophage activity by decreasing the expression of inflammatory cytokines and chemokines including TNF-α, IL-1α, and certain matrix metalloproteinases (MMPs), ultimately suppressing the production of nitric oxide.[53,55] Low levels of IL-13 are thus associated with macrophage activation and subsequent production of inducible nitric oxide synthetase by pro-inflammatory cytokines and chemokines. High levels of nitric oxide strongly suppress RANTES protein production despite elevated TNF-α, which would normally serve to upregulate RANTES protein production.[56]

There are 2 important conclusions that can be drawn from these results. First, wounds that dehisce demonstrate a unique biomarker profile that is similar to that seen in chronic inflammation. Second, the concentration of cytokines and chemokines was universally higher in the effluent when compared to the serum, further suggesting local, extracirculatory production and supporting the theory that effluent analysis may be more representative of local wound conditions.

Hawksworth and coauthors[31] further investigated the inflammatory profile of acute wounds. In addition to the local wound environment, they hypothesized that the systemic inflammatory response may affect the local wound inflammatory response and thereby indirectly influence wound healing. They subsequently postulated that because wound healing depends on the appropriate balance of pro- and anti-inflammatory mediators,[57] profiling both the local and systemic inflammatory response may provide prognostic wound healing inflammation. Fifty-seven high-energy war-time extremity wounds in 35 consecutive patients were studied. Serum, wound effluent, and tissue specimens were collected at each surgical debridement and again at the time of wound closure. Study subjects were then followed longitudinally for 30 days. Wounds requiring a return to the operating room for wound dehiscence or more than 50% skin graft loss were considered failures. Serum and effluent samples were measured for 22 cytokines and chemokines IL 1-8, 10, 12, 13, and 15; EIP; eotaxin; IFN-γ; GM-CSF; MCP-1α; RANTES; and TNF-α.

This study was able to define, for the first time, the time courses of these biomarkers over the debridement process. In wounds that dehisced, IL-6, a proinflammatory cytokine, as well as IL-8 and MIP-1α, proinflammatory chemokines, remained persistently elevated in the serum throughout the debridement process. This cytokine and chemokine profile suggests persistent systemic inflammation. Within the local wound environment, however, the response was more mixed, as evidenced by elevated concentrations of IL-6 and lower concentrations of IL-2 and IP-10. The gene transcript expression also differed between wounds that failed and those that healed. In dehisced wounds, the expression of pro-inflammatory (IL-1α, IL-1β, IL-8, MCP-1, MIP-1α, GM-CSF) was upregulated and the expression of anti-inflammatory (IL-4, IL-5, IL-13) cytokines and chemokines was downregulated compared to wounds that healed normally. These data support the study's hypothesis that the systemic inflammatory response may, in fact, adversely influence the local wound inflammatory response.

This study also noted that the expression of IL-2, IFN-γ, IP-10, and RANTES, considered to be proinflammatory cytokines and chemokines, was downregulated in wounds that failed compared to wounds that healed normally. Importantly, the serum from these patients demonstrated persistently elevated pro-inflammatory IL-6, IL-8, and MIP-1α, with an absence of anti-inflammatory cytokines and chemokines. This interesting finding suggests that tissue expression and systemic production of pro- and anti-inflammatory mediators is mixed. However, this pattern appears dysregulated because, in normal and even delayed wound healing, one would expect a more transient period of unchecked inflammation tempered by a predictable increase in anti-inflammatory protein concentration. It is this dysregulated inflammatory response that may enable persistent inflammation to continue and thus prevent the wound from progressing through the normal phases of wound healing.

Matrix Metalloproteinases

MMPs are essential to wound healing and the restoration of normal tissue architecture.[58] Depending on their primary substrate, MMPs are generally classified into 5 classes: collagenases, gelatinases, stromelysins, matrilysins, and membrane-type MMPs. Within the wound healing process, MMPs perform several critical functions related to inflammatory signaling and wound remodeling[58-60] and can positively or negatively[61] influence the wound healing process. Although 9 principal MMPs are involved in wound remodeling (MMPs 1-3, 7-10, 12, and 13), it is likely that all MMPs play essential or supporting roles in the wound healing process.[58,59,62-66] In fact, recent evidence continues to suggest that many MMPs have overlapping functions.[64,67]

Utz and colleagues summarized the functions of many applicable MMPs.[32] In short, MMP-1, MMP-8, and MMP-13 are referred to as collagenases and are active early in the wound healing process. Their function is to cleave types I, II, and III fibrillar collagen present in the extracellular matrix. This activity facilitates keratinocyte migration, important for wound remodeling.[58,59,68] Next, MMP-2 and MMP-9, the gelatinases, participate in wound remodeling by cleaving types IV, V, VII, and X collagen, elastin, and other basement-membrane proteins.[58-60] MMP-2 and MMP-9 also recruit inflammatory cells by establishing chemotactic gradients that direct immune cell migration.[58] The stromelysins (MMP-3, MMP-10, and MMP-11) further prepare the wound bed by degrading elastin as well as collagens IV, V, and X.[58,59] Similar to MMPs 2 and 9, MMP-3 also regulates chemokine signaling, plays a critical role in the maturation phase of wound healing, and is involved in both re-epithelialization and wound contraction.[58] Matrilysin (MMP-7), like MMP-3, is essential for wound bed re-epithelialization, but also shares similarities with MMP-2 and MMP-9 by its enhanced chemotactic ability, following the activation of osteopontin.[58] Membrane-type MMPs 14-17 function by binding other MMPs to cell surfaces, effectively activating and stimulating wound re-epithelialization.[59] Elevated concentrations of MMPs 2 and 3 have been observed in the effluent of chronic wounds.[66] Furthermore, persistent elevation of MMPs without a proportionate increase in their corresponding inhibitor expression has been implicated in chronic wounds.[57,60,69,70]

Having already observed that wound dehiscence is the result of an inflammatory dysregulation of the systemic and local wound molecular environment,[31] the same collaborative group also sought to evaluate MMP expression in high-energy war-time extremity wounds.[32] The goal was to, for the first time, characterize the MMP expression in these types of wounds and, more importantly, to identify patterns in MMP expression that may be indicative or predictive of wound failure. Thirty-eight wounds in 25 patients were studied. In contrast to the previous studies that defined wound failures as those requiring a surgical debridement for dehiscence or infection,[14,31] Utz et al compared wounds that healed uneventfully to those that exhibited impaired healing (ie, wounds that had not been definitively closed within 21 days or dehisced after surgical closure).[32] Serum concentrations of MMPs 2, 3, 7, 9, and 13 were measured at the time of each surgical debridement procedure, then at the time of definitive wound closure or flap coverage. As with cytokine and chemokine expression,[31] it is hypothesized that MMP expression could be used as an objective marker of wound status and could be useful to more appropriately time definitive wound closure or flap coverage.[32]

Utz and colleagues found that the concentrations of serum MMPs 2 and 7, both considered pro-inflammatory, were significantly elevated in impaired wounds.[32] This, again, implicated systemic inflammation as a major influence in wound outcome. MMP-2 cleaves the basement membrane and collagen, as well as establishes chemotactic gradients for inflammatory cell migration. MMP-7 similarly processes the extracellular matrix and enhances the ability of neutrophils to migrate to areas in need of repair.[58] Conversely, concentrations of MMP-3, critical for the maturation and ultimate healing of the acute wound, were lower.[32]

Conclusion

These studies highlight the importance of the systemic inflammatory response as it relates to wound healing. In addition to the protein and RNA data, all of these discussed studies observed risk factors for wound failure that are directly related to the degree of systemic inflammation. Traumatic brain injury,[14] APACHE II score,[31] vascular injury,[14,31,32] and the Injury Severity Score all correlated with local wound outcomes.[31,32] Perhaps most importantly, these studies identified systemic and local wound biomarker profiles associated with wound failure. These easily measured proteins may provide much-needed objective measures of wound status and the resultant capacity to heal. This information has great potential for use in guiding surgical decision making, reducing the number of debridement procedures, and appropriately timing the definitive closure or flap coverage in patients with high-energy extremity war wounds for optimum wound healing through individualized patient care.

References

1. Manring MM, Hawk A, Calhoun JH, Andersen RC. Treatment of war wounds: a historical review. *Clin Orthop Relat Res.* 2009;467(8):2168-2191.
2. London PS. Medical lessons from the Falkland Islands' campaign. Report of a meeting of the united services section of the royal society of medicine held at the royal college of surgeons on February 17 and 18, 1983. *J Bone Joint Surg Br.* 1983;65(4):507-510.
3. Gofrit ON, Leibovici D, Shapira SC, Shemer J, Stein M, Michaelson M. The trimodal death distribution of trauma victims: military experience from the Lebanon war. *Mil Med.* 1997;162(1):24-26.
4. Mabry RL, Holcomb JB, Baker AM, et al. United States army rangers in Somalia: an analysis of combat casualties on an urban battlefield. *J Trauma.* 2000;49(3):515-528; discussion 528-529.
5. Islinger RB, Kuklo TR, McHale KA. A review of orthopedic injuries in three recent U.S. Military conflicts. *Mil Med.* 2000;165(6):463-465.
6. Covey DC. Blast and fragment injuries of the musculoskeletal system. *J Bone Joint Surg Am.* 2002;84-A(7):1221-1234.
7. Champion HR, Bellamy RF, Roberts CP, Leppaniemi A. A profile of combat injury. *J Trauma.* 2003;54(5 Suppl):S13-S19.
8. Lin DL, Kirk KL, Murphy KP, McHale KA, Doukas WC. Evaluation of orthopaedic injuries in Operation Enduring Freedom. *J Orthop Trauma.* 2004;18(8 Suppl):S48-S53.
9. Patel TH, Wenner KA, Price SA, Weber MA, Leveridge A, McAtee SJ. A U.S. Army forward surgical team's experience in Operation Iraqi Freedom. *J Trauma.* 2004;57(2):201-207.
10. Covey DC. Combat orthopaedics: a view from the trenches. *J Am Acad Orthop Surg.* 2006;14(10 Spec No.):S10-S17.
11. Hofmeister EP, Mazurek M, Ingari J. Injuries sustained to the upper extremity due to modern warfare and the evolution of care. *J Hand Surg [Am].* 2007;32(8):1141-1147.
12. Fox CJ, Gillespie DL, Cox ED, et al. Damage control resuscitation for vascular surgery in a combat support hospital. *J Trauma.* 2008;65(1):1-9.
13. Hayda RA, Mazurek MT, Powell ET IV, et al. From Iraq back to Iraq: modern combat orthopaedic care. *Instr Course Lect.* 2008;57:87-99.
14. Forsberg JA, Elster EA, Andersen RC, et al. Correlation of procalcitonin and cytokine expression with dehiscence of wartime extremity wounds. *J Bone Joint Surg Am.* 2008;90(3):580-588.
15. Forsberg JA, Pepek JM, Wagner S, et al. Heterotopic ossification in high-energy wartime extremity injuries: prevalence and risk factors. *J Bone Joint Surg Am.* 2009;91(5):1084-1091.

16. Potter BK, Burns TC, Lacap AP, Granville RR, Gajewski D. Heterotopic ossification in the residual limbs of traumatic and combat-related amputees. *J Am Acad Orthop Surg*. 2006;14(10 Spec No.):S191-S197.

17. Potter BK, Burns TC, Lacap AP, Granville RR, Gajewski DA. Heterotopic ossification following traumatic and combat-related amputations. Prevalence, risk factors, and preliminary results of excision. *J Bone Joint Surg Am*. 2007;89(3):476-486.

18. Nesti LJ, Jackson WM, Shanti RM, et al. Differentiation potential of multipotent progenitor cells derived from war-traumatized muscle tissue. *J Bone Joint Surg Am*. 2008;90(11):2390-2398.

19. Atala A. The clinician scientist and medical advances. *J Urol*. 2008;180(2):431-432.

20. Chambers SK. The gynecologic oncology model: research. *Surg Oncol Clin N Am*. 1998;7(2):255-262.

21. Rigby MR. The role of the physician-scientist in bridging basic and clinical research in type 1 diabetes. *Curr Opin Endocrinol Diabetes Obes*. 2010;17(2):131-142.

22. Rosenblum ND, Bazett-Jones DP, O'Brodovich H. A scientist track investigator program to support early career outcomes for clinician scientists. *J Pediatr*. 2009;155(5):603-604.e1.

23. Sullivan R. Cancer research in the UK: a policy review of the junior academic clinical faculty. *Mol Oncol*. 2008;1(4):366-373.

24. Clark RAF. *The Molecular and Cellular Biology of Wound Repair*. New York, NY: Springer; 1996.

25. Assoian RK, Komoriya A, Meyers CA, Miller DM, Sporn MB. Transforming growth factor-beta in human platelets. Identification of a major storage site, purification, and characterization. *J Biol Chem*. 1983;258(11):7155-7160.

26. Shimokado K, Raines EW, Madtes DK, Barrett TB, Benditt EP, Ross R. A significant part of macrophage-derived growth factor consists of at least two forms of pdgf. *Cell*. 1985;43(1):277-286.

27. Baird A, Mormede P, Bohlen P. Immunoreactive fibroblast growth factor in cells of peritoneal exudate suggests its identity with macrophage-derived growth factor. *Biochem Biophys Res Commun*. 1985;126(1):358-364.

28. Singer AJ, Clark RA. Cutaneous wound healing. *N Engl J Med*. 1999;341(10):738-746.

29. Dinarello CA. Interleukin 1 as mediator of the acute-phase response. *Surv Immunol Res*. 1984;3(1):29-33.

30. Robson MC, Steed DL, Franz MG. Wound healing: biologic features and approaches to maximize healing trajectories. *Curr Probl Surg*. 2001;38(2):72-140.

31. Hawksworth JS, Stojadinovic A, Gage FA, et al. Inflammatory biomarkers in combat wound healing. *Ann Surg*. 2009;250(6):1002-1007.

32. Utz ER, Elster EA, Tadaki DK, et al. Metalloproteinase expression is associated with traumatic wound failure. *J Surg Res*. 2009;159(2):633-639.

33. Damas P, Ledoux D, Nys M, et al. Cytokine serum level during severe sepsis in human il-6 as a marker of severity. *Ann Surg*. 1992;215(4):356-362.

34. Damas P, Reuter A, Gysen P, Demonty J, Lamy M, Franchimont P. Tumor necrosis factor and interleukin-1 serum levels during severe sepsis in humans. *Crit Care Med*. 1989;17(10):975-978.

35. Hack CE, De Groot ER, Felt-Bersma RJ, et al. Increased plasma levels of interleukin-6 in sepsis. *Blood*. 1989;74(5):1704-1710.

36. Pinzur MS, Smith D, Osterman H. Syme ankle disarticulation in peripheral vascular disease and diabetic foot infection: the one-stage versus two-stage procedure. *Foot Ankle Int*. 1995;16(3):124-127.

37. Pinzur MS, Stuck RM, Sage R, Hunt N, Rabinovich Z. Syme ankle disarticulation in patients with diabetes. *J Bone Joint Surg Am*. 2003;85-A(9):1667-1672.

38. Robbins GM, Masri BA, Garbuz DS, Duncan CP. Evaluation of pain in patients with apparently solidly fixed total hip arthroplasty components. *J Am Acad Orthop Surg*. 2002;10(2):86-94.

39. Shih LY, Wu JJ, Yang DJ. Erythrocyte sedimentation rate and c-reactive protein values in patients with total hip arthroplasty. *Clin Orthop Relat Res*. 1987;225:238-246.

40. Song KM, Sloboda JF. Acute hematogenous osteomyelitis in children. *J Am Acad Orthop Surg*. 2001;9(3):166-175.

41. Spangehl MJ, Masri BA, O'Connell JX, Duncan CP. Prospective analysis of preoperative and intraoperative investigations for the diagnosis of infection at the sites of two hundred and two revision total hip arthroplasties. *J Bone Joint Surg Am*. 1999;81(5):672-683.

42. Spangehl MJ, Younger AS, Masri BA, Duncan CP. Diagnosis of infection following total hip arthroplasty. *Instr Course Lect*. 1998;47:285-295.

43. van Deuren M, Dofferhoff AS, van der Meer JW. Cytokines and the response to infection. *J Pathol*. 1992;168(4):349-356.

44. Zorrilla P, Gomez LA, Salido JA, Silva A, Lopez-Alonso A. Low serum zinc level as a predictive factor of delayed wound healing in total hip replacement. *Wound Repair Regen*. 2006;14(2):119-122.

45. Zorrilla P, Salido JA, Lopez-Alonso A, Silva A. Serum zinc as a prognostic tool for wound healing in hip hemiarthroplasty. *Clin Orthop Relat Res*. 2004;420:304-308.

46. Pallister I, Empson K. The effects of surgical fracture fixation on the systemic inflammatory response to major trauma. *J Am Acad Orthop Surg*. 2005;13(2):93-100.

47. Zedler S, Faist E. The impact of endogenous triggers on trauma-associated inflammation. *Curr Opin Crit Care*. 2006;12(6):595-601.

48. Carrel A. Effet d'un abcès à distance sur la cicatrisation d'une plaie aseptique. *CR Soc Biol*. 1924;90:333-335.

49. Clark MA, Plank LD, Hill GL. Wound healing associated with severe surgical illness. *World J Surg*. 2000;24(6):648-654.

50. Goodson WH, Lopez-Sarmiento A, Jensen JA, West J, Granja-Mena L, Chavez-Estrella J. The influence of a brief preoperative illness on postoperative healing. *Ann Surg*. 1987;205(3):250-255.

51. Muller B, White JC, Nylen ES, Snider RH, Becker KL, Habener JF. Ubiquitous expression of the calcitonin-I gene in multiple tissues in response to sepsis. *J Clin Endocrinol Metab*. 2001;86(1):396-404.

52. Bassim CW, Redman RS, DeNucci DJ, Becker KL, Nylen ES. Salivary procalcitonin and periodontitis in diabetes. *J Dent Res*. 2008;87(7):630-634.

53. Viallon A, Zeni F, Pouzet V, et al. Serum and ascitic procalcitonin levels in cirrhotic patients with spontaneous bacterial peritonitis: diagnostic value and relationship to pro-inflammatory cytokines. *Intensive Care Med*. 2000;26(8):1082-1088.

54. Morgenthaler NG, Struck J, Chancerelle Y, et al. Production of procalcitonin (pct) in non-thyroidal tissue after lps injection. *Horm Metab Res*. 2003;35(5):290-295.

55. Harris IR, Yee KC, Walters CE, et al. Cytokine and protease levels in healing and non-healing chronic venous leg ulcers. *Exp Dermatol*. 1995;4(6):342-349.

56. Frank S, Kampfer H, Wetzler C, Stallmeyer B, Pfeilschifter J. Large induction of the chemotactic cytokine rantes during cutaneous wound repair: a regulatory role for nitric oxide in keratinocyte-derived rantes expression. *Biochem J*. 2000;347(Pt 1):265-273.

57. Eming SA, Krieg T, Davidson JM. Inflammation in wound repair: molecular and cellular mechanisms. *J Invest Dermatol*. 2007;127(3):514-525.

58. Gill SE, Parks WC. Metalloproteinases and their inhibitors: regulators of wound healing. *Int J Biochem Cell Biol*. 2008;40(6-7):1334-1347.

59. Armstrong DG, Jude EB. The role of matrix metalloproteinases in wound healing. *J Am Podiatr Med Assoc*. 2002;92(1):12-18.

60. Li J, Chen J, Kirsner R. Pathophysiology of acute wound healing. *Clin Dermatol*. 2007;25(1):9-18.

61. Sigurdson L, Sen T, Hall LR, et al. Possible impedance of luminal reepithelialization by tracheal cartilage metalloproteinases. *Arch Otolaryngol Head Neck Surg.* 2003;129(2):197-200.

62. Beidler SK, Douillet CD, Berndt DF, Keagy BA, Rich PB, Marston WA. Multiplexed analysis of matrix metalloproteinases in leg ulcer tissue of patients with chronic venous insufficiency before and after compression therapy. *Wound Repair Regen.* 2008;16(5):642-648.

63. Maclauchlan S, Skokos EA, Agah A, et al. Enhanced angiogenesis and reduced contraction in thrombospondin-2-null wounds is associated with increased levels of matrix metalloproteinases-2 and -9, and soluble vegf. *J Histochem Cytochem.* 2009;57(4):301-313.

64. Ra HJ, Parks WC. Control of matrix metalloproteinase catalytic activity. *Matrix Biol.* 2007;26(8):587-596.

65. Simeon A, Monier F, Emonard H, et al. Expression and activation of matrix metalloproteinases in wounds: modulation by the tripeptide-copper complex glycyl-l-histidyl-l-lysine-cu2+. *J Invest Dermatol.* 1999;112(6):957-964.

66. Stechmiller JK, Kilpadi DV, Childress B, Schultz GS. Effect of vacuum-assisted closure therapy on the expression of cytokines and proteases in wound fluid of adults with pressure ulcers. *Wound Repair Regen.* 2006;14(3):371-374.

67. Sternlicht MD, Werb Z. How matrix metalloproteinases regulate cell behavior. *Annu Rev Cell Dev Biol.* 2001;17:463-516.

68. Pilcher BK, Dumin JA, Sudbeck BD, Krane SM, Welgus HG, Parks WC. The activity of collagenase-1 is required for keratinocyte migration on a type I collagen matrix. *J Cell Biol.* 1997;137(6):1445-1457.

69. Blakytny R, Jude E. The molecular biology of chronic wounds and delayed healing in diabetes. *Diabet Med.* 2006;23(6):594-608.

70. Menke NB, Ward KR, Witten TM, Bonchev DG, Diegelmann RF. Impaired wound healing. *Clin Dermatol.* 2007;25(1):19-25.

71. Sims JE, Smith DE. The IL-1 family: regulators of immunity. *Nat Rev Immunol.* 2010;10(2):89-102.

72. Kaplan E, Dinarello CA, Gelfand JA. Interleukin-1 and the response to injury. *Immunol Res.* 1989;8(2):118-129.

73. Smith KA, Gilbride KJ, Favata MF. Lymphocyte activating factor promotes t-cell growth factor production by cloned murine lymphoma cells. *Nature.* 1980;287(5785):853-855.

74. Smith KA, Lachman LB, Oppenheim JJ, Favata MF. The functional relationship of the interleukins. *J Exp Med.* 1980;151(6):1551-1556.

75. Wagemaker G, Burger H, van Gils FC, van Leen RW, Wielenga JJ. Interleukin-3. *Biotherapy.* 1990;2(4):337-345.

76. Ihle JN. Interleukin-3 and hematopoiesis. *Chem Immunol.* 1992;51:65-106.

77. Howard M. Interleukins for b lymphocytes. *Immunol Res.* 1983;2(3):210-212.

78. Sideras P, Noma T, Honjo T. Structure and function of interleukin 4 and 5. *Immunol Rev.* 1988;102:189-212.

79. Yokota T, Arai N, de Vries J, et al. Molecular biology of interleukin 4 and interleukin 5 genes and biology of their products that stimulate b cells, t cells and hemopoietic cells. *Immunol Rev.* 1988;102(137-187.

80. Dubucquoi S, Desreumaux P, Janin A et al. Interleukin 5 synthesis by eosinophils: association with granules and immunoglobulin-dependent secretion. *J Exp Med.* 1994;179(2):703-708.

81. Kishimoto T. Interleukin-6: from basic science to medicine: 40 years in immunology. *Annu Rev Immunol.* 2005;23:1-21.

82. Mengozzi M, Bertini R, Sironi M, Ghezzi P. Inhibition by interleukin 1 receptor antagonist of in vivo activities of interleukin 1 in mice. *Lymphokine Cytokine Res.* 1991;10(5):405-407.

83. Khaled AR, Durum SK. Lymphocide: cytokines and the control of lymphoid homeostasis. *Nat Rev Immunol.* 2002;2(11):817-830.

84. O'Garra A, Vieira P. T(h)1 cells control themselves by producing interleukin-10. *Nat Rev Immunol.* 2007;7(6):425-428.

85. Moroguchi A, Ishimura K, Okano K, Wakabayashi H, Maeba T, Maeta H. Interleukin-10 suppresses proliferation and remodeling of extracellular matrix of cultured human skin fibroblasts. *Eur Surg Res.* 2004;36(1):39-44.

86. D'Andrea A, Aste-Amezaga M, Valiante NM, Ma X, Kubin M, Trinchieri G. Interleukin 10 (il-10) inhibits human lymphocyte interferon gamma-production by suppressing natural killer cell stimulatory factor/il-12 synthesis in accessory cells. *J Exp Med.* 1993;178(3):1041-1048.

87. Tripp CS, Wolf SF, Unanue ER. Interleukin 12 and tumor necrosis factor alpha are costimulators of interferon gamma production by natural killer cells in severe combined immunodeficiency mice with listeriosis, and interleukin 10 is a physiologic antagonist. *Proc Natl Acad Sci U S A.* 1993;90(8):3725-3729.

88. Goriely S, Neurath MF, Goldman M. How microorganisms tip the balance between interleukin-12 family members. *Nat Rev Immunol.* 2008;8(1):81-86.

89. Zurawski G, de Vries JE. Interleukin 13, an interleukin 4-like cytokine that acts on monocytes and B cells, but not on T cells. *Immunol Today.* 1994;15(1):19-26.

90. Minty A, Chalon P, Derocq JM, et al. Interleukin-13 is a new human lymphokine regulating inflammatory and immune responses. *Nature.* 1993;362(6417):248-250.

91. Lee YB, Satoh J, Walker DG, Kim SU. Interleukin-15 gene expression in human astrocytes and microglia in culture. *Neuroreport.* 1996;7(5):1062-1066.

92. Fehniger TA, Caligiuri MA. Interleukin 15: biology and relevance to human disease. *Blood.* 2001;97(1):14-32.

93. Schroder K, Hertzog PJ, Ravasi T, Hume DA. Interferon-gamma: an overview of signals, mechanisms and functions. *J Leukoc Biol.* 2004;75(2):163-189.

94. Schroder JM, Christophers E. The biology of nap-1/il-8, a neutrophil-activating cytokine. *Immunol Ser.* 1992;57:387-416.

95. Koch AE, Polverini PJ, Kunkel SL, et al. Interleukin-8 as a macrophage-derived mediator of angiogenesis. *Science.* 1992;258(5089):1798-1801.

96. Angiolillo AL, Sgadari C, Taub DD, et al. Human interferon-inducible protein 10 is a potent inhibitor of angiogenesis in vivo. *J Exp Med.* 1995;182(1):155-162.

97. Gasperini S, Marchi M, Calzetti F, et al. Gene expression and production of the monokine induced by ifn-gamma (mig), ifn-inducible t cell alpha chemoattractant (I-tac), and ifn-gamma-inducible protein-10 (ip-10) chemokines by human neutrophils. *J Immunol.* 1999;162(8):4928-4937.

98. Jiang Y, Beller DI, Frendl G, Graves DT. Monocyte chemoattractant protein-1 regulates adhesion molecule expression and cytokine production in human monocytes. *J Immunol.* 1992;148(8):2423.

99. Bischoff SC, Krieger M, Brunner T, Dahinden CA. Monocyte chemotactic protein 1 is a potent activator of human basophils. *J Exp Med.* 1992;175(5):1271-1275.

100. Leonard EJ, Yoshimura T. Human monocyte chemoattractant protein-1 (mcp-1). *Immunol Today.* 1990;11(3):97-101.

101 Yoshimura T, Leonard EJ. Human monocyte chemoattractant protein-1: structure and function. *Cytokines.* 1992;4:131-152.

102. Demetri GD, Griffin JD. Granulocyte colony-stimulating factor and its receptor. *Blood.* 1991;78(11):2791-2808.

103. Ruef C, Coleman DL. Granulocyte-macrophage colony-stimulating factor: pleiotropic cytokine with potential clinical usefulness. *Rev Infect Dis.* 1990;12(1):41-62.

104. Jing H, Yen JH, Ganea D. A novel signaling pathway mediates the inhibition of ccl3/4 expression by prostaglandin e2. *J Biol Chem.* 2004;279(53):55176-55186.

Chapter **10**

HETEROTOPIC OSSIFICATION

MAJ Benjamin K. Potter, MD and LCDR Jonathan Agner Forsberg, MD

The term *heterotopic ossification* (HO) refers to the formation of mature lamellar bone in nonosseous tissue. Crudely translated, HO literally refers to bone formation in other location. In the civilian setting, HO is usually associated with severe systemic inflammation stemming from spinal cord injury, traumatic brain injury, or neoplasm.[1-9] HO also complicates the wounds of total hip arthroplasty, as well as fractures of the acetabulum and elbow, particularly those requiring operative fixation. This implies a relationship between HO and muscle trauma, whether due to high-energy injury or operative dissection.[10-25] Genetic causes of heterotopic bone formation include fibrodysplasia ossificans progressiva and progressive osseous heteroplasia.[26-28] Although both proven risk factors and genetic predispositions exist, the underlying cause(s) of HO is largely unknown, and the entity itself remains a source of limb pain, stiffness, and subsequent disability.

The incidence of HO in combat-wounded servicemembers has been reported as high as 63% to 64.6%,[29,30] far greater than that described in civilian trauma centers. Formation of HO in this patient population is significantly associated with patients who have sustained a blast injury, a combat-related amputation within the zone of injury, and Injury Severity Scores (ISSs) greater than 16.[29,30] In contrast, the largest civilian series found that HO complicated the extremities in 11% of severe traumatic brain-injured patients and 20% of spinal cord injuries.[31] Earlier work reported rates of ectopic bone growth in various long-bone fractures, including forearm fractures (20%),[17] femoral shaft fractures (52%),[32] and tibial

shaft fractures (0%),[33] all in the setting of significant head injury.

Few case series evaluating both head-injured and nonhead-injured patients with fractures contain a control group for comparison. Spencer[34] compared the healing times and radiographic callus appearance in 82 fractures in 53 patients with head injuries to 30 patients with extremity fractures and no head injury. An exuberant healing response was present in 53% of tibia fractures, 60% of femur fractures, and 36% of humerus fractures in patients with head injuries compared to an average of 10% across the 3 fracture sites in patients without head injury. He also demonstrated a decreased time to union in the head-injured group and concluded that the term HO may be more appropriate in describing exuberant fracture callus. Giannoudis and coauthors[35] reported similar findings in patients with femur fractures, noting a shorter time to union and a higher callus-to-diaphyseal bone diameter ratio in patients with a head injury when compared to nonhead-injured controls. More recent literature corroborates these findings, reporting a 2-fold shorter time to union but, more importantly, a linear relationship between the amount of radiographically apparent (exuberant) callus and the in vitro proliferation rates of a human osteoblastic cell line in response to sera from study participants.[36] There is no apparent consensus regarding the rate of HO in civilian long-bone extremity trauma without head injury. Nevertheless, the incidence of clinically relevant or symptomatic HO in this setting is generally considered to be low.[6,34,35,37]

Owens BD, Belmont PJ Jr, eds. *Combat Orthopedic Surgery: Lessons Learned in Iraq and Afghanistan (pp 85-92)*
© 2011 SLACK Incorporated

Other estimates of injury severity and subsequent systemic inflammation can be used to predict HO. The occurrence of autonomic dysfunction or evidence of systemic infection correlates with an increased risk of HO formation. The ISS has also been shown to predict the development of HO.[29,38] Critics of ISS utility as a prognostic factor for HO growth argue that head-injured patients score higher and therefore are inherently more likely to develop heterotopic bone. However, Steinberg and Hubbard[37] reported that the ISS, independent of a head injury, remained an important predictor of the development of HO following intramedullary nailing of femoral fractures. These findings add to the growing body of evidence suggesting that systemic factors, arguably related to the degree of systemic inflammation, initiate or contribute to an exaggerated osteogenic response that may ultimately be responsible for the development of heterotopic bone.

The association between heterotopic bone growth and the number and method of surgical debridement procedures, including the use of intermediate-pressure pulsatile lavage irrigation devices and negative pressure wound therapy, is not well understood. Two recent studies reported trends toward an association between HO formation and the number of debridement procedures as well as the duration of negative pressure dressing therapy.[29,30] However, these results should be interpreted with caution because the increases in both the number of debridement procedures and the duration of negative pressure dressing therapy are ostensibly also indicators of greater local injury severity; therefore, establishment of a causal linkage between local ectopic bone and these wound care modalities is difficult and fraught with confounding factors.

The type of definitive fracture treatment (internal fixation, external fixation, or amputation) appears unrelated to the formation of HO in extremity trauma, despite an historic association with certain surgical approaches to the hip and acetabulum.[15,20,24,39-44] This theoretical concern has not been borne out in clinical studies of extremity trauma.[29]

Amputees

The predilection of heterotopic bone for growth within the residual limbs of amputees is an important observation.[29,30] In combat-wounded servicemembers, serial debridement procedures are performed every 24 to 72 hours prior to definitive wound closure or coverage in an effort to remove devitalized tissue and gross contamination. Antibiotic-impregnated polymethylmethacrylate beads are routinely used to reduce the bacterial bioburden, as are negative pressure wound dressings. Definitive amputations are often performed within or near the zone of injury (which is extensive in blast injuries) in an effort to preserve residual limb length, joint levels, and subsequent function. As a result, there exists a strong association between these injuries and the subsequent development of both radiographic and symptomatic HO.[30]

Several grading classification systems exist to classify HO formation about the hip, knee, and elbow.[4,20,24,45-48] These were later extrapolated to other joints, but none are directly applicable or adaptable to the residual limbs of amputees. For these patients, a classification system,[30] originally described by one of the authors (BKP), has been adopted. The severity of HO is graded using a single radiographic projection (anteroposterior, lateral, or oblique) that maximizes the extent of the ectopic bone within the soft tissues of the residual limb. For example, ectopic bone formation is considered to be *mild* if it occupies less than 25%, *moderate* if it occupies 25% to 50%, and *severe* if it occupies more than 50% of the soft tissues on a single radiographic projection (Figure 10-1).

Though the formation of HO in these patients is theorized to stem from a prolonged inflammatory response, the cause of HO is largely unknown. Considerable efforts are underway to define the mechanistic pathways responsible for this unique phenomenon. Animal models have been developed to evaluate pathways associated with the expression of bone morphogenetic protein (BMP), a member of the transforming growth factor super-family. Despite this seemingly appropriate approach, the cell(s) that ultimately differentiate into osteoblasts at extraosseous locations also need to be identified and characterized.

Shafritz and others[49] have identified genetic mutations localizing to chromosome 4q 27-31 related to HO formation. Though the BMP4 gene itself does not harbor a genetic mutation, overexpression of BMP4 and its receptor BMPRIA coupled with underexpression of its antagonists are thought to be required for HO formation.[49-52] This phenomenon, first identified in patients with fibrodysplasia ossificans progressiva, firmly establishes a link between HO and traditional osteoblastic signaling. Davis, in association with Gannon and others, further defined the microenvironment by identifying the presence of brown (hypoxic) adipocytes in the early stages of HO development.[53] The hypoxic environment induces both chondrogenesis and neovascularization. The result is an increase in oxygen tension enabling endochondral ossification to occur. Nesti and coauthors[54] isolated a population of mesenchymal progenitor cells present in traumatized muscle. The authors concluded, based on their ability to demonstrate pluripotency, that these cells may play a central role in the pathologic osteogenic response. However, in a more recent study, Lounev and others[55] implicate progenitor cells of a vascular lineage.

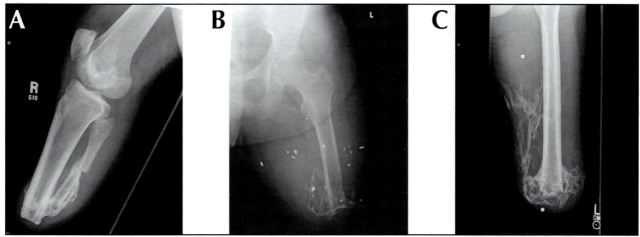

Figure 10-1. Walter Reed classification of HO in the residual limbs of amputees. (A) Mild (0% to 25%). (B) Moderate (25% to 50%). (C) Severe (>50%).

Ongoing studies from our own institutions examine sera, tissue, and wound effluent from high-energy war-time extremity wounds. We have developed predictive biomarker and gene-based profiles for HO formation in these patients. These profiles will permit the early identification of patients most at risk for HO via computer-based algorithms, potentially allowing aggressive and personalized primary prophylaxis. Additionally, we have successfully induced stem cell production of bone in vitro using patient sera, with the composite goals of identifying molecular triggers of HO production, evaluating therapeutic targets, and developing and testing novel preventative treatments.

Primary and Secondary Prophylaxis

Numerous randomized studies have documented the efficacy of primary prophylaxis to prevent HO in patients at risk. This type of prophylaxis is given after high-risk index procedures, such as total hip arthroplasty or operative fixation of acetabular fractures.[56-66] Typically, 5 to 10 Gy of local radiation therapy is dosed in a single fraction, with or without nonsteroidal anti-inflammatory drugs (NSAIDs). NSAIDs alone can be expected to provide a cost-effective, dose-related decrease in heterotopic bone formation, though the risk of complications, gastrointestinal and otherwise, appears higher.[57,67] Although some randomized series have demonstrated no difference in ectopic bone formation between nonsteroidal treatment and radiation therapy,[56,62,65] the bulk of the existing literature, including 2 meta-analyses, modestly favors radiation therapy, arguably related to compliance issues with medical treatment.[60,66,68,69] Two randomized series

found no difference between preoperative and postoperative radiation when dosing single fraction of 7 to 10 Gy, provided it is given less than 4 hours prior to or 48 hours after surgery.[58,64]

Evidence supporting secondary prophylaxis following excision of symptomatic HO is lacking. To our knowledge, there exist no randomized trials of any secondary prevention modality. Nevertheless, the rate of recurrence in the appropriate surgical candidate is generally accepted to be low, and the theoretical benefit of secondary prophylaxis outweighs the risks of symptomatic recurrence for most patients.

Novel means of primary prophylaxis are currently being developed. Acknowledging that the endochondral ossification observed in HO first requires chondrocytic differentiation from chondrogenic precursor cells and that the retinoid signaling pathway is active early in this process,[70] Pacifici and colleagues[70,71] sought to determine whether this pathway would be susceptible for targeted therapy. The authors established a murine HO model by injecting rhBMP-2 in the subcutaneous tissue. They then evaluated whether an oral α-specific retinoic acid receptor antagonist dosed daily for 20 days resulted in less ectopic bone formation. This experiment yielded several important results. First, the α-agonist-treated mice developed significantly less ectopic bone by micro-computed tomography. Second, angiogenesis was also suppressed in the treated mice as evidenced by a dramatic visual difference in blood vessel size and number, as well as a significant decrease in vascular endothelial growth factor α gene expression. Finally, and perhaps most importantly, the treated mice demonstrated marked downregulation of key genes involved in chondrogenesis and later osteogenesis, including Sox9 and Runx2, as well as the BMP signaling system.

Complications of Prophylaxis

Unfortunately, the use of HO prophylaxis is not without consequence. Following radiation therapy, wound- and implant-related complications have been reported.[41,66] For this reason, close consultation with a radiation oncologist will help ensure that the skin incision is protected and any press-fit implants are properly shielded. Patients with high-energy penetrating extremity wounds exhibit a relatively high baseline incidence of wound and fracture-related complications. The use of radiation therapy on these complex wounds is highly controversial and is theorized to result in an unacceptably high wound complication rate, in addition to logistic and treatment-timing concerns. Considering this, radiation as primary prophylaxis for HO is not currently recommended in this patient population.

NSAIDs may also be problematic in certain patient populations. Cyclooxygenase-2 is required for endochondral bone formation, a mechanism critical to the development of HO, as well as early fracture healing.[53] Concerns about NSAIDs in an orthopedic population stem from this blunting of "helpful" inflammation necessary for endochondral ossification,[72-76] leading to increased time to union and increase in the number of delayed unions in several studies.[72,73,75-78] The potential benefit of NSAIDs for HO prophylaxis must be weighed heavily against potential fracture-related complications.

Etidronate is the only Food and Drug Administration-approved drug for the primary prophylaxis of HO and thus deserves consideration as well as a complete discussion. The FDA label states that etidronate is indicated following total hip replacement or spinal cord injury, though the drug has been evaluated off-label in other settings such as civilian trauma and burns. Etidronate blocks the aggregation, growth, and mineralization of hydroxyapatite crystals necessary for the formation of heterotopic bone. Early randomized and pseudo-randomized trials demonstrated efficacy,[79-84] but only as long as the drug was administered. "Rebound" formation of HO following cessation of therapy was common,[79-82,84] and follow-up studies failed to corroborate the earlier results.[85-87] In fact, a recent Cochrane database review did not demonstrate pharmacologic efficacy and could not recommend etidronate treatment for the primary prophylaxis of HO.[88]

Treatment of Symptomatic Heterotopic Ossification

The treatment of HO is individualized. Most cases are mild, minimally symptomatic or asymptom- atic, and result in little or no functional impairment.[13-16,18,20,22,38,39,43-48,59-61,63,64,67,89-94] Moderate to severe cases can be highly debilitating, particularly in peri-articular locations or in the residual limbs of amputees.[16,30,95] Once HO has been identified radiographically, an assessment should be made as to the impact on the patient's level of function and activities of daily living. In amputees, it is important to identify and treat other sources of residual limb pain such as painful bursae, myodesis failure, and neuromata.[96,97] Conservative management including rest, local and systemic medications, activity modification, and prosthetic socket/suspension modifications require close consultation with skilled prosthetists, physical therapists, and physiatrists. Likewise, in nonamputees, alternative causes of pain and functional limitations including infection, fracture nonunion, and neuropathic pain syndromes should be evaluated and treated. Surgical excision is reserved for pain, ulceration, or joint stiffness attributable to HO that remains refractory to exhaustive conservative measures.

The timing of excision HO is controversial. Historically, excision was advocated only after prolonged observation, ensuring that the ectopic bone was "mature," as evidenced by quiescent 3-phase bone scans and normalization of the serum alkaline phosphatase.[98-100] This practice has recently been called into question, as these measures do not accurately predict recurrence.[4] Numerous studies support earlier excision based on the roentgenographic appearance of the lesion.[30,101-111] This approach allows earlier range of motion and return of functional mobility and a recurrence rate similar to late excision.[102] Garland et al[4] identified other prognostic factors for HO excision in patients with head injuries, using a classification system based on the patient's cognitive and physical disability (Table 10-1). In this series, motion-related outcomes and recurrence rates were excellent in classes I and II and uniformly poor, with a 100% recurrence rate, in class V. They theorized that the latter group of patients possessed a systemic osteogenic stimulus that may persist for years after the initial injury. Knowledge of this can help set patient and family expectations, particularly in cases involving severe traumatic brain injury. After appropriate patient selection and preoperative counseling, we advocate surgical excision as soon as symptoms warrant, following appropriate efforts at conservative management. Regarding the amputee with variable cognitive and minimal other physical disability, excellent results of excision can be achieved. In one series of 25 combat-related amputations, an 8% recurrence rate of mild, asymptomatic ectopic bone has been reported with secondary prophylaxis treatment in 84% of cases.[30]

Table 10-1	
Garland Classification/ Prognostic Factors of Heterotopic Ossification Excision	
Class	*State of Disability*
I	Minimum cognitive and physical disability
II	Minimum cognitive, but moderate physical disability
III	Minimum cognitive with severe physical disability
IV	Moderate to severe cognitive deficits with minimal physical deficits
V	Moderate to severe cognitive deficits with severe physical disability

Conclusion

HO is a complex disorder with numerous proven and putative risk factors and varied initiating external stimuli, ultimately resulting from both local and systemic internal biologic factors. Lesions are often asymptomatic but can result in significant patient disability due to pain, ulceration, and joint stiffness. When practicable, primary prophylaxis via radiation therapy or NSAIDs is effective in a majority of patients at risk. After an appropriate trial of conservative measures, operative excision of symptomatic heterotopic bone provides generally good results with low recurrence rates in appropriately selected patients treated with secondary prophylaxis. Future research regarding biomarker-based prognostication and identification of initiating chemokines, genes, and cellular origin of ectopic bone may permit expanded early prophylaxis and development of novel targeted therapies to prevent or limit HO.

References

1. Kaplan FS, Glaser DL, Hebela N, Shore EM. Heterotopic ossification. *J Am Acad Orthop Surg.* 2004;12(2):116-125.
2. Hoffer MM, Garrett A, Brink J, Perry J, Hale W, Nickel VL. The orthopaedic management of brain-injured children. *J Bone Joint Surg Am.* 1971;53(3):567-577.
3. Garland DE, Razza BE, Waters RL. Forceful joint manipulation in head-injured adults with heterotopic ossification. *Clin Orthop Relat Res.* 1982;169:133-138.
4. Garland DE, Hanscom DA, Keenan MA, Smith C, Moore T. Resection of heterotopic ossification in the adult with head trauma. *J Bone Joint Surg Am.* 1985;67(8):1261-1269.
5. Garland DE, Keenan MA. Orthopedic strategies in the management of the adult head-injured patient. *Phys Ther.* 1983;63(12):2004-2009.
6. Garland DE. A clinical perspective on common forms of acquired heterotopic ossification. *Clin Orthop Relat Res.* 1991;263:13-29.
7. Como JJ, Yowler CJ, Malangoni MA. Extensive heterotopic mesenteric ossification after penetrating abdominal trauma. *J Trauma.* 2008;65(6):1567.
8. Kypson AP, Morphew E, Jones R, Gottfried MR, Seigler HF. Heterotopic ossification in rectal cancer: rare finding with a novel proposed mechanism. *J Surg Oncol.* 2003;82(2):132-136; discussion 137.
9. Mansoor A, Beals RK. Enchondral ossification of muscles of the calf: a case report on a new form of heterotopic ossification. *J Pediatr Orthop B.* 2008;18:2.
10. Sanchez-Sotelo J, Torchia ME, O'Driscoll SW. Complex distal humeral fractures: internal fixation with a principle-based parallel-plate technique. *J Bone Joint Surg Am.* 2007;89(5):961-969.
11. Rama KR, Vendittoli PA, Ganapathi M, Borgmann R, Roy A, Lavigne M. Heterotopic ossification after surface replacement arthroplasty and total hip arthroplasty: a randomized study. *J Arthroplasty.* 2009;24(2):256-262.
12. Mikic ZD, Vukadinovic SM. Late results in fractures of the radial head treated by excision. *Clin Orthop Relat Res.* 1983;181:220-228.
13. Kreder HJ, Rozen N, Borkhoff CM, et al. Determinants of functional outcome after simple and complex acetabular fractures involving the posterior wall. *J Bone Joint Surg Br.* 2006;88(6):776-782.
14. Kamineni S, Morrey BF. Distal humeral fractures treated with noncustom total elbow replacement. *J Bone Joint Surg Am.* 2004;86-A(5):940-947.
15. Giannoudis PV, Grotz MR, Papakostidis C, Dinopoulos H. Operative treatment of displaced fractures of the acetabulum. A meta-analysis. *J Bone Joint Surg Br.* 2005;87(1):2-9.
16. Garland DE, Blum CE, Waters RL. Periarticular heterotopic ossification in head-injured adults. Incidence and location. *J Bone Joint Surg Am.* 1980;62(7):1143-1146.
17. Garland DE, Dowling V. Forearm fractures in the head-injured adult. *Clin Orthop Relat Res.* 1983;176:190-196.
18. Garland DE, O'Hollaren RM. Fractures and dislocations about the elbow in the head-injured adult. *Clin Orthop Relat Res.* 1982;168:38-41.
19. Dias DA. Heterotopic para-articular ossification of the elbow with soft tissue contracture in burns. *Burns Incl Therm Inj.* 1982;9(2):128-134.
20. Brooker AF, Bowerman JW, Robinson RA, Riley LHJ. Ectopic ossification following total hip replacement. Incidence and a method of classification. *J Bone Joint Surg Am.* 1973;55(8):1629-1632.
21. Broberg MA, Morrey BF. Results of treatment of fracture-dislocations of the elbow. *Clin Orthop Relat Res.* 1987;216:109-119.
22. Back DL, Smith JD, Dalziel RE, Young DA, Shimmin A. Incidence of heterotopic ossification after hip resurfacing. *ANZ J Surg.* 2007;77(8):642-647.
23. Ahrengart L. Periarticular heterotopic ossification after total hip arthroplasty. Risk factors and consequences. *Clin Orthop Relat Res.* 1991;263:49-58.
24. Morrey BF, Adams RA, Cabanela ME. Comparison of heterotopic bone after anterolateral, transtrochanteric, and posterior approaches for total hip arthroplasty. *Clin Orthop Relat Res.* 1984;188:160-167.
25. Ozer H, Solak S, Turanli S, Baltaci G, Colakoglu T, Bolukbasi S. Intercondylar fractures of the distal humerus treated with the triceps-reflecting anconeus pedicle approach. *Arch Orthop Trauma Surg.* 2005;125(7):469-474.

26. Kaplan FS, Hahn GV, Zasloff MA. Heterotopic ossification: two rare forms and what they can teach us. *J Am Acad Orthop Surg.* 1994;2(5):288-296.
27. Kaplan FS, McCluskey W, Hahn G, Tabas JA, Muenke M, Zasloff MA. Genetic transmission of fibrodysplasia ossificans progressiva. Report of a family. *J Bone Joint Surg Am.* 1993;75(8):1214-1220.
28. Kaplan FS, Shore EM. Progressive osseous heteroplasia. *J Bone Miner Res.* 2000;15(11):2084-2094.
29. Forsberg JA, Pepek JM, Wagner S, et al. Heterotopic ossification in high-energy wartime extremity injuries: prevalence and risk factors. *J Bone Joint Surg Am.* 2009;91(5):1084-1091.
30. Potter BK, Burns TC, Lacap AP, Granville RR, Gajewski DA. Heterotopic ossification following traumatic and combat-related amputations. Prevalence, risk factors, and preliminary results of excision. *J Bone Joint Surg Am.* 2007;89(3):476-486.
31. Garland DE. Clinical observations on fractures and heterotopic ossification in the spinal cord and traumatic brain injured populations. *Clin Orthop Relat Res.* 1988;233:86-101.
32. Garland DE, Rothi B, Waters RL. Femoral fractures in head-injured adults. *Clin Orthop Relat Res.* 1982;166:219-225.
33. Garland DE, Toder L. Fractures of the tibial diaphysis in adults with head injuries. *Clin Orthop Relat Res.* 1980;150:198-202.
34. Spencer RF. The effect of head injury on fracture healing. A quantitative assessment. *J Bone Joint Surg Br.* 1987;69(4):525-528.
35. Giannoudis PV, Mushtaq S, Harwood P, et al. Accelerated bone healing and excessive callus formation in patients with femoral fracture and head injury. *Injury.* 2006;37(Suppl 3):S18-S24.
36. Cadosch D, Gautschi OP, Thyer M, et al. Humeral factors enhance fracture-healing and callus formation in patients with traumatic brain injury. *J Bone Joint Surg Am.* 2009;91(2):282-288.
37. Steinberg GG, Hubbard C. Heterotopic ossification after femoral intramedullary rodding. *J Orthop Trauma.* 1993;7(6):536-542.
38. Brumback RJ, Wells JD, Lakatos R, Poka A, Bathon GH, Burgess AR. Heterotopic ossification about the hip after intramedullary nailing for fractures of the femur. *J Bone Joint Surg Am.* 1990;72(7):1067-1073.
39. Griffin DB, Beaule PE, Matta JM. Safety and efficacy of the extended iliofemoral approach in the treatment of complex fractures of the acetabulum. *J Bone Joint Surg Br.* 2005;87(10):1391-1396.
40. Oh CW, Kim PT, Park BC, et al. Results after operative treatment of transverse acetabular fractures. *J Orthop Sci.* 2006;11(5):478-484.
41. Petsatodis G, Antonarakos P, Chalidis B, Papadopoulos P, Christoforidis J, Pournaras J. Surgically treated acetabular fractures via a single posterior approach with a follow-up of 2-10 years. *Injury.* 2007;38(3):334-343.
42. Rath EM, Russell GVJ, Washington WJ, Routt MLJ. Gluteus minimus necrotic muscle debridement diminishes heterotopic ossification after acetabular fracture fixation. *Injury.* 2002;33(9):751-756.
43. Schara K, Herman S. Heterotopic bone formation in total hip arthroplasty: predisposing factors, classification and the significance for clinical outcome. *Acta Chir Orthop Traumatol Cech.* 2001;68(2):105-108.
44. Triantaphillopoulos PG, Panagiotopoulos EC, Mousafiris C, Tyllianakis M, Dimakopoulos P, Lambiris EE. Long-term results in surgically treated acetabular fractures through the posterior approaches. *J Trauma.* 2007;62(2):378-382.
45. Lazansky MG. Complications revisited. The debit side of total hip replacement. *Clin Orthop Relat Res.* 1973;95:96-103.
46. Riegler HF, Harris CM. Heterotopic bone formation after total hip arthroplasty. *Clin Orthop Relat Res.* 1976;117:209-216.
47. Ritter MA, Vaughan RB. Ectopic ossification after total hip arthroplasty. Predisposing factors, frequency, and effect on results. *J Bone Joint Surg Am.* 1977;59(3):345-351.
48. Dalury DF, Jiranek WA. The incidence of heterotopic ossification after total knee arthroplasty. *J Arthroplasty.* 2004;19(4):447-452.
49. Shafritz AB, Shore EM, Gannon FH, et al. Overexpression of an osteogenic morphogen in fibrodysplasia ossificans progressiva. *N Engl J Med.* 1996;335(8):555-561.
50. de la Pena LS, Billings PC, Fiori JL, Ahn J, Kaplan FS, Shore EM. Fibrodysplasia ossificans progressiva (fop), a disorder of ectopic osteogenesis, misregulates cell surface expression and trafficking of bmpria. *J Bone Miner Res.* 2005;20(7):1168-1176.
51. Roush W. Protein builds second skeleton. *Science.* 1996;273(5279):1170.
52. Feldman G, Li M, Martin S, et al. Fibrodysplasia ossificans progressiva, a heritable disorder of severe heterotopic ossification, maps to human chromosome 4q27-31. *Am J Hum Genet.* 2000;66(1):128-135.
53. Olmsted-Davis E, Gannon FH, Ozen M, et al. Hypoxic adipocytes pattern early heterotopic bone formation. *Am J Pathol.* 2007;170(2):620-632.
54. Nesti LJ, Jackson WM, Shanti RM, et al. Differentiation potential of multipotent progenitor cells derived from war-traumatized muscle tissue. *J Bone Joint Surg Am.* 2008;90(11):2390-2398.
55. Lounev VY, Ramachandran R, Wosczyna MN, et al. Identification of progenitor cells that contribute to heterotopic skeletogenesis. *J Bone Joint Surg Am.* 2009;91(3):652-663.
56. Burd TA, Lowry KJ, Anglen JO. Indomethacin compared with localized irradiation for the prevention of heterotopic ossification following surgical treatment of acetabular fractures. *J Bone Joint Surg Am.* 2001;83-A(12):1783-1788.
57. Fransen M, Neal B. Non-steroidal anti-inflammatory drugs for preventing heterotopic bone formation after hip arthroplasty. *Cochrane Database Syst Rev.* 2004;3:CD001160.
58. Gregoritch SJ, Chadha M, Pelligrini VD, Rubin P, Kantorowitz DA. Randomized trial comparing preoperative versus postoperative irradiation for prevention of heterotopic ossification following prosthetic total hip replacement: preliminary results. *Int J Radiat Oncol Biol Phys.* 1994;30(1):55-62.
59. Knelles D, Barthel T, Karrer A, Kraus U, Eulert J, Kolbl O. Prevention of heterotopic ossification after total hip replacement. A prospective, randomised study using acetylsalicylic acid, indomethacin and fractional or single-dose irradiation. *J Bone Joint Surg Br.* 1997;79(4):596-602.
60. Kolbl O, Knelles D, Barthel T, Kraus U, Flentje M, Eulert J. Randomized trial comparing early postoperative irradiation vs. the use of nonsteroidal antiinflammatory drugs for prevention of heterotopic ossification following prosthetic total hip replacement. *Int J Radiat Oncol Biol Phys.* 1997;39(5):961-966.
61. Kolbl O, Knelles D, Barthel T, Raunecker F, Flentje M, Eulert J. Preoperative irradiation versus the use of nonsteroidal anti-inflammatory drugs for prevention of heterotopic ossification following total hip replacement: the results of a randomized trial. *Int J Radiat Oncol Biol Phys.* 1998;42(2):397-401.
62. Moore KD, Goss K, Anglen JO. Indomethacin versus radiation therapy for prophylaxis against heterotopic ossification in acetabular fractures: a randomised, prospective study. *J Bone Joint Surg Br.* 1998;80(2):259-263.
63. Pakos EE, Pitouli EJ, Tsekeris PG, Papathanasopoulou V, Stafilas K, Xenakis TH. Prevention of heterotopic ossification in high-risk patients with total hip arthroplasty: the experience of a combined therapeutic protocol. *Int Orthop.* 2006;30(2):79-83.
64. Pellegrini VDJ, Konski AA, Gastel JA, Rubin P, Evarts CM. Prevention of heterotopic ossification with irradiation after total hip arthroplasty. Radiation therapy with a single dose of eight hundred centigray administered to a limited field. *J Bone Joint Surg Am.* 1992;74(2):186-200.

65. Seegenschmiedt MH, Keilholz L, Martus P, et al. Prevention of heterotopic ossification about the hip: final results of two randomized trials in 410 patients using either preoperative or postoperative radiation therapy. *Int J Radiat Oncol Biol Phys.* 1997;39(1):161-171.

66. Sell S, Willms R, Jany R, et al. The suppression of heterotopic ossifications: radiation versus NSAID therapy—a prospective study. *J Arthroplasty.* 1998;13(8):854-859.

67. Matta JM, Siebenrock KA. Does indomethacin reduce heterotopic bone formation after operations for acetabular fractures? A prospective randomised study. *J Bone Joint Surg Br.* 1997;79(6):959-963.

68. Blokhuis TJ, Frolke JP. Is radiation superior to indomethacin to prevent heterotopic ossification in acetabular fractures? A systematic review. *Clin Orthop Relat Res.* 2009;467(2):526-530.

69. Pakos EE, Ioannidis JP. Radiotherapy vs. nonsteroidal anti-inflammatory drugs for the prevention of heterotopic ossification after major hip procedures: a meta-analysis of randomized trials. *Int J Radiat Oncol Biol Phys.* 2004;60(3):888-895.

70. Pacifici M, Cossu G, Molinaro M, Tato F. Vitamin a inhibits chondrogenesis but not myogenesis. *Exp Cell Res.* 1980;129(2):469-474.

71. Shimono K, Morrison TN, Tung WE, et al. Inhibition of ectopic bone formation by a selective retinoic acid receptor alpha-agonist: a new therapy for heterotopic ossification? *J Orthop Res.* 2010;28(2):271-277.

72. Bergenstock M, Min W, Simon AM, Sabatino C, O'Connor JP. A comparison between the effects of acetaminophen and celecoxib on bone fracture healing in rats. *J Orthop Trauma.* 2005;19(10):717-723.

73. Herbenick MA, Sprott D, Stills H, Lawless M. Effects of a cyclooxygenase 2 inhibitor on fracture healing in a rat model. *Am J Orthop.* 2008;37(7):E133-E137.

74. Mullis BH, Copland ST, Weinhold PS, Miclau T, Lester GE, Bos GD. Effect of cox-2 inhibitors and non-steroidal anti-inflammatory drugs on a mouse fracture model. *Injury.* 2006;37(9):827-837.

75. Simon AM, Manigrasso MB, O'Connor JP. Cyclo-oxygenase 2 function is essential for bone fracture healing. *J Bone Miner Res.* 2002;17(6):963-976.

76. Simon AM, O'Connor JP. Dose and time-dependent effects of cyclooxygenase-2 inhibition on fracture-healing. *J Bone Joint Surg Am.* 2007;89(3):500-511.

77. Macfarlane RJ, Ng BH, Gamie Z, et al. Pharmacological treatment of heterotopic ossification following hip and acetabular surgery. *Expert Opin Pharmacother.* 2008;9(5):767-786.

78. O'Connor JP, Lysz T. Celecoxib, NSAIDs and the skeleton. *Drugs Today (Barc).* 2008;44(9):693-709.

79. Banovac K. The effect of etidronate on late development of heterotopic ossification after spinal cord injury. *J Spinal Cord Med.* 2000;23(1):40-44.

80. Banovac K, Gonzalez F, Renfree KJ. Treatment of heterotopic ossification after spinal cord injury. *J Spinal Cord Med.* 1997;20(1):60-65.

81. Banovac K, Gonzalez F, Wade N, Bowker JJ. Intravenous disodium etidronate therapy in spinal cord injury patients with heterotopic ossification. *Paraplegia.* 1993;31(10):660-666.

82. Spielman G, Gennarelli TA, Rogers CR. Disodium etidronate: Its role in preventing heterotopic ossification in severe head injury. *Arch Phys Med Rehabil.* 1983;64(11):539-542.

83. Finerman GA, Stover SL. Heterotopic ossification following hip replacement or spinal cord injury. Two clinical studies with ehdp. *Metab Bone Dis Relat Res.* 1981;3(4-5):337-342.

84. Stover SL, Niemann KM, Miller JM. Disodium etidronate in the prevention of postoperative recurrence of heterotopic ossification in spinal-cord injury patients. *J Bone Joint Surg Am.* 1976;58(5):683-688.

85. Garland DE, Alday B, Venos KG, Vogt JC. Diphosphonate treatment for heterotopic ossification in spinal cord injury patients. *Clin Orthop Relat Res.* 1983;176:197-200.

86. Hu HP, Kuijpers W, Slooff TJ, van Horn JR, Versleyen DH. The effect of biphosphonate on induced heterotopic bone. *Clin Orthop Relat Res.* 1991;272:259-267.

87. Thomas BJ, Amstutz HC. Results of the administration of diphosphonate for the prevention of heterotopic ossification after total hip arthroplasty. *J Bone Joint Surg Am.* 1985;67(3):400-403.

88. Haran M, Bhuta T, Lee B. Pharmacological interventions for treating acute heterotopic ossification. *Cochrane Database Syst Rev.* 2004;4:CD003321.

89. Ebraheim NA, Patil V, Liu J, Haman SP. Sliding trochanteric osteotomy in acetabular fractures: a review of 30 cases. *Injury.* 2007;38(10):1177-1182.

90. Grohs JG, Schmidt M, Wanivenhaus A. Selective cox-2 inhibitor versus indomethacin for the prevention of heterotopic ossification after hip replacement: a double-blind randomized trial of 100 patients with 1-year follow-up. *Acta Orthop.* 2007;78(1):95-98.

91. Higo T, Mawatari M, Shigematsu M, Hotokebuchi T. The incidence of heterotopic ossification after cementless total hip arthroplasty. *J Arthroplasty.* 2006;21(6):852-856.

92. Kasetti RJ, Shetty AA, Rand C. Heterotopic ossification after uncemented hydroxyapatite-coated primary total hip arthroplasty. *J Arthroplasty.* 2001;16(8):1038-1042.

93. Saudan M, Saudan P, Perneger T, Riand N, Keller A, Hoffmeyer P. Celecoxib versus ibuprofen in the prevention of heterotopic ossification following total hip replacement: a prospective randomised trial. *J Bone Joint Surg Br.* 2007;89(2):155-159.

94. van der Heide HJ, Rijnberg WJ, Van Sorge A, Van Kampen A, Schreurs BW. Similar effects of rofecoxib and indomethacin on the incidence of heterotopic ossification after hip arthroplasty. *Acta Orthop.* 2007;78(1):90-94.

95. Hendricks HT, Geurts AC, van Ginneken BC, Heeren AJ, Vos PE. Brain injury severity and autonomic dysregulation accurately predict heterotopic ossification in patients with traumatic brain injury. *Clin Rehabil.* 2007;21(6):545-553.

96. Potter BK, Granville RR, Bagg MR, et al. Special surgical considerations for the combat casualty with limb loss. In: Pasquina CR, ed. *Rehabilitation of Combat Casualties With Limb Loss.* Washington, DC: Borden Institute, 2008:153-190.

97. Ehde DM, Smith DG. Chronic pain management. In: Smith DG, Michael JW, Bowker JH, eds. *Atlas of Amputations and Limb Deficiencies: Surgical, Prosthetic, and Rehabilitation Principles.* 3rd ed. Rosemont, IL: American Academy of Orthopaedic Surgeons; 2004:711-726.

98. Furman R, Nicholas JJ, Jivoff L. Elevation of the serum alkaline phosphatase coincident with ectopic-bone formation in paraplegic patients. *J Bone Joint Surg Am.* 1970;52(6):1131-1137.

99. Hsu JD, Sakimura I, Stauffer ES. Heterotopic ossification around the hip joint in spinal cord injured patients. *Clin Orthop Relat Res.* 1975;112:165-169.

100. Pittenger DE. Heterotopic ossification. *Orthop Rev.* 1991;20(1):33-39.

101. Beingessner DM, Patterson SD, King GJ. Early excision of heterotopic bone in the forearm. *J Hand Surg [Am].* 2000;25(3):483-488.

102. Chalidis B, Stengel D, Giannoudis PV. Early excision and late excision of heterotopic ossification after traumatic brain injury are equivalent: a systematic review of the literature. *J Neurotrauma.* 2007;24(11):1675-1686.

103. Ellerin BE, Helfet D, Parikh S, et al. Current therapy in the management of heterotopic ossification of the elbow: a review with case studies. *Am J Phys Med Rehabil.* 1999;78(3):259-271.

104. Freebourn TM, Barber DB, Able AC. The treatment of immature heterotopic ossification in spinal cord injury with combination surgery, radiation therapy and NSAID. *Spinal Cord.* 1999;37(1):50-53.

105. Garland DE, Orwin JF. Resection of heterotopic ossification in patients with spinal cord injuries. *Clin Orthop Relat Res.* 1989;242:169-176.

106. McAuliffe JA, Wolfson AH. Early excision of heterotopic ossification about the elbow followed by radiation therapy. *J Bone Joint Surg Am.* 1997;79(5):749-755.

107. Mitsionis GI, Lykissas MG, Kalos N, et al. Functional outcome after excision of heterotopic ossification about the knee in ICU patients. *Int Orthop.* 2009;33(6):1619-1625.

108. Moritomo H, Tada K, Yoshida T. Early, wide excision of heterotopic ossification in the medial elbow. *J Shoulder Elbow Surg.* 2001;10(2):164-168.

109. Tsionos I, Leclercq C, Rochet JM. Heterotopic ossification of the elbow in patients with burns. Results after early excision. *J Bone Joint Surg Br.* 2004;86(3):396-403.

110. Viola RW, Hanel DP. Early "simple" release of posttraumatic elbow contracture associated with heterotopic ossification. *J Hand Surg [Am].* 1999;24(2):370-380.

111. Wysocki RW, Cohen MS. Radioulnar heterotopic ossification after distal biceps tendon repair: results following surgical resection. *J Hand Surg [Am].* 2007;32(8):1230-1236.

Chapter **11**

IRRIGATION AND DEBRIDEMENT

MAJ Scott Waterman, MD; CDR Mark E. Fleming, DO; and
LTC Brett D. Owens, MD

As with previous conflicts, open extremity wounds sustained in Operation Enduring Freedom (OEF) and Operation Iraqi Freedom (OIF) require irrigation and debridement. Improvements in the evacuation process and forward deployment of surgical units have allowed for more rapid surgical intervention, often within 1 hour of sustaining the injury.[1] US servicemembers who sustain open wounds typically undergo irrigation and debridement prior to skeletal stabilization with external fixation, if required, before evacuation from the theater of operation to reduce the chance of developing wound infection.

Several factors influence the development of wound infections in the wounded warrior, including the size and severity of the wounds, the quantity of dead tissue present within the wound, and the presence of foreign material. When nonviable tissue or foreign matter is present within a war wound, irrigation and debridement combined with early antibiotic administration and tetanus prophylaxis can significantly reduce the risk of wound infection. The goals of irrigation and debridement are removal of foreign material, detection and removal of nonviable tissue, reduction of bacterial contamination, and the creation of a healthy wound bed. With a greater amount of necrotic tissue and foreign material within a wound, there is a greater likelihood of infection. Nonviable tissue serves as a medium for bacterial proliferation. Initial combat-related wounds are typically contaminated with gram-positive bacteria with more multi-drug-resistant gram-negative bacteria contaminating the wound further along in the evacuation process.[1,2] One of the central tenets of war wound management

is to never primarily close a war wound. War wounds are contaminated, and early wound closure frequently results in the development of frank purulence with deleterious effects on limb viability and long-term outcome.[3]

Epidemiology

During OEF and OIF, 36,757 servicemembers have been injured, and 5380 have died.[4] Of this total, 46% to 54% of injuries sustained involve the extremities.[5,6] While the highest profile extremity injuries of this conflict are open tibia fracture and traumatic amputations and a majority of wounds are in the lower extremity, 40% of injuries sustained are in the upper extremity.[5] Almost 68% to 87% of all injuries sustained are from an explosive mechanism.[5,7,8]

Basic Science Research

While debridement was first described by Desault in the 18th century,[9] irrigation and debridement has evolved to become the standard treatment for open wounds sustained in both civilian and military settings. While irrigation and debridement has been performed for almost 2 centuries, many of the principles that are currently taught have had limited basic science or clinical research supporting their use. These include the need for surgical treatment within 6 hours of injury, irrigation with 10 L of irrigant, the use of high-pressure lavage, as well as the use of antibiotics and antiseptics in the irrigant. Recently, many of these

Owens BD, Belmont PJ Jr, eds. *Combat Orthopedic Surgery: Lessons Learned in Iraq and Afghanistan* (pp 93-100)
© 2011 SLACK Incorporated

teachings on irrigation have been tested using a novel large animal contaminated fracture model developed at the US Army Institute of Surgical Research.[10] This model uses a bioluminescent bacteria that allows for real-time quantitative assessment of wound bacterial counts (Figure 11-1). There has been considerably less research on the quality or quantity of debridement, as this can be challenging to measure in a scientific manner. The teaching on debridement has focused on the removal of all foreign and necrotic debris and the four Cs: contractility, color, consistency, and capacity to bleed.[11]

Wound Assessment/ Debridement

Not all wounds require surgical debridement and irrigation. No specific guidelines exist, and clinical judgment must be used to determine which wounds require operative intervention versus nonoperative management.

Superficial fragment wounds typically will not require surgical intervention. Bowyer published a series of 83 casualties who sustained 1200 fragment wounds in Afghanistan. A series of 850 small-fragment wounds affecting only the skin and muscle were treated nonoperatively with only 2 patients developing localized abscesses.[12] The wounds that were considered for nonoperative management were classified according to the Red Cross wound classification as grade 1 type ST (small, simple, soft tissue wounds) without fracture or vascular involvement or breach of the perineum or pleura. The nonoperative management consisted of cleansing and dressing the wound and administering IV antibiotics. Surgeons should resist the temptation to perform surgery in an attempt to remove all small fragments.[13,14]

Civilian literature suggests that selected low-energy small arms gunshot wounds can be managed nonoperatively. A series of studies from a US-based, busy Level I trauma center reported on their management of minor gunshot wounds and rate of infection. In this study of more than 3300 patients, 62 developed wound infections.[15] Only 1% underwent local debridement. These authors suggested that wound debridement and antibiotics are often unnecessary unless the wounds are grossly contaminated, are large, have significant tissue devitalization, or had a delay in treatment.

Timing of Operative Procedure

Traditionally, irrigation and debridement has been recommended within 6 hours of sustaining open frac-

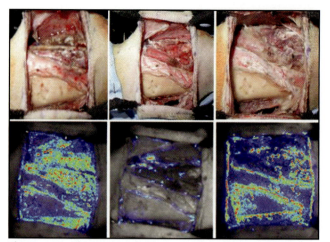

Figure 11-1. This series of images was taken from the bioluminescent large animal model used in quantifying the bacterial load in contaminated wounds. The top images are gross photographs, and the bottom images are the corresponding coupled photon-captured images in the following order: pre-irrigation, immediate post-irrigation, and 48 hours post-irrigation.

tures. This 6-hour timeframe is based on the time at which biofilm formation begins, with maturation of biofilm at 10 hours. Biofilm formation decreases the effectiveness of host defenses and increases bacterial antibiotic resistance.[16,17] Bacteria may develop a biofilm that can essentially shield them from the host defenses or antibiotics as early as 5 hours after inoculation. Timing of surgical intervention in a combat environment is dependent on the duration of evacuation and the quantity of servicemembers injured. There have been limited studies evaluating timing of intervention in combat-related injuries, which are distinct from civilian trauma secondary to the mechanism and severity of injury. Testing in a caprine open fracture model demonstrated improved bacterial clearance with earlier surgical intervention with significant difference comparing surgery at 70% of baseline bacterial count at 3 hours, 52% at 6 hours, and 37% at 12 hours.[18] Current civilian clinical literature has been mixed, but a recent study noted that the severity of injury is more of a factor than timing of surgical intervention.[19-22] A recent study by Pollak and colleagues suggests that the time from injury to operative debridement is not a significant independent predictor of the risk of infection.[23] This study evaluated 315 patients who sustained severe high-energy lower extremity injuries and underwent aggressive debridement, antibiotic administration, fracture stabilization, and timely soft tissue coverage. A total of 27% developed an infection, and time to surgery was not a factor. Another study that evaluated the effect of time on the rate of infection of open fractures reviewed 227 patients with 241 open long-bone fractures in which 20 patients developed a deep infection.[20] This study found that, up to

13 hours from the time of injury to surgical intervention, there was no increased rate of infection when early prophylactic antibiotics were administered. This differs from 3 combat-related case series, with the American experience in Somalia and Panama and the British experience in the Falkland Campaign, delayed evacuation was necessary, which both showed increased infections following delay of more than 6 hours.[24-26] All of these studies are retrospective, and there are no prospective studies on combat injuries.

With mixed clinical results in infection rates for wounds treated before or after 6 hours and an animal study suggesting increased difficulty with bacterial eradication at time points further out from wound inoculation, irrigation and debridement should be undertaken as soon as possible.[1]

Irrigant

The austere conditions and remoteness encountered by some units in Iraq and Afghanistan often do not offer the sterile conditions or readily available supplies available in civilian trauma centers. This necessitated the investigation of alternative irrigants and additives. Svoboda and colleagues noted no differences in bacterial burden after irrigation with potable water and sterile saline in a caprine model, offering an alternative when sterile fluid is not available.[27] These findings were further supported by a randomized clinical trial comparing tap water and sterile saline for lacerations and noted no difference in infection rates.[28] Anglen studied the use of Castile soap and noted a decrease in culture-positive *Staphylococcus aureus*.[29,30] Another study showed Castile soap to have a rebound in bacterial quantity above baseline at 48 hours post-debridement.[31] In this same study, benzalkonium chloride and bacitracin solution irrigation were noted to have a more significant rebound when compared to normal saline. Conroy and colleagues also noted increased wound complications when treating *Pseudomonas aeruginosa* with benzalkonium chloride.[30] Anglen, in a clinical study, compared Castile soap with bacitracin solution and noted no difference in infection rate, but noted a significantly increased risk of wound healing problems with the bacitracin solution.[30] This study unfortunately did not have a normal saline group for comparison. Bhandari evaluated multiple additives, ethanol, povidone-iodine, chlorhexidine gluconate, liquid soap, and bacitracin in a mice calvarial model and noted a decrease in osteoblast and osteoclast viability compared with saline.[32] With mixed results often showing improved initial results and both bac-

terial rebound and wound healing problems, irrigation with normal saline (or potable water if sterile saline is not available) is currently recommended and used in Iraq and Afghanistan, Landstuhl, and Echelon V military treatment facilities in the continental United States.[1,33]

Method of Delivery

There are multiple methods of irrigation, which include bulb syringe, gravity flow, pulse lavage, and parallel flow irrigation. The optimal delivery system has yet to be determined. Bulb syringe was compared to gravity flow, and there was no difference between the bacterial count or wound healing.[34,35] Bulb syringe and pulse lavage have been compared in multiple studies with mixed results. The initial studies documented that pulse lavage initially cleared more bacteria than bulb syringe with less quantity of irrigation.[10,36-38] In the same model, Owens and colleagues noted a significant rebound to almost initial bacterial level in the pulse lavage group, which was not seen in the bulb syringe group.[31] Other studies have documented that irrigation with high-pressure pulse lavage resulted in increased wound tissue, increased residual inorganic tissue, damage to bone and fracture healing, and deeper penetration of bacteria following treatment.[36,39-42] Recently, a parallel flow irrigation system was introduced with a few animal studies and comparative clinical trials.[43] Lalliss and colleagues noted that this device was able to remove more bacteria with less volume when compared to bulb syringe.[44] The vast majority of these studies are completed in animal models, and there is not a well-done clinical study comparing these options. With studies demonstrating mixed results using high-pressure pulse lavage and limited studies on the parallel flow irrigation system, low-pressure irrigation, between 1 and 15 psi, is currently recommended.[1]

Volume

As with the irrigant and delivery device, this area is poorly researched. Irrigation volume has empirically recommended 3 L for grade 1 fractures, 6 L for grade 2 fractures, and 9 L for grade 3 fractures.[33,45] There have been multiple small animal studies evaluating fluid quantity, which are difficult to extrapolate to humans.[46,47] To obtain the same amount of bacterial clearance using a large animal model requires 9 L of irrigant via bulb syringe, 3 L via pulse lavage, and 1.25 L via parallel flow irrigation.[10,31,44]

Clinical Recommendations

IN THEATER

Initial extremity surgical care is provided by forward surgical teams and combat support hospitals, which focuses on damage control surgery.[48] The wounded warrior should be initially assessed in the triage process. Care should be initiated with the overall assessment per the *Emergency War Surgery* and Advance Trauma Life Support protocol.[48,49] The orthopedic procedure begins with the evaluation of the extremity wounds to assess the number, severity, and contamination of all wounds. A tourniquet should be applied and may be used to limit exsanguination in patients with massive wounds and prevent further blood loss.[8] Incisions should be made through skin, and possibly fascia, in line proximally to distally in line with the long axis of the extremity to allow for exposure of the depth of the wounds and debridement. Debridement should be performed from superficial to deep to remove all necrotic debris, nonviable tissue, and readily removable foreign material. Multiple incisions to locate small fragments should be avoided. Pre- and post-debridement cultures are not routinely obtained at the lower echelon facilities, with good evidence to support a recommendation against its use.[1]

Only nonviable skin edges should be excised to preserve length.[48] Vital structures, such as nerves and vascular structures, should be identified and protected. Debridement should include excision of nonviable subcutaneous fat and muscle. Muscle viability is assessed by the capacity of the muscle to bleed and its color, consistency, and ability to contract. Contractility can be assessed by using electrocautery or pinching the muscle with a forceps. The clinical utility of the characteristics of muscle viability has been evaluated.[50] The rationale for excision of nonviable muscle is to minimize the risk of infection by decreasing the contamination. Encountered foreign debris should be removed.

WOUNDS INVOLVING FRACTURES

Bone fragments without soft tissue attachments can essentially serve as a nidus for infection. Therefore, all unattached bone fragments should be removed. If the periosteum appears viable, preservation may facilitate later bony healing.

WOUNDS INVOLVING AMPUTATIONS

The principles remain the same. However, surgeons should avoid the temptation to excise what appears to be excess tissue. If the tissue appears viable, it may be preserved and used as a fillet flap.[51,52]

IRRIGATION

Following debridement, irrigation should be performed within 6 hours, if possible, for open wounds. Irrigation with normal saline or potable water, when sterile water is unavailable, should follow Anglen recommendations of 3 L for grade 1 fractures, 6 L for grade 2 fractures, and 9 L for grade 3 fractures using bulb syringe or gravity flow. Irrigation and debridement should be followed with fracture stabilization as needed. The wounds should be left open and covered with sterile dressings. Repeat irrigation and debridements should be repeated every 48 to 72 hours.

ECHELON V

After evacuation from the theater of conflict and treatment at Landstuhl Regional Medical Center, the wounded warriors are received at multiple Echelon V facilities, having undergone irrigation and debridement every 48 to 72 hours since injury. Many of the same techniques used in theater continued to be applied once the patient arrives in the continental United States. All wounded warriors should undergo a tertiary survey assessing the patient's overall status and assessing each wound individually on arrival. As expected, wounds caused by high-energy mechanisms with large amounts of contamination typically "progress." Despite a perceived or reportedly adequate initial debridement, the receiving surgeon should thoroughly reassess the wounds and perform repeat irrigation and debridement as needed. Many of the wounds are being treated with negative pressure wound therapy, and these dressings are typically removed in the operating room prior to irrigation and debridement the day after transfer. A tourniquet should be applied to the affected extremity, but it is infrequently used. Debridement commences with an evaluation of all tissues from superficial to deep to include skin, subcutaneous fat, fascia, and muscle, making sure to protect all vital structures.

Illustrative Case Presentation

Figures 11-2 through 11-6 illustrate a large surface area soft tissue wound requiring multiple irrigation and debridements. Due to the appearance of the initial wound upon presentation to an Echelon V facility, pre-debridement cultures were obtained, revealing the presence of mold as well as gram-negative bacteria. Initial debridement required the excision of more than 1 kg of nonviable soft tissue. Figures 11-3

Figure 11-2. Initial pre-debridement of wound on residual limb.

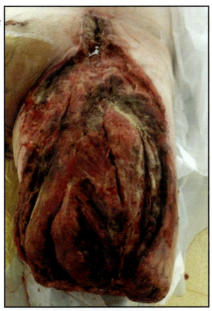

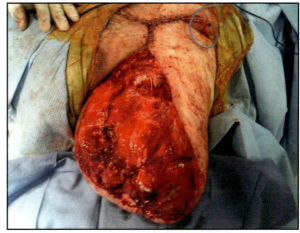

Figure 11-4. Post-debridement wound following V-Y advancement.

Figure 11-5. Wound following placement of Integra.

Figure 11-3. Post-debridement wound following excision of necrotic tissue.

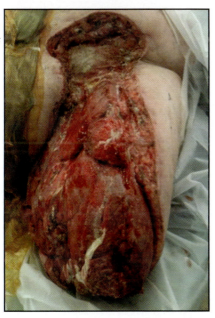

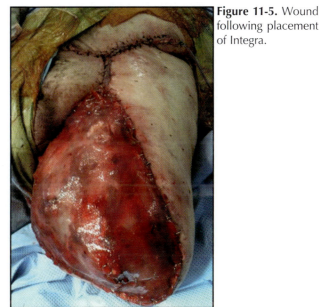

Figure 11-6. Wound following split-thickness skin grafting.

through 11-6 reveal repeated irrigations and debridements followed by coverage with Integra (Integra LifeSciences, Plainsboro, NJ) and eventual split-thickness skin grafts.

Conclusion

Irrigation and debridement of combat-related injuries remains a mainstay of treatment to decrease the incidence of infection. Current animal research and clinical literature have reported mixed results with regard to the type, volume, and method of irrigation, as well as timing of surgery. Open combat wounds and fractures should be irrigated and

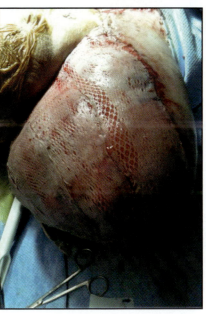

debrided as soon as possible to decrease bacterial adherence and biofilm formation. Debridement should focus on the surgical removal of necrotic tissue, easily removable foreign bodies, and decreasing bacterial burden. Low-pressure irrigation with normal saline or potable water should also be performed to aid debridement.

References

1. Adib N, Davies K, Grahame R, Woo P, Murray KJ. Joint hypermobility syndrome in childhood. A not so benign multisystem disorder? *Rheumatology (Oxford)*. 2005;44:744-750.

2. Aronson NE, Sanders JW, Moran KA. In harm's way: infections in deployed American military forces. *Clin Infect Dis*. 2006;43:1045-1051.

3. Coupland RM, Howell PR. An experience of war surgery and wounds presenting after 3 days on the border of Afghanistan. *Injury*. 1988;19:259-262.

4. Anderson JM. Multinucleated giant cells. *Curr Opin Hematol*. 2000;7:40-47.

5. Masini BD, Waterman SM, Wenke JC, Owens BD, Hsu JR, Ficke JR. Resource utilization and disability outcome assessment of combat casualties from Operation Iraqi Freedom and Operation Enduring Freedom. *J Orthop Trauma*. 2009;23:261-266.

6. Owens BD, Kragh JF Jr, Macaitis J, Svoboda SJ, Wenke JC. Characterization of extremity wounds in Operation Iraqi Freedom and Operation Enduring Freedom. *J Orthop Trauma*. 2007;21:254-257.

7. Belmont PJ Jr, Goodman GP, Zacchilli M, Posner M, Evans C, Owens BD. Incidence and epidemiology of combat injuries sustained during "the surge" portion of operation Iraqi Freedom by a U.S. Army brigade combat team. *J Trauma*. 2010;68:204-210.

8. Owens BD, Kragh JF Jr, Wenke JC, Macaitis J, Wade CE, Holcomb JB. Combat wounds in Operation Iraqi Freedom and Operation Enduring Freedom. *J Trauma*. 2008;64:295-299.

9. Helling TS, Daon E. In Flanders fields: the Great War, Antoine Depage, and the resurgence of debridement. *Ann Surg*. 1998;228:173-181.

10. Owens BD, Wenke JC, Svoboda SJ, White DW. Extremity trauma research in the United States Army. *J Am Acad Orthop Surg*. 2006;14:S37-S40.

11. Simovitch R, Sanders B, Ozbaydar M, Lavery K, Warner JJ. Acromioclavicular joint injuries: diagnosis and management. *J Am Acad Orthop Surg*. 2009;17:207-219.

12. Bowyer GW. Management of small fragment wounds: experience from the Afghan border. *J Trauma*. 1996;40:S170-S172.

13. Coupland RM. Hand grenade injuries among civilians. *JAMA*. 1993;270:624-626.

14. Covey DC, Lurate RB, Hatton CT. Field hospital treatment of blast wounds of the musculoskeletal system during the Yugoslav civil war. *J Orthop Trauma*. 2000;14:278-286; discussion 277.

15. Ordog GJ, Sheppard GF, Wasserberger JS, Balasubramanium S, Shoemaker WC. Infection in minor gunshot wounds. *J Trauma*. 1993;34:358-365.

16. Gristina AG, Naylor PT, Myrvik QN. Mechanisms of musculoskeletal sepsis. *Orthop Clin North Am*. 1991;22:363-371.

17. Harrison-Balestra C, Cazzaniga AL, Davis SC, Mertz PM. A wound-isolated Pseudomonas aeruginosa grows a biofilm in vitro within 10 hours and is visualized by light microscopy. *Dermatol Surg*. 2003;29:631-635.

18. Owens BD, Wenke JC. Early wound irrigation improves the ability to remove bacteria. *J Bone Joint Surg Am*. 2007;89:1723-1726.

19. Bednar DA, Parikh J. Effect of time delay from injury to primary management on the incidence of deep infection after open fractures of the lower extremities caused by blunt trauma in adults. *J Orthop Trauma*. 1993;7:532-535.

20. Harley BJ, Beaupre LA, Jones CA, Dulai SK, Weber DW. The effect of time to definitive treatment on the rate of nonunion and infection in open fractures. *J Orthop Trauma*. 2002;16: 484-490.

21. Khatod M, Botte MJ, Hoyt DB, Meyer RS, Smith JM, Akeson WH. Outcomes in open tibia fractures: relationship between delay in treatment and infection. *J Trauma*. 2003;55:949-954.

22. Patzakis MJ, Wilkins J. Factors influencing infection rate in open fracture wounds. *Clin Orthop Relat Res*. 1989;243:36-40.

23. Pollak AN, Jones AL, Castillo RC, Bosse MJ, MacKenzie EJ. The relationship between time to surgical debridement and incidence of infection after open high-energy lower extremity trauma. *J Bone Joint Surg Am*. 2010;92:7-15.

24. Jacob E, Erpelding JM, Murphy KP. A retrospective analysis of open fractures sustained by U.S. military personnel during Operation Just Cause. *Mil Med*. 1992;157:552-556.

25. Mabry RL, Holcomb JB, Baker AM, et al. United States Army Rangers in Somalia: an analysis of combat casualties on an urban battlefield. *J Trauma*. 2000;49:515-528; discussion 528-529.

26. Mishra MB, Ryan P, Atkinson P, et al. Extra-articular features of benign joint hypermobility syndrome. *Br J Rheumatol*. 1996;35:861-866.

27. Svoboda SJ, Owens BD, Gooden HA, Melvin ML, Baer DG, Wenke JC. Irrigation with potable water versus normal saline in a contaminated musculoskeletal wound model. *J Trauma*. 2008;64:1357-1359.

28. Moscati RM, Mayrose J, Reardon RF, Janicke DM, Jehle DV. A multicenter comparison of tap water versus sterile saline for wound irrigation. *Acad Emerg Med*. 2007;14:404-409.

29. Anglen JO. Comparison of soap and antibiotic solutions for irrigation of lower-limb open fracture wounds. A prospective, randomized study. *J Bone Joint Surg Am*. 2005;87:1415-1422.

30. Conroy BP, Anglen JO, Simpson WA, et al. Comparison of castile soap, benzalkonium chloride, and bacitracin as irrigation solutions for complex contaminated orthopedic wounds. *J Orthop Trauma*. 1999;13:332-337.

31. Owens BD, White DW, Wenke JC. Comparison of irrigation solutions and devices in a contaminated musculoskeletal wound survival model. *J Bone Joint Surg Am*. 2009;91:92-98.

32. Bhandari M, Adili A, Schemitsch EH. The efficacy of low-pressure lavage with different irrigating solutions to remove adherent bacteria from bone. *J Bone Joint Surg Am*. 2001;83-A:412-419.

33. Hospenthal DR, Murray CK, Andersen RC, et al. Guidelines for the prevention of infection after combat-related injuries. *J Trauma*. 2008;64:S211-S220.

34. Brown GA, Tan JL, Kirkley A. The lax shoulder in females. Issues, answers, but many more questions. *Clin Orthop Relat Res*. 2000;372:110-122.

35. Hamer ML, Robson MC, Krizek TJ, Southwick WO. Quantitative bacterial analysis of comparative wound irrigations. *Ann Surg*. 1975;181:819-822.

36. Bhandari M, Schemitsch EH, Adili A, Lachowski RJ, Shaughnessy SG. High and low pressure pulsatile lavage of contaminated tibial fractures: an in vitro study of bacterial adherence and bone damage. *J Orthop Trauma*. 1999;13:526-533.

37. Keblish DJ, DeMaio M. Early pulsatile lavage for the decontamination of combat wounds: historical review and point proposal. *Mil Med*. 1998;163:844-846.

38. Moussa FW, Gainor BJ, Anglen JO, Christensen G, Simpson WA. Disinfecting agents for removing adherent bacteria from orthopedic hardware. *Clin Orthop Relat Res*. 1996;329:255-262.

39. Boyd JI 3rd, Wongworawat MD. High-pressure pulsatile lavage causes soft tissue damage. *Clin Orthop Relat Res.* 2004;427: 13-17.

40. Dirschl DR, Duff GP, Dahners LE, Edin M, Rahn BA, Miclau T. High pressure pulsatile lavage irrigation of intraarticular fractures: effects on fracture healing. *J Orthop Trauma.* 1998;12:460-463.

41. Draeger RW, Dahners LE. Traumatic wound debridement: a comparison of irrigation methods. *J Orthop Trauma.* 2006;20:83-88.

42. Hassinger SM, Harding G, Wongworawat MD. High-pressure pulsatile lavage propagates bacteria into soft tissue. *Clin Orthop Relat Res.* 2005;439:27-31.

43. Sainsbury DC. Evaluation of the quality and cost-effectiveness of Versajet hydrosurgery. *Int Wound J.* 2009;6:24-29.

44. Lalliss SJ, Wenke JC, Branstetter J. High pressure parallel flow and bulb syringe irrigation in a bioluminescent wound model. In American Academy of Orthopedic Surgeons 2008 Annual Meeting. San Francisco, CA, 2008.

45. Anglen JO. Wound irrigation in musculoskeletal injury. *J Am Acad Orthop Surg.* 2001;9:219-226.

46. Gainor BJ, Hockman DE, Anglen JO, Christensen G, Simpson WA. Benzalkonium chloride: a potential disinfecting irrigation solution. *J Orthop Trauma.* 1997;11:121-125.

47. Peterson LW. Prophylaxis of wound infection: studies with particular reference to soaps and irrigation. *Arch Surg.* 1945;50: 177-183.

48. Szul AC, Davis LB, Walter Reed Army Medical Center Borden Institute, eds. *Emergency War Surgery.* 3rd US rev. Washington, DC: Walter Reed Army Medical Center Borden Institute; 2004.

49. American College of Surgeons. *Advanced Trauma Life Support for Doctors Student Course Manual.* 8th ed. Chicago, IL: Author; 2008.

50. Crockett HC, Gross LB, Wilk KE, et al. Osseous adaptation and range of motion at the glenohumeral joint in professional baseball pitchers. *Am J Sports Med.* 2002;30:20-26.

51. Kasabian AK, Glat PM, Eidelman Y, et al. Salvage of traumatic below-knee amputation stumps utilizing the filet of foot free flap: critical evaluation of six cases. *Plast Reconstr Surg.* 1995;96:1145-1153.

52. Kuntscher MV, Erdmann D, Homann HH, Steinau HU, Levin SL, Germann G. The concept of fillet flaps: classification, indications, and analysis of their clinical value. *Plast Reconstr Surg.* 2001;108:885-896.

Chapter 12

TISSUE ENGINEERING AND REGENERATION

LCDR Jared A. Vogler, DO; Wesley Jackson, PhD; and
MAJ Leon J. Nesti, MD, PhD

As with previous large-scale military conflicts, the recent campaigns in Iraq and Afghanistan have led to advances in medical science. The treatment of complex injury patterns encountered in these wars, arguably the most severe yet survivable injuries ever sustained in combat, coupled with seemingly fictional technology has resulted in what many may deem a medical marvel. These wars will likely be characteristic of future military conflicts in terms of scope, tactics, strategies, and casualties, and the difficulty in treating these complex injury patterns will no doubt pressure the medical community to continue to make advances in treatment options.

Unprecedented battlefield survivability has been heralded as one of the many medical success stories emerging from the current wars, and it is the result of advancements on many fronts. Today's servicemember goes into battle wearing body armor and a uniform that is second to none: improved, lightweight Kevlar (DuPont, Wilmington, DE) helmet; ballistic eye protection; high-collared flak vest with groin protector; protective ceramic insert shielding vital structures of the torso; and fire-resistant, breathable clothing are some of the key features in these uniforms. Additionally, the first aid kit is complete with battle-tested tourniquets and hemostatic agents, and servicemembers trained in rendering basic life-saving procedures are often at the scene of injury to provide immediate care. The "golden hour" that revolutionized civilian emergency medicine has been brought to the battlefield, resulting in a highly effective medical evacuation (MEDEVAC) system capable of transporting the critically wounded to well-placed medical support units able to provide care in incrementally more advanced levels—the next

higher echelon of care. Once stabilized, the MEDEVAC system continues to transport the injured out of theater to facilities capable of definitive care. From the personal protective equipment issued to the soldiers to the advanced medical systems designed for their care after injury, those injured on the battlefield have a much higher likelihood of survival.

The higher battlefield survival rate leads to a higher number of patients with severe, complex extremity wounds.[1] Now that servicemembers are surviving what were previously thought to be lethal injuries, a host of new, complex, traumatic wounds have resulted in significant functional limitations and decreased quality of life for a number of young, highly active people. To treat these complex wounds, surgeons rely on fundamental wound care strategies augmented with novel treatment options and technology (Figure 12-1).

The human body's incredible capacity to repair and regenerate damaged musculoskeletal tissue is overwhelmed by the injuries sustained on the battlefield. Hence, there is an immediate need for tissue repair, regeneration, and replacement strategies (ie, the fields of tissue engineering and regenerative medicine). Unfortunately, many of these strategies are still in the experimental or design phase. As with much of the biological sciences, tissue engineering and regenerative medicine has seen incredible growth during the past decade. Many theories once thought fanciful are now being tested, and many devices once thought theoretical are now being constructed. Undoubtedly, this is an exciting time to be at the scientific frontier, especially when that frontier lies at the intersection of biology, engineering, chemistry, physics, and medicine: tissue engineering and regenerative medicine.

Owens BD, Belmont PJ Jr, eds. ***Combat Orthopedic Surgery:***
Lessons Learned in Iraq and Afghanistan (pp 101-108)
© 2011 SLACK Incorporated

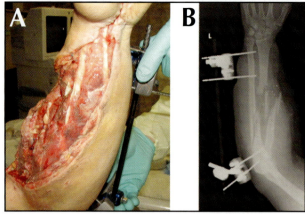

Figure 12-1. Traumatic war wound. Extremity war injuries in the recent military conflicts are a result of high-energy injuries and often include damage to multiple tissue types (ie, bone, muscle, tendon, fat, cartilage, vessels, nerves).

Current Surgical Options for Tissue Defects

All fractures with severe soft tissue injury require the same treatment course: re-establishment of stability, adequate soft tissue coverage with an adequate blood supply, and a barrier against infection. Traditionally, these processes begin with internal or external fixation to achieve skeletal stability followed by varying degrees of reconstruction, proportionate to the wound severity, to achieve sufficient soft tissue coverage and subsequent skin coverage. As a means of discussing wound management, we use a concept popularized by Levin: the "reconstructive ladder."[2] This treatment paradigm begins with a respect and recognition for the "soft tissue envelope," multiple and distinct tissue layers surrounding the skeleton.

The most superficial layer, the skin, is composed of an epidermal layer and a deeper dermis. It is important to note that violation of this layer defines an open fracture, and therefore restoration of the skin's proper function and assurance of its integrity must be appreciated as a major goal of soft tissue management. Skin's unique properties allow it to be harvested and grafted on nearly any body surface with sufficient vascularity, but often traumatic war wounds do not provide such an environment. Skin closure, whether through primary or secondary means, or via a skin graft, is the most basic step on the reconstructive ladder. Conventional bandages attempt to function as a temporary "skin" to retain moisture and resist infection, often with disappointing results. Recently, materials engineered with the needs of the tissue in mind closed the gap between native skin and temporary dressings by maintaining more moisture and providing a better barrier to infection. Examples of these

newer "biological dressings" include Integra (Integra LifeSciences, Plainsboro, NJ), a cross-linked bovine collagen matrix, and Apligraf (Organogenesis, Canton, MA), a cell-based bioengineered skin bilayer using neonatal foreskin fibroblasts and a collagen matrix.[3,4]

Subcutaneous tissue and fascia are the next deepest layers. Subcutaneous tissue is less vascular than the dermis but provides cushioning to the underlying structures. Insufficiency here may lead to pressure damage in an adjacent layer. The fascial layer, which envelops muscle, is quite vascular. It allows shear between tissue planes and sometimes serves as a basic supporting layer for skin flaps.

Muscle lies deep to fascia. It is intensely vascular, often containing large vessels and associated perforators. This layer can be manipulated and rearranged for soft tissue coverage as it is in transposition flaps, pedicle flaps, and free-tissue transfer (free flaps). The level of complexity involved in each flap procedure determines its position on the reconstructive ladder. Free flaps require an in-depth understanding of anatomy as well as special technical skills in microvascular repair to freely transfer the tissue from one region of the body to another. Although free flaps are at the top of the reconstructive ladder, the many variations of free flaps can add even greater complexity.

The last soft tissue layer prior to reaching bone is the highly vascular periosteum. It, too, can be used as part of a flap often in an effort to augment bone grafting as the periosteum has osteogenic potential.[5]

Significant, segmental bone defects are challenging to treat, especially when complicated by a compromised soft tissue envelope. It is this type of injury that will likely benefit greatly from advances made in tissue engineering and regenerative medicine. One of the most successful methods that is currently used to treat these injuries is the Ilizarov method or distraction osteogenesis.[6-9] This process of mechanically induced bone and soft tissue regeneration requires temporary shortening of the extremity to reapproximate the bone ends, thus allowing for bony bridging. Once callus has bridged the gap, the limb is slowly lengthened, thereby distracting the callus between the bone ends as new bone forms. Such a process is time consuming in that the distraction rate must not exceed new callus formation nor must it exceed the ability of the soft tissue to adapt to lengthening of the limb, which is a particular concern for the peripheral nerves.[10,11] One could argue that this technique may be one of our first attempts at tissue regeneration.

The varying degrees of heroic measures involved in limb salvage, from skin grafts to flaps to bone transport, are necessary because currently no other modality can offer the reliability and function of human tissue. Human tissue is a minimally renewable resource that requires sacrificing healthy tissue to replace missing tissue. However, these reconstructive techniques require the use of native tissue taken from previously unaffected regions of the body and result in significant co-morbidity. If an allograft is chosen in order to avoid additional donor site morbidity, then the patient is exposed to risks of infection, rejection, and questionable tissue integrity.

Regenerative Medicine and Tissue Engineering

The fields of tissue engineering and regenerative medicine have evolved from this unmet need to repair or replace critically damaged tissue and restore or optimize function (Figure 12-2). Although the fields are similar (the terms are often used interchangeably) and there are degrees of interdependence, there are some subtle differences that define each discipline.

Both disciplines are based on 3 pillars: cells, signals, and scaffolds. Cells are needed to populate the tissue and perform biologic functions (such as extracellular matrix production, growth factor production, hormone production, etc). The most familiar of the 3 components, cells, often provides the most tangible characteristics of a tissue. However, in actuality, in vivo cellular function is largely dependent on the surrounding chemical and physical environment. Biochemical signaling factors are cells' primary means of communicating with their macro- and microenvironments. A wide variety of cellular effects can result based on the timing, concentration, and presence of synergistic and/or antagonistic signals. Chemotactic factors, which promote cellular migration, and trophic factors, which promote growth and development, are fundamental to cellular function and regeneration.[12] It is this incredible variation that enables the cell to express precise cellular functions in response to environmental cues, as well as tremendous consternation in any attempt to engineer specific cellular functions.[13,14]

A scaffold is the tissue engineering equivalent to an extracellular matrix and therefore is the greatest determinant of cellular perception. It determines the structural microenvironment through which the reparative cells interact and the regenerating tissue develops. Its composition and structure will determine what biochemical signals reach the cell and what mechanical forces the cell experiences. In addition to the scaffold's interaction with the cells, it is possible to engineer the interaction of the scaffold with its environment. For example, it is possible to control the ability of the scaffold to integrate into the surrounding tissue by controlling its biodegradability, and mechanical properties will determine how much stress shielding it may impart on nearby supporting structures. Only

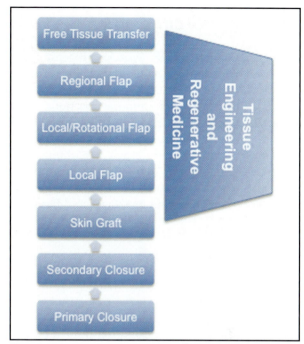

Figure 12-2. Tissue engineering and regenerative medicine in the reconstructive ladder. Schematic of escalating soft tissue reconstructions from simple to complex. Tissue engineering and regenerative medicine may provide more options for more complex wounds. (Adapted from Levin LS. The reconstructive ladder. An orthoplastic approach. *Orthop Clin North Am.* 1993;24:393-409.)

when cells, their signals, and the scaffold function in concert will they function properly as a tissue.

Regenerative medicine borrows many of the concepts and strategies from tissue engineering, but places a greater emphasis on incorporating the body's native repair and regenerative mechanisms to create a relevant and improved replacement tissue.[15,16] In other words, the therapeutic construct does not necessarily need to be a perfect replacement upon implantation, but must attain certain minimum requirements that are tissue and location specific. However, it should provide the necessary cells, signals, and preliminary scaffold that can capitalize on the body's ability to regenerate damaged or missing tissue.

Tissue engineering focuses on the in vitro production of a replacement tissue that is biocompatible and often biodegradable. The intention is that, following implantation, the tissue construct will integrate into the surrounding native tissue and provide a functional role (and remodel if biodegradable).[17] The advantages of this strategy are that it could yield an "off the shelf" modular product and that it could be "plugged into" a defect to provide an immediate function. This is appealing from both a treatment perspective and a business/marketing perspective. The major challenge, however, is creating a tissue substitute that can fulfill all these requirements.[18]

Stem Cells

Mesenchymal stem cells (MSCs), progenitor cells, and embryonic stem cells are the focus of intense research with the goal of having one's own cells heal oneself, thereby avoiding immune reactions, avoiding sacrifice of healthy tissue, and replacing lost tissue with precisely the same type of tissue. Such an achievement would help to reach the ultimate goal of restoring the anatomy and function to limbs that might otherwise not be salvaged. Using developmental biology as both a guide and model, science has begun to unravel the countless interactions a cell has with its surrounding chemical (growth factors, cytokines, etc), biological (extracellular matrix, surrounding cells, etc), and physical (compressive, tensile, shear, hydrostatic, osmotic forces) microenvironment and coupling those stimuli with its intracellular genetic blueprint.[19] These intra- and extracellular stimuli act in concert to ultimately dictate cell fate. Determining how to harness, or at least understand, cell fate will be a large step forward. Once the fate of a pluripotent cell can be reliably and predictably controlled, then tissue regeneration will have arrived.

At this time, multipotent cells can be isolated from multiple tissues throughout the adult body: adipose, ligament, bone marrow, blood, muscle, etc. Once isolated, these cells can be induced to differentiate into an alternative lineage. For instance, MSCs are well-characterized adult stem cells that have been isolated from the bone marrow and can be induced to differentiate into osteoblasts, adipocytes, and chondrocytes under defined induction conditions (Figure 12-3).[20]

During the recent conflicts, several bone graft substitutes have been used in an effort to obviate the need for iliac crest bone graft harvest. Such products include osteoconductive void fillers and bone graft extenders, osteoinductive signaling molecules and grafts, and most recently, MSC grafts, which possibly add osteogenic potential to the graft product. A recent product, Trinity MSC matrix (Blackstone Medical Inc, Baltimore, MD), has been used at our institution with some early signs of success, but it is still too early to determine its exact role in tissue regeneration.

An investigation of soft tissues debrided following combat trauma in Iraq and Afghanistan yielded a novel population of mesenchymal progenitor cells (MPCs).[21] Similar to MSCs, the MPCs are capable of differentiation (ie, into osteocytes, adipocytes, and chondrocytes) and have demonstrated proregeneration functions to promote immunosuppression and angiogenesis.[22] Unfortunately, as mentioned above, in vivo cell fate is not strictly an intracellular phenomenon predetermined by the cell's nuclear blueprint, but rather a multifactorial process with a significant portion of the

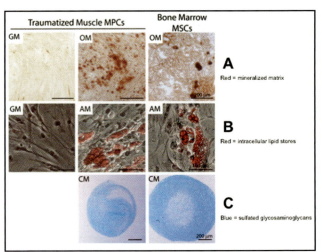

Figure 12-3. Multilineage differentiation with induction media. Muscle-derived MPCs after exposure to various induction media resulting in (A) osteogenic, (B) adipogenic, and (C) chondrogenic differentiation. (Reprinted with permission from Jackson WM, Aragon F, Djouad Y, et al. Mesenchymal progenitor cells derived from traumatized human muscle. *J Tissue Eng Regen Med.* 2009;3:129-138.)

ultimate fate determined by the extracellular milieu. Therefore, controlling the fate of these multipotent cells in vivo is a delicate task; the requirements of which we have only recently begun to fully resolve.

Stem cell differentiation can often be successfully manipulated in vitro through specialized induction media. Previous work using human bone marrow-derived MSCs has been successful in engineering intervertebral discs, cartilage, and adipose tissue.[23-25] Current work on the aforementioned muscle-derived MPCs has led to reliable MPC neurotrophic induction via treatment with defined media (Figure 12-4). This has allowed work on potential stem cell applications to proceed while significant hurdles facing controlled in vivo cell differentiation are addressed. In our lab, in vitro work has been fruitful thus far and has contributed to the development of novel peripheral nerve and bone regeneration strategies.

Truly, controlling stem cell fate will have far-reaching consequences and impressive applications. The capability of simple composite tissues or even single tissues may render current complex and tedious procedures obsolete. Although more directly affecting the surgical fields, regenerative medicine technology will ultimately affect nearly every field of medicine, from the treatment of diabetes and heart disease to the reconstruction of traumatic wounds or malformations.

Cellular Signals

In addition to the replacement of tissue, there are several growth factors and cytokines available

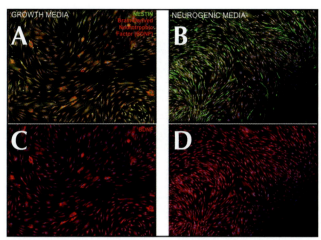

Figure 12-4. Immunofluorescence images of MPC enhancement of neurotrophic induction. Muscle-derived MPCs in (A) standard growth media and (B) neurogenic media with immunofluorescence staining for brain-derived neurotrophic factor (BDNF), Nestin and the cell body (Hoechst). MPCs in (C) standard growth media and (D) neurogenic media with Nestin immunofluorescence subtracted to highlight the difference in BDNF expression with neurogenic media. Also of note is BDNF's perinuclear accumulation.

that assist with wound healing and tissue regeneration on the cellular level via their action on chemotaxis, cell proliferation, matrix production, and cell differentiation. Their actions are often difficult to discern due to their complexity, subtleties, and incredible number. However, techniques of molecular biology are elucidating these complex and transient subcellular proteins and their interdependence. Growth factor and cytokine pathways are being continually described and modeled in greater detail on online databases, allowing widespread access to the information (Table 12-1). Of the many known trophic factors, cytokines, and signaling mediators, bone morphogenetic protein-2 (BMP-2) and to a lesser extent osteogenic protein-1 (OP-1, or BMP-7) were used in various forms to assist in bony fusion of problematic fractures.[26]

An alternative to using recombinant growth factors, platelet-rich plasma (PRP) consists of platelet α granules, which are rich in growth factors associated with healing.[27] Although the mechanism through which PRP acts is still poorly understood, its relative ease of use and outcomes thus far are very promising. As an autologous blood product, concerns for disease transmission and immunogenicity are avoided. Also, because it is derived from the patient's whole blood, it is a renewable source of growth factors. As with all new modalities, defining PRP is fundamental to the standardization necessary before it becomes an accepted treatment modality. PRP is defined as the volume of the plasma fraction of autologous blood having a platelet concentration above baseline.[28,29]

Platelets begin secreting growth factors within 10 minutes of clotting. By 1 hour, 95% of these presynthesized proteins are secreted. In vitro application of PRP has shown a significant relationship between PRP and proliferation of fibroblasts, adult MSCs, and the production of extracellular matrix.[30-33] At this time, however, there are no Level I data supporting PRP use for clinical purposes.

Scaffolds

Scaffolds comprise the third pillar of tissue engineering and regenerative medicine. They function as the extracellular matrix in tissue and provide the appropriate niche for cellular function. Of the 3 pillars, scaffolds are arguably the easiest to synthesize in the laboratory, although replicating the extracellular matrix complexity has proven to be significantly more and more difficult. Most obviously, a scaffold supports cells, allowing them to take on a 3-dimensional orientation, and as Thompson described in 1917, tissue structure is a "diagram of underlying forces" to which they respond.[34] In other words, the spatial arrangement of each tissue is related to its function and therefore affects the characteristics of each tissue type. Additionally, the cell-to-cell interaction is largely determined by the cellular arrangement: the distance cell signals must diffuse; the amount of shear, tensile, compressive, osmotic, electrostatic, or hydrostatic force that is transmitted to each cell; the freedom of movement permitted; the ease of diffusion of extracellular substances; and the ability of the construct to integrate into native tissue.[35] Recapitulating such a fine balance poses a substantial challenge to both those studying scaffolds as well as those creating them.

Despite these challenges, advances have been made. Cell matrices have taken many forms, including mesh, fleece, hydrogel, nanofiber, and those customized layer by layer.[36] Many of these constructs are manufactured using biodegradable polymers, and most investigators use polymers that have received Food and Drug Administration approval, typically variations of polylactic acid or polyglycolic acid.[37] Although many of the scaffolds' basic components are similar and the manufacturing techniques have familiar themes, there are still a great variety of scaffolds. Scaffolding models designed for a spinal cord injury will certainly have much different characteristics than for skin or cartilage, and yet the fundamentals mentioned above remain similar.[38-42]

Although there are multiple techniques to create scaffolding depending on its intended purpose, a technique that currently is receiving great interest is the process of electrospinning nanofibers. In this

Table 12-1

Common Growth Factors and Their Effects

Growth Factor	Effects
Bone morphogenetic proteins (BMP)	<ul><li>Osteoinductive BMPs: BMP-2, -4, -7.</li><li>BMP-12 (growth and differentiation factor 7, GDF-7) and BMP-13 (GDF-6) are expressed at embryonic development at sites that form tendons and their insertions. Rat studies with these factors have led to improved tendon healing after laceration.[43-45]</li><li>Compose only 0.1% by weight of all bone proteins and are not accessible until the bone matrix has been demineralized.[26]</li></ul>
Platelet-derived growth factor (PDGF)	<ul><li>Most important specific activities are angiogenesis, fibroblast proliferation[46] and chemotaxis, collagen synthesis.[47]</li><li>Potentially enhances ligament and tendon healing via its action as a mitogen and chemotactic cytokine.[48]</li></ul>
Transforming growth factor (TGF)	<ul><li>TGF-β is released from degranulating platelets during wound healing and is secreted by many of the cells involved in the healing process (inflammatory cells, fibroblasts, endothelial and epithelial cells, smooth muscle cells).[49]</li><li>One of many growth factors in a "superfamily" of growth and differentiation factors that includes BMP.[50]</li><li>There are 3 isoforms: β1, β2, β3.[51]</li><li>Promotes extracellular matrix production,[52] enhances fibroblast proliferation,[46] stimulates type I collagen production, and induces bone matrix deposition.[53]</li><li>May favor bone formation by inhibiting osteoclast.[54]</li><li>TGF-β3 is thought to be associated with the scarless wound and TGF-β1 results in exuberant scar[55] formation but ultimately weaker tissue.</li></ul>
Vascular endothelial growth factor (VEGF)	<ul><li>Subfamily of PDGF.</li><li>Important and potent signaling protein involved in angiogenesis thereby enhancing healing and is expressed in high concentrations in healing tendons following repair.[56,57]</li></ul>
Basic fibroblast growth factor (bFGF)	<ul><li>Stimulates fibroblasts to produce collagenase and stimulates the proliferation of capillary endothelial cells and helps initiate wound granulation.</li></ul>

process, a chosen polymer is expressed onto a charged collection plate or rotating drum to produce nano-scale fibers that are on the same order of magnitude as a collagen fibril—one of the fundamental components of many extracellular matrices. It is possible to fabricate several different types of nanofiber constructs by changing the polymer, the orientation of the fibers, the configuration of the collection plate, and/or varying the speed of the drum. Additionally, fiber diameter can be controlled as well as the construct's overall porosity. In our lab, we have used this strategy to create tissue-engineered scaffolds for a variety of tissues, such as bone, fat, cartilage, intervertebral disc, and peripheral nerve (Figure 12-5).

Conclusion

The current military conflicts in Iraq and Afghanistan have presented the orthopedic community with incredibly challenging musculoskeletal

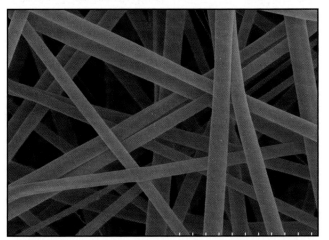

Figure 12-5. Nanofibrous scaffolds. Electrospun collagen fiber scaffold, with an average diameter of 250 nm. The nanofiber network was created by applying a large electrical potential across an extruding collagen solution, electrostatically depositing the resulting jet as a nonwoven fiber mesh. Glutaraldehyde vapor cross-linking stabilizes the substrate, making it suitable for cell applications. (Micrograph courtesy of Dr. Gregory Christopherson. Reprinted with permission.)

injuries. The common component of many of these injuries is the significant loss or complete destruction of multiple tissue types. The lack of satisfying treatment options has prompted clinicians and scientists to devise newer, more sophisticated solutions that, for the most part, have yet to be realized. Many of these novel treatment options will likely arise from the fields of tissue engineering and regenerative medicine, aiming at the repair, replacement, and/or regeneration of functional tissue.

Using history as a guide, we can safely assume that the medical challenges encountered during these conflicts will yield to medical advances that society as a whole can enjoy. This is only the beginning in the new chapter of advanced orthopedic reconstruction.

References

1. Champion HR, Holcomb JB, Young LA. Injuries from explosions: physics, biophysics, pathology, and required research focus. *J Trauma*. 2009;66:1468-1477; discussion 1477.
2. Levin LS. The reconstructive ladder. An orthoplastic approach. *Orthop Clin North Am*. 1993;24:393-409.
3. DeCarbo WT. Special segment: soft tissue matrices—bilayered bioengineered skin substitute to augment wound healing. *Foot Ankle Spec*. 2009;2:303-305.
4. Helgeson MD, Potter BK, Evans KN, Shawen SB. Bioartificial dermal substitute: a preliminary report on its use for the management of complex combat-related soft tissue wounds. *J Orthop Trauma*. 2007;21:394-399.
5. Schantz JT, Hutmacher DW, Chim H, Ng KW, Lim TC, Teoh SH. Induction of ectopic bone formation by using human periosteal cells in combination with a novel scaffold technology. *Cell Transplant*. 2002;11:125-138.
6. Ilizarov GA. The tension-stress effect on the genesis and growth of tissues: part II. The influence of the rate and frequency of distraction. *Clin Orthop Relat Res*. 1989:263-285.
7. Ilizarov GA. The tension-stress effect on the genesis and growth of tissues: part I. The influence of stability of fixation and soft-tissue preservation. *Clin Orthop Relat Res*. 1989:249-281.
8. Ilizarov GA. Clinical application of the tension-stress effect for limb lengthening. *Clin Orthop Relat Res*. 1990:8-26.
9. Aronson J. Limb-lengthening, skeletal reconstruction, and bone transport with the Ilizarov method. *J Bone Joint Surg Am*. 1997;79:1243-1258.
10. Johnson EE. Acute lengthening of shortened lower extremities after malunion or non-union of a fracture. *J Bone Joint Surg Am*. 1994;76:379-389.
11. Noonan KJ, Price CT, Sproul JT, Bright RW. Acute correction and distraction osteogenesis for the malaligned and shortened lower extremity. *J Pediatr Orthop*. 1998;18:178-186.
12. Karalaki M, Fili S, Philippou A, Koutsilieris M. Muscle regeneration: cellular and molecular events. *In Vivo*. 2009;23:779-796.
13. Langer R. Tissue engineering: perspectives, challenges, and future directions. *Tissue Eng*. 2007;13:1-2.
14. Chen FH, Rousche KT, Tuan RS. Technology insight: adult stem cells in cartilage regeneration and tissue engineering. *Nat Clin Pract Rheumatol*. 2006;2:373-382.
15. Corsi KA, Schwarz EM, Mooney DJ, Huard J. Regenerative medicine in orthopaedic surgery. *J Orthop Res*. 2007;25:1261-1268.
16. Vats A, Tolley NS, Buttery LD, Polak JM. The stem cell in orthopaedic surgery. *J Bone Joint Surg Br*. 2004;86:159-164.
17. Cowan CM, Soo C, Ting K, Wu B. Evolving concepts in bone tissue engineering. *Curr Top Dev Biol*. 2005;66:239-285.
18. Khademhosseini A, Vacanti JP, Langer R. Progress in tissue engineering. *Sci Am*. 2009;300:64-71.
19. Tuan RS. Biology of developmental and regenerative skeletogenesis. *Clin Orthop Relat Res*. 2004;(427 Suppl):S105-S117.
20. Caterson EJ, Nesti LJ, Danielson KG, Tuan RS. Human marrow-derived mesenchymal progenitor cells: isolation, culture expansion, and analysis of differentiation. *Mol Biotechnol*. 2002;20:245-256.
21. Nesti LJ, Jackson WM, Shanti RM, et al. Differentiation potential of multipotent progenitor cells derived from war-traumatized muscle tissue. *J Bone Joint Surg Am*. 2008;90:2390-2398.
22. Djouad F, Jackson WM, Bobick BE, et al. Activin A expression regulates multipotency of mesenchymal progenitor cells. *Stem Cell Research & Therapy*. 2010;1:11.
23. Nesti LJ, Li WJ, Shanti RM, et al. Intervertebral disc tissue engineering using a novel hyaluronic acid-nanofibrous scaffold (HANFS) amalgam. *Tissue Eng Part A*. 2008;14:1527-1537.
24. Caterson EJ, Li WJ, Nesti LJ, Albert T, Danielson K, Tuan RS. Polymer/alginate amalgam for cartilage-tissue engineering. *Ann N Y Acad Sci*. 2002;961:134-138.
25. Shanti RM, Janjanin S, Li WJ, et al. In vitro adipose tissue engineering using an electrospun nanofibrous scaffold. *Ann Plast Surg*. 2008;61:566-571.
26. Miyazaki M, Tsumura H, Wang JC, Alanay A. An update on bone substitutes for spinal fusion. *Eur Spine J*. 2009;18:783-799.
27. Alsousou J, Thompson M, Hulley P, Noble A, Willett K. The biology of platelet-rich plasma and its application in trauma and orthopaedic surgery: a review of the literature. *J Bone Joint Surg Br*. 2009;91:987-996.
28. Marx RE. Platelet-rich plasma (PRP): what is PRP and what is not PRP? *Implant Dent*. 2001;10:225-228.
29. Marx RE. Platelet-rich plasma: evidence to support its use. *J Oral Maxillofac Surg*. 2004;62:489-496.
30. Schliephake H. Application of bone growth factors—the potential of different carrier systems. *Oral Maxillofac Surg*. 2010;14:17-22.
31. Lucarelli E, Fini M, Beccheroni A, et al. Stromal stem cells and platelet-rich plasma improve bone allograft integration. *Clin Orthop Relat Res*. 2005:62-68.
32. Slater M, Patava J, Kingham K, Mason RS. Involvement of platelets in stimulating osteogenic activity. *J Orthop Res*. 1995;13:655-663.
33. Liu Y, Kalen A, Risto O, Wahlstrom O. Fibroblast proliferation due to exposure to a platelet concentrate in vitro is pH dependent. *Wound Repair Regen*. 2002;10:336-340.
34. Thompson DA. *On Growth and Form*. Cambridge, UK: Cambridge University Press; 1917.
35. Mammoto T, Ingber DE. Mechanical control of tissue and organ development. *Development*. 2010;137:1407-1420.
36. Wan AC, Ying JY. Nanomaterials for in situ cell delivery and tissue regeneration. *Adv Drug Deliv Rev*. 2010;62:731-740.
37. Dorozhkin SV, Schmitt M, Bouler JM, Daculsi G. Chemical transformation of some biologically relevant calcium phosphates in aqueous media during a steam sterilization. *J Mater Sci Mater Med*. 2000;11:779-786.
38. Hadlock T, Elisseeff J, Langer R, Vacanti J, Cheney M. A tissue-engineered conduit for peripheral nerve repair. *Arch Otolaryngol Head Neck Surg*. 1998;124:1081-1086.
39. Park H, Cannizzaro C, Vunjak-Novakovic G, Langer R, Vacanti CA, Farokhzad OC. Nanofabrication and microfabrication of functional materials for tissue engineering. *Tissue Eng*. 2007;13:1867-1877.
40. Teng YD, Lavik EB, Qu X, et al. Functional recovery following traumatic spinal cord injury mediated by a unique polymer scaffold seeded with neural stem cells. *Proc Natl Acad Sci U S A*. 2002;99:3024-3029.

41. Horch RE, Kopp J, Kneser U, Beier J, Bach AD. Tissue engineering of cultured skin substitutes. *J Cell Mol Med*. 2005;9:592-608.

42. Christenson EM, Anseth KS, van den Beucken JJ, et al. Nanobiomaterial applications in orthopedics. *J Orthop Res*. 2007;25:11-22.

43. Wolfman NM, Hattersley G, Cox K, et al. Ectopic induction of tendon and ligament in rats by growth and differentiation factors 5, 6, and 7, members of the TGF-beta gene family. *J Clin Invest*. 1997;100:321-330.

44. Lou J, Tu Y, Burns M, Silva MJ, Manske P. BMP-12 gene transfer augmentation of lacerated tendon repair. *J Orthop Res*. 2001;19:1199-1202.

45. Aspenberg P, Forslund C. Enhanced tendon healing with GDF 5 and 6. *Acta Orthop Scand*. 1999;70:51-54.

46. Oates TW, Rouse CA, Cochran DL. Mitogenic effects of growth factors on human periodontal ligament cells in vitro. *J Periodontol*. 1993;64:142-148.

47. Matsuda N, Lin WL, Kumar NM, Cho MI, Genco RJ. Mitogenic, chemotactic, and synthetic responses of rat periodontal ligament fibroblastic cells to polypeptide growth factors in vitro. *J Periodontol*. 1992;63:515-525.

48. Letson AK, Dahners LE. The effect of combinations of growth factors on ligament healing. *Clin Orthop Relat Res*. 1994:207-212.

49. Molloy T, Wang Y, Murrell G. The roles of growth factors in tendon and ligament healing. *Sports Med*. 2003;33:381-394.

50. Celeste AJ, Iannazzi JA, Taylor RC, et al. Identification of transforming growth factor beta family members present in bone-inductive protein purified from bovine bone. *Proc Natl Acad Sci U S A*. 1990;87:9843-9847.

51. ten Dijke P, Hansen P, Iwata KK, Pieler C, Foulkes JG. Identification of another member of the transforming growth factor type beta gene family. *Proc Natl Acad Sci U S A*. 1988;85:4715-4719.

52. Wrana JL, Maeno M, Hawrylyshyn B, Yao KL, Domenicucci C, Sodek J. Differential effects of transforming growth factor-beta on the synthesis of extracellular matrix proteins by normal fetal rat calvarial bone cell populations. *J Cell Biol*. 1988;106:915-924.

53. Bonewald LF, Mundy GR. Role of transforming growth factor-beta in bone remodeling. *Clin Orthop Relat Res*. 1990:261-276.

54. Mohan S, Baylink DJ. Bone growth factors. *Clin Orthop Relat Res*. 1991:30-48.

55. Kim HM, Lee YM. Role of TGF-beta 1 on the IgE-dependent anaphylaxis reaction. *J Immunol*. 1999;162:4960-4965.

56. Ferrara N, Gerber HP. The role of vascular endothelial growth factor in angiogenesis. *Acta Haematol*. 2001;106:148-156.

57. Wurgler-Hauri CC, Dourte LM, Baradet TC, Williams GR, Soslowsky LJ. Temporal expression of 8 growth factors in tendon-to-bone healing in a rat supraspinatus model. *J Shoulder Elbow Surg*. 2007;16:S198-S203.

Chapter 13

INFECTION IN ORTHOPEDIC EXTREMITY INJURIES

LTC Clinton K. Murray, MD

Infections of wounds have complicated the care of combat-related injuries throughout history.[1,2] During the Vietnam War, there was a 3.69% early infection rate of 7106 upper extremity injuries and a 5.04% rate among 8838 lower extremity injuries, but this did not include the longitudinal care of the 68% of casualties that were evacuated out of Vietnam.[3] A study of 84 open tibial shaft fractures evacuated from Vietnam to the United States revealed 1 of the 23 (4.3%) high-velocity wounds developed an infection, notably with *Staphylococcus aureus*, whereas 6 (9.8%) fractures associated with lower velocity injuries developed infections with *Pseudomonas* (3), *S. aureus* (2), and *Aerobacter* (1).[4] Nine of 37 (24%) open fractures became infected in Operation Just Cause in Panama.[5]

During the current wars in Iraq and Afghanistan, casualties are surviving their combat-related injuries in part due to the use of body armor, better-trained combat medics and corpsmen providing care at the point of injury, rapid evacuation of the wounded to medical care, early tourniquet use, hemostatic dressings, and the presence of forward surgical assets. A review of the Joint Theater Trauma Registry revealed that approximately one-third of casualties develop an infectious complication.[6] These infections are concerning as they are increasingly associated with multidrug-resistant (MDR) bacteria such as methicillin-resistant *S. aureus* (MRSA), extended spectrum beta-lactamase producing gram-negative rods such as *Klebsiella pneumoniae* and *Escherichia coli*, and MDR such as *Acinetobacter baumannii* and *P. aeruginosa*.[7] The source of these bacteria is likely multifactorial and includes colonization of the patient prior to injury, inoculation of the wound at the time of injury, and, especially for the MDR gram-negative rods, nosocomial transmission.[7,8]

Epidemiology

Extremity injuries are the most commonly encountered pattern of combat-related injuries, similar to previous US conflicts; however, despite our extensive knowledge of wounding patterns, the infectious complications and their associated outcomes in the war wounded from Operation Iraqi and Enduring Freedom (OIF/OEF) are not currently well described. Infectious complications of extremity injuries are often associated with co-morbidities and are reflective of the degree of injury.[9] Military personnel are typically young adults lacking co-morbidities; therefore, the injury pattern is likely a better predictor of infectious complications. Gustilo and Anderson classified open fractures into 3 types, which correlate relatively well with rate of infectious complications in civilian extremity trauma.[10-13] The percentage of patients who develop infection is approximately 0% to 2% in type I, 2% to 5% in type II, 5% to 10% in type IIIA, 10% to 50% in type IIIB, and 25% to 50% in type IIIC. While type III tibial fractures have the highest infection rates (between 6% and 39%), the amputation rate has been less than 10%.[14-17] The infecting bacteria of open fractures include staphylococci and gram-negative rods.[10,11,18-20] One of the more recent studies of severe high-energy lower extremity injuries, the Lower Extremity Assessment Program (LEAP), revealed a 28% infection rate and 7.7% osteomyelitis rate at 8 Level I US trauma centers.[21]

Current published studies looking at infections among casualties in Iraq and Afghanistan are frequently single-site studies and typically focus on a specific anatomical site or intervention (Table 13-1).

Owens BD, Belmont PJ Jr, eds. *Combat Orthopedic Surgery:
Lessons Learned in Iraq and Afghanistan (pp 109-120)*
© 2011 SLACK Incorporated

Table 13-1

Review of Combat-Related Extremity Injury Papers With Associated Injury Patterns and Infectious Complications From Operation Iraqi Freedom and Operation Enduring Freedom in Afghanistan

Reference	Time Frame	Combat Zone(s)	Treating Facility	Focus of Study	Subjects	Infectious Information	Bacteria
Helgeson et al[94]	9/2001 to 6/2006	Iraq and Afghanistan	WRAMC/BAMC	Calcium sulfate carrier for antibiotics and bone graft substitute	15 patients (17 fractures)	Postoperatively, 4 of 18 grafting procedures showed clinical infection with 13 of 17 having positive intraoperative bacteria 22% rate of osteomyelitis	Intraoperative cultures—11 Acinetobacter, 5 Staphylococcus, 2 Klebsiella, 2 Pseudomonas, 1 each with Bacteroides, Bacillus, or Corynebacterium
Lin et al[78]	12/2001 to 1/2003	Afghanistan	WRAMC	Extremity injuries	52 (15 with traumatic amputations)	No infections in fracture only group; 2 infections among amputee patients	Pseudomonas and methicillin-resistant S. aureus (MRSA) + Acinetobacter
Yun et al[25]	2/2003 to 8/2006	Iraq and Afghanistan	BAMC	Orthopedic injuries with osteomyelitis	2854 admission with 664 admitted to orthopedics and 103 with osteomyelitis 2:1 ratio of lower to upper extremities injuries with osteomyelitis	84 (83%) of these patients did not relapse during a follow-up that ranged from 2 to 36 weeks Gram-positive organisms were more likely during recurrences; S. aureus (13% versus 53%)	A. baumannii, K. pneumoniae, and P. aeruginosa isolated during an original episode
Enad and Headrick[103]	3/2003 to 5/2003	Iraq	USNS Comfort	Orthopedic injuries	58 total service-members, 30 fractures and 14 total with battle injury	No perioperative infections	None listed
Hinsley et al[104]	3/2003 to 5/2003	Iraq	British military	90% Iraqi	39 patients with 50 ballistic fractures (17 upper and 33 lower extremity)	43 evaluable wounds—13/43 became infected with 5 of 43 deep infections Infection occurred significantly more often with gunshot fractures, wound closed primarily and intra-articular fractures	None listed
Peterson et al[105]	3/2003 to 5/2003	Iraq	USNS Comfort		211 patients (179 Iraqi)	44 of 56 extremities injuries developed infection; no fracture data	Most common bacteria—Acinetobacter, E. coli, Pseudomonas species, Enterobacter species

(continued)

Table 13-1 (continued)

Review of Combat-Related Extremity Injury Papers With Associated Injury Patterns and Infectious Complications From Operation Iraqi Freedom and Operation Enduring Freedom in Afghanistan

Reference	Time Frame	Combat Zone(s)	Treating Facility	Focus of Study	Subjects	Infectious Information	Bacteria
Johnson et al[24]	3/2003 to 9/2006	Iraq and Afghanistan	BAMC	Type III tibial fractures	62 open tibial fractures with 40 type III, 35 with data	27 with at least 1 organism—deep wound culture. None of the initially recovered gram-negative bacteria were cultured again after being treated for a deep infection or osteomyelitis. 5 of 35 patients ultimately required limb amputation with infectious complications cited as the reason in 4	Acinetobacter species, Enterobacter spp. and P. aeruginosa were the most commonly recovered bacteria initially. Staphylococcal organisms were found in every wound at the time of repeat operation along with P. aeruginosa in 3 samples
Mack et al[106]	3/2003 to 1/2007	Iraq and Afghanistan	NNMC/ WRAMC	Open peri-articular shoulder	44 (33 type IIIA, 1 type IIIB, 10 type IIIC)	31 of 44 initially cultured of which 22 were positive; At 1 or more year of follow-up, 5/35 became infected—4 IIIA and 1 IIIC	Of 22 initial cultures, 14 were A. baumannii; 3 were acute infections—K. pneumoniae (1), polymicrobial (1), Candida (1); 2 were Chronic—1 MRSA and 1 E. coli
Possley et al[107]	3/2003 to 6/2007	Iraq and Afghanistan	BAMC	Safety of external fixation	55 type III tibia fractures	No cases of pin tract osteomyelitis 8 cases of osteomyelitis at fracture site. An additional 22 tibias were clinically diagnosed and treated for osteomyelitis at the fracture site without a positive bone culture, 2 soft tissue infections	Not listed
Geiger et al[108]	3/2003 to 12/2005	Iraq and Afghanistan	NNMC	Plastic surgery care	42 patients with lower extremity injury, 20 with upper extremity, and 10 with both	15 of 62 developed acute osteomyelitis and 1 of 62 developed chronic osteomyelitis	9 A. baumannii, 5 Enterobacter, 4 coagulase-negative Staphylococcus, 3 Enterococcus, 2 MRSA, 1 Bacillus, 1 Klebsiella
Brown et al[36]	8/2003 to 5/2008	Iraq and Afghanistan	British hospital	Mangled extremity	84 casualties (85 extremities)	24% developed infection with 6% developed osteomyelitis. Fasciotomy, antibiotics during air evacuation and P. aeruginosa were significantly associated with infectious complications	S. aureus were recovered later in casualties' clinical course in contrast to early recovery of Acinetobacter
Brown et al[109]	12/2003 to 4/2008	Iraq and Afghanistan	British hospitals	Vascular injury	37 total (29 with fracture)	20 of 29 limbs with a fracture developed superficial infection and 2 of 8 limbs without a fracture developed a superficial infection; 3 of 29 with fracture developed deep infection	None listed

(continued)

Table 13-1 (continued)

Review of Combat-Related Extremity Injury Papers With Associated Injury Patterns and Infectious Complications From Operation Iraqi Freedom and Operation Enduring Freedom in Afghanistan

Reference	Time Frame	Combat Zone(s)	Treating Facility	Focus of Study	Subjects	Infectious Information	Bacteria
Clasper and Phillips[89]	2003	Iraq	British field hospital	External fixation use	15 external devices (14 patients)	3 fixators developed pin track infections and failed despite antibiotics	None listed
Mody et al[26]	2003 to 2007	Iraq and Afghanistan	WRAMC	Damage control orthopedics	58 patients—34 type IIIA, 9 type IIIB, 3 type IIIC	Fracture site infection 40% and suspected osteomyelitis 17%	23 surgical site infections—polymicrobial 44%, gram-negative 65%, and gram-positive 44%; 13 early infections—9 gram-positive, 5 gram-negative; 9 late infection—5 gram-positive, 6 gram-negative
Orr et al[72]	2003 to 2008	Iraq and Afghanistan	BAMC	Sural artery flap foot and ankle	10 type IIIB	3 deep wound infections with osteomyelitis	Multidrug-resistant Klebsiella and Acinetobacter
Keeling et al[91]	4/2004 to 1/2007	Iraq and Afghanistan	NNMC	Ring external fixation	67 type III tibial shaft fractures with 45 tibia fixations with 36 cases reviewable	Standardized treatment protocol—3 of 38 tibia infected and all treated successfully with debridement and antibiotics without frame removal	None listed
Leininger et al[51]	9/2004 to 5/2005	Iraq	Field hospital—non-US personnel	Negative pressure wound therapy study	Soft tissue infections—20 upper and 38 lower extremity	No fracture data present; no infections described with standard debridement and use of negative pressure wound therapy	None listed
Kumar et al[73]	2004 to 2007	Iraq and Afghanistan	NNMC	Upper extremity flaps	23 patients with 26 upper extremity injuries	46% of wound colonized at admission; 2 flaps early postop infections with no sequelae	75% A. baumannii
Kumar et al[74]	9/2004 to 2/2007	Iraq and Afghanistan	NNMC	Lower extremity flap reconstruction	43 patients all with type IIIB and type IIIC fractures—22% upper extremity, 52% tibia/fibula, 22% ankle/foot	50% of wounds colonized at admission; 8 flaps early infection with no sequelae	57% A. baumannii
Keeney et al[92]	9/2005 to 1/2006	Iraq	Echelon III facility	Immediate nailing or staged treatment of closed femoral fracture	22 patients (23 femoral fractures) with 16 type IIIA open fractures	Follow-up 2 months for 8 and 6 months for 5; no infections	None listed

BAMC = Brooke Army Medical Center, NNMC = National Naval Medical Center, USNS = United States Naval Ship, WRAMC = Walter Reed Army Medical Center.

At the time of injury in a combat zone, the bacteria contaminating the wound are typically gram-positive.[22] However, further back in the evacuation chain, more resistant gram-negative pathogens are recovered, likely influenced by the administration of broad-spectrum systemic antibiotic prophylaxis and nosocomial transmission.[7,8,23] Proposed risk factors associated with infectious complications have included mechanisms of injury, severity of injury, and presence of retained foreign material including fragments, debris, and clothing.[6,24,25] Relapses often occur with gram-positive bacteria, notably *S. aureus*, although this is not consistent between various military treatment facilities, possibly reflective of differing management strategies.[24-26]

Management Strategies to Mitigate Infectious Complications

The current therapy of extremity injuries is to prevent infection, promote fracture healing, and restore function. For maximal success, management includes wound debridement and irrigation, initial stabilization, systemic antimicrobial therapy, timely wound closure, rehabilitation, and appropriate follow-up. In addition, certain adjuvants including local antibiotic therapy, open wound management, flap closure, and bone grafting may also be implemented. A consensus conference held in June 2007 reviewed the literature to produce evidence-based recommendations for improving extremity trauma outcomes.[27,28] These documents address the utility of microbial culture, antimicrobial therapy, irrigation solutions and techniques, timing of operative procedures, fixation, antibiotic beads, wound closure, and wound coverage. The major findings and data supporting these recommendations are addressed in the following sections (Table 13-2).

UTILITY OF PRE- AND POST-DEBRIDEMENT CULTURE

Studies assessing the utility of cultures obtained from combat casualties at the time of injury are limited. Cultures from 30 marines with 63 extremity injuries during the Vietnam War revealed a mixture of gram-positive and gram-negative bacteria at the time of injury, which transitioned to mostly gram-negative rods by 5 days after injury.[29] The one study from OIF/OEF revealed a predominance of gram-positive bacteria including occasional MRSA at the time of injury, but recovered no MDR gram-negative bacteria.[22]

Available civilian data support similar findings with gram-positive bacteria predominating at the time of injury and a transition to gram-negative bacteria causing ultimate infection. Empiric therapy can modify the bacteria recovered, and it does not appear that pre- or post-debridement cultures are predictive of infection.[12,19,20,30]

Based upon available literature regarding combat-related and civilian open fractures, routine collection of pre- or post-debridement cultures is not recommended at any level of care for combat-related extremity injuries except when there is evidence of ongoing infection as assessed by local signs and symptoms of infections or abnormal laboratory parameters.

ANTIBIOTICS

The administration of antimicrobial agents at the time of injury is considered standard of care; however, the best agent to use and its duration of use is not clearly defined. A panel of military trauma experts published a list of antibiotics that were recommended as part of tactical combat care or care provided at the time of injury.[31,32] The International Committee of the Red Cross recommends intravenous penicillin for compound fractures, amputations, and major soft tissue wounds for 48 hours and then orally until delayed primary closure, typically 5 days after injury.[33] If repeat debridement is performed instead of delayed primary closure, antibiotics should be stopped if there are no signs of infection or local inflammation. If patients present after 72 hours or are injured as a result of antipersonnel land mines, metronidazole is added for 48 hours followed by oral therapy until delayed primary closure. The British military also have differing opinions on pre-hospital antibiotic administration.[34-36] A recent study revealed that enhanced anaerobic coverage might be associated with higher infection rates.[36] An in-theater study evaluated the effect of systemic antibiotic prophylaxis and irrigation.[37] Although the results supported the importance of irrigation as the primary treatment modality more so than antibiotics, the assessment excluded all patients who needed evacuation.

The use of antibiotics in the management of open fractures in the civilian community has been extensively analyzed. A Cochrane review published in 2004 revealed that antibiotics had a protective effect against early infection compared to no antibiotics.[38] The EAST Practice Management Guidelines Working Group concluded that antibiotics were useful but that further work was needed, especially with regard to type IIIB fractures.[39] The Surgical Infection Society concluded that the current standard of care for implementation of antibiotic prophylaxis is based on very limited data with no direct evidence in some cases.[40]

One of the major areas of controversy includes which antibiotics are to be provided and the role of enhanced gram-negative coverage at the time of injury.

Table 13-2

Evidence-Based Recommendations for Management/Prevention of Combat-Related Infections Complicating Extremity Injuries by Level of Care[28]

	Echelon IIB/III (Combat Zone Surgical Care)	Echelon IV (Germany)	Echelon V (United States)	Comments
Utility of pre- and post-debridement culture	EII	EII	EII	Management should not be based upon cultures at Echelons IV, V
Antibiotic agent	AI—First generation cephalosporin; DIII—Enhanced gram-negative activity	AI—First-generation cephalosporin perioperatively	AI—First-generation cephalosporin perioperatively	Echelon IIB/III—wound pre-emptive therapy; Echelon IV—treat infected wounds; avoid use of vancomycin and broad-spectrum antibiotics; Echelons IV and V—treat infections and use standard of care perioperative antibiotic recommendations
Antibiotic timing	AII—Initiate therapy within 3 hours of injury	AI—Initiate therapy 0.5 to 1 hour prior to procedures	AI—Initiate therapy 0.5 to 1 hour prior to procedures	At initial damage control surgery or if surgery is delayed
Antibiotic duration	BII—Pre-emptive therapy for 3 days and reassess wound	AI—Perioperative not to exceed 24 hours	AI—Perioperative not to exceed 24 hours	No evidence to continue antibiotics during evacuation if that occurs after initial 72 hours with no evidence of infection; no need to continue antibiotics awaiting wound closure
Irrigation—type of fluid	AI	AI	AI	Irrigate wound with available fluid (NS, LR, or potable water)
Irrigation—volume of fluid	BIII	BIII	BIII	Type I—3 L; Type II—6 L; Type III—9 L
Irrigation—delivery methods	BIII	BIII	BIII	Low pressure irrigation
Irrigation—additives	DII	DII	DII	
Timing of operative procedure	CIII	N/A	N/A	Surgery performed within 6 hours
Immediate primary closure	EII	N/A	N/A	No primary closure during transport or evacuation
Negative pressure wound therapy	BII	CIII	BII	
Fixation	AII			External fixation
Antibiotic beads	BII	BII	BII	
Retained extremity metal fragment	BII—One dose of first-generation cephalosporin	N/A	N/A	Wound characteristics: entrance/exit wound size (<2 cm), no high-risk etiology such as mines, no bone or joint involvement, no breach of pleura or peritoneum, no major vascular injury

LR = lactate ringers, N/A = not applicable, NS = normal saline.
Evidence grade: Strength of recommendation—A = Good evidence to support a recommendation for use, B = Moderate evidence to support a recommendation for or against use, C = Poor evidence to support a recommendation for or against use, D = Moderate evidence to support recommendation against use, E = Good evidence to support a recommendation against use.
Quality of evidence—I = Evidence from at least one properly randomized controlled trial (RCT), II = Evidence from at least one well-designed clinical trial without randomization or from cohort or case-controlled studies, III = Expert opinion.
Levels of care—Echelon I = Care at time of injury, immediate stabilization, and evacuation to an initial aid station, Echelon II = Short-term holding capacity and initial resuscitation with (a) or without (b) capacity for acute, life-saving surgical care, Echelon III = Presence of multiple surgical specialties and support equivalent to a well-staffed community hospital, Echelon IV = Definitive surgical and intensive care outside the combat zone, Echelon V. = Most definitive rehabilitative and tertiary level of care in US military and Veterans Affairs medical centers.

Given the MDR nature of the gram-negative bacteria found to be subsequently infecting combat casualties' injuries after broad-spectrum regimens are used (eg, cefazolin and levofloxacin), it is currently not clear if the use of fluoroquinolones with enhanced gram-negative activity or aminoglycosides are resulting in the selection of these resistant pathogens. Worse yet, this practice may be leading to the development of resistance.[12,40,41] Overall, cephalosporins alone performed as well as cephalosporins or penicillin in combination with aminoglycosides.[12,41] Ciprofloxacin monotherapy had higher failure rates in comparison to cephalosporin in combination with an aminoglycoside for type III fractures.[42] Overall, it is unclear if additional gram-negative coverage is required or if it is potentially complicating wound care. Gathered from data derived from the Yom Kippur War (although not rigorously evaluated), one group proposed that overly broad-spectrum antimicrobial agents had led to the development of infections with resistant bacteria due to a reliance on antibiotics to "sterilize" the wound instead of relying on surgical debridement and irrigation.[43]

Other controversial issues include the use of penicillin in addition to standard therapy for open fractures to prevent clostridial infections. Of increasing concern is the rise of in vitro resistance to penicillin of the bacteria that cause gas gangrene and limited animal data revealing no improved outcome for gas gangrene in comparison to untreated controls.[44]

Although the timing of antibiotics has not been rigorously studied, one study noted a higher infection rate (7.4%, 49 of 661 patients) if antibiotics were given after 3 hours versus a lower infection rate (4.7%, 17 of 364) when antibiotics were given within 3 hours.[12] This 3-hour window was supported during the Falklands Campaign in 1982.[45] Although the number of type III injuries was not reported, 0 of 17 patients with extremity injuries who received antibiotics within 3 hours became infected. In contrast, 6 of 18 casualties who received antibiotics between 4 and 9 hours after injury became infected. Earlier administration of the first dose of antibiotics was not supported in an OIF/OEF British extremity infection study focusing on in-theater care.[36]

The ideal duration of antibiotics is also not currently clear. Prospective studies have revealed therapy as short as 1 day may be as effective as the traditionally recommended 5 days of therapy.[46-48] There are data suggesting that prolonged courses of antibiotics are associated with resistant systemic infections that developed later in a patient's hospital course.[49,50] Further assessments of antimicrobial agents also need to be conducted to determine the potential adverse effect of antimicrobial therapy on wound healing. Some agents have effects on cartilage, fracture healing, and inhibitory effects on bone in vitro.

Enhanced gram-negative therapy even for type III fractures is discouraged. At Echelon IV or V military medical facilities, antibiotics should include those agents started earlier in the evacuation chain, but these should be stopped after 72 hours if there is no evidence of infection upon evaluation of the wound. Overall, therapy in the combat zone should emphasize wound pre-emptive therapy, while at Echelon IV or V facilities, physicians should be treating only infected wounds and using periprocedure antibiotics as part of routine care. There is also no evidence to support continuing antibiotics during evacuation or continuing antibiotics until the wound is covered or until all drains are removed.

IRRIGATION

A hallmark of combat casualty wound management is aggressive surgical debridement and wound irrigation. Although not the primary focus of a study evaluating the use of negative pressure wound therapy performed on casualties in Iraq, the use of pulsatile jet irrigation with at least 3 L of saline was part of the very successful management strategies that decreased combat-related injury infection rate.[51] In a study looking at wounds in Iraq that were not evacuated, irrigation was the most important factor in preventing infections.[37] One review of the literature assessing irrigation of wounds in open fractures indicated that normal saline was recommended for irrigation with limited use of additives and the use of low-pressure irrigation.[52] Overall there does not appear to be a difference between normal saline versus tap water for simple lacerations; however, some additives as adjunctive measures, such as bacitracin, might interfere with wound healing.[53,54] In animal models, higher volumes delivered at lower pressure earlier after injury with normal saline or potable water are appropriate.[55-59] In addition, high-pressure pulsed lavage has been shown to be associated with macroscopic bone and soft tissue damage.[57,60]

Based upon the currently available data, the traditional volumes should be used to irrigate a wound with normal saline or Lactated Ringer's while avoiding the use of additives to the fluid. Potable water may be used if the other fluids are not available. The utility of high-pressure pulsatile lavage needs further assessment and is not recommended, while low-pressure lavage is recommended.

TIMING OF OPERATIVE PROCEDURE

Traditionally, it has been recommended that open fractures undergo operative procedures within 6 hours of injury. Among those with extremity injuries during the Falkland Campaign, there were 2 septic patients among 20 who underwent surgery within 6 hours in contrast to 7 of the 29 patients treated after

6 hours. Nine of those 29 went to surgery after 15 hours, 3 became septic.[45] The US military experience in Somalia revealed 14 of the 16 casualties that developed infection were treated either outside of Somalia or were treated after 6 hours.[61] During US military operations in Panama, of the 9 type III open fractures debrided in Panama, only 2 became infected.[5] In contrast, 6 of the 9 type III open fractures first debrided after being transported to the United States became infected.[5] Timing did not appear to have an effect upon severe extremity injuries managed by the British; however, their overall evacuation times were very rapid.[36]

There are a number of publications addressing time to surgery in the civilian trauma literature, and most indicate that timing to surgical procedure does not greatly impact outcome.[62-66] In the LEAP study, 84 of 315 (27%) patients with severe high-energy lower extremity injuries developed an infection within 3 months after injury.[67] Timing from injury to first debridement, from admission to first debridement, or from first debridement to soft tissue coverage was not associated with infection. Of note though, the timing from injury to admission to a definitive trauma treatment center was an independent predictor of the likelihood of infection with those admitted after 2 hours being 3.1 (95% CI 1.4 to 7.0) times more likely to develop a major infection. Those patients transferred after 11 to 24 hours were 2.6 (95% CI 1.1 to 6.2) times more likely to develop a major infection in comparison to those transferred within 3 hours of injury to a Level I trauma center.

Although data support that delayed surgical procedures may be acceptable, these studies are limited by their retrospective nature and are not adequately representative of military-type high-energy injuries. Therefore, patients should be evacuated to surgical care as soon as possible based upon a thorough risk-benefit analysis of the combat environment with a goal of initial evaluation by a surgeon within 6 hours.

COVERAGE AND CLOSURE OF WOUNDS

It is currently recommended that closure of wounds in combat environments be delayed because of the high contamination rate and the risk of *Clostridium* infection.[33] There have been an increased number of civilian trauma centers evaluating early closure of wounds due to the findings that nosocomial bacteria are typically infecting wounds. A retrospective evaluation of early closure of wounds after standard irrigation and antibiotics revealed no difference in immediate closure versus those with second-look closures or delayed primary closure.[68] Only 1 of 19 type IIIA fractures developed an infection after immediate primary closure in contrast to 0 of 5 that

underwent delayed primary closure. Another study evaluating type IIIB and IIIC fractures revealed 10 of 84 patients developed deep bone infection.[69] One of the 33 patients who underwent immediate closure (<24 hours), 3 of the 30 treated with early closure (>24, <72 hours), and 6 of 21 with late closure (>72 hours) developed deep infection.

Wound coverage with negative pressure wound therapy has become a standard of care in many facilities. In a prospective study, the density of nonfermentative gram-negative bacilli significantly decreased in negative pressure wound therapy-treated wounds in contrast to *S. aureus*, which significantly increased in negative pressure wound therapy-treated wounds.[70] A prospective randomized study of severe fractures revealed a 28% infection rate within the control group and 5.4% in the negative pressure wound therapy group ($P = 0.024$).[71]

Wound coverage through flaps has been implemented during the management of combat-related injuries with relative success. In an assessment of sural artery flap for foot and ankle wounds, 3 of the 10 patients developed deep infections with chronic osteomyelitis.[72] Separate studies by Kumar looking at upper and lower extremity battle injuries requiring flap reported early infections (8% and 17% respectively), but no resultant sequelae.[73,74]

Overall, negative pressure wound therapy and flaps appear effective; however, delayed primary closure of combat-related extremity injuries is still standard of care.

FIXATION

Fixation of open fractures has a number of beneficial effects, including protecting against further damage of soft tissue, improved wound care, improving pain control, facilitating transportation, tissue healing, and possibly reducing infection despite the presence of foreign material.[75] There are a number of methods used for bony stabilization, although internal fixation has traditionally been contraindicated in war surgery.[33,76] Based upon an analysis of the conflict in Somalia, external fixation was the preferred stabilization method.[77] External fixation has been used in many instances with success in combat-related injuries; however, no trials have been performed.[78-85] A study assessing the use of the Ilizarov method of 30 war-injured grade IIIB tibial injuries resulted in good outcomes without chronic infections.[86] Two reviews assessing the use of fixation in the management of war wounds have been published emphasizing the role of external fixation.[87,88] Recently, an evaluation of the complications of fixation during OIF reported a high rate of early complications with external fixation and cautioned against its universal acceptance.[89] A series of 24 patients with combat-related type III open tibia fractures were treated with circular (Ilizarov) external fixation. One of these patients went on to amputation (4.2%), and another developed a deep infection (4.2%).[90] Moreover, a recent review of 38 severe open tibia fractures sustained during OIF/OEF and treated in circular fixators to completion at a military hospital showed a moderate (7.9%) deep infection rate and a 97% union rate with the benefit of no retained hardware.[91] Of note, one study assessed closed intramedullary nailing of femoral shaft fractures in a combat support hospital in Iraq with good success; however, the study had limited follow-up.[92]

There is ongoing concern of early internal fixation of combat-related extremity injuries because of potential increased infection risk so this is discouraged. There is also debate of the impact external fixation has on pin tract infection and subsequent surgical stabilization, but this is considered standard of care within the US military.

ANTIBIOTIC BEADS

The utility of antibiotic-impregnated beads has not been adequately evaluated in combat casualties but are widely used as part of civilian care. Antibiotic-impregnated beads develop very high local drug levels but maintain low systemic concentrations.[93] One study has assessed the use of antibiotic-impregnated calcium sulfate in combat-related open fractures in 15 patients with 17 fractures with only 2 infections, all occurring in the 5 patients who underwent amputations.[94] Given the resistant bacteria infecting these wounds, finding the ideal antimicrobial agent was challenging. Although civilian data support the use of aminoglycoside-impregnated beads in the treatment of open fractures, many of these studies are limited by their retrospective nature or small sample size. In a retrospective evaluation of tobramycin-impregnated beads, those patients who received the beads had a lower infection rate (31 of 845 [3.7%] patients) in contrast to those without beads (29 of 240 [12.1%] patients).[95] This was especially true for type IIIB and IIIC fractures. The patients with impregnated beads were closed earlier, introducing a potential bias. A prospective randomized trial comparing local administration of tobramycin-eluting beads to systemic antimicrobial therapy with a first-generation cephalosporin for type II, IIIA, and IIIB fractures until wound closure revealed no difference in infection rates between the 2 arms of the study (2 infections in 24 [8.3%] treated with local therapy and 2 infections of 38 [5.3%] treated with systemic).[96]

There has been concern over use of antimicrobial beads in theater due to evacuation policies of casualties, but they appear to be effective for the temporary management of complex combat wounds, especially those with associated dead-spaces.

ADDITIONAL MANAGEMENT STRATEGIES

Retained Fragments

Many currently employed weaponry systems can result in numerous fragments being lodged into the body. Often, due to the sheer numbers of fragments, these are not amenable to complete removal. An assessment of 63 casualties with 866 fragments managed nonoperatively with antibiotics and dressings found only 2 infectious complications, both superficial abscesses.[97] Criteria for nonoperative management included soft tissue injuries only (no fractures, no major vascular involvement, and no break of pleura or peritoneum), wound entry/exit size less than 2 cm in maximum dimension, wounds not frankly infected, and exclusion of mine wounds.

Inflammatory Biomarkers

Current laboratory parameters such as white blood cell count, C-reactive protein, and erythrocyte sedimentation rate have not been reliable to predict infection in extremity wounds. A number of studies have evaluated alternative inflammatory biomarkers with some encouraging results.[98-100] Of these markers, only procalcitonin is currently available in clinical laboratories.

Infection Control Strategies

The MDR bacteria that currently infect combat-related injuries appear to be associated with nosocomial transmission. There has been substantial emphasis on improving infection control interventions within the combat zone and within US military treatment facilities.[101] Continued focus on simple strategies such as hand hygiene, appropriate isolation and cohorting, and appropriate use of antibiotics are necessary to mitigate ongoing transmission.[102]

Conclusion

Open fractures are a challenge to manage especially in a combat environment with high-energy explosive injuries, high contamination rates, challenging environmental constraints, different levels of medical care, and varying evacuation procedures and times. The management of these combat-related wounds has not substantially changed during the past 50 years with early surgical debridement and stabilization, antibiotic administration, and delayed primary closures still the standard of care. While the civilian community has tried to advance the understanding of open fracture care during peace time, there are still many unanswered questions with regard to the optimal management of these casualties.

References

1. Manring MM, Hawk A, Calhoun JH, Andersen RC. Treatment of war wounds. A historical review. *Clin Orthop Relat Res.* 2009;467(8):2168-2169.

2. Murray CK, Hinkle MK, Yun HC. History of infections associated with combat-related injuries. *J Trauma.* 2008;64(3 Suppl): S221-S231.

3. Hardaway RM III. Vietnam wound analysis. *J Trauma.* 1978;18(9):635-643.

4. Witschi TH, Omer GE Jr. The treatment of open tibial shaft fractures from Vietnam War. *J Trauma.* 1970;10(2):105-111.

5. Jacob E, Erpelding JM, Murphy KP. A retrospective analysis of open fractures sustained by U.S. military personnel during Operation Just Cause. *Mil Med.* 1992;157(10):552-556.

6. Murray CK, Wilkins K, Molter NC, et al. Infections in combat casualties during Operations Iraqi and Enduring Freedom. *J Trauma.* 2009;66(4 Suppl):S138-S144.

7. Murray CK. Epidemiology of infections related to combat-related injuries in Iraq and Afghanistan. *J Trauma.* 2008;64(3 Suppl): S232-S238.

8. Murray CK. Infectious disease complications of combat-related injuries. *Crit Care Med.* 2008;36(7 Suppl):S358-S364.

9. Bowen TR, Widmaier JC. Host classification predicts infection after open fracture. *Clin Orthop Relat Res.* 2005;433:205-211.

10. Gustilo RB, Anderson JT. Prevention of infection in the treatment of one thousand and twenty-five open fractures of long bones: retrospective and prospective analyses. *J Bone Joint Surg Am.* 1976;58(4):453-458.

11. Gustilo RB, Mendoza RM, Williams DN. Problems in the management of type III (severe) open fractures: a new classification of type III open fractures. *J Trauma.* 1984;24(8):742-746.

12. Patzakis MJ, Wilkins J. Factors influencing infection rate in open fracture wounds. *Clin Orthop Relat Res.* 1989;243:36-40.

13. Gustilo RB, Gruninger RP, Davis T. Classification of type III (severe) open fractures relative to treatment and results. *Orthopedics.* 1987;10(12):1781-1788.

14. Parrett BM, Matros E, Pribaz JJ, Orgill DP. Lower extremity trauma: trends in the management of soft-tissue reconstruction of open tibia-fibula fractures. *Plast Reconstr Surg.* 2006;117(4):1315-1322; discussion 1323-1314.

15. Rajasekaran S, Naresh Babu J, Dheenadhayalan J, et al. A score for predicting salvage and outcome in Gustilo type-IIIA and type-IIIB open tibial fractures. *J Bone Joint Surg Br.* 2006;88(10):1351-1360.

16. Naique SB, Pearse M, Nanchahal J. Management of severe open tibial fractures: the need for combined orthopaedic and plastic surgical treatment in specialist centres. *J Bone Joint Surg Br.* 2006;88(3):351-357.

17. Giannoudis PV, Papakostidis C, Roberts C. A review of the management of open fractures of the tibia and femur. *J Bone Joint Surg Br.* 2006;88(3):281-289.

18. Sen C, Eralp L, Gunes T, Erdem M, Ozden VE, Kocaoglu M. An alternative method for the treatment of nonunion of the tibia with bone loss. *J Bone Joint Surg Br.* 2006;88(6):783-789.

19. Lee J. Efficacy of cultures in the management of open fractures. *Clin Orthop Relat Res.* 1997;339:71-75.

20. Carsenti-Etesse H, Doyon F, Desplaces N, et al. Epidemiology of bacterial infection during management of open leg fractures. *Eur J Clin Microbiol Infect Dis.* 1999;18(5):315-323.

21. Harris AM, Althausen PL, Kellam J, Bosse MJ, Castillo R, and the LEAP. Complications following limb-threatening lower extremity trauma. *J Orthop Trauma.* 2009;23(1):1-6.

22. Murray CK, Roop SA, Hospenthal DR, et al. Bacteriology of war wounds at the time of injury. *Mil Med.* 2006;171(9):826-829.

23. Aronson NE, Sanders JW, Moran KA. In harm's way: infections in deployed American military forces. *Clin Infect Dis.* 2006;43(8):1045-1051.

24. Johnson EN, Burns TC, Hayda RA, Hospenthal DR, Murray CK. Infectious complications of open type III tibial fractures among combat casualties. *Clin Infect Dis.* 2007;45(4):409-415.

25. Yun HC, Branstetter JG, Murray CK. Osteomyelitis in military personnel wounded in Iraq and Afghanistan. *J Trauma.* 2008;64(2 Suppl):S163-S168.

26. Mody RM, Zapor M, Hartzell JD, et al. Infectious complications of damage control orthopedics in war trauma. *J Trauma.* 2009;67(4):758-761.

27. Hospenthal DR, Murray CK, Andersen RC, et al. Guidelines for the prevention of infection following combat-related injuries. *J Trauma.* 2008;64(3 Suppl):S211-S220.

28. Murray CK, Hsu JR, Solomkin JS, et al. Prevention and management of infections associated with combat-related extremity injuries. *J Trauma.* 2008;64(3 Suppl):S239-S251.

29. Tong MJ. Septic complications of war wounds. *JAMA.* 1972;219(8):1044-1047.

30. Valenziano CP, Chattar-Cora D, O'Neill A, Hubil EH, Cudjoe EA. Efficacy of primary wound cultures in long bone open extremity fractures: are they of any value? *Arch Orthop Trauma Surg.* 2002;122(5):259-261.

31. Butler F, O'Connor K. Antibiotics in tactical combat casualty care 2002. *Mil Med.* 2003;168(11):911-914.

32. Murray CK, Hospenthal DR, Holcomb JB. Antibiotics use and selection at the point of injury in tactical combat casualty care for casualties with penetrating abdominal injury, shock, or unable to tolerate an oral agent. *J Special Op Med.* 2005;5(3):56-61.

33. Dufour D, Jensen SK, Owen-Smith M, et al. *Surgery for Victims of War.* 3rd ed. Geneva, Switzerland: International Committee of the Red Cross; 1998.

34. Parker PJ. Pre-hospital antibiotic administration. *J R Army Med Corps.* 2008;154(1):5-6.

35. Green AD, Hutley EJ. Pre-hospital antibiotic administration: a response. *J R Army Med Corps.* 3008;154(1):6-9.

36. Brown KV, Murray CK, Clasper J. Infectious complications of combat-related mangled extremity injuries in the British Military. *J Trauma.* 2010;69(Suppl 1):S109-S115.

37. Gerhardt RT, Matthew JM, Sullivan SG. The effect of systemic antibiotic prophylaxis and wound irrigation on penetrating combat wounds in a return-to-duty population. *Prehosp Emerg Care.* 2009;13(4):500-504.

38. Gosselin RA, Roberts I, Gillespie WJ. Antibiotics for preventing infection in open limb fractures. *Cochrane Database Syst Rev.* 2004:CD003764.

39. Luchetter FA, Bone LB, Born CT, et al. EAST practice management guidelines work group: practice management guidelines for prophylactic antibiotic use in open fractures. http://www.east.org/tpg/openfrac.pdf. Accessed September 21, 2007.

40. Hauser CJ, Adams CA Jr, Eachempati SR. Surgical Infection Society guideline: prophylactic antibiotic use in open fractures: an evidence-based guideline. *Surg Infect (Larchmt).* 2006;7(4):379-405.

41. Patzakis MJ, Harvey JP Jr, Ivler D. The role of antibiotics in the management of open fractures. *J Bone Joint Surg Am.* 1974;56(3):532-541.

42. Patzakis MJ, Bains RS, Lee J, et al. Prospective, randomized, double-blind study comparing single-agent antibiotic therapy, ciprofloxacin, to combination antibiotic therapy in open fracture wounds. *J Orthop Trauma.* 2000;14(8):529-533.

43. Klein RS, Berger SA, Yekutiel P. Wound infection during the Yom Kippur war: observations concerning antibiotic prophylaxis and therapy. *Ann Surg.* 1975;182(1):15-21.

44. Stevens DL, Maier KA, Laine BM, Mitten JE. Comparison of clindamycin, rifampin, tetracycline, metronidazole, and penicillin for efficacy in prevention of experimental gas gangrene due to *Clostridium perfringens. J Infect Dis.* 1987;155(2):220-228.

45. Jackson DS. Sepsis in soft tissue limbs wounds in soldiers injured during the Falklands Campaign 1982. *J R Army Med Corps.* 1984;130(2):97-99.

46. Dellinger EP, Caplan ES, Weaver LD, et al. Duration of preventive antibiotic administration for open extremity fractures. *Arch Surg.* 1988;123(3):333-339.

47. Merritt K. Factors increasing the risk of infection in patients with open fractures. *J Trauma.* 1988;28(6):823-827.

48. Sloan JP, Dove AF, Maheson M, Cope AN, Welsh KR. Antibiotics in open fractures of the distal phalanx? *J Hand Surg [Br].* 1987;12(1):123-124.

49. Hoth JJ, Franklin GA, Stassen NA, Girard SM, Rodriguez RJ, Rodriguez JL. Prophylactic antibiotics adversely affect nosocomial pneumonia in trauma patients. *J Trauma.* 2003;55(2):249-254.

50. Velmahos GC, Toutouzas KG, Sarkisyan G, et al. Severe trauma is not an excuse for prolonged antibiotic prophylaxis. *Arch Surg.* 2002;137(5):537-541; discussion 541-542.

51. Leininger BE, Rasmussen TE, Smith DL, Jenkins DH, Coppola C. Experience with wound VAC and delayed primary closure of contaminated soft tissue injuries in Iraq. *J Trauma.* 2006;61(5):1207-1211.

52. Crowley DJ, Kanakaris NK, Giannoudis PV. Irrigation of the wounds in open fractures. *J Bone Joint Surg Br.* 2007;89(5):580-585.

53. Moscati RM, Mayrose J, Reardon RF, Janicke DM, Jehle DV. A multicenter comparison of tap water versus sterile saline for wound irrigation. *Acad Emerg Med.* 2007;14(5):404-409.

54. Anglen JO. Comparison of soap and antibiotic solutions for irrigation of lower-limb open fracture wounds. A prospective, randomized study. *J Bone Joint Surg Am.* 2005;87(7):1415-1422.

55. Svoboda SJ, Bice TG, Gooden HA, Brooks De, Thomas DB, Wenke JC. Comparison of bulb syringe and pulsed lavage irrigation with use of a bioluminescent musculoskeletal wound model. *J Bone Joint Surg Am.* 2006;88(10):2167-2174.

56. Hassinger SM, Harding G, Wongworawat MD. High-pressure pulsatile lavage propagates bacteria into soft tissue. *Clin Orthop Relat Res.* 2005;439:27-31.

57. Boyd JI 3rd, Wongworawat MD. High-pressure pulsatile lavage causes soft tissue damage. *Clin Orthop Relat Res.* 2004;427:13-17.

58. Owens BD, White DW, Wenke JC. Comparison of irrigation solutions and devices in a contaminated musculoskeletal wound survival model. *J Bone Joint Surg.* 2009;91(1):92-98.

59. Bhandari M, Schemitsch EH, Adili A, Lachowski RJ, Shaughnessy SG. High and low pressure pulsatile lavage of contaminated tibial fractures: an in vitro study of bacterial adherence and bone damage. *J Orthop Trauma.* 1999;13(8):526-533.

60. Owens BD, Wenke JC. Early wound irrigation improves the ability to remove bacteria. *J Bone Joint Surg Am.* 2007;89(8):1723-1726.

61. Mabry RL, Holcomb JB, Baker AM, et al. United States Army Rangers in Somalia: an analysis of combat casualties on an urban battlefield. *J Trauma.* 2000;49(3):515-528; discussion 528-529.

62. Charalambous CP, Siddique I, Zenios M, et al. Early versus delayed surgical treatment of open tibial fractures: effect on the rates of infection and need of secondary surgical procedures to promote bone union. *Injury.* 2005;36(5):656-661.

63. Harley BJ, Beaupre LA, Jones CA, Dulai SK, Weber DW. The effect of time to definitive treatment on the rate of nonunion and infection in open fractures. *J Orthop Trauma.* 2002;16(7):484-490.

64. Skaggs DL, Friend L, Alman B, et al. The effect of surgical delay on acute infection following 554 open fractures in children. *J Bone Joint Surg Am.* 2005;87(1):8-12.

65. Khatod M, Botte MJ, Hoyt DB, Meyer RS, Smith JM, Akeson WH. Outcomes in open tibia fractures: relationship between delay in treatment and infection. *J Trauma.* 2003;55(5):949-954.

66. Lowry KF, Curtis GM. Delayed suture in the management of wounds; analysis of 721 traumatic wounds illustrating the influence of time interval in wound repair. *Am J Surg.* 1950;80(3):280-287.

67. Pollak AN, Jones AL, Castillo RC, Bosse MJ, MacKenzie EJ. LEAP. The relationship between time to surgical debridement and incidence of infection after open high-energy lower extremity trauma. *J Bone Joint Surg Am.* 2010;92(1):7-15.

68. DeLong WG Jr, Born CT, Wei SY, Petrik ME, Ponzio R, Schwab CW. Aggressive treatment of 119 open fracture wounds. *J Trauma.* 1999;46(6):1049-1054.

69. Gopal S, Majumder S, Batchelor AG, Knight SL, De Boer P, Smith RM. Fix and flap: the radical orthopaedic and plastic treatment of severe open fractures of the tibia. *J Bone Joint Surg Br.* 2000;82(7):959-966.

70. Moues CM, Vos MC, van den Bemd GJ, Stijnen T, Hovius SE. Bacterial load in relation to vacuum-assisted closure wound therapy: a prospective randomized trial. *Wound Repair Regen.* 2004;12(1):11-17.

71. Stannard JP, Volgas DA, Stewart R, McGwin G, Alonso JE. Negative pressure wound therapy after severe open fractures: a prospective randomized study. *J Orthop Trauma.* 2009;23(8):552-555.

72. Orr J, Kirk KL, Antunez V, Ficke J. Reverse sural artery flap for reconstruction of blast injuries of the foot and ankle. *Foot Ankle Int.* 2010;31(1):59-64.

73. Kumar AR, Grewal NS, Chung TL, Bradley JP. Lessons from the modern battlefield: successful upper extremity injury reconstruction in the subacute period. *J Trauma.* 2009;67(4):752-757.

74. Kumar AR, Grewal NS, Chung TL, Bradley JP. Lessons from Operation Iraqi Freedom: successful subacute reconstruction of complex lower extremity battle injuries. *Plast Reconstr Surg.* 2009;123(1):218-229.

75. Worlock P, Slack R, Harvey L, Mawhinney R. The prevention of infection in open fractures: an experimental study of the effect of fracture stability. *Injury.* 1994;25(1):31-38.

76. Weapons effects and parachute injuries. In: Szul AC, Davis LB, Walter Reed Army Medical Center Borden Institute, eds. *Emergency War Surgery.* 3rd US rev. Washington, DC: Walter Reed Army Medical Center Borden Institute; 2004:1.1-1.4.

77. McHenry T, Simmons S, Alitz C, et al. Forward surgical stabilization of penetrating lower extremity fractures: circular casting versus external fixation. *Mil Med.* 2001;166(9):791-795.

78. Lin DL, Kirk KL, Murphy KP, McHale KA, Doukas WC. Evaluation of orthopaedic injuries in Operation Enduring Freedom. *J Orthop Trauma.* 2004;18(8 Suppl):S48-S53.

79. Zinman C, Norman D, Hamoud K, Reis ND. External fixation for severe open fractures of the humerus caused by missiles. *J Orthop Trauma.* 1997;11(7):536-539.

80. Davis TP, Alexander BA, Lambert EW, et al. Distribution and care of shipboard blast injuries (USS Cole DDG-67). *J Trauma.* 2003;55(6):1022-1027; discussion 1027-1028.

81. Beekley AC, Watts DM. Combat trauma experience with the United States Army 102nd Forward Surgical Team in Afghanistan. *Am J Surg.* 2004;187(5):652-654.

82. Cho JM, Jatoi I, Alarcon AS, Morton TM, King BT, Hermann JM. Operation Iraqi Freedom: surgical experience of the 212th Mobile Army Surgical Hospital. *Mil Med.* 2005;170(4):268-272.

83. Rich NM, Metz CW Jr, Hutton JE Jr, Baugh JH, Hughes CW. Internal versus external fixation of fractures with concomitant vascular injuries in Vietnam. *J Trauma.* 1971;11(6):463-473.

84. Has B, Jovanovic S, Wertheimer B, Mikolasevic I, Brdic P. External fixation as a primary and definitive treatment of open limb fractures. *Injury.* 1995;26(4):245-248.

85. Dubravko H, Zarko R, Tomislav T, Dragutin K, Vjenceslav N. External fixation in war trauma management of the extremities—experience from the war in Croatia. *J Trauma.* 1994;37(5):831-834.

86. Bumbasirevic M, Tomic S, Lesic A, Molosevic I, Atkinson HDE. War-related infected tibial nonunion with bone and soft-tissue loss treated with bone transport using the Ilizarov method. *Arch Orthop Trauma Surg.* 2010;130(6):739-749. Epub 2009 Nov 28.

87. Coupland RM. War wounds of bones and external fixation. *Injury.* 1994;25(4):211-217.

88. Zinman C, Reis ND. External fixation in wartime limb surgery. *Isr J Med Sci.* 1984;20(4):308-310.

89. Clasper JC, Phillips SL. Early failure of external fixation in the management of war injuries. *J R Army Med Corps.* 2005;151(2):81-86.

90. Lerner A, Fodor L, Soudry M. Is staged external fixation a valuable strategy for war injuries to the limbs? *Clin Orthop Relat Res.* 2006;448:217-224.

91. Keeling JJ, Gwinn DE, Tintle SM, Andersen RC, McGuigan FX. Short-term outcomes of severe open wartime tibial fractures treated with ring external fixation. *J Bone Joint Surg Am.* 2008;90(12):2643-2651.

92. Keeney JA, Ingari JV, Mentzer KD, Powell ET. Closed intramedullary nailing of femoral shaft fractures in an echelon III facility. *Mil Med.* 2009;174(2):124-128.

93. Wininger DA, Fass RJ. Antibiotic-impregnated cement and beads for orthopedic infections. *Antimicrob Agents Chemother.* 1996;40(12):2675-2679.

94. Helgeson MD, Potter BK, Tucker CJ, Frisch HM, Shawen SB. Antibiotic-impregnated calcium sulfate use in combat-related open fractures. *Orthop.* 2009;32(5):323.

95. Ostermann PA, Seligson D, Henry SL. Local antibiotic therapy for severe open fractures. A review of 1085 consecutive cases. *J Bone Joint Surg Br.* 1995;77(1):93-97.

96. Moehring HD, Gravel C, Chapman MW, Olson SA. Comparison of antibiotic beads and intravenous antibiotics in open fractures. *Clin Orthop Relat Res.* 2000;372:254-261.

97. Bowyer GW. Management of small fragment wounds: experience from the Afghan border. *J Trauma.* 1996;40(3 Suppl):S170-S172.

98. Forsberg JA, Elster EA, Andersen RC, et al. Correlation of procalcitonin and cytokine expression with dehiscence of wartime extremity wounds. *J Bone Joint Surg Am.* 2008;90(3):580-588.

99. Hawksworth JS, Stojadinovic A, Gage FA, et al. Inflammatory biomarkers in combat wound healing. *Ann Surg.* 2009;250(6):1002-1007.

100. Hunziker S, Hugle T, Schuchardt K, et al. The value of serum procalcitonin level for differentiation of infectious from noninfectious causes of fever after orthopaedic surgery. *J Bone Joint Surg Am.* 2010;92(1):138-148.

101. Hospenthal DR, Crouch HK. Infection control challenges in deployed US military treatment facilities. *J Trauma.* 2009;66(4 Suppl):S120-S128.

102. Hospenthal DR, Crouch HK, English JF, et al. Response to infection control challenges in the deployed setting—Operations Iraqi and Enduring Freedom. *J Trauma.* (In press.)

103. Enad JG, Headrick JD. Orthopedic injury in U.S. casualties treated on a hospital ship during Operation Iraqi Freedom. *Mil Med.* 2008;173(10):1008-1013.

104. Hinsley DE, Phillips SL, Clasper JS. Ballistic fractures during the 2003 Gulf Conflict—early prognosis and high complication rate. *J R Army Med Corp.* 2006;152(2):96-101.

105. Peterson K, Riddle MS, Danko JR, et al. Trauma-related infections in battlefield casualties from Iraq. *Ann Surg.* 2007;245(5):803-811.

106. Mack AW, Groth AT, Frisch HM, Doukas WC. Treatment of open periarticluar shoulder fractures sustained in combat-related injuries. *Am J Orthop.* 2008;37(3):130-135.

107. Possley DR, Burns TC, Stinner DJ, Murray CK, Wenke JC, Hsu JR. External fixation is safe for damage control orthopaedics in a combat environment. *J Trauma.* (In press.)

108. Geiger S, McCormick F, Chou R, Wandel AG. War wounds: lessons learned from Operation Iraqi Freedom. *Plast Reconstr Surg.* 2008;122(1):146-153.

109. Brown KV, Ramasany A, Tai N, MacLeod J, Midwinter M, Clasper JC. Complications of extremity vascular injuries in conflict. *J Trauma.* 2009;66(4 Suppl):S145-S149.

TOURNIQUETS

COL John F. Kragh Jr, MD

Emergency tourniquet use is the most obvious combat orthopedic advance of the current war, and a definitive academic record of lessons learned in Iraq and Afghanistan is due. Tourniquet treatment practices in combat casualty care are plainly different from routine civilian care, especially regarding the rate of casualties seen with tourniquets.[1,2] Emergency tourniquets are one of the most controversial topics in first aid and orthopedics, and recommendations have changed recently since military services have evidenced major life-saving benefits with minor morbidity if the right devices are used at the right time for the right casualties in the right way.[2-6] However, until recently, most opinions have been that tourniquet use is best avoided or used as a last resort,[7] and so few providers have compiled experience with hundreds of cases except for a few forward military surgeons.

The aim of this chapter is to report the emergency tourniquet lessons learned from a large emergency tourniquet program and, in particular, offer recommendations for clinical use.

Historical Background of Emergency Tourniquet Use

The historical record of tourniquet use has been poorly documented from the Neolithic Era until recently, and much of the controversy was rooted in a paucity or absence of evidence on whether tourniquets should be used emergently. Given so little evidence, any plausible argument could not be refuted. Key historical developments in emergency tourniquet use include the first definite recorded use of a battlefield tourniquet by Étienne J. Morel at the siege of Besançon in 1674, Jean-Louis Petit's demonstration of his screw tourniquet for surgical amputation in Paris in 1718, Joseph Lister's tourniquet use in elective surgery in Britain in 1864, and Lorenz Bohler's detailed lessons learned in Austria in the World Wars.[8,9] Wolff and Adkins in World War II noted 200 cases and generally gave favorable outcomes and offered pearls and pitfalls, but there was little depth to the data reported.[10] Although Wolff and Adkins' report had little data, it was the largest case series reported to that date. Later, the US military analyzed preventable causes of death in the Vietnam War and then again in Somalia, and tourniquets were thought to be the most practical way to prevent the most common cause of preventable battlefield death.[11-16]

In 2003, the Israelis reported their experience, and although their report on 91 cases was smaller than Wolff and Adkins' 200, the data were broader and deeper.[17] The Israeli study showed that all cases survived and had infrequent morbidity. The 2003 Israeli study brought emergency tourniquet knowledge up to the current wars, in which the knowledge was to soon pivot.

Situation in 2001 at the Beginning of the Current Wars

When the current wars began in 2001, there was no good tourniquet available for the battlefield. A compelling scientific case was made over time in

Owens BD, Belmont PJ Jr, eds. *Combat Orthopedic Surgery: Lessons Learned in Iraq and Afghanistan (pp 121-128)* © 2011 SLACK Incorporated recent wars that battlefield hemorrhage was a leading cause of death, limb exsanguination was plausibly preventable with hemorrhage control devices like tourniquets, and isolated limb exsanguination was the foremost preventable cause of death on the battlefield.[11] Epidemiologically, the frequency of isolated limb exsanguination has appeared to be about 7% in a few wars where it was estimated[11,12,18]; and so in combat, this lethal problem is common. Until recently in war, surgeons rarely offered substantial evidence that emergency hemorrhage control of limb exsanguination improves survival.[6,19] In the mid-1980s, the Israelis issued emergency tourniquets widely to their soldiers and evidenced that there were few adverse events, but they were criticized for their inability to show life-saving benefit.[17,20,21]

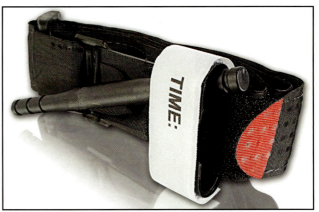

Figure 14-1. Standard issue tourniquet for US soldiers deploying to war, the Combat Application Tourniquet (CAT). The CAT is a strap and windlass design field tourniquet and has the highest effectiveness rate for prehospital devices. (© 2009 North American Rescue, LLC. Used with permission.)

Preclinical Work Related to Emergency Tourniquet Use

Recent scientific developments have permitted a better understanding of the problem of hemorrhagic shock, hemorrhage control techniques, safety of tourniquet designs, tourniquet effectiveness, and the pathophysiology of ischemia-reperfusion.[8,22-25] The main cause of shock in battle trauma was unclear until the primary role of hemorrhage was elucidated.[26,27] Hemorrhagic shock prevention and treatment has focused mainly on transfusion practices, but tourniquets were occasionally evidenced to control hemorrhage in trauma patients.[19] The safety and effectiveness of tourniquet designs evolved in elective surgery, particularly with the development of pneumatic tourniquets, and the studies indicated that device width and edge shape affected both safety and effectiveness.[23,24,28-36] The gains in knowledge during the past few decades about limb ischemia-reperfusion helped in understanding the risks of tourniquet use, especially the duration of ischemia.[37,38] These multiple and concurrent scientific developments permitted a reappraisal of the burden of injury detailed in the above paragraph on epidemiology so that more tools were available to engineer a solution set to the problem at hand—namely, preventable battlefield deaths from limb exsanguination.[6,8]

Throughout history, many tourniquets of varied designs have been used, such as Petit's screw tourniquet, Morel's block tourniquet, and the strap and windlass tourniquet.[3,8] Many tourniquets have been designed by trial and error from materials at hand without recognition or analysis of the lengthy record of historical designs dating more than 2 millennia; thus, many of the devices we are asked to review are actually similar to prior devices inadvertently reinvented or redesigned. Currently, the standard

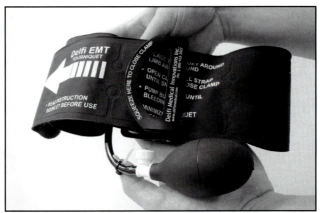

Figure 14-2. The Emergency and Military Tourniquet ([EMT] Delfi Medical Innovations, Vancouver, British Columbia, Canada). The EMT is a pneumatic tourniquet that was the most effective device used in the Army clinical trial. (Photograph used with permission of Delfi Medical Innovations.)

issue tourniquet for US soldiers deploying to war is the Combat Application Tourniquet ([CAT] licensed and manufactured by Composite Resources Inc, Rock Hill, SC, and distributed mainly by North American Rescue [NAR], Greer, SC). The CAT (National Stock Number 6515-01-521-7976), shown in Figure 14-1, is a strap and windlass design field tourniquet that is 38 mm wide. The US Department of Defense ran a large clinical trial in a combat support hospital in Baghdad (National Clinical Trial NCT00517166 at ClinicalTrials. gov) that showed the CAT was the field tourniquet with the highest effectiveness rate (79% of limbs where only a single CAT was used).[3] The hospital tourniquet that was evidenced to have the highest effectiveness rate was the Emergency and Military Tourniquet ([EMT] Delfi Medical Innovations, Vancouver, British Columbia, Canada), shown in Figure 14-2. The EMT

Table 14-1

Current Emergency Tourniquet Recommendations and Findings

If one device does not stop the bleeding, then use a wider device or use 2 side by side.
With good tourniquet designs, use on 2-boned segments has the *highest*, not the lowest, effectiveness.
Tourniquet design should account for all relevant science, including casualty anthropometry.
One-handed tourniquet application is desirable but not essential to success in general use.
Different devices have different components that wear or break depending on use or misuse.
Specific devices are single-use or designed for reuse, and the steward should test devices.
Users should understand how devices work best in order to attain optimal outcomes.
Designs should meet user expectations if scientifically grounded by care setting.
When user expectations mismatch the device science, problems abound.
When user expectations match the device science, optimal care is more easily attained.
Leaders should select devices most appropriate for their users based on the best data available.
The steward of a hospital tourniquet service should have experience or training.

is a pneumatic tourniquet that is 88 mm wide, which was effective in 92% of limbs with only one EMT used in the clinical trial.[3] The limb segment where ineffectiveness was most encountered was the thigh, which confirms the challenges of compressing larger amounts of tissue as evidenced in the elective surgery literature.[23,24,39] Device design should account for a broad range of knowledge to include anthropometry, safety data, and effectiveness data.[40-45] Specific devices are single use or designed for reuse. If necessary, a steward for the hospital's emergency tourniquet service should test, clean, and restore devices or remove them from use (Table 14-1). Obviously, the steward of a hospital tourniquet service should have adequate experience or training.

Improvised tourniquets usually are strap-and-stick constructs but in practice have included a broad spectrum of items: strings, intravenous tubes, bungee cords, bands (engineer tape), waist belts, screwdrivers, scissors, tree limbs, and rifle cleaning rods. The effectiveness of improvised tourniquets is generally inferior to well-designed tourniquets but measurably better than no tourniquet at all.[3] The wider improvised tourniquets (cravats and windlass type, especially when 2 were used side by side) were effective in 42% of limbs in the clinical trial, whereas the narrower ones were effective in 25% of limbs. The width of improvised tourniquets has been associated with their effectiveness, which indicates that the width of the device applied to the limb is an important design feature.[3] We have noted that improvised devices often function as venous tourniquets and so are ineffective, and this is particularly true when the device is narrow.

Emergency Tourniquet Use: Implementation, Policy Changes, and Resultant Outcomes

Given a plausible solution to a pressing need, a large-scale fielding of tourniquets to individual deploying US soldiers was executed rapidly in April 2005; the clinical impact of this logistical and medical effort was prompt and positive.[3,6] Furthermore, the recent emergence of clear and specific needs of those rescuers using tactical combat casualty care has permitted a reconsideration of tenets of such a trauma system, which can differ substantially from routine civilian systems.[13,14,46,47] The Emergency Tourniquet Program leaders who ran the recent clinical trial in Baghdad (National Clinical Trial NCT00517166 at ClinicalTrials.gov) reconciled the last resort versus first aid conflict by changing the question from whether we should use tourniquets to how should we use tourniquets.[3] The compiled subject matter expertise came from the detailed analyses of hundreds of cases from that performance improvement project that has been an academic focus these past few years for us.[3,6,9,15,48-51]

The US Army experience in the current war has shown that if tourniquets are used in casualties at risk of limb exsanguination, the survival rate is higher with use than without use.[6,9] The Army clinical trial has also evidenced that use is associated with longer survival, which permits more life-saving interventions and better resuscitation.[9] The Army trial also evidenced that if the tourniquets are used before shock onset, the majority of the life-saving benefit is maintained and that if the tourniquets are first used after shock onset, then most of the life-saving benefit is lost.[6,9] The trial also evidenced that morbidity with tourniquet use was uncommon, temporary, and minor.[3] Because very few first aid devices are ever evidenced to improve survival rates, the emergency tourniquet was the prehospital medical breakthrough of the current war.

Clinical Settings for Emergency Tourniquet Use

The main setting is prehospital for emergency tourniquet use in war in that 85% of casualties with tourniquets used emergently have their first one applied before arrival at the emergency department of the first hospital.[3] The remaining 15% have their first tourniquet applied in the emergency department, but experienced providers judged that the entire 15% should have had prehospital use.[3,6] The emergency department of busy military trauma centers acts as the funnel—the one place where the majority, if not all, of casualties in an area flow through. Such an emergency department can accrue rapidly high case counts in an epidemic of war casualties. The Army trial case accrual rate recently was 29 times that of the prior record of the Israelis. Therefore, although most use of tourniquets is prehospital, the experience gained in these referral patterns has been most concentrated in a busy trauma emergency department. The Army trial also evidenced that if the tourniquets are used prehospital, the survival rate is higher than if the first tourniquet is used in the emergency department. This geographic categorization by care setting, however, was a weaker association than the strong physiologic categorization by time of hemorrhagic shock onset.[6,9] The prehospital setting is often where casualties can be treated for their major limb trauma before shock onset; so shock prevention appears to be the main benefit of tourniquet use.[9]

Tourniquet Use Indications, Contraindications, and Management in Theater

The indication for emergency tourniquet use is any compressible limb bleeding that the rescuer thinks may be life threatening; this indication can be categorized into situations or lesions.[52] The main war situational indication is care under fire in that the rescuer and the casualty are under gunfire or similar danger;

the benefit of getting the casualty and the rescuer to safety decreases the risk of casualty death and probably rescuer death.[3] Another situation can be mass casualty events where scores of casualties occur at one place and time, such as the recent incidents at Fort Hood and Virginia Tech, and need simultaneous hemorrhage control quickly by a few rescuers.[53] Another situation can be a casualty with multiple injuries who needs hemorrhage control at the same time as other life-saving procedures, such as airway control, when under care of few rescuers.[53] Lesions that indicate tourniquets are major bleeding, often uncontrolled by prior means such as wound compression, limb elevation, or pressure dressings. If one device does not stop the bleeding, then a wider device or 2 devices side by side should be used.[3]

The contraindications for emergency tourniquet use are many but are not clearly evidenced. Apparently, many lesions need not have a tourniquet and can be managed by simpler and less risky ways to control hemorrhage. Direct wound compression, limb elevation, or pressure dressings may work, but each of these is not evidenced to improve survival. Limb splinting for an open fracture such as a femur is rarely evidenced to improve survival but may help control hemorrhage and ease transport.[54-56] Wound compression and pressure dressings have sound scientific underpinnings and clearly are popular. They likely have clinical merit although their role has not been delimited clearly, especially for specific lesions or situations.[57,58] Pressure point control of hemorrhage has been studied, but the models are limited and the results have been mixed.[59,60] The real world with situations and lesions being present simultaneously, the difficulty of accurately assessing bleeding (estimating blood loss volume, differentiating arterial from venous bleeding), and the lack of adequate hemorrhage control data sets make differentiating indications and contraindications based on evidence difficult.

The use of tourniquets in emergent settings does not appear to have an obvious effect on the management of the individual casualty later on in the trauma system except for a higher casualty survival rate. A minor effect is a general increase in the severity of injuries to limbs seen in survivors during the span of the war. The Injury Severity Scores for limb-injured casualties surviving to evacuation to the US tertiary care (Echelon IV facility) in Germany has doubled from 2003 to 2007 from 6 to 12, mostly because of the severity of the limb injury. Another minor effect is that the surviving casualties after tourniquet use require more care, like fasciotomy, probably because of the more severe injuries.[3] The rate of fasciotomy has been associated with both injury severity and the duration of tourniquet use.[3] The tourniquet use emergently does have an ischemia-reperfusion phenomenon, but this effect is not obvious and is transitory; there are many other causes of ischemia-reperfusion in war casualties such as shock, vessel injuries, compartment syndromes, and hypoxia.[3]

Emergency Tourniquet Use Techniques, Misuse, Complications, and Abuse

Analysis of recovered devices provides evidence of how tourniquets should be used and how they should not be used. When recovered devices are systematically analyzed in the context of use as in the clinical trial, it is clear that one-handed tourniquet application is desirable but not essential to success in general use and that hospital devices are neither self-applied nor used one-handedly. Therefore, the specifications of devices should account for a broad range of clinical settings. Forcing the makers of a hospital device to make it self-applied with one hand is a useless constraint not based on any practical need but is just inadvertently constraining hospital device designs to the specifications of ideal prehospital devices.

Designers with special experience use that experience in their designs. For example, a design team with a track record of making ski boot buckles has made a tourniquet that looks similar to such buckles, the Ratcheting Medical Tourniquet ([RMT] sometimes known as the Burke RMT, M2 Inc, Winooski, VT). A design team that includes a clinical engineer with a long track record of developing surgical tourniquets and generating knowledge on tourniquet use developed a precision instrument, the EMT. Furthermore, tourniquet design should account for all relevant science, including casualty anthropometry, because devices that do not account for the size of the limbs of the casualties do not fit. For example, the US Army anthropometry study of 1998 gives a good approximation of what the current needs of soldiers are.[61] However, the clinical needs of others, such as children or obese adults, remain plainly different. Device wear analysis indicates that different devices have different components that wear or break depending on use or misuse. In other words, the weakest links vary by design, and how a device is used determines, in part, its effectiveness. Devices that are misused are ineffective. In an example of misuse, if a pneumatic bladder has a needle or knife puncture, then the device fails. Abuse of a device is rare but has included soldiers testing tourniquets on pipes by twisting the devices until the windlass breaks as if there were no consequences to overtwisting and limbs were winch drums of hoisting machines. Overtwisting is needed

to make a device effective when the slack is not taken out before twisting, and the taking out of slack is one of the first steps of application after deciding to apply a tourniquet. The users of the devices we have observed and interviewed have tried to apply the devices lightly and with little limb manipulation by not pulling the device tight before twisting (contrary to the written instructions and training), and this inadvertently makes the device less effective and at risk for breakage. The unintended consequence of trying to be gentle is to be late or lethal in failing to control hemorrhage. In general, the order of the steps in application is the order of importance in survival in that the most important is deciding whether to use a device, the second is the time of application, and the third is taking out the slack before tightening. The latter steps are evidently less important to survival.

Emergency Tourniquet Training, Knowledge, and Recurring Misconceptions

There are several important issues concerning the interrelated topics of emergency tourniquet training, knowledge, and misconceptions. The US military has found a cultural difference between how Afghans and Iraqis perform first aid with tourniquets. Afghan soldiers rarely improvise when needed to save lives with tourniquets, and if a bandage or tourniquet is unavailable, they let their wounded comrade die unaided.[62] On the other hand, at the same time, Iraqis improvise tourniquets commonly with any imaginable material while the Afghans rarely did so despite similar materials being available while exposed to the same tourniquet doctrines. In a larger sense, user "cultures" and expectations vary; if users know that hemorrhage control can save lives, that they have practical experience in training and education specifically in how to use tourniquets, and that they have adequate devices or materials, they can and do save lives.[6,9] However, if users have little knowledge, experience, or training, then casualties can frequently die.

US Army training in 2009 is dramatically different than in 2002 regarding tourniquet use. The depth, breadth, and repetition of tourniquet training are more extensive today, and the doctrine, refined through several years of laboratory and clinical research, is more specific and now evidence based. These widespread training and doctrine improvements are one of the reasons that the casualty survival rate on the battlefield is at an all-time high despite the increasingly severe injuries, particularly to the limbs.[63]

There is a broad knowledge set developed in elective surgery about the principles of tourniquet use,[25,64] and many of these principles apply to emergency tourniquet use as well.[3] For example, the main tissue vulnerable to the duration of tourniquet use is skeletal muscle, which is the limb tissue most sensitive to ischemia-reperfusion; whereas the main tissue vulnerable to the pressure gradient under a tourniquet is peripheral nerve.[3,65-67]

Despite a broad and growing knowledge base available to tourniquet users, misconceptions persist.[5] Recent articles have produced practical tourniquet findings that have refined training and doctrine, and those refinements appear to be important to performance improvement in trauma systems.[3,5,6,49] However, misconceptions often reappear despite such knowledge production and refinements.[5] A recent 2008 publication perpetuated the 2-bone segment misconception, for example, as the authors reviewed 11 casualties in Boston over 7 years and felt that 2-boned body segments such as the forearm or leg would have less tourniquet effectiveness than 1-boned segments like the arm and thigh.[67] However, given adequate device designs, the 2-boned segments actually have the *highest*, not the lowest, effectiveness; and a large body of knowledge indicates this has been so for some time.[3,5,23-25] The reason this misconception persists is based on an oversimplification: effectiveness is not due to 1 or 2 bones but to a complex relationship among pressure, device width, and limb circumference.[3,23] Another reason that misconceptions recur is that rarely are civilian emergency tourniquet cases compiled for study. The Boston study findings were supportive of more civilian use, but other misconceptions were fostered and not dispelled. (The authors noted that pressure was associated with effectiveness but had no consideration of device width or limb circumference. The authors assumed that observers can reliably tell arterial from venous bleeding without regard for contrary evidence.[68]) Users should understand how devices work best in order to attain optimal outcomes. Designs should meet user expectations by care setting if expectations are scientifically grounded because when user expectations mismatch the device science, problems abound. When user expectations match the device science, optimal care is more easily attained.

Emergency Tourniquet Use Doctrines, Policies, Positions, and Algorithms

Trauma systems may or may not have a doctrine (even policies or practices) on emergency tourniquet use. The US military has organized itself to put surgical capabilities forward and close to the point of injury, which is crucial to preventing complications and to translate early prevention of blood loss into improved outcome. The military currently does have a coherent, evidenced-based clinical doctrine on the emergency use of tourniquets, but in the past, the doctrine was unclear and lacked evidence. The US military has taken a trauma systems approach to battlefield survival, and important, long-term efforts of military medics like Sergeant First Class (now retired) Robert Miller of the US Army Rangers and surgeon-leaders like Captain (now retired) Frank Butler of the US Navy and Colonel (now retired) John Holcomb of the US Army helped marshal the systematic analysis. Taking a performance improvement strategy, they looked for opportunities to improve casualty survival and helped develop tactical combat casualty care, one of the key differences between civilian and military trauma care. The frequency of tactical casualty care in combat is high, but in civilian care, it is low. Therefore, the military efforts in tactical casualty care took the lead; and the refinement in hemorrhage control by use of emergency tourniquets required an analysis of historical perspective, candidate devices, development of a clear doctrine, an overhaul of training, clinical research, and integrated feedback for system improvement.[13,14]

Despite the growing evidence that limb exsanguination was the leading cause of preventable death on the battlefield upon entry into the current wars, there was a need to broadcast that knowledge to key leaders in order to inform the decisions needed for logistical acquisition and fielding of devices. The media and legislative processes helped in the lead up to the decision of the US Army Surgeon General to recommend the issuance of an emergency tourniquet to deploying servicemembers in April 2005. The policy enactment therefore was not with a stroke of a pen but rather was an integrated, complex set of actions aimed at providing a suitable solution. These policies were concordant with the medical evidence that was becoming manifest through the refined doctrine and training.

Organizations that deal with emergency trauma are currently challenged in integrating the new tourniquet knowledge into their policies and practices.[69] For example, some emergency medicine authors have advocated more consideration and study of tourniquet use in civilian settings or have made position statements.[52,70] Some authors have tried to set the use of emergency tourniquets into algorithms in order to simplify the complexities and guide treatment. Examples include the protocols of Taillac and Doyle,[70] which are not developed from any stated data set, and the algorithm developed by the US Army Rangers, which has been developed over several years and many casualties.[71] Each algorithm is aimed at 2 populations at risk, and the Rangers have their specific and evidenced needs, which are not obviously similar or comparable to the general population at which the other authors aim.

Research Gaps: Dressings, Pressure Points, and Proximal Bleeding

Future directions for research are numerous as there are many items to confirm, develop, or refine. Tourniquet alternatives including elevation, pressure dressings, and pressure points are without clear and practical data sets evidencing hemorrhage control, so these are candidates of further study. Enough data have been published recently to consider decision analysis, medico-legal, or actuarial studies or models of emergency tourniquet use in order to model whether or how they are used. Such study may help trauma system leaders decide whether their system's constituents need tourniquets available or whether they know how best to use them.

If tourniquets solved the limb exsanguination death problem after we picked it as the lowest lying fruit in combat casualty care, then the next fruit to be picked requires a longer reach. Bleeding from very proximal extremities may require new or different tourniquets in order to compress the groin or axilla because conventional tourniquets are less effective there. We currently label such hemorrhage *junctional bleeding*. Similarly, abdominal or aortic tourniquets may be studied in order to determine if or when these devices might be used to gain hemorrhage control.[60,72]

Acknowledgments

Dr. Kragh thanks Otilia Sanchez for assistance in manuscript preparation.

References

1. Bailey H. *Surgery of Modern Warfare*. Edinburgh, UK: Livingstone; 1941:273-279.
2. Beekley AC, Sebesta JA, Blackbourne LH, et al. Prehospital tourniquet use in Operation Iraqi Freedom: effect on hemorrhage control. *J Trauma*. 2008;64(2):S28-S37.
3. Kragh JF Jr, Walters TJ, Baer DG, et al. Practical use of emergency tourniquets to stop bleeding in major limb trauma. *J Trauma*. 2008;64:S38-S50.
4. Tien HC, Jung V, Rizoli SB, Acharya SV, MacDonald JC. An evaluation of tactical combat casualty care interventions in a combat environment. *J Am Coll Surg*. 2008;207(2):174-178.
5. Brodie S, Hodgetts TJ, Ollerton J, McLeod J, Lambert P, Mahoney P. Tourniquet use in combat trauma: UK military experience. *J Royal Army Med Corps*. 2007;153(4):310-333.
6. Kragh JF Jr, Walters TJ, Baer DG, et al. Survival with emergency tourniquet use to stop bleeding in major limb trauma. *Ann Surg*. 2009;249(1):1-7.
7. American College of Surgeons, Committee on Trauma. *Advanced Trauma Life Support for Doctors*. 7th ed. Chicago, IL: Author; 2004.
8. Mabry RL. Tourniquet use on the battlefield. *Mil Med*. 2006;171(5):352-356.
9. Kragh JF Jr, Littrel ML, Jones JA, et al. Battle casualty survival with emergency tourniquet use to stop limb bleeding. *J Emerg Med*. E-pub ahead of print. Aug 28, 2009.
10. Wolff LH, Adkins TF. Tourniquet problems in war injuries. *Bulletin of the US Army Medical Department*. 1945;87:77-84.
11. Bellamy RF. The causes of death in conventional land warfare: implications for combat casualty care research. *Mil Med*. 1984;149(2):55-62.
12. Mabry RL, Holcomb JB, Baker AM, et al. United States Army Rangers in Somalia: an analysis of combat casualties on an urban battlefield. *J Trauma*. 2000;49(3):515-528; discussion 528-529.
13. Butler FK Jr, Hagmann J, Butler EG. Tactical combat casualty care in special operations. *Mil Med*. 1996;161(Suppl):3-16.
14. Butler FK Jr. Tactical medicine training for SEAL mission commanders. *J Special Oper Med*. 2004;4(1):40-51.
15. Walters TJ, Wenke JC, Kauvar DS, et al. Effectiveness of self-applied tourniquets in human volunteers. *Prehosp Emerg Care*. 2005;9(4):416-422.
16. Office of the Surgeon General, US Army, Health Plans & Security Directorate, All Army Action message (ALARACT). *Individual Soldier Tourniquets—Combat Application Tourniquet*. March 2005.
17. Lakstein D, Blumenfeld A, Sokolov T, et al. Tourniquets for hemorrhage control on the battlefield: a 4-year accumulated experience. *J Trauma*. 2003;54(5 Suppl):S221-S225.
18. Conzelmann FJ. Improvised Esmarch bandage. The military surgeon. *J Assoc Mil Surg US*. 1907;30:62.
19. Artz CP, Howard JM, Sako Y, Bronwell AW, Prentice T. Clinical experiences in the early management of the most severely injured battle casualties. *Ann Surg*. 1955;141(3):285-296.
20. Navein J, Coupland R, Dunn R. The tourniquet controversy. *J Trauma*. 2003;54(5 Suppl):S219-S220.
21. Husum H, Gilbert M, Wisborg T, Pillgram-Larsen J. Prehospital tourniquets: there should be no controversy. *J Trauma*. 2004;56(1):214-215.
22. Holcomb JB. Damage control resuscitation. *J Trauma*. 2007;62(6 Suppl):S36-S37.
23. Graham B, Breault MJ, McEwen JA, McGraw RW. Occlusion of arterial flow in the extremities at subsystolic pressures through the use of wide tourniquet cuffs. *Clin Orthop*. 1993;286:257-261.
24. Graham B, Breault MJ, McEwen JA, McGraw RW. Perineural pressures under the pneumatic tourniquet in the upper extremity. *J Hand Surg (Br)*. 1992;17(3):262-266.
25. Klenerman L. *The Tourniquet Manual*. London, UK: Springer; 2003.
26. Grant RT, Reeve EB. Observations on the general effects of injury in man: with special reference to wound shock. *Medical Research Council Special Report Series No. 277*. London: HM Stationery Office; 1951:3-67.
27. Wiggers CJ. *Physiology of Shock*. New York, NY: Commonwealth Fund; 1950:95-120.
28. Anonymous. Editorial: the tourniquet, instrument or weapon? *Can Med Assoc J*. 1973;109(9):827.

29. Anonymous. Recommended practices. Use of the pneumatic tourniquet. AORN Recommended Practices Coordinating Committee. *AORN Journal.* 1990;52(5):1041-1044.

30. Sanders R. The tourniquet: instrument or weapon? *Hand.* 1973;5(2):119-123.

31. Bussani CR, McEwen JA. Improved tracking of limb occlusion pressure for surgical tourniquets. *IEEE Trans Biomed Eng.* 1988;35(4):221-229.

32. Crenshaw AG, Hargens AR, Gershuni DH, Rydevik B. Wide tourniquet cuffs more effective at lower inflation pressures. *Acta Orthop Scand.* 1988;59(4):447-451.

33. Hargens AR, McClure AG, Skyhar MJ, Lieber RL, Gershuni DH, Akeson WH. Local compression patterns beneath pneumatic tourniquets applied to arms and thighs of human cadavers. *J Orthop Res.* 1987;5(2):247-252.

34. Moore MR, Garfin SR, Hargens AR. Wide tourniquets eliminate blood flow at low inflation pressures. *J Hand Surg.* 1987;12A(6):1006-1011.

35. McEwen J. Complications of and improvements in pneumatic tourniquets used in surgery. *Med Instrum.* 1981;15(4):253-257.

36. Younger AS, McEwen JA, Inkpen K. Wide contoured thigh cuffs and automated limb occlusion measurement allow lower tourniquet pressures. *Clin Orthop.* 2004;428:286-293.

37. van der Meer C, Valkenburg PW, Ariens AT, van Benthem RM. Cause of death in tourniquet shock in rats. *Am J Physiol.* 1966;210(3):513-525.

38. Blaisdell FW. The pathophysiology of skeletal muscle ischemia and the reperfusion syndrome: a review. *Cardiovasc Surg.* 2002;10(6):620-630.

39. Shaw JA, Murray DG. The relationship between tourniquet pressure and underlying soft-tissue pressure in the thigh. *J Bone Joint Surg.* 1982;64A(8):1148-1152.

40. Thomson AE, Doupe J. Some factors affecting the auscultatory measurement of arterial blood pressures. *Can J Res.* 1949;27(E):72-80.

41. McGraw RW, McEwen JA. The tourniquet. In: McFarlane RM, ed. *Unsatisfactory Results in Hand Surgery.* New York, NY: Churchill Livingstone; 1987:5-13.

42. Middleton RW, Varian JP. Tourniquet paralysis. *Aust N Z J Surg.* 1974;44(2):124-128.

43. Russell AE, Wing LM, Smith SA, et al. Optimal size of cuff bladder for indirect measurement of arterial pressure in adults. *J Hypertension.* 1989;7(8):607-613.

44. McEwen JA, Inkpen K. Surgical tourniquet technology adapted for military and prehospital use. NATO Research and Technology Organization, RTO-MP-HFM-109, 19-1-12, 16-18, August 2004. Symposium on "Combat Casualty Care in Ground Based Tactical Situations: Trauma Technology and Emergency Medical Procedures," St. Pete Beach, FL.

45. McEwen JA, Casey V. Measurement of hazardous pressure levels and gradients produced on human limbs by non-pneumatic tourniquets. 32nd Can Med Biol Eng Soc Conf; 2009.

46. Mucciarone JJ, Llewellyn CH, Wightman JM. Tactical combat casualty care in the assault on Punta Paitilla airfield. *Mil Med.* 2006;171:687-690.

47. Parsons DL, Walters TJ. Tourniquets: lifesavers on the battlefield. *J Spec Oper Med.* 2004;4(4):51-53.

48. Walters TJ, Wenke JC, Baer DG. Research on tourniquet related injury for combat casualty care. NATO Research and Technology Organization, RTO-MP-HFM-109, P33 – 1-8, 16-18 August 2004. Symposium on "Combat Casualty Care in Ground Based Tactical Situations: Trauma Technology and Emergency Medical Procedures," St. Pete Beach, FL.

49. Walters TJ, Wenke JC, Greydanus, DJ, Kauvar DS, Baer DG. Laboratory evaluation of battlefield tourniquets in human volunteers. *US Army Institute of Surgical Research Technical report 2005-05.* 2005.

50. Kragh JF Jr, Baer DG, Walters TJ. Extended (16-hour) tourniquet application after combat wounds: a case report and review of the current literature. *J Orthop Trauma.* 2007;21(4):274-278.

51. Kragh JF Jr. Emergency tourniquet use. *Ann Surg.* 2009;250(3):497.

52. National Association of Emergency Medical Technicians. *PHTLS Prehospital Trauma Life Support: Military Version.* 6th ed. St. Louis, MO: Mosby; 2007.

53. Cain JS. From the battlefield to our streets: how combat medicine is revolutionizing civilian prehospital care. *J Emerg Med Serv.* The War on Trauma Supplement. 2008:16-23.

54. Gray HMW. *The Early Treatment of War Wounds.* London, UK: Oxford University Press; 1919:49-63.

55. Sinclair M. *The Thomas Splint and Its Modifications in the Treatment of Fractures.* New York, NY: Oxford University Press; 1927.

56. Kirkup J. Fracture care of friend and foe during World War I. *Aust N Z J Surg.* 2003;73(6):453-459.

57. Wangensteen SL, Eddy DM, Ludewig RM. The hydrodynamics of arterial hemorrhage. *Surg.* 1968;64(5):912-921.

58. Wangensteen SL, Deoll JD, Ludewig RM, Madden JJ Jr. The detrimental effect of the G-suit in hemorrhagic shock. *Ann Surg.* 1969;170(2):187-192.

59. Swan KG Jr, Wright DS, Barbagiovanni SS, Swan BC, Swan KG. Tourniquets revisited. *J Trauma.* 2009;66(3):672-675.

60. Blaivas M, Shiver S, Lyon M, Adhikari S. Control of hemorrhage in critical femoral or inguinal penetrating wounds: an ultrasound evaluation. *Prehosp Disast Med.* 2006;21(6):379-382.

61. Gordon CC, Churchill T, Clauser CE, et al. *Anthropometric Survey of U.S. Army Personnel: Methods and Summary Statistics.* Yellow Springs, OH: Anthropology Research Project Inc; 1989.

62. Center of Army Lessons Learned Bulletin 09-41. The Combat Application Tourniquet (CAT). 3: 91-94, 2009.

63. Holcomb JB, Stansbury LG, Champion HR, Wade C, Bellamy RF. Understanding combat casualty care statistics. *J Trauma.* 2006;60(2):397-401.

64. Noordin S, McEwen JA, Kragh JF Jr, Eisen A, Masri BA. Surgical tourniquets in orthopaedics. *J Bone Joint Surg Am.* 2009;91:2958-2967.

65. Ochoa J, Danta G, Fowler TJ, Gilliatt RW. Nature of the nerve lesion caused by a pneumatic tourniquet. *Nature.* 1971;233(5317):265-266.

66. Ochoa J, Fowler TJ, Gilliatt RW. Anatomical changes in peripheral nerves compressed by a pneumatic tourniquet. *J Anat.* 1972;113(Pt 3):433-455.

67. Dayan L, Zinmann C, Stahl S, Norman D. Complications associated with prolonged tourniquet application on the battlefield. *Mil Med.* 2008;173(1):63-66.

68. Kalish J, Burke P, Feldman J, et al. The return of tourniquets. Original research evaluates the effectiveness of prehospital tourniquets for civilian penetrating extremity injuries. *J Emerg Med Serv.* 2008;33(8):44-54.

69. Fludger S, Bell A. Tourniquet application in a rural Queensland HEMS environment. *Air Med J.* 2009;28(6):291-293.

70. Taillac PP, Doyle GS. Tourniquet first! Safe & rational protocols for prehospital tourniquet use. *J Emerg Med Serv JEMS.* The War on Trauma Supplement. 2008:24-27.

71. *Ranger Medic Handbook.* Las Vegas, NV: Cielo Azul Publications; 2007.

72. Coule PL Calhoun DJ. Evaluation and comparison of tourniquets for hemorrhage control. *Abstracts of 16th World Congress on Disaster and Emergency Medicine Prehospital and Disaster Medicine.* 2009;24(Suppl 1):54-55.

Chapter **15**

EXTERNAL FIXATION PRINCIPLES

LCDR Joseph Carney, MD and CAPT D.C. Covey, MD

External fixation has become a mainstay in the treatment of battlefield fractures.[1] It was first used during the early part of World War II, and American casualties treated with this technique in a stable environment had favorable outcomes.[2] However, external fixation fell out of favor as the war progressed due to an unacceptably high complication rate, probably resulting from inappropriate use or lack of familiarity with principles of external fixation.[2,3] However, its use has dramatically increased both in and out of the combat zone since that time.

Brief History of External Fixation

Although use of external fixation for treatment of fractures may be considered by some as a relatively recent development, Hippocrates (c. 460 to 380 BC) described an external technique for achieving fracture reduction more than 2000 years ago.[4] The modern era of external fixation dates from the 1840s when Malgaigne invented the "pointe métallique," a nail placed through a semicircular metallic band that was percutaneously nailed into the fracture fragment, and a "griffe métallique," literally and figuratively a metallic claw for compression and immobilization of patella fractures.[5]

In 1893, Keetley was the first to use percutaneous bicortical pins with a special external fixation device for the treatment of long-bone fractures.[6]

Subsequently in 1897, Parkhill developed the modern concept of unilateral external fixation with 2 half pins above and 2 below the fracture site joined by a unique clamp for fracture reduction and immobilization.[6] In 1902, Lambotte described a construct consisting of 2 pins proximal and 2 pins distal to the fracture that were fixed between 2 heavy metal plates, making the apparatus rigid and thus more suitable for early limb mobilization.[5]

During the first half of the 20th century, many others made significant contributions to the development of the external fixator. Notable advancements were made by Codvilla in 1904, Crile in 1919, and Conn in 1931.[5] Also in 1931, Pitkin and Blackfield developed the first bilateral frame.[6] In the 1930s, Roger Anderson developed an external fixator device that consisted of a series of rods and pins interconnected by moveable clamps that permitted multiplanar adjustment of fracture fragments.[7,8] His device was used in the US Army in World War II, while the US Navy used an external fixator developed by Stader in 1937 that facilitated fracture reduction in 2 planes. Both were used guardedly.[5]

Beginning in the 1930s, Hoffmann worked on developing an external fixator with ball-and-socket joints that could swivel, thus permitting the rigid bar and the entire frame to move in continuity, and this allowed the surgeon to complete fracture reduction in 3 spatial planes independently.[9] Although today's external fixators may incorporate some advanced modifications, the basic principles, technique, and indications for their use were first described by Hoffmann.[5]

Owens BD, Belmont PJ Jr, eds. *Combat Orthopedic Surgery:*
Lessons Learned in Iraq and Afghanistan (pp 129-134)
© 2011 SLACK Incorporated

External Fixation Categories: Large Pin Longitudinal Bar Versus Small Wire Circular Frame

External fixation systems can be categorized according to the type of bone anchorage used and are typically divided into large-diameter threaded pin systems or small-diameter transfixation wire systems. These pins or wires are then connected to each other through the use of longitudinal bars or circular rings. Longitudinal bar fixation employs the use of only large-diameter threaded pins while circular fixators may use either threaded pins or small tensioned wires to attach bone to the frame. The application of circular small wire frames has certain biomechanical principles specific to this technique of external fixation. For example, the use of circular or semicircular fixators allows for multiple planes of fixation, producing frame behavior that can eliminate cantilever loading and shear forces to a great degree while accentuating axial micro motion that can promote fracture healing and bone formation.[10-13] Circular small wire fixation systems are typically not available in the war theater and when used are commonly done at the highest echelons of care outside of the war theater for definitive treatment of extremity injuries. Consequently, we will focus on the biomechanical principles of large pin longitudinal fixation techniques and defer discussion of circular small wire fixation systems to later chapters discussing the definitive treatment of specific extremity injuries.

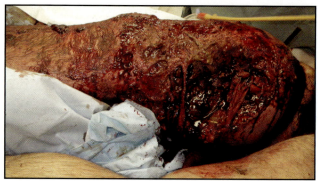

Figure 15-1. Extensive right thigh soft tissue wound from an IED. This soldier sustained extensive right thigh soft tissue wounds when he was struck by an IED while dismounting in Afghanistan.

Table 15-1

External Fixator Variables That Improve Biomechanical Stability

Injury Site	Anatomical reduction
	Fracture compression
Component Elements	Increased diameter
	Increase number
	Stiffer material
Frame Geometry	Pins placed in bending plane
	Pins placed in multiple planes (ie, orthogonal pin placement)
	Increased pin spread
	Increased rod to bone distance

Biomechanics of External Fixation for the War Surgeon

Typically, the application of external fixation in the war theater occurs early after injury. In most cases, fractures are fresh, and soft tissue damage is extensive (Figure 15-1). Thus, the use of external fixation by the war surgeon has a specific purpose to stabilize fractures and protect soft tissue compromise as patients travel through the medical evacuation (MEDEVAC) system. The application of external fixation attempts to impart rigid stability to the fracture construct in an effort to maintain reduction and avoid collapse. In essence, the external fixation system can be considered as "portable traction" and improves the ability to mobilize patients as fragment motion is reduced, pain control is improved, and nursing care is facilitated. Following specific biomechanical principles when using the technique can increase the effectiveness of its use in war surgery.

The mechanical properties of external fixation systems can be improved by affecting 3 main categories: 1) fracture site, 2) fixation system components, and 3) the geometry of the fixation system (Table 15-1).[14-16] In cases where interfragmentary compression can be achieved via external fixation, the stability of the fracture site is greatly improved. Unfortunately, most war theater injuries are of such a high-energy nature that comminution and bone and soft tissue loss are common, and interfragmentary compression is not possible (Figure 15-2). Therefore, in most instances of external fixation application in the war theater, the mechanical properties of the external fixation system are optimized solely by increasing stiffness of the apparatus through component interventions and geometry improvements in the construct.

Optimization of external fixation system components focuses on material properties, number, and size of components used. In general, the goal is to improve the stiffness of the construct by using components

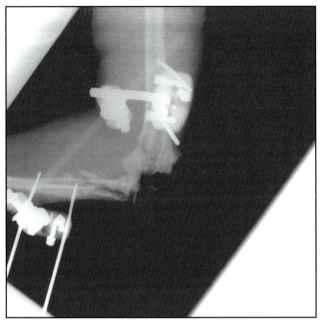

Figure 15-2. Radiograph of external fixation of a severely comminuted elbow fracture caused by an IED. Navy servicemember injured by an IED while on patrol, sustaining an open, type IIIB left elbow fracture and a radial nerve palsy.

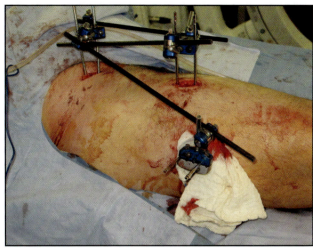

Figure 15-3. Biplanar external fixation spanning a hip joint for an unstable posterior wall acetabular fracture. This patient sustained a large posterior wall acetabulum fracture in a tactical vehicle rollover resulting in a grossly unstable hip joint in extension requiring external fixation as temporary traction for MEDEVAC to a higher echelon where he underwent internal fixation of the fracture dislocation.

made of the stiffest materials available. In deployed situations, there is rarely an option to choose from multiple components of different stiffness as the austere environment precludes opportunities for robust supply reserve. Therefore, the components available for use are usually of constant material properties. Subsequently, component interventions to improve external fixation systems in the war theater focus on increasing the number and/or size of the components used.

In general, increasing the number of pins or rods is less desirable than increasing their diameter.[14,17] Improvement in stiffness of the fixation system can be achieved by increasing the diameter of the components. Bending stiffness improves by the fourth power and resistance to torsion by the third power with this augmentation.[18] However, increasing pin size too much can risk fracture through the pin site, and it is generally recommended that pin size be limited to 20% of the diameter of the bone.[16] When pins of larger sizes are desired but not available, advancing the wider shaft of the pin into the proximal "near" cortex increases the stiffness of most pins, provides a tighter pin-bone fit, and can decrease stress at the pin-bone interface.[18-20] This technique is not recommended in situations where it would be necessary to advance the pin excessively into the distal "far" soft tissues in order to engage the shaft of the pin into the proximal "near" cortex if neurovascular structures are at risk opposite the far cortex.

The stability of large pin longitudinal bar external fixation systems can be improved through augmentations of the geometry of the fixation construct. External fixation systems that require optimization of stability and stiffness can be improved with application of fixation pins orthogonal to each other (Figure 15-3).[15] Pin placement in 2 or more planes allows for biplanar stabilization of the injured region. Biplanar stabilization protects from bending forces in more than one plane and is inherently more stable. However, this construct can come at the cost of more pins and a bulkier frame. The addition of more pins increases the potential for pin site infections, and the addition of longitudinal bars in multiple planes enlarges the "footprint" of the external fixation system, which can make patient positioning, patient transfers, and patient mobility more of a challenge.

External Fixation Application Technique

The war-injured patient requiring external fixation often is a polytrauma patient with wounds that are grossly contaminated. Advanced Trauma Life Support guidelines are followed, and a multidisciplinary team approach is used. Once the patient is transferred to the surgical theater, the recommended patient position is supine on a radiolucent operating table, which allows for full access to most regions of the body that may need surgical attention. Specifically, the chest, abdomen, pelvis, head, neck, and extremities can all be accessed and, if available, fluoroscopy can be used from head to toe. When addressing limb injuries, the proximal and distal joints surrounding the injured region should be included in the surgical field to facilitate correct alignment, and, in some instances, including the opposite uninjured limb can be helpful as well.

Most war wounds are grossly contaminated, and debridement is recommended prior to performing external fixator application. Pin insertion should be carefully planned to decrease potential complications related to pin placement technique, keeping in mind that the pins often need to be left in place for several weeks and complications could compromise future fixation decisions. Pin locations are determined by the size, severity, inherent stability, and relationship of the injury to important structures. If possible, pins should be inserted outside of the zone of injury and in safe regions that do not contain important neurovascular structures or musculotendinous units. Pins should not violate joint spaces. In general, pins are placed percutaneously using soft tissue sleeves with the aid of fluoroscopy if available. Pins should be placed to avoid over- or underpenetration of the opposite cortex, and clustering of multiple pins should be avoided as this may increase risk for fracture through these stress riser holes. Pins should avoid open wounds, blisters, burns, and severe abrasions if possible. When the frame is constructed, it should be adapted to optimally accommodate surgical access routes, repeated debridements, and the application of future internal fixation while not risking inadequate construct stiffness.

At the time of pin insertion, fluoroscopy should be used if available. The lowest echelons of surgical care in theater likely will not have fluoroscopy available, but plain film radiography can be used to check pin placement when complete. When radiography is limited, the technique of making small incisions for pin placement in risky limb segments and the pelvis can be used to ensure safer insertion of pins (Figure 15-4). At the completion of external fixator application, sterile dressings should be applied to the pin sites with care to avoid excessive bandage pressure that may cause necrosis.

Complications Associated With External Fixation

Most early complications that occur with the use of external fixation have a physician component to them. The most significant complications occur with improper insertion of pins causing injury to nerves, vessels, intra-articular joint structures, and musculotendinous

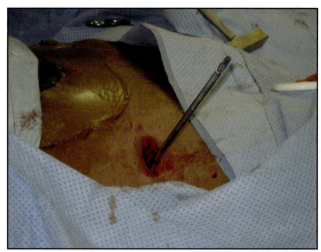

Figure 15-4. Incision for the safe placement of supra-acetabular pelvic fixation pin.

structures. Furthermore, the iatrogenic damage to tissue that occurs with improper pin insertion can increase the risk of compartment syndrome, which is inherently a concern in the war-injured patient due to the prevalence of high-energy injuries and the unique risk factors intrinsic in the MEDEVAC process. Most of these complications are preventable when technically proficient pin insertion techniques are used and the surgeon maintains a clear understanding of the relevant anatomy. Pin insertion techniques that can minimize risk include the use of small incisions for pin placement in regions where neurovascular structures are at risk, such as the lateral distal humerus, the iliac crest, and the radial aspect of the distal forearm. Furthermore, drill guides with trochars can be used to accurately place fixation pins on the bone of interest with minimal disruption of surrounding tissue.

Common late complications that occur with external fixation include infection and component failure causing loss of stability. Most instances of component failure are due to inadequate stiffness of the construct. When component failure occurs, it is most often the result of surgeons not following the basic biomechanical principles of external fixation outlined previously in this chapter. Infection complications that occur with external fixation use are often multifactorial in nature. In the war theater environment, most wounds present with gross contamination that is often deep. Subsequently, these injuries are at an increased risk of infection when compared to the civilian injured patient. Predictable practices that can contribute to the already increased risk of pin site drainage, pin tract infection, and pin loosening include insertion of pins through a thick soft tissue sleeve, excessive motion at the pin-soft tissue interface, and placement of pins near or in a focus of potential contamination.[14] Pin placement technique can also contribute to the late presentation of infection after conversion of external fixation to internal fixation. Specifically, the placement of pins within a zone of injury and/or near future planned internal fixation sites can increase future postoperative infections when conversion to internal fixation is performed.

Steps should be taken to ensure that the risks associated with external fixation application are minimized regardless of the resources available and the environment in which the procedure is performed. At the lowest echelons of care in the war theater, intraoperative fluoroscopy may not be available. Therefore, the surgeon's surgical training and thorough understanding of applied surgical anatomy prior to working in the combat theater is of paramount importance. Additionally, surgeons should have adequate experience with applying external fixators either in the civilian trauma or laboratory setting prior to their deployment. Specifically, the surgeon should be familiar with safe and unsafe zones of the limbs and pelvis for placing external fixation pins. Typically, safe zones do not include important neurovascular structures nor musculotendinous units.

Conclusion

Application of the external fixator is the most common orthopedic fixation procedure performed in the war theater. The use of external fixation by the war surgeon typically serves the purpose of stabilizing fractures and protecting soft tissue injuries as patients travel through the MEDEVAC system. The application of external fixation attempts to impart rigid stability to the fracture construct in an effort to maintain reduction and avoid collapse. In essence, the external fixation system can be considered as "portable traction" and improves the ability to mobilize patients, control pain, and provide nursing care. Adequate preparation by the war surgeon prior to entering the war theater, safe pin insertion techniques, and following specific biomechanical principles when applying external fixation systems can maximize the effectiveness of its use in war surgery and decrease potential complications.

References

1. Covey DC. Combat orthopaedics: a view from the trenches. *J Am Acad Orthop Surg.* 2006;14:S10-S17.
2. Dougherty PJ, Carter PR, Seligson D, Benson DR, Purvis JM. Orthopaedic surgery advances resulting from World War II. *J Bone Joint Surg Am.* 2004;86:176-181.
3. Covey DC. From the frontlines to the homefront: the crucial role of military orthopaedic surgeons. *J Bone Joint Surg Am.* 2009;91:998-1006.
4. Hippocrates, Adams F. On fractures: part 30. *The Internet Classics Archives.* 2009. http://classics.mit.edu/Hippocrates/fractur.30.30.html. Accessed June 30, 2010.
5. Schwechter EM, Swan KG. Raoul Hoffmann and his external fixator. *J Bone Joint Surg Am.* 2007;89:672-678.
6. Wood GW. General principles of fracture treatment. In: Canale ST, Beaty JH, eds. *Campbell's Operative Orthopaedics.* 11th ed. Philadelphia, PA: Mosby Elsevier; 2008:3063.
7. Anderson R. An automatic method for treatment for fractures of the tibia and fibula. *Surg Gynecol Obstet.* 1934;58:639-646.
8. Grana WA, Kopta JA. The Roger Anderson device in the treatment of the distal end of the radius. *J Bone Joint Surg Am.* 1979;61:1234-1238.
9. Hoffmann R. "Closed osteosynthesis," with special reference to war surgery. *Acta Chir Scand.* 1942;86:235-266.
10. Fisher DA. Skeletal stabilization with a multiplane external fixation device. Design rationale and preliminary clinical experience. *Clin Orthop.* 1983;180:50-62.
11. Williams EA, Rand JA, An KN, et al. The early healing of tibial osteotomies stabilized by one-plane or two-plane external fixation. *J Bone Joint Surg Am.* 1987;69(3):355-365.
12. McCoy MT, Chao EY, Kasman RA. Comparison of mechanical performance in four types of external fixation. *Clin Orthop.* 1983;180:23-33.
13. Aronson J, Harrison B, Boyd CM. Mechanical induction of osteogenesis: the importance of pin rigidity. *J Pediatr Orthop.* 1988;8(4):396-401.
14. Behrens F. General theory and principles of external fixation. *Clin Orthop.* 1989;241:15-23.
15. Etter C, Burri C, Claes L, Kinzl L, Raible M. Treatment of external fixation of open fractures associated with severe soft tissue damage of the leg. *Clin Orthop.* 1983;178:80-88.
16. Vidal J. External fixation. *Clin Orthop.* 1983;180:7-14.
17. Briggs BT, Chao EY. The mechanical performance of the standard Hoffmann-Vidal external fixation apparatus. *J Bone Joint Surg Am.* 1982;64A:566-573.
18. Behrens F, Johnson WD, Koch TW, Kovacevic N. Bending stiffness of unilateral and bilateral fixator frames. *Clin Orthop.* 1983;178:103-110.
19. Evan M, Kenwright J, Tanner KE. Analysis of single sided fracture fixation. *Eng Med.* 1979;8:133-137.
20. Hyldahl C, Pearson S, Tepic S, Perren SM. Induction and prevention of pin loosening in external fixation: an in vivo study on sheep tibiae. *J Orthop Trauma.* 1991;5(4):485-492.

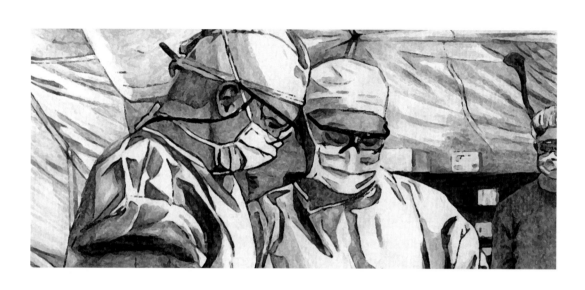

SECTION III
UPPER EXTREMITY

Chapter 16

UPPER EXTREMITY NERVE INJURIES

CAPT Eric P. Hofmeister, MD; LT Kathryn H. Hanna, MD; and
LCDR Leo T. Kroonen, MD

Modern warfare has seen an increase in the destructiveness of enemy weaponry. In contrast, the fatality rates during the Iraq and Afghanistan Wars are at a historic low. Advances in US military personnel protective measures to include Kevlar helmets, individual body armor, protective eyewear, and vehicular body armor; strategic placement of skilled surgical teams; and rapid medical evacuation times have reduced the case fatality rate to only 8% to 10%.[1,2] Despite these improvements, the percentage of injured extremities has continued to account for approximately half of all battlefield injuries.[1,3] Injuries to the accompanying nerves of the upper extremity are common, often difficult to treat, and usually associated with severe injury to the surrounding soft tissue and bone. Treatment of these injuries requires a thorough understanding of the anatomy and biology of the upper extremity nerves, familiarity with multiple surgical techniques, and meticulous handling of the associated injuries.

Historical Background

Prior to World War II, little specialized consideration was given to the surgical management of injuries to the upper extremity in the combat casualty. This changed when Dr. Sterling Bunnell was appointed as the hand surgery consultant to the Surgeon General of the US Army in 1944. Over the course of the next year, 9 hand centers were established throughout the United States. This was the first time hand surgery was recognized as a specialty. Interestingly, during World War II, almost all peripheral nerve injuries were referred to

neurosurgical specialty centers.[4] Data collected at these centers revealed that nerve injuries were associated with 15% of all upper and lower combat extremity wounds.[5] It was not until the Vietnam War that more extremity nerve injuries were referred to hand centers.[4]

One such hand center established in support of the Vietnam War was located at Brooke Army Medical Center (BAMC). Omer reported on the collective experience at BAMC dealing with peripheral nerve injuries during the Vietnam War and found that 22% of all patients with upper extremity combat wounds during the war had associated major peripheral nerve injuries.[4] Twenty years after the BAMC study, Stanec and colleagues described their experience treating peripheral nerve war wounds during the Croatian War. Their series described a 25% incidence of peripheral nerve injuries in all extremity war wounds.[5] The wars in Iraq and Afghanistan have continued to produce extremity wounds with associated nerve injuries.

Upper extremity nerve injuries from modern day combat are often complex, devastating injuries. In addition to the deficits from the nerve injury, there is often a large zone of injury that includes the surrounding skin, muscle, fascia, vessels, and nerves. In these situations, the nerve gap can become quite large. The goal in treating these injuries is to restore protective sensation and motor function to the affected extremity. Direct repair, without tension, is the optimal treatment whenever possible. However, segmental loss of nerves requires grafting, resulting in the sacrifice of small cutaneous nerves of the forearm, redundant muscular nerve branches, or the sural nerve. The consequence of donor site morbidity in harvesting these nerve grafts is sensory deficits at the donor sites.

Owens BD, Belmont PJ Jr, eds. *Combat Orthopedic Surgery:
Lessons Learned in Iraq and Afghanistan (pp 137-146)*
© 2011 SLACK Incorporated

Fractures and bone loss, tendon lacerations or defects, and soft tissue coverage concerns often accompany traumatic peripheral nerve injuries, adding to the difficulty in treating these combat casualties. These concomitant injuries must be treated by procedures to include bony stabilization, bone grafting, tendon repairs and transfers, and soft tissue coverage procedures, which range from skin grafting to free flaps. Although delays in treatment after denervation lead to muscle atrophy, adequate time must be allowed for the zone of injury to be identifiable during surgery.

Epidemiology

Musculoskeletal extremity injuries have been reported to comprise approximately 50% of all combat wounds during the Iraq and Afghanistan Wars.[1,3] During the course of the 20th century, a generalized trend has occurred, whereby the number of casualties due to explosions has increased relative to those due to gunshot. The 77% to 84% casualty figure for explosive mechanisms of injury during the Iraq and Afghanistan Wars represents the highest proportion in history.[1,3] Secer et al examined data from war injuries and reported that peripheral nerve injuries make up 10% to 15% of all injuries and up to 30% of extremity injuries.[6] During the Croatian War, combat-injured soldiers with high-energy fractures caused by gunshot had associated nerve lesions 25% of the time.[5]

In a 16-year retrospective review of 456 patients with 557 peripheral nerve injuries in a civilian population in Brazil, it was demonstrated that the upper limb is most commonly involved (73.5% of cases) and that the ulnar nerve is the most commonly injured nerve, either isolated or in combination, usually with the median nerve.[7]

Current US military personnel protective measures, rapid medical evacuation, and close proximity of surgical assets have resulted in a decreased percentage of lethal thoracic injuries, while extremity injuries have decreased only minimally compared to previous US conflicts and continue to be prevalent.[1,3] Currently, 54% of all combat wounds from the US Joint Theater Trauma Registry are to the extremities. Eighty-one percent of these injuries are caused by explosion, whereas only 19% are caused by gunshot.[8]

Management in Theater

The initial treatment of any patient begins with ensuring the area is safe and with the initiation of Advanced Trauma Life System (ATLS) protocols. If at all possible, a thorough neurologic exam, including sensation testing and a motor exam, should be performed. Just as crucial to performing the neurologic exam is to sufficiently document the findings and ensure the information is available to the definitive treating surgeon.

At the time of surgical exploration, a thorough wound irrigation and debridement should occur. Transected or lacerated nerves should be tagged with dyed, nonabsorbable sutures for easier location at the time of definitive treatment. If this is not performed in theater, a considerable amount of time and dissection of scar tissue may be required to isolate the nerve lesion, and damage to accompanying nerve branches and vessels may occur.

Splinting of the extremity is usually dictated by the associated bone or soft tissue injuries, but in the rare case of isolated nerve injuries, splinting is recommended. Splinting helps prevent the development of distal joint contracture from muscle imbalance, aids in pain control, allows the soft tissue to rest, and potentially prevents migration of nerve ends or further damage to partially inured nerves.

The early and continued management of nerve injuries also involves the control of pain. Early use of long-acting catheters for regional blocks is very useful, minimizes the amount of narcotics required, and may be employed at an Echelon III facility. These regional blocks provide excellent pain control during the evacuation from the battlefield while allowing the combat casualty to be more alert and less sedated en route to more definite medical centers. Despite the success of these catheters, combat casualties must be carefully observed to ensure that a compartment syndrome does not develop.

Communication, transfer, and referral to a specialist should be done early. This allows for continued serial exams by the same provider or team; thorough education of the patient; proper timing of all surgical interventions; optimization of pain management; enrollment in appropriate splinting, therapy, and desensitization programs; and ensuring correct timing of electrodiagnostic nerve studies, if required.

Definitive Management

Definitive management of peripheral nerve injuries is based upon the nature of the injury. Nerves can be injured by traction (most common in civilian nerve injuries), penetrating trauma, crush, ischemia, or a collection of less common etiologies like vibration, thermal, percussion, radiation, and electric shock.[9,10] It has been demonstrated that, in high-velocity gunshot wounds, the pulsating temporary cavity left by the missile can damage peripheral nerves and vessels, even if they are not directly hit by the projectile.[5] The reconstructive ladder for nerve surgery begins with direct repair and progresses to autograft, conduits, and allograft, followed by nerve transfers.

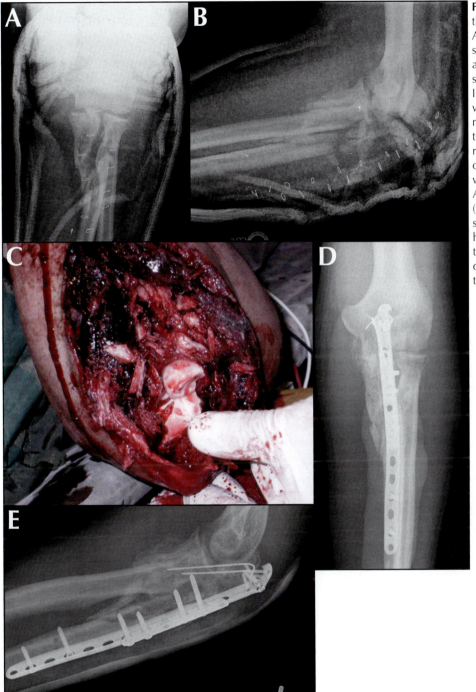

Figure 16-1. Case demonstrating the resiliency of an ulnar nerve. A 21-year-old servicemember sustained an open elbow injury and complete motor and sensory ulnar nerve deficit after an IED blast (A,B). After multiple washouts, he underwent a formal ulnar nerve exploration and transposition in addition to open reduction and internal fixation of his left olecranon, coronoid, with iliac crest bone grafting. Although he had a large wound (C), he recovered nearly full ulnar sensation and motor function. He healed his fractures (D,E) and soft tissue injuries, but was ultimately discharged from the service due to his restricted elbow motion.

TIMING

Contusions/Closed Injuries

Nerves in continuity can regenerate by axonal sprouting either from surviving axons or from the site of injury; therefore, close observation is warranted (Figure 16-1). Improvement in motor or sensation, a progressing or "traveling" Tinel's sign, and improvement on electrodiagnostic studies can all assist with assessment.

Lacerations/Sharp Injuries

In most cases, assuming the soft tissues can tolerate further surgery, we attempt direct repair or grafting as soon as possible. Sharp transections and lacerations should be reconstructed immediately by primary end-to-end neurorrhaphy. This decreases the amount of cell death; maximizes use of natural landmarks for repair, such as epineural blood vessels; and minimizes the amount of retraction.[11-13]

			Table 16-1

Classification of Nerve Injury and Recovery

Seddon	Sunderland	Mackinnon	Injury	Recovery
Neuropraxia	Degree I	Degree I	Conduction block	Spontaneous, rapid
Axonotmesis	Degree II	Degree II	Axonal rupture with intact basal lamina	Spontaneous
	Degree III	Degree III	Axonal and basal lamina rupture	Spontaneous but variable
	Degree IV	Degree IV	Complete scar block	Surgery required
Neurotmesis	Degree V	Degree V	Complete transection	Surgery required
		Degree VI	Mixed/combination of I-V	Surgery required, sparing normal fascicles

Blast

In cases where there has been severe damage to the nerve, initial treatment is directed at the soft tissue to allow for demarcation of the zone of injury. Nerve grafting is usually delayed and done in conjunction with definitive bony fixation and final wound coverage. For proximal injuries in which innervation to the distal muscles is of great length, concomitant nerve or tendon transfer can be undertaken simultaneously.

TECHNIQUE OF DIRECT REPAIR

A primary direct repair should always be performed when the clinical situation allows. In order for direct end-to-end repair to be successful, the nerve repair must be tension free. Optimally, the repair should be performed with joints in a neutral position.[14] Tension-free repair accomplished only by postural positioning of the extremity will risk the integrity of the repair if the position is changed prior to nerve regeneration. Ideally, an intraneural grouped fascicular repair should be performed, unless the fascicles are primarily mixed motor and sensory without well-defined groups of fascicles, in which case an epineurial repair should be performed.[14] If the nerve is repaired without a clear understanding of the interneural anatomy and the repair causes sensory and motor disorganization, the nerve may regenerate without functional recovery.

Basic principles of nerve injury management have expanded upon Sunderland's original complex relationship between motor and sensory nerve fascicles in the extremity.[15] Anatomic studies have demonstrated that in the more distal section of nerves, the complex sorting between the fascicles has stabilized, and fascicle segments no longer have intercommunications.[14] This allows for easier intrafascicular dissection and interneural repair.

The technique of end-to-end neurorrhaphy becomes complicated when patients present with mixed-degree injuries (Table 16-1). First-, second-, and third-degree injuries where some degree of fascicular arrangement is preserved recover spontaneously with results superior to surgical intervention.[14] In the peripheral nerve injury with mixed degrees of fascicle injury, the surgeon must separate the fourth- and fifth-degree injured fascicles for repair while being careful to protect the normal and less injured fascicles.

Good functional outcome after primary repair of peripheral nerves is observed in younger aged patients as well as in more distal peripheral nerve injuries, as the shorter distance required to regenerate and the more discrete motor and sensory bundles facilitate an easier repair.[9] Additionally, early primary repair of peripheral nerves has proven superior.[12,13,16] Although muscle damage is irreversible after about 18 months, sensory fibers and receptors stay alive much longer, suggesting that even a late repair may restore protective sensation to an affected limb.

NERVE AUTOGRAFTING/CABLE GRAFTS

Although the gold standard for peripheral nerve repair is tension-free end-to-end neurorrhaphy, there are many situations when this is not possible. For these cases, an intrafascicular nerve graft using a cable-graft technique is a viable option.[14,17] Cable grafting is a technique where one or more cutaneous nerves are attached by suture or adhesive to create a graft of the same diameter as the recipient nerve. Multiple sites of graft selection are possible, including sural, terminal branch of posterior interosseous, and medial brachial cutaneous nerves (Figure 16-2). Considerations for autograft nerve gap repair must be weighed against the donor site morbidity, the need for a second incision site for harvest (especially in the

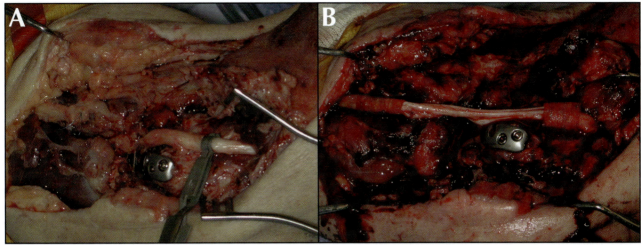

Figure 16-2. While on patrol in Iraq, this 20-year-old servicemember sustained a blast injury to the elbow from an IED, resulting in a distal humerus fracture and complete transection with segmental loss to his ulnar nerve. At the time of his definitive humerus fixation, the ulnar nerve was grafted with autograft sural nerve. Although he regained protective sensation in his ulnar digits, he failed to regain any intrinsic function to his hand and ultimately required a tendon transfer procedure.

multiply injured combat casualty), and the prolonged duration of surgery to harvest the graft.[18]

NERVE CONDUITS

To avoid the donor-site deficit, another available option is a hollow nerve conduit. Autogenous venous grafts were first performed in humans in the early 1920s.[19] Since that time, the search for the perfect material has led to the development of autogenous and exogenous materials, as well as artificial and biodegradable conduits.[20-23] Currently, a number of different nerve conduits are available, including conduits made of collagen or synthetic materials.

Nerve conduits are designed to bridge the gap between injured nerve stumps. By directing the growth of axonal sprouting, they prevent neuroma formation and provide a conduit for the diffusion of neurotropic and neurotrophic factors released by the nerve endings.[19] The effect of the conduit is 2-pronged, allowing for both contact guidance and neurotropism, which have been shown to be important for nerve regeneration.[19]

Interposition autogenous vein nerve conduits (AVNC) are an appealing choice because they do not require implanting foreign material.[24] However, their poor handling properties have led us to use the more rigid and easy-to-work-with materials. Our current conduit of choice is a collagen conduit for its easy handling characteristics.

Conduits have been reported in the literature with successful results for nerve gaps between 4 and 17 mm.[16,25] However, the absolute maximum length for which a conduit can be used has yet to be determined. In an experimental animal model, rabbit peroneal nerve injuries treated with AVNCs of up to 3 cm in length have been shown to support good axonal growth, while gaps of 3.5 to 5.25 cm showed only rare regrowth, and gaps of 6 cm of more showed only 1.45 cm of axonal growth.[20] These authors did not advocate AVNC lengths of greater than 3 cm. In our practice, we limit the use of any nerve conduit to defects less than 2.5 cm in length. If the defect is longer than this, we prefer the use of autogenous nerve graft or nerve transfer.

NERVE TRANSFERS

The final technique to be considered in the treatment of traumatic peripheral nerve injuries is the use of nerve transfers. Similar to the way tendon transfers are used to restore function after a proximal injury, nerve transfers can be used as well. In these transfers, a donor nerve can be selected to serve as the axonal supply for the injured nerve. It has been recognized that motor function is unlikely to return if the regenerating nerve has not reached the motor endplates of the muscle by about 18 months. The general premise of nerve transfers is to supply neurologic input (axons) at a location closer to the motor endplates than the level of the injury, thus improving the chances of re-innervating the muscle prior to the death of the motor endplates.

The donor nerve must be an "expendable" nerve, either in that its distal function is redundant (ie, served by another nerve or nerve branch) or will not result in an unacceptable sensory or motor deficiency. The donor nerve is then dissected out along with the distal end of the injured nerve. The proximal donor is anastomosed to the distal portion of the injured nerve at a location as near as possible to the motor end. In

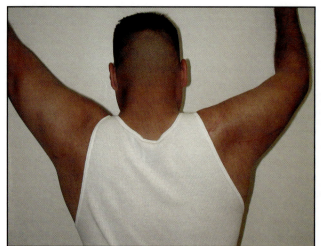

Figure 16-3. A 28-year-old man sustained ipsilateral clavicle, acromion, and coracoid fractures in addition to an axillary nerve palsy. Five months after his medial triceps to axillary nerve transfer, he was able to demonstrate greatly improved deltoid function without any appreciable loss of triceps strength.

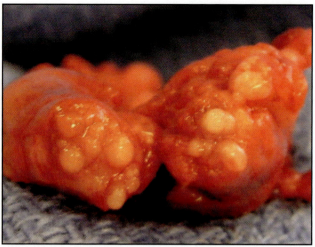

Figure 16-4. A hard nerve, when cut, has intraneural scarring and lack of blood or protrusion of fascicular contents as opposed to this normal nerve.

selecting a nerve transfer site, therefore, a more distal neurorrhaphy decreases the recovery time to ensure the "deadline" of 18 months is not exceeded (Figure 16-3).

Nerve transfers have been most widely used in the surgical treatment of brachial plexus injuries, and their use has been extrapolated to more peripheral nerve injuries. The Oberlin transfer[26] is commonly used to restore elbow flexion in a C5-C6 brachial plexus lesion. In this transfer, 1 or 2 fascicles of the ulnar nerve that supply the flexor carpi ulnaris are taken in an area adjacent to the branch of the musculocutaneous nerve branches into the biceps and/or the brachialis. They are then sutured to these small motor branches close to the motor endplates of the biceps and/or brachialis. This technique has been found to reliably restore elbow flexion without significantly disturbing distal hand function. Another commonly studied nerve transfer uses the distal portion of the anterior interosseous nerve to supply the deep motor branch of the ulnar nerve after a high ulnar nerve laceration. Providing an axonal input to the fibers of the deep motor branch of the ulnar nerve nearer to the hand allows for intrinsic hand muscle innervation to occur much sooner, thus increasing the likelihood of recovery of their function.

Surgical Techniques and Algorithm

The decision to proceed with surgical repair of nerve injuries can occur once the zone of injury and the surrounding soft tissues are healthy enough to

provide vascularization and protection for the repair. Meticulous handling of the soft tissues is necessary to preserve the integrity of these soft tissues that have already sustained recent trauma.

Careful dissection is used to identify both the proximal and distal ends of the severed nerve. Ideally, the proximal and distal ends of the upper extremity peripheral nerve injury would have been previously identified and tagged with a colored, nonabsorbable monofilament suture. Once these ends have been identified, the dissection must be carried back until the nerve tissue is normal in consistency and appearance, both grossly and using the microscope. Attempts should be made to preserve as much healthy tissue as possible. Traumatized nerve will take on a hardened and "rubbery" consistency and will often demonstrate hemorrhage externally. We use a combination of gentle palpation with fingers and gentle compression with microforceps to evaluate the consistency of the nerve. Any nerve that is not normal in consistency should be resected. While there are commercially available nerve-cutting guides, our preference is to make the nerve cuts using a fresh scalpel blade onto a sterile tongue depressor. Healthy nerve will take on a "sprouting" appearance (Figure 16-4).

Once nontraumatized, normal-appearing nerve has been identified and determined both proximally and distally, the appropriate repair technique is selected. Of primary importance is the length of any segmental defect between healthy ends, as this will play the principal role in determining which technique for repair will be used. In larger nerves, under the microscope or high-power loupes, fascicles can be seen traveling in groups. When possible, matching these fascicles proximally and distally is attempted. Accompanying vessels can also be used to properly match the 2 segments. Sometimes a gentle, short segment neurolysis of these fascicles can facilitate making these grouped fascicular repairs.

For cases in which there is minimal gap and in which nerves can easily be mobilized, we prefer a primary nerve repair. Gentle dissection with the aid of the operating microscope is used to mobilize the nerve ends just enough to allow for a tensionless repair. Once the nerve ends are approximated, microsurgical instruments and 8-0 or 9-0 nylon sutures are used to perform the nerve repairs, taking special care to grab only the epineurium with the suture. Under the microscope, special attention is paid to ensuring circumferential approximation of the epineurium, with no fascicles extruding.

For nerve defects of 1 cm or less, our preference is to use a hollow conduit to facilitate the repair. A simple ruler or a commercial cutting guide can be used to measure the diameter of the proximal and distal end of the nerve. An appropriate-sized conduit is then selected. If there is any question, we err toward a larger conduit. Once the conduit is prepared (soaked) and on the field, it is secured into one end of the nerve using a nylon suture. A suture is placed from outside the conduit into the lumen about 2 to 3 mm in from the edge of the conduit. The needle is then passed in horizontal mattress fashion through the epineurium only, about 4 to 5 mm in from the cut end of the nerve. Once this suture is placed back through the conduit from inside to out, it is tied down, pulling the cut end of the nerve into the conduit. A second simple nylon suture is then added to secure the nerve to the conduit 180 degrees from the first suture. The conduit is then cut to an appropriate length to prevent any kinking of the conduit once the repair is complete. A syringe with a 22-gauge needle is inserted into the center of the remaining conduit and is used to instill saline into the conduit to flush out any clot that has accumulated. Once this has been completed, a similar suture technique is used to bring the other nerve end into the conduit, and the repair is complete. Final flushing is performed prior to tying the first suture.

For nerve deficits between 1 and 2.5 cm, we prefer either a nerve conduit, cable graft, or an acellular nerve allograft. Nerve allograft, once defrosted, is easy to handle and is very much like native nerve tissue. The nerve tissue is then secured to the proximal and distal nerve ends with 8-0 nylon suture. If there is any concern with a size mismatch at the distal end (with the allograft having a larger diameter than the distal end of the native nerve), we do not hesitate to supplement the neurorrhapy with a nerve conduit. In these cases, we will sometimes split the conduit and wrap it around the neurorrhapy, securing it in place with nylon suture.

Currently, our preference for segmental loss of nerve greater than 2.5 cm is for autograft nerve. Our most commonly used donor nerve is the sural nerve, as it is easy to harvest and the sensory deficit associated with its harvest is well tolerated by the patient. The terminal branch of the anterior or posterior interosseous nerve can also be considered for donor nerves. For cases in which the defect is greater than 2.5 cm and the diameter of the injured nerve is greater than that of the donor, we use the cable grafting technique.

The sural nerve is easily harvested from either leg, or both, depending upon the length that is needed (Figure 16-5). We begin our dissection with a longitudinal incision located halfway between the lateral edge of the Achilles tendon and the lateral malleolus. Blunt dissection in this area will usually promptly reveal the sural nerve. While multiple techniques for harvest have been described from several stab incisions to endoscopic, our preference is still to use an open incision that we progressively make from distal to proximal along the course of the sural nerve. For cases in which a large segmental loss is present, we take special care to maximize the length of our sural nerve donor. Our incision not infrequently ends near the popliteal fossa.

Once the donor nerve has been harvested, the sural nerve is cut into as many "cables" as needed to match the diameter of the injured nerve. These individual cables are then secured proximally and distally on the injured nerve using nylon suture, taking time to match individual cables to grouped fascicles if this is feasible. Fibrin glue or a nerve conduit can also be used to supplement each neurorrhapy and insulate it from surrounding tissues.

For cases in which direct nerve repair is unlikely to reach distal motor endplates prior to 18 months, we advocate the use of nerve transfers. The nerve repairs for these transfers are performed in the same fashion as the direct repairs mentioned above. It is imperative that these repairs are made under no tension.

Outcomes

DIRECT REPAIR

Omer's large series in 1974 was one of the first comprehensive studies on nerve injuries and their outcomes.[4] He reported on 917 war wounds with major nerve injuries distal to the axilla and proximal to the volar carpal ligament that were admitted to BAMC. Six hundred forty-eight of the nerve lesions were in continuity, and 70% of these injuries went on to spontaneous recovery. Of the 269 nerve injuries that did not remain in continuity,

Figure 16-5. Typical incision from harvesting of a sural nerve graft with cable grafting of a common peroneal nerve palsy following no recovery after a knee dislocation. The grafting was done in conjunction with revision of the lateral collateral ligament reconstruction 6 months after his primary reconstruction. Visible are the contributions of the lateral cutaneous nerve (from the common peroneal nerve) and the medial cutaneous nerve (from the sciatic nerve).

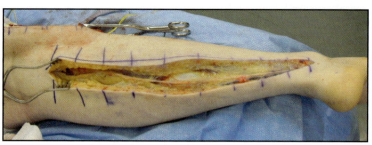

183 were treated with direct suture repair. These injuries were from a mix of gunshot wounds and trauma due to fracture-dislocations. Nerve injuries caused by gunshot wounds above the elbow took longer to return to function than nerve injuries below the elbow, with a range of 3 to 9 months for recovery. Nerves injured secondary to fracture-dislocations took 1 to 4 months to recover.[4] Fifty of the 183 nerves recovered good function. Seventy percent of these were nerve injuries that underwent early neurorrhapy (within the first 6 weeks). Nerve repairs below the elbow did better than the anastomoses above the elbow.

In a report on their experience treating nerve injuries during the Croatian War, Stanec and colleagues noted that 37% of patients with nerve injuries had associated vascular injuries caused by weapons of war, and all nerves required microsurgical procedures for repair.[5] Their average time from injury to secondary nerve repair was 5.6 months (range of 1 to 9 months). A variety of microsurgical techniques were used, including direct repair, internal neurolysis, use of nerve conduits, sural nerve cable grafting, and free vascularized nerve grafts. Only 3 out of 58 injured nerves were amenable to direct neurorrhaphy secondary to the nature of the nerve injury. Functional upper extremity movement was obtained in only 45% of the cases. This low rate of functional upper extremity movement was attributed to insufficient vascularization, proximal extent of the injury, and long nerve defects.

A large portion of wartime-specific data comes from lower extremity peripheral nerve injuries, which may be extrapolated to peripheral nerves in general. In a study of 157 patients with missile-induced peroneal nerve injuries, nerve repairs were followed prospectively based upon their level of injury: high-level, above the middle thigh; intermediate-level, above the popliteal crease; and low-level.[27] Successful outcomes were obtained in 10.8% of high-level, 31.1% of intermediate-level, and 56.7% of low-level repairs. Nerve defects larger than 4 cm and a delay of surgical intervention longer than 3 months led to worse outcomes. In a separate study looking at tibial nerve injury, significantly worse outcomes were related to nerve defects larger than 5 cm and delays of surgery longer than 4 months.[28] Similar to other studies, successful outcomes were more common in low-level

injuries (such as of the tibial nerve), with an 85.7% success rate.

In a retrospective analysis of surgical outcomes in patients with ulnar nerve injuries, 42 of 58 (72%) patients who received end-to-end repair had functional recoveries of grade 3 motor and sensory. Primary repairs performed within 72 hours of injury were more likely to obtain grade 3 or better recovery.[29]

CABLE GRAFTING

Seddon first reported on using multiple grafts to solve the dilemma of diameter differences.[30] Early success using this technique was reported by Haase on complete transections of 39 median nerve injuries and 26 ulnar nerve lesions treated with intrafascicular cable nerve grafting with autologous sural nerve.[17] At a 2.5- to 5-year follow-up, recovery was graded using the British Medical Research Council grading system. Useful motor recovery of M3 or better was obtained in 84% of median nerve lesions and motor recovery of M2+ or better in 73% of ulnar nerves. Sensory recovery of S3+ was found in 63% of median and 50% of ulnar low-level lesions. Outcomes were dependent on length of graft and age of the patient. Grafts 2.5 to 5 cm did better than longer grafts, and patient age less than 20 years led to more successful outcomes. Median nerve lesions at a low-level did better overall than ulnar nerve injuries at the same level.

More recently, Kim and colleagues reported on 654 surgical outcomes in patients with ulnar nerve entrapments, injuries, and tumors. In a subgroup of 33 patients with ulnar nerve injury who received a graft repair, it was reported that 70% (23/33) recovered to a LSUHSC grade 3 or better.[29] The lengths of grafts were not specified.

Varying lengths of nerve autograft can be used and still result in a successful outcome. In another study, 47.1% of patients with grafts 3 cm or less had the most successful outcome.[6] The least successful outcomes were in the 9.1- to 15-cm group. More successful outcomes were demonstrated with shorter grafts and the shorter preoperative periods.

NERVE CONDUITS

Current evidence suggests that bioabsorbable nerve conduits can be used as an alternative to nerve autograft for digital nerve injuries, with no clear evidence to show any superiority of one material over another. Nerve conduits give clinical results comparable to classic nerve graft techniques in patients with nerve deficits less than 3 cm while sparing the morbidity associated with a second harvest site. To date, no studies are available to recommend their use in greater than 3-cm gaps.

In a case series of secondary nerve reconstructions with polyglycolic acid (PGA) conduits after failed digital nerve repairs, results of 15 patients with nerve gaps ranging from 0.5 to 3.0 cm were reported.[31] At a mean follow-up of 22 months, good to excellent sensory function (S3 or greater) was seen in 86% of patients. The authors concluded that PGA conduits gave clinical results at least comparable to classic nerve graft techniques in patients with nerve deficits less than 3 cm. These data were confirmed in a more recent randomized, prospective trial that followed 98 patients with 136 digital nerve injuries reconstructed with PGA conduits or autograft.[25] Nerve gaps in the PGA conduit group were longer (7 mm) compared to the autograft nerve graft (4.3 mm). The authors found sensory recovery was better in the PGA conduit group in gaps less than 4 mm and that PGA nerve conduits produced comparable results to autograft at short and moderate lengths. Other studies found similar comparable results to autograft using caprolactone conduits.[32,33] Semi-permeable collagen conduits have also been studied and were found to provide good to excellent results in 2 studies.[34,35]

NERVE ALLOGRAFT

At the present time, the use of nerve allograft is in its infancy. Hollow nerve conduits are presently limited to gaps of 3 cm or less; however, nerve allograft could potentially allow for longer lengths of regeneration, similar to that seen with cable grafts. To date, few published series of patients treated with acellular nerve allograft can be found. In one study, decellularized nerve allograft was used in 7 patients with 10 peripheral sensory nerve injuries. The mean length of allograft used was 2.23 cm (range, 0.5 cm to 3 cm). These patients averaged static 2-point discrimination recovery to 5.5 mm and moving 2-point discrimination recovery to 4.4 mm. More intriguing is that the researchers went back to re-explore 2 of their repairs for unrelated reasons (flexor tendon injuries) and were able to visually confirm incorporation of the allograft in both cases.[36] As of yet, no published literature has documented effective use of nerve allograft for defects greater than 3 cm.

NERVE TRANSFERS

Most of the literature on nerve transfers presents case reports and techniques. Limited data are available reporting outcomes of these procedures. Hattori and colleagues[37] reported their results restoring sensory function to the hand in patients with complete brachial plexus injuries. Using intercostal nerve transfers, they were able to restore Semmes-Weinstein monofilament sensation to at least the 6.65 level in all of their 17 patients. None of these patients regained 2-point discrimination. Eight could perceive warmth, and 13 patients could appreciate cold.

In a case series of 8 patients undergoing an anterior interosseous nerve to deep motor branch of ulnar nerve transfer for intrinsic hand muscle function, all 8 patients regained intrinsic function, improved lateral pinch, and grip strength.[38] A number of other techniques with associated small case series have been described in the literature, supporting the use of nerve transfers, but no higher level studies exist to date.

Complications

Complications in nerve surgery are not well documented in the literature, in part due to the fact that it is difficult to differentiate a complication from poor outcome because our understanding of nerve repair and regeneration is incomplete. When counseling patients prior to surgery, time should be taken to discuss the likely possibility of incomplete recovery. Currently, there is no simple method for determining partial nerve injury. Thus, if intraneural scarring is present (a so-called sixth-degree nerve injury), it might not be appreciated. The net outcome in this scenario could be incomplete recovery of distal function.

Donor site morbidity should be fully disclosed to any patient undergoing nerve autografting. While the underlying premise is that the donor nerve is "expendable," it is vital to specifically discuss the projected sensory or motor deficit with the patient so he or she is not surprised postoperatively.

Extrusion of the nerve from a conduit, extrusion of fascicles from the epineurium in a primary repair, and even extrusion of the conduit itself from the wound are all reported complications. Extrusion of nerve fascicles from within a repair can result in painful neuroma. It is not possible to calculate the prevalence of such events without re-exploring all of the repairs. It is likely, however, that some cases that do not regain function have had graft extrusion as the underlying cause. Weber and colleagues[25] reported that 3 of 46 nerve conduit repairs had conduit extrusion. All of these were in cases with poor soft tissue surroundings in the digit; none had any sensation distal to their injury. Finally, infection and foreign body reactions are possible in nerve repairs but are not commonly reported.

References

1. Belmont PJ Jr, Goodman GP, Zacchilli M, Posner M, Evans C, Owens BD. Incidence and epidemiology of combat injuries sustained during "The Surge" portion of Operation Iraqi Freedom by a U.S. Army Brigade Combat Team. *J Trauma*. 2010;68(1):204-210.

2. Covey DC. From the frontlines to the home front. The crucial role of military orthopaedic surgeons. *J Bone Joint Surg*. 2009;91(4):998-1006.

3. Owens BD, Kragh JF Jr, Macaitis J, Svoboda SJ, Wenke JC. Characterization of extremity wounds in Operation Iraqi Freedom and Operation Enduring Freedom. *J Orthopaedic Trauma*. 2007;21(4):254-257.

4. Omer GE. Injuries to the nerves of the upper extremity. *J Bone Joint Surg*. 1974;56:1615-1624.

5. Stanec S, Tonkovic I, Stance Z, Tonkovic C, Dzepina I. Treatment of upper limb nerve war injuries associated with vascular trauma. *Injury*. 1997;28(7):463-468.

6. Secer HI, Daneyemez M, Gonul E, Izci Y. Surgical repair of ulnar nerve lesions caused by gunshot and shrapnel: results in 407 lesions. *J Neurosurg*. 2007;107:776-783.

7. Kouyoumdjian JA. Peripheral nerve injuries: a retrospective survey of 456 cases. *Muscle and Nerve*. 2006;34(6):785-788.

8. Ecklund JM, Ling GSF. Peripheral nerve surgery in modern day warfare. *Neurosurg Clin N Am*. 2009;20:107-110.

9. Campbell WW. Evaluation and management of peripheral nerve injury. *Clin Neurophys*. 2008;119:1951-1965.

10. Robinson LR. Traumatic injury to peripheral nerves. *Adv Clin Neurophys*. 2004;57S:173-186.

11. Brushart T. Nerve repair and grafting. In: Green DP, Hotchkiss RN, Pederson WC, eds. *Green's Operative Hand Surgery*. 4th ed. Philadelphia, PA: Churchill Livingstone; 1999:1381-1403.

12. Ma J, Novikov LN, Kellerth JO, Wiberg M. Early nerve repair after injury to the postganglionic plexus: an experimental study of sensory and motor neuronal survival in adult rats. *Scand J Plast Reconstr Surg Hand Surg*. 2003;37:1-9.

13. Trumble TE, McCallister WV. Repair of peripheral nerve defects in the upper extremity. *Hand Clin*. 2000;16:37-52.

14. MacKinnon SE. New directions in peripheral nerve surgery. *Ann Plas Sur*. 1989;22(3):257-273.

15. Sunderland S. *Nerves and Nerve Injuries*. 2nd ed. New York, NY: Churchill Livingstone; 1978:133-138.

16. Lundborg G. *Nerve Injury and Repair*. 2nd ed. Philadelphia, PA: Elsevier Churchill Livingstone; 2004.

17. Haase J, Bjerre P, Simseen K. Median and ulnar nerve transections treated with microsurgical interfasicular cable grafting with autogenous sural nerve. *J Neurosurg*. 1980;53(1):73-84.

18. Siemionow M, Brezicki G. Current techniques and concepts in peripheral nerve repair. *Int Rev Neurobiol*. 2009;87:141-172.

19. Taras JS, Nanavati V, Steelman P. Nerve conduits. *J Hand Ther*. 2005;18(2):191-197.

20. Strauch B, Ferder M, Lovelle-Allen S, Moore K, Kim DJ, Llena J. Determining the maximal length of a vein conduit used as an interposition graft for nerve regeneration. *J Reconstr Microsurg*. 1996;12(8):521-527.

21. Strauch B. Use of nerve conduits in peripheral nerve repair. *Hand Clin*. 2000;16(1):123-130.

22. Lundborg G, Dahlin LB, Danielsen N, et al. Nerve regeneration in silicone chambers: influence of gap length and of the distal stump components. *Exp Neurol*. 1982;76(2):361-375.

23. Lundborg G, Rosen B, Dahlin L, Danielson N, Holmberg J. Tubular versus conventional repair of median and ulnar nerves in the human forearm: early results from a prospective, randomized, clinical study. *J Hand Surg*. 1997;22(1):99-106.

24. Stahl S, Rosenburg N. Digital nerve repair by autogenous vein graft in high-velocity gunshot wounds. *Mil Med*. 1999;164:603-604.

25. Weber RA, Breidenbach WC, Brown RE, Jabaley ME, Mass DP. A randomized prospective study of polyglycolic acid conduits for digital nerve reconstruction in humans. *Plast Reconstr Surg*. 2000;106(5):1036-1045.

26. Oberlin C, Beal D, Leechavengvongs S, Salon A, Dauge MC, Sarcy JJ. Nerve transfer to biceps muscle using a part of ulnar nerve C5-6 avulsion of the brachial plexus; anatomical study and report of four cases. *J Hand Surg (Am)*. 1994;19:232-237.

27. Roganovic Z. Missile-caused complete lesions of the peroneal nerve and peroneal division of the sciatic nerve: results of 157 repairs. *Neurosurgery*. 2005;57(6):1201-1212.

28. Roganovic Z, Pavlicevic G, Petkovic S. Missile-induced complete lesions of the tibial nerve and tibial division of the sciatic nerve: results of 119 repairs. *J Neurosurg*. 2005;103(4):622-629.

29. Kim DH, Han K, Tiel RL, Murovic JA, Kline DG. Surgical outcomes of 654 ulnar nerve lesions. *J Neurosurg*. 2003;98:993-1004.

30. Seddon HJ. Nerve grafting. *J Bone Joint Surg (Br)*. 1963;45(3):446-461.

31. MacKinnon SE, Dellon AL. Clinical nerve reconstruction with bioabsorbable polyglycolic acid tube. *Plast Reconstr Surg*. 1990;85:419-424.

32. Bertleff MJOE, Meek M, Nicolai JA. A prospective clinical evaluation of biodegradable Neurolac nerve guides for sensory nerve repair in the hand. *J Hand Surg*. 2005;30A(3):513-518.

33. Shin RH, Friedrich P, Crum BA, Bishop AT, Shin AY. Treatment of a segmental nerve defect in the rat with use of bioabsorbable synthetic nerve conduits: a comparison of commercially available conduits. *J Bone Joint Surg*. 2009;91:2194-2204.

34. Bushnell BD, McWilliams AD, Whitener GB. Early clinical experience with collagen nerve tubes in digital nerve repair. *J Hand Surg*. 2008;33A:1080-1087.

35. Cheng CJ. Synthetic nerve conduits for digital nerve reconstruction. *J Hand Surg*. 2009;34A(19):1718-1721.

36. Karabekmex FE, Duymaz A, Moran S. Early clinical outcomes with the use of decellularized nerve allograft for repair of sensory defects within the hand. *Hand*. 2009;4(3):245-249.

37. Hattori Y, Doi K, Sakamoto S, Yukata K. Sensory recovery of the hand with intercostal nerve transfer following complete avulsion of the brachial plexus. *Plast Reconstruct Surg*. 2009;123(1):276-283.

38. Novak CB, Mackinnon SE. Distal anterior interosseous nerve transfer to the deep motor branch of the ulnar nerve for reconstruction of high ulnar nerve injuries. *J Reconstr Microsurg*. 2002;18(6):459-464.

Chapter **17**

UPPER EXTREMITY AMPUTATIONS

LTC(P) Kenneth F. Taylor, MD and COL Gerald L. Farber, MD

The most basic tenet of military surgery has long been to preserve life and limb. As we progress in our understanding of injury patterns and the apparent life-saving application of body armor, we can now definitively add to this tenet the preservation of function. This process begins with early, aggressive, and repeated wound debridement in order to prevent infection and to decrease the systemic effects of necrotic muscle tissue. When mangling wounds are severe, amputation may be necessary. Amputations of the upper extremity often carry with them significant social stigma.[1-4] Much of a person's self-identity, the capacity to return to gainful employment, and the ability to participate in recreational activities depends significantly on the function and appearance of the hand and upper extremity. When necessary, a well-planned and carefully performed amputation should not be considered a defeat, but rather the next positive step in a servicemember's path to recovery.

The indications and techniques of surgical amputation have been described for as long as surgeons have followed armies into battle. Where speed once was paramount, careful surgical technique now reigns. Each surgical procedure, during the course of medical evacuation and ultimate definitive care, must consider the functional end state of the upper extremity. Important factors include the patient's age and overall health, occupation and avocation, as well as resources available throughout the course of treatment and rehabilitation.

Epidemiology

The overall incidence of combat-related amputations has declined from 8.5% in the American Civil War to approximately 2% in the Vietnam War.[5] Likewise, the proportion of amputations involving the upper extremity has also declined from 40.4% during the Civil War to 13.9% during the Vietnam War.[5] In a series of 300 Vietnam War amputees, a similar rate of 12% involved the upper extremity. Eighty-one percent of all amputees sustained single limb loss.[6] Similar rates were reported for 3 low-intensity conflicts: Grenada, Desert Shield/Storm, and Somalia. Fourteen percent of those evacuated to a tertiary care stateside facility sustained combat-related amputations. Of the 31 amputees, only one had an upper extremity amputation.[7]

During the period from October 2001 through January 2005 (Operation Iraqi Freedom and Operation Enduring Freedom), 54% of all combat-related wounds involved the extremities. The upper limbs accounted for 51% (1838/3575) of all extremity wounds. The overall incidence of amputations involving either upper or lower extremities was only 4% of the full spectrum of injuries.[8] In a comparison between peace-time (1998-2001) and war-time (2001-2006) years, the overall incidence of injuries to the upper extremities increased only 3%. Conversely, the incidence of war-time amputations to the upper extremity increased dramatically by 47% compared to the peace-time years.[9]

A review of the military's Joint Theater Trauma Registry from the onset of current hostilities on

Owens BD, Belmont PJ Jr, eds. *Combat Orthopedic Surgery:
Lessons Learned in Iraq and Afghanistan (pp 147-156)*
© 2011 SLACK Incorporated

October 1, 2001 through June 1, 2006 reviewed the incidence of severe trauma and the subset of those resulting in amputation proximal to the wrist or ankle.[10] Of 8058 casualties requiring admission for at least 72 hours, 5684 (70%) involved at least one severe extremity injury. There were 423 individuals with at least one major limb amputation, resulting in an incidence of 5.2% of overall serious injury and 7.4% of serious injuries to the extremities. Of those with severe upper extremity injuries, the incidence of amputation was 3.1% (105/3349). Conversely, 8.5% (328/3854) of severe lower extremity injuries resulted in amputation. This difference has been attributed to the mechanism of injury in which ground-deployed explosive devices predominate. The authors of this study[10] caution against the direct comparison of their data to previous reports as the method of reporting previous injury incidence may often be diluted by the inclusion of relatively minor traumatic wounds.

Management in Theater

Evaluation of the combat-injured soldier can often be daunting. The initial assessment should proceed with the basic principles and protocols of Advanced Trauma Life Support.[11] Management of the severely injured upper extremity begins once the initial evaluation and treatment of these associated life-threatening injuries is accomplished. The upper extremity should be assessed systematically and the injuries documented as accurately as possible. This evaluation should address the 6 major tissues: skin, muscle, tendon, bone, vessel, and nerve.[12] Awareness of nerve and vascular injuries is of critical importance during the evacuation of the combat casualty through multiple echelons of care.[13]

The decision to amputate in theater can be a difficult one for the uninitiated surgeon. In many cases, the decision has already been made when the patient presents with a traumatic amputation. In other cases, the evaluation of a severely injured upper extremity is extremely challenging. Some authors suggest that an amputation should be performed if 4 or more of the 6 basic tissue components are injured.[12] If there is any question that the limb is potentially salvageable, we recommend debridement and stabilization with rapid evacuation to the next level of care. The limb can then be re-evaluated and amputation performed if indicated. The surgeon performing the definitive reconstruction is in the best position to make a decision regarding amputation of a viable but likely unsalvageable digit or limb.

Several things should be considered during the initial surgical debridement. The surgeon should maintain as much soft tissue distally as practically possible. Open circular amputations performed at the lowest possible skin level were initially described in the American Civil War. This remained the technique of choice through the Vietnam War as it allowed for drainage, prevention of infection, and maintenance of length for later revision.[5] We recommend, when possible, to avoid circular-type amputations that sacrifice viable distal muscle and skin. The resulting atypical flaps can be useful during subsequent procedures to avoid the need to resort to a shorter than necessary amputation level during definitive revision and closure. The surgeon should also maintain as much skeletal length and as many joints as possible. One should not arbitrarily amputate through a fracture if there is a viable distal fragment and soft tissue envelope.

The hand warrants some special considerations. The initial debridement of hand injuries should be conservative. Only obvious necrotic skin and soft tissue should be removed. Questionable tissue should be left for reassessment at the next debridement. Bony debridement should follow the same principle. Only obvious small loose fragments void of soft tissue attachment are excised. Larger bony fragments are preserved if possible for later use during reconstruction. Even unreconstructable but viable tissues should be maintained, as they can be used as sources of skin cover, bone, tendon, or nerve grafting during later definitive reconstruction.[12,13]

There is a temptation, at the time of initial debridement, to revise and close traumatic war wounds to measured levels performed for definitive elective amputations. There are several problems with this approach. Most importantly, early closure of war wounds, particularly contaminated amputations with unpredictable and wide zones of injury, significantly increases the risk of deep infection. Subsequent debridements would further shorten the limb. Early determination of final amputation levels also has potential implications in limiting future options for prosthetic suspension and wear. It may also adversely sacrifice length in situations in which the patient ultimately decides against prosthetic use altogether. These decisions should therefore be delayed until the final phases of surgical care far from the war zone.

Definitive Management

Definitive management is generally accomplished once the injured soldier reaches a tertiary care facility and the wounds are considered clean and stable. Again, the residual limb should be kept as long as practically possible. The orthopedic surgeon should have a close working relationship with the prosthetists and should discuss optimal amputation levels for both function and prosthetic fitting. The surgeon is cautioned not to sacrifice length solely for the sake of ease of prosthetic fitting. Greater length offers greater function when the patient is not wearing the prosthesis. This can be especially true in above-elbow amputees, who often do not wear their prostheses and can use a longer residual limb to assist with carrying objects, body positioning while lying down, and for transfers.

Once the appropriate amputation level is determined and the bones are cut to the appropriate lengths, the ends should be fashioned so that they are smooth without sharp edges. Myodesis of the extensors and flexors to the bone ends is preferred for transhumeral, through elbow, transradial, and wrist disarticulation levels. This helps prevent co-contraction and aids in myoelectric control of the prosthesis. Myoplasty, or suturing of the flexors to the extensors over the bone ends, should be avoided. In addition to complicating wear of this particular prosthesis type, it can lead to painful bursa formation over the bone ends.[14,15]

Early prosthetic fitting occurs ideally within 30 days of the amputation, before the patient learns to function one-handed. It assists with remodeling of the residual limb and facilitates early functional use of the prosthesis for daily activities. Residual phantom limb pain does not appear to be a limiting factor in prosthetic utilization in most cases,[16] but should be addressed early when present.

Complications should be anticipated in the significant injuries of the combat casualty. Gross contamination is common when zones of injury are extensive. Infection, heterotopic bone formation, joint contracture, soft tissue breakdown due to inadequate skin, insensitivity, and prosthetic wear are but a few problems encountered. Many of these potential pitfalls and suggestions for their management are described in the following case examples.

ILLUSTRATIVE CASE EXAMPLES

Case 1—Sacrifice of Unsatisfactory Digit

A 23-year-old soldier sustained a penetrating injury to his nondominant middle finger. He had comminution of the proximal phalanx with bone loss and extensor mechanism involvement. His flexor tendons were intact, and his distal finger was neurovascularly viable. There was an attempt to salvage the digit. An external fixator maintained length during serial debridements. Once his wounds were stable, he underwent bone grafting and internal fixation of the proximal phalanx. This eventually healed, but with extensive adhesions of the extensor mechanism and flexor tendons with a fixed proximal interphalangeal

joint. Subsequent extensor tenolysis did not improve motion, and the patient underwent arthrodesis. The arthrodesis healed, but the patient found that he was unable to return to his previous job because of difficulty gripping with his uninjured fingers due to the quadrigia effect in which the stiff finger precludes full flexion of the adjacent digits. After discussion of the treatment options, the patient elected to undergo ray amputation of the middle finger. After his recovery from surgery and rehabilitation, his hand function was markedly improved. The patient was able to remain in the military in his pre-injury occupational specialty.

The decision to salvage or amputate a compromised digit includes factors such as cosmesis as well as function. In the advent of durable and anatomically acceptable prostheses, cosmesis and function are not mutually exclusive. Consideration for amputation includes those instances in which prosthetic function is predicted to be superior to that of the salvaged hand.[17] This determination can be facilitated by the irreversible involvement of greater than 3 of the 6 critical tissues.[12] Other measureable factors include the presence of deep infection, significant pain, and individual functional requirements. Economic factors such as the need to return to work and psychological issues such as appearance and body image are also considered.[17]

Several studies have examined the functional outcomes associated with digital amputation. A large clinical series of digital amputations demonstrated relatively low disability in patients with well-constructed amputations involving 1 or 2 digits.[18] Complications encountered in this series included those due to the nail remnant; digital joint stiffness, in particular the proximal interphalangeal joint; and symptomatic neuroma. Infection was thought to be attributable more to tight wound closure than to bacterial contamination. Retraction of transected flexor tendons often resulted in palmar tenderness. Interestingly, the authors noted no instances of paradoxical extension of the residual digit. Predictors of successful outcome included selection of amputation level providing tensionless closure and distal soft tissue coverage of adequate bulk. Post-amputation therapy was stressed. The priority for hand amputation was digital function, not simply maximal length. While this article questioned the indications for any replantation in middle-aged laborers, this must be placed in proper context as the series was reported at the onset of early microvascular surgical technique.

A frequently referenced clinical review of active surgeons who, for either congenital or acquired causes, sustained an amputation of at least one digit confirmed that an individual's motivation remains more important than the specific amputation level or part. Many surgeons in fact requested amputation of painful or otherwise nonfunctional digits, thereby improving overall hand function.[19] A seemingly minor trauma can have a profound effect on the overall function of the limb. This case demonstrates the intimate relationship between a patient and his reconstructive surgeon. This relationship affords the ability to share the educated decision to sacrifice a viable yet otherwise useless digit. This decision should not be made in the acute setting.

Case 2—Biceps Release and Proximal Radius Excision for Short Below-Elbow Amputation Coverage

A 19-year-old soldier sustained traumatic bilateral below-elbow amputations secondary to a blast. His left upper extremity amputation was fairly short. After initial debridements, he underwent revision and closure of his amputations. The right upper extremity amputation was addressed with myodesis and standard closure with skin flaps. The left upper extremity was noted to be extremely short with inability to close the wound without significant further shortening of the limb. There was concern that he would not be able to be fitted with a below-elbow prosthesis and may require revision to the transhumeral level.

At surgery, the residual limb was debrided one final time. The distal biceps tendon was transected and tenodesed to the brachialis. The proximal radius was excised, preserving the lateral ulnar collateral ligaments. After excising the radius, the wound was closed primarily with the exception of a small area, which was treated with a split-thickness skin graft. He later returned to the operating room for excision of the friable skin graft with primary closure. The patient was able to be fitted with a below-elbow prosthesis instead of requiring revision to a transhumeral amputation.

Very short transradial amputations present a significant challenge for prosthesis suspension while maintaining a functional elbow. One viable solution is biceps tendon sectioning. This procedure, initially described in 1946, is based on the experience of the amputation centers established during World War II.[20] The minimal functional length of the residual forearm necessary to suspend and activate a prosthesis was determined to be 1.5 inches distal to the intact biceps insertion measured with the elbow flexed at 90 degress against resistance. Excising 1 inch of the distal biceps tendon effectively increased the length of the forearm by 2 inches. Remaining soft tissues were debrided to further decrease the bulk of the limb. The authors noted resulting elbow flexion strength to be minimally affected. The brachialis, which is the primary motor for elbow flexion, remained intact

just distal to the coronoid process. Loss of forearm supination, otherwise provided by an intact biceps, is inconsequential.

This technique was subsequently modified to include reattachment of the biceps tendon to the proximal ulna and removal of the residual radius entirely.[21] The authors state that 4 to 5 cm of ulnar length are required to suspend a prosthesis with retention of elbow flexion, though the exact landmarks used to measure this were not described. Care should be taken to avoid reattachment of the biceps too far distally. The resulting long biceps moment arm could otherwise result in an elbow flexion contracture.

The technique we advocate addresses each of the noted concerns. Tenodesis of the transected biceps tendon to brachialis may improve flexion torque without the concern of increasing the biomechanical moment arm. Excision of the residual radius facilitates decreasing bulk of the residual limb. Preservation of ulnohumeral ligaments provides stability of the elbow joint. When possible, the presence of friable soft tissue coverage, such as that seen in split-thickness skin grafts, should be minimized in order to avoid complications with weight-bearing devices. Primary closure also improves sensitivity of the residual limb.

Case 3—Spare Parts

A 22-year-old soldier sustained traumatic index finger amputation at the metacarpophalangeal joint level. In addition, he had loss of the proximal third of the middle finger proximal phalanx and loss of the extensor tendon. He underwent debridement, provisional fixation, and closure during his treatment in theater. His middle finger was neurovascularly viable and had intact flexor tendons and intrinsic function for interphalangeal joint extension. His index metacarpal had been preserved during his initial treatment. His wounds were allowed to heal prior to consideration for reconstruction.

A decision was made to reconstruct his middle finger in order to optimize hand width and function. He was taken to surgery where his index metacarpal was removed as in a ray amputation. This metacarpal was then reversed and used as an intercalary bone graft to lengthen the middle finger and allow for metacarpophalangeal joint fusion. The arthrodesis healed well, facilitating his ability to grasp, pinch, and function with his dominant hand. He was able to remain on active duty and ultimately returned to his unit.

The concept of "spare parts" forms the basis for well-described tissue transfer techniques. The use of local nonvascularized free tissue from areas otherwise nonviable or of little functional use is also well described though perhaps underused. In situations where native tissue is not repairable, the surgeon faces the decision to amputate or reconstruct. Allograft or distant autograft tissues are commonly used in reconstructive efforts. In the presence of mutilating injuries in which multiple digits are involved, the creative reconstructive surgeon has the added availability of local soft and bony tissue. The surgeon must carefully survey individual and composite tissue systems to determine appropriate candidates for transfer.[22,23] In the case described here, sacrifice of the index metacarpal served 2 purposes. It provided a structural autograft to replace segmental bone loss and provide for stable fixation. Conversion to a border ray amputation also functioned to deepen the web space between the thumb and now adjacent middle finger with a stable metacarpophalangeal arthrodesis.

Case 4—Peri-Articular Heterotopic Ossification

A 21-year-old marine sustained traumatic right below-elbow amputation with an associated open elbow fracture with partial loss of the medial condyle and ulnohumeral articulation. The patient was having difficulty with prosthetic fitting and use because of limited elbow motion. He was transferred for possible revision to a transhumeral amputation level. On examination, his elbow was fixed in approximately 60 degrees of flexion. He had a well-healed residual limb. Radiographs were significant for heterotopic ossification bridging the joint, as well as post-traumatic changes to the ulnohumeral articulation. A computed tomography scan was obtained. A 3-dimensional model was fabricated from these images (Figure 17-1). The patient underwent excision of the heterotopic bone and capsular release in an attempt to preserve a transradial-level amputation and elbow function. The model was very helpful in ensuring removal of the significant heterotopic bone. His motion improved to a 30 to 95 degree flexion arc. His elbow remained stable to varus and valgus stress. Postoperative radiographs demonstrated the extent of heterotopic bone excision (Figure 17-2). The patient was treated postoperatively with a single 700 centigray dose of radiation. He was subsequently fitted with a below-elbow prosthesis and obtained good function.

Heterotopic ossification is one of the more common complications encountered in combat-related amputations. A recent series reported a prevalence of 63%.[24] A blast mechanism and final amputation within the original zone of injury were both predictive of occurrence. While the prevalence was relatively high, only 19% of these were symptomatic. Heterotopic bone has been noted at the terminal portion of the residual limb, as well as in peri-articular areas. Its presence can cause problems with range of motion as well as soft tissue and skin breakdown. Skin-grafted areas are

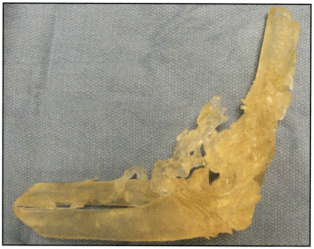

Figure 17-1. Three-dimensional resin model fabricated from computed tomography scan demonstrating the extent of ulno-humeral joint loss and heterotopic bone.

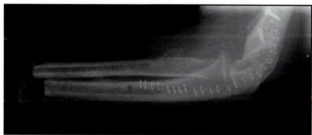

Figure 17-2. Postoperative radiograph following excision of heterotopic bone.

at significant risk due to their friability and relative insensitivity. This is usually managed with excision of the heterotopic bone and revision of the soft tissue coverage as indicated.

Much of how we treat heterotopic ossification about the elbow and forearm is based upon the experience derived about the hip and pelvis. When encountered in the elbow and forearm, treatment may be guided by a functional classification system based upon symptomatology.[25] Controversy remains concerning the timing of excision of heterotopic ossification. While excision has typically been delayed for longer than 12 months to prevent recurrence, a small series of patients undergoing excision at an average of 4 months from the onset of ossification resulted in no recurrences.[26] Of note, each patient in this series received both perioperative radiation and treatment with 25 mg oral indomethacin 3 times daily for 6 weeks. There is some hesitation concerning the potential side-effect profile of high-dose nonsteroidal anti-inflammatory medications. Use of a single low-dose irradiation has been shown to be effective, without risk of gastrointestinal complication.[27]

Case 5—Maintain Long Soft Tissue Flaps

A 32-year-old soldier sustained a traumatic right upper extremity transhumeral amputation with irregular skin loss proximal to the level of amputation. At his initial treatment in theater, his soft tissue flaps were maintained with as much length as possible. He had some necrosis at the very distal end of the soft tissue flap by the time he arrived in the United States (Figure 17-3). The remainder of his wounds were clean and well debrided. The atypical soft tissue flap facilitated simple coverage at the time of final revision and closure. The preserved length of skin and soft tissue made it possible to primarily close the more proximal skin loss without the need to shorten the bone further (Figure 17-4).

Classic fishmouth closures over the terminal aspect of traumatic amputations often require further shortening of bone. This in turn may compromise function by shortening lever arms and making prosthetic suspension more difficult. In the case of transhumeral amputations, where the patient often does not use a prosthesis, preservation of length is of critical importance to avoid muscle imbalance pulling the shoulder into abduction. It also maximizes use of the upper arm in holding objects to the side, and it facilitates trunk mobility. Preservation of well perfused yet atypically long flaps may therefore optimize ultimate function of the limb.

Case 6—Atypical Distal Pedicle Flaps

A 20-year-old marine sustained a traumatic transradial amputation. His treatment through the evacuation system consisted of multiple surgical debridements and ultimately a latissimus muscle flap with a split-thickness skin graft in an effort to maintain his short below-elbow amputation. He was subsequently transferred to our medical treatment facility. Distal wound breakdown with exposed bone was noted during early prosthetic training. Faced with the possibility of conversion to a shorter amputation level, we elected to revise the coverage to retain his below-elbow amputation. We also sought not to further compromise shoulder function by pursuing more traditional proximal flaps. He underwent debridement of the distal wound to include the surrounding split-thickness skin graft site in favor of a more durable soft tissue flap. An anteriorly based thoracoepigastric pedicled flap was chosen to cover this defect. The flap was divided and inset 3 weeks later. This flap provided durable surface and facilitated preservation of a functional below-elbow amputation level to accommodate his prosthesis. The patient has subsequently done very well with his prosthesis and has not had soft tissue complication.

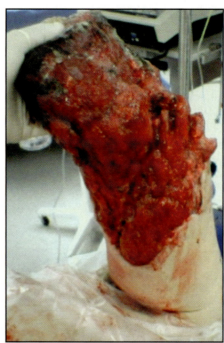

Figure 17-3. Intraoperative view of a traumatic transhumeral amputation with maintenance of long soft tissue flaps. Note some necrosis at the very end of the flap.

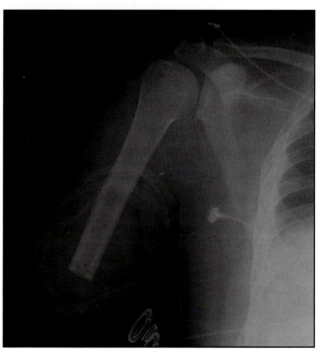

Figure 17-4. Radiograph of the final bony length of the amputation.

Thoracoabdominal pedicle flaps were initially described as a means to reconstruct friable and extensive scar tissue resulting from extremity wounds encountered during World War II.[28,29] Since the advent of successful microvascular reconstruction, they have been given little attention beyond that afforded by surgical textbooks,[30,31] anatomic descriptions, and case reports.[32-34]

Free vascularized tissue coverage of the residual limb has been used successfully to preserve amputation levels,[35] but may require vascular grafts to create an anastamosis outside the zone of injury. We have in fact effectively applied this concept to appropriate surgical situations. We have also used pedicled latissimus flaps with success; however, they are often much larger than necessary. Furthermore, the most distal portion of the flap critical for coverage is at the greatest risk for necrosis as demonstrated in this case. Traditional approaches do not work in all instances. These include multi-extremity mutilating injuries in which conventional flaps may not be readily available or cases in which they may further compromise function. For instance, other periscapular flaps were not used in this patient so as not to interfere with utilization of his body-powered prosthesis.

We have performed 7 pedicled thoracoabdominal flaps to cover elbow peri-articular wounds with good success.[36] One application is outlined here. To date, none of our patients has required a delay of flap division. There have been no flap failures, and none has required revision or defatting. Pedicled thoracoabdominal flaps have several disadvantages, including the residual donor site scar and the need to attach the patient's arm to his or her torso for approximately 3 weeks. The patient's inability to mobilize his or her extremity for so long provides several challenges, such as personal hygiene and the potential of graft dislodgement due to tension during ambulation and movement. Additionally, the flap is insensate. Therefore, pressure and temperature precautions must be emphasized.

All this considered, the judicious use of pedicled thoracoabdominal flaps has several significant advantages. The flaps can be based anteriorly or posteriorly to accommodate soft tissue wounds anywhere about the elbow. The flap dimensions can be adjusted to cover defects of small to significant size. These fasciocutaneous flaps are relatively thick and durable and therefore can withstand joint motion and prosthetic wear. Finally, these flaps can be employed during scar revision or as definitive initial soft tissue coverage of clean wounds. While we prefer microvascular techniques when appropriate, there are instances that place their viability at risk. We have found pedicled thoracoabdominal flaps to be a durable and reliable option for coverage of large soft tissue wounds about the elbow. As such, they should be included in the clinical armamentarium of surgeons who might encounter this potentially devastating injury pattern.

Case 7—Local Pedicle Flaps

A 21-year-old marine sustained a severe crush injury to his nondominant hand. He underwent provisional skeletal fixation and repair of the superficial

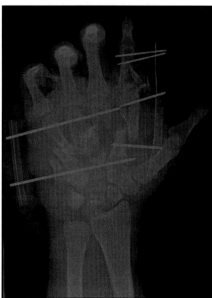

Figure 17-5. Posterior-anterior radiograph upon presentation, demonstrating malreduction of multiple fractures.

palmar arch with autologous vein graft at a local civilian facility prior to his evacuation (Figure 17-5). Upon arrival, he underwent repeated debridement and revision pin fixation of multiple comminuted metacarpal fractures. His viable index finger was placed in a spanning external fixator (Figure 17-6). Significant distal palm degloving injury was noted. Marginal tissue was preserved in anticipation of a staged reconstruction. He returned to the operating room 3 days later. Upon repeat examination, the distal palmar skin was determined to be nonviable (Figure 17-7). Additionally, the palmar arch vein graft was thrombosed. Digital arteries were weakly dopplerable. The thumb and index finger were dependent solely upon radial artery inflow, whereas the middle, ring, and small fingers were supplied entirely by the ulnar artery. Necrotic tissue was debrided. By the fifth surgical intervention, the remaining tissue appeared sufficiently healthy to undergo definitive coverage. While the index finger continued to be well vascularized, the extent of skeletal injury precluded its functional utility. In light of palmar skin loss, the index finger was used as a fillet flap. The remaining uncovered tissue was left to epithelialize. At 1 year from the time of his injury, he remained on active duty and was able to perform 6 pull-ups (Figure 17-8).

The fillet flap is an excellent option for soft tissue coverage in reconstruction of the hand. It is developed from a well-vascularized digit whose injury otherwise precludes its functional use. Patency of the digital vessels is determined prior to planning the fillet flap. The circumferential distance from the web space is roughly equal to the distance to a point just proximal

Figure   17-6.
Posterior-anterior
radiograph after revision open reduction
pin fixation of multiple metacarpal fractures and spanning
external fixation to
maintain length of
index finger ray.

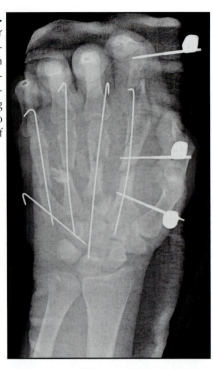

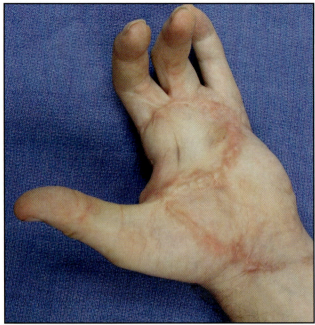

Figure 17-8. Clinical photograph 1 year from injury.

Figure   17-7.
Clinical photograph demonstrating nonviable distal palmar skin.

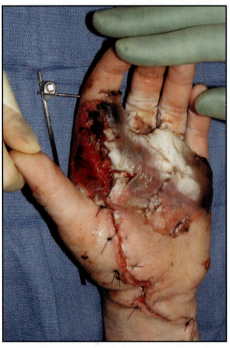

The advantages of this local pedicle flap are readily apparent. Restoration of resilient and densely innervated composite tissue is difficult to achieve with flaps obtained from elsewhere in the body.[38] The flap can easily survive on either vascular pedicle. The recipient area enjoys sensation at least equal to the surrounding tissue.[39] The area of potential coverage is significant and durable,[40] making this a valuable usage of an otherwise functionally compromised digit.

Conclusion

This chapter discussed the management of amputation of the upper extremity resulting from wounds sustained on the battlefield. In this patient population, special emphasis must be placed upon considerations of associated injuries, resources available to the combat surgeon, and the evacuation process. Higher survivability rates present new challenges in surgical and rehabilitative management of these complex wounds. Further work is required in areas such as prosthetic choice, suspension, and control. This in turn will continue to influence surgical decisions made throughout the course of treatment to positively effect rapid return to vocational and recreational activities in this previously high-functioning patient population.

to the nail fold, making this a highly dependable axial pattern flap. Measuring this distance provides a rough estimate of its area of potential coverage as the digit to be used is often itself compromised by scar tissue limiting its flexibility. Overstretching its tissue may compromise the vascularity.[37] Once the flap is adequately planned, an appropriate longitudinal incision is made. Skeletal and tendinous elements are then removed, leaving the remaining soft tissues on one or both intact vascular pedicles.

References

1. Copuroglu C, Ozcan M, Yilmaz B, Gorgulu Y, Abay E, Yainiz E. Acute stress disorder and post-traumatic stress disorder following traumatic amputation. *Acta Orthop Belg*. 2010;76(1):90-93.

2. Ferguson AD, Richie BS, Gomez MJ. Psychological factors after traumatic amputation in landmine survivors: the bridge between physical healing and full recovery. *Disabil Rehabil*. 2004;26(14-15):931-938.

3. Hamill R, Carson S, Dorahy M. Experiences of psychosocial adjustments within 18 months of amputation: an interpretative phenomenological analysis. *Disabil Rehabil*. 2010;32(9):729-740.

4. van der Sluis CK, Hartman PP, Schoppen T, Dijkstra PU. Job adjustments, job satisfaction and health experience in upper and lower limb amputees. *Prosthet Orthot Int*. 2009;33(1):41-51.

5. Dougherty PJ. Wartime amputations. *Mil Med*. 1993;158(12):755-763.

6. Wilber MC, Willett L, Buono F. Combat amputees. *Clin Orthop*. 1970;68:10-13.

7. Islinger RB, Kuklo TR, McHale KA. A review of orthopedic injuries in three recent U.S. military conflicts. *Mil Med*. 2000;165(6):463-465.

8. Owens BD, Kragh JF, Macaitis J, Svovoda SJ, Wenke JC. Characterization of extremity wounds in Operation Iraqi Freedom and Operation Enduring Freedom. *J Orthop Trauma*. 2007;21(4):254-257.

9. Brininger TL, Antczak A, Breland HL. Upper extremity injuries in the U.S. military during peacetime years and wartime years. *J Hand Therapy*. 2008;Apr-Jun:115-122.

10. Stansbury LG, Lalliss SJ, Branstetter JG, Bagg MR, Holcomb JB. Amputations in U.S. military personnel in the current conflicts in Afghanistan and Iraq. *J Orthop Trauma*. 2008;22(1):43-46.

11. American College of Surgeons. *Advanced Trauma Life Support for Doctors Student Course Manual*. Chicago, IL: Author; 2008:1-24.

12. Eardley WGP, Stewart PM. Early management of ballistic hand trauma. *J Am Acad Orthop Surg*. 2010;18:118-126.

13. Burkhalter WE. Wounds of the hand. In: Burkhalter WE, ed. *Medical Department, United States Army, Surgery in Vietnam, Orthopedic Surgery*. Washington, DC: Office of the Surgeon General and Center of Military History; 1994:55-81.

14. Baumgartner RF. The surgery of arm and forearm amputations. *Ortho Clin North Am*. 1981;12(4):805-817.

15. Beasley RW, de Bese GM. Upper limb amputations and prostheses. *Ortho Clin North Am*. 1986;17(3):395-405.

16. Pinzur MS, Angelats J, Light TR, Izuierdo R, Pluth T. Functional outcome following traumatic upper limb amputation and prosthetic fitting. *J Hand Surg*. 1994;19A:836-839.

17. Brown PW. Sacrifice of the unsatisfactory hand. *J Hand Surg*. 1979;4(5):417-423.

18. Conolly WB, Goulston E. Problems of digital amputations: a clinical review of 260 patients and 301 amputations. *Aust NZ J Surg*. 1973;43(2):118-123.

19. Brown PW. Less than ten—surgeons with amputated fingers. *J Hand Surg*. 1982;7(1):31-37.

20. Blair HC, Morris HD. Conservation of short amputation stumps by tendon section. *J Bone Joint Surg*. 1946;28(3):427-433.

21. Owens P, Ouellette EA. Wrist disarticulation and transradial amputation: surgical management. In: Smith DG, Michael JW, Bowker JH, eds. *Atlas of Amputations and Limb Deficiencies, Surgical, Prosthetic, and Rehabilitation Principles*. Rosemont, IL: American Academy of Orthopaedic Surgeons; 2004:219-222.

22. Brown RE, Wu TYT. Use of "spare parts" in mutilated upper extremity injuries. *Hand Clin*. 2003;19:73-87.

23. Russell RC, Neumeister MW, Ostric SA, Engineer NJ. Extremity reconstruction using nonreplantable tissue ("spare parts"). *Clin Plast Surg*. 2007;34:211-222.

24. Potter BK, Burns TC, Lacap AP, Granville RR, Gajewski DA. Heterotopic ossification following traumatic and combat-related amputations. Prevalence, risk factors, and preliminary results of excision. *J Bone Joint Surg*. 2007;89A:476-486.

25. Hastings H II, Graham TJ. The classification and treatment of heterotopic ossification about the elbow and forearm. *Hand Clin*. 1994;10:417-451.

26. Beingessner DM, Patterson SD, King GJW. Early excision of heterotopic bone in the forearm. *J Hand Surg*. 2000;25A(3):483-488.

27. Cullen JP, Pellegrini VD, Miller RJ, Jones JA. Treatment of traumatic radioulnar synostosis by excision and postoperative low-dose irradiation. *J Hand Surg*. 1994;19A:394-401.

28. Brown JB, Cannon B, Graham WC, et al. Direct flap repair of defects of the arm and hand: preparation of gunshot wounds for repair of nerves, bones and tendons. *Ann Surg*. 1945;122(4):706-715.

29. Cannon B, Trott AW. Expeditious use of direct flaps in extremity repairs. *Plast Reconstr Surg*. 1949;4:415-419.

30. Lewis VL. Thoraco-epigastric skin flap to the arm. In: Strauch B, ed. *Grabb's Encyclopedia of Flaps*. 1st ed. Boston, MA: Little, Brown and Co; 1990:1149-1153.

31. Zook EG, Russell RC. Lateral trunk flaps. In: Strauch B, ed. *Grabb's Encyclopedia of Flaps*. 1st ed. Boston, MA: Little, Brown and Co; 1990:1154-1157.

32. Brown RG, Vasconez LO, Jurkiewicz MJ. Transverse abdominal flaps and the deep epigastric arcade. *Plast Reconstr Surg*. 1975;55(4):416-421.

33. Davis WM, McCraw JB, Carraway JH. Use of a direct, transverse, thoracoabdominal flap to close difficult wounds of the thorax and upper extremity. *Plast Reconstr Surg*. 1977;60(4):526-533.

34. Lewis VL, Cook JQ. The nondelayed thoracoepigastric flap: coverage of an extensive electric burn defect of the upper extremity. *Plast Reconstr Surg*. 1980;65:492-493.

35. Baccarani A, Follmar KE, De Santis G, et al. Free vascularized tissue transfer to preserve upper extremity amputation levels. *Plast Reconstr Surg*. 2007;120(4):971-981.

36. Farber GL, Taylor KF, Smith AC. Pedicled thoracoabdominal flap coverage about the elbow in traumatic war injuries. *Hand*. 2010;5(1):43-48.

37. Pederson WC, Lister G. Skin flaps. In: Green DP, Hotchkiss RN, Pederson WC, Wolfe SW, eds. *Green's Operative Hand Surgery*. Philadelphia, PA: Elsevier Inc; 2005:1648-1704.

38. Peacock EE. Reconstruction of the hand by the local transfer of composite tissue island flaps. *Plast Reconstr Surg*. 1960;25:298-311.

39. Koegel AM, Banducci DR, Kahler SH, Hauck RM, Manders EK. Sensibility of finger fillet flaps on late follow-up evaluation. *J Hand Surg*. 1995;20A:679-682.

40. Küntscher MV, Erdmann D, Homann HH, Steinau HU, Levin SL, Germann G. The concept of fillet flaps: classification, indications, and analysis of their clinical value. *Plast Reconstr Surg*. 2001;108:885-896.

Chapter 18

UPPER EXTREMITY COVERAGE: MANAGEMENT OF COMBAT-RELATED SOFT TISSUE INJURY OF THE UPPER EXTREMITY

CDR (Ret) Anand R. Kumar, MD; CAPT Alan A. Lim, MD; LT Scott Tintle, MD; and James P. Bradley, MD

Extremity trauma has always been a demoralizing feature of warfare, and modern conflicts have seen even greater rates of extremity injuries.[1-5] Despite the progression of modern combat weaponry leading to the increased rate of extremity wounds, the fields of plastic, orthopedic, and vascular surgery have likewise progressed, leading to an overall decreased rate of extremity amputation with each major military conflict. The one exception to this generalization is the Vietnam War, which saw a dramatic increase in the destructive nature of high-velocity firearms, landmines, and booby-traps. These weapons along with increased patient survivability led to increasingly worse extremity injuries.[6,7] The introduction of body armor and improved medical evacuation capabilities were likely responsible for the increased survival as well as the increase in the amputation rates seen during the Vietnam War.[8,9] During Operation Iraqi Freedom/Operation Enduring Freedom (OIF/OEF), despite another dramatic progression in the violence of modern weaponry, the major extremity amputation rate has little changed at between 7% and 10% for all combat casualties with extremity injuries who were unable to return to duty within 72 hours of injury.[8,10] This is in large part due to the continued advancement of battlefield medicine, body armor, and limb salvage surgery. Additionally, the ability to provide safe, vascularized wound coverage in the form of rotational, pedicled, and free tissue transfer in the subacute or late time periods are likely responsible for maintaining the current limb salvage rates.[11-14]

Upper extremity combat injuries present a significant challenge to reconstructive surgeons. The composite nature of these blast and projectile wounds frequently accompanied by other injuries and systemic compromise demands that a cooperative effort amongst trauma, orthopedic, and plastic surgeons takes place in order to achieve optimal outcomes. The blast mechanism frequently leaves large soft tissue and bone voids with disrupted vascular supply. These large zones of injury, coupled with the complex microflora seen in battlefield extremity wounds and concurrent injuries, make soft tissue reconstruction challenging.

These upper extremity combat injuries often require prolonged reconstruction over many months and multiple surgical interventions. For this reason, the soft tissue coverage must be durable and well vascularized in order to allow for multiple surgical procedures. The ultimate goal of achieving a supple extremity with healed fractures, a functional range of motion, and protective sensation must be equally embraced by all members of the reconstructive team. This chapter outlines the principles of management and describes a reconstruction algorithm for these complex upper extremity wounds based upon our experiences at an Echelon V treatment facility.

Owens BD, Belmont PJ Jr, eds. *Combat Orthopedic Surgery: Lessons Learned in Iraq and Afghanistan* (pp 157-168)
© 2011 SLACK Incorporated

Epidemiology

During the Vietnam War, 65% of casualties sustained extremity trauma.[1] In more recent conflicts, the rates of extremity injury have increased. During the 1993 Somali conflict, 84% of the US wounded had penetrating extremity injuries.[2] Approximately 49% to 54% of all soldiers wounded in action during OIF/OEF sustained a musculoskeletal injury to the extremity.[5] The most recent large study looking at OIF/OEF indicated that 82% of patients sustaining extremity fractures sustained open injuries.[5] This study also found that the distribution of upper to lower extremity fractures was equal.[5] Current combat-related literature does not adequately document the percentage of extremity wounds requiring soft tissue coverage with skin grafts, rotational flaps, pedicled flaps, or free tissue transfers. Our experience at the National Naval Medical Center has found these rates to be very high, and therefore it is recommended that military orthopedic and plastic surgeons should be familiar with these techniques.

A previously published review of our experience with upper extremity flap procedures over a 30-month period during OIF/OEF provided the following specific epidemiologic data: patient age ranged from 19 to 43 years (mean, 25 years old), 13% of the patients required 2 simultaneous flap procedures, and the average number of pre-reconstructive washouts was 6 (range of 3 to 22). The average time to flap reconstruction was 31 days (range of 9 to 161). The sites of flap coverage were as follows: upper arm and elbow (23%), forearm (27%), and hand (50%). Blast injuries or high-velocity gunshot wounds accounted for 88% of the injuries. All injuries requiring upper extremity flap procedures were associated with upper extremity fractures, and 46% were culture positive upon admission to the Echelon V treatment facility (Tables 18-1 through 18-3).[13]

Management in Theater

Upper extremity limb salvage considerations differ significantly from the lower extremity. The functional capabilities of a normal hand are appreciably better than the most advanced upper extremity prosthesis. There is even functional advantage of a severely injured replanted upper extremity over an amputation and prosthesis.[15] For this reason, all possible attempts at upper extremity limb salvage should be exhausted in theater and at progressive echelons of care. Despite these efforts, it is imperative in the management of severe upper extremity trauma that an early frank evaluation and discussion with the patient (if possible)

about upper extremity limb salvage versus amputation takes place so that unreasonable expectations of wound coverage and limb preservation are avoided.

The ability of negative pressure wound therapy to safely prolong the time to soft tissue coverage remains equivocal in the literature. Despite this, we believe that the use of negative pressure wound therapy likely contributes to eventual flap success. It has been shown to decrease edema, stimulate fibroblast proliferation, remove destructive proteinases from the wound, facilitate bacterial clearance from the wound, and limit cross contamination from the patient's environment, all of which likely contribute to eventual wound coverage success.[16,17] Recent literature with a large number of combat casualties has determined that the use of negative pressure wound therapy is safe during intercontinental flight, and as such we believe that it should be used as early as possible in the medical evacuation chain.[18]

While the specific early management of combat wounds has been described previously in this text, we will highlight the National Naval Medical Center Limb Salvage Protocol[12]:

- Combat-injured patients with open wounds are rapidly assessed and evacuated to local medical treatment facilities.

- The initial treatment at these facilities includes gross decontamination of foreign material and the debridement of nonviable tissue. Following adequate early debridement, copious amounts of irrigation are used.

- Vascular repair and fasciotomies are performed if necessary, and if indicated monoplanar external fixation is applied.

- Wound debridement and irrigation are then performed every 48 to 72 hours following the initial debridement and stabilization until arrival to the United States.

- Upon arrival to the tertiary care center in the United States, trauma surgery, orthopedic surgery, and plastic surgery thoroughly evaluate each patient.

- Broad-spectrum antibiotics are initiated (if they have not been already) and are continued until all wounds are closed.

- Patients return to the operating room every 48 to 72 hours until definitive wound closure or coverage. Aggressive debridement is performed at every procedure. Loosening of the external fixation device to facilitate fracture site delivery into the wound and debridement followed by reduction and reapplication of external fixation is an invaluable adjunct to thorough wound debridement. Due to the high rate of bacterial

Table 18-1

Fasciocutaneous Flap Reconstruction

Age	IED Injury	Time to Flap (Days)	# Prior Washouts	Flap Type	Flap Failure/ Connection	Comments	Associated Fracture	Associated Injury	Wound Culture
25	No	21	4	Abdominal flap	Pedicled	Partial flap loss	Open metacarpal		*Acinetobacter calcoaceticus baumannii*
43	No	43	3	Contralateral radial forearm flap	Free		Open carpals Distal radius	Radial artery Digital nerve	*Stenotrophomonas maltophilia*
24	Yes	16	4	Reverse radial forearm flap	Pedicled		Open metacarpal	Digital nerve	*Acinetobactor calcoaceticus baumannii Klebsiella pneumoniae*
37	No	53	12	Groin flap	Pedicled		Open metacarpal		
27	Yes	161	9	Reverse radial forearm flap	Pedicled	Elective amputation	Open metacarpal		*Staphlococcus epidermidis*
28	Yes	9	3	Radial forearm flow-through flap	Free		Open metacarpal	Ulnar nerve Median nerve	
23	No	11	4	Local flap, STSG	Bipedicled		Open distal radius		
24	No	15	3	Reverse radial forearm flap	Pedicled		Open type III distal ulna		
22	Yes	25	10	Anterolateral thigh flap, STSG	Free		Open metacarpal	Median and radial arteries Superficial palmar arch	*Enterococcus faecalis Acinetobactor calcoaceticus baumannii*
30	Yes	31	10	Fibula-oseocutaneous flap	Free		Open radius		*Acinetobactor calcoaceticus baumannii*
21	Yes	27	5	Anterolateral thigh flap	Free		Open ulna	Ulnar nerve	
19	Yes	17	5	Latissimus flap	Pedicled	Total flap loss	Open elbow Humerus	Ulnar nerve	*Acinetobactor calcoaceticus baumannii Enterococcus coli Enterococcus faecium Clostridia Scedosporium* spp. (fingers)
22	Yes	22	7	Oblique rectus abdominus flap	Pedicled		Open radius		
22	Yes	22	7	Groin flap	Pedicled		Open metacarpals Open phalanges		
21	No	22	7	Anterolateral thigh flap, STSG	Free	Partial flap loss	Open ulna		
22	No	19	4	A flap	Pedicled		Open ulna		
22	No	19	4	Epigastric flap	Pedicled		Open metacarpals		

IED = improvised explosive device, STSG = split-thickness skin graft.

Table 18-2

Musculocutaneous Flap Reconstruction

Age	IED Injury	Time to Flap (Days)	# Prior Washouts	Flap Type	Connection	Flap Failure/ Comments	Associated Fracture	Associated Injury	Wound Culture
25	No	14	4	Latissimus flap, STSG	Pedicled		Open humerus		Acinetobacter calcoaceticus baumannii
25	Yes	82	22	Latissimus flap, STSG	Pedicled		Open humerus	Radial nerve Ulnar nerve	MDR Pseudomonas aeruginosa Acinetobacter calcoaceticus baumannii
27	Yes	15	3	Triceps flap, STSG	Pedicled		Open humerus		Acinetobacter calcoaceticus baumannii Coagulase negative Staph
21	No	11	3	Triceps flap, STSG	Pedicled		Open elbow	Radial nerve	Bacillus spp.
25	Yes	28	6	Latissimus flap, STSG	Pedicled		Open humerus		Acinetobacter calcoaceticus baumannii

IED = improvised explosive device, STSG = split-thickness skin graft.

Table 18-3

Adipofascial Flap Reconstruction

Age	IED Injury	Time to Flap (Days)	# Prior Washouts	Flap Type	Connection	Flap Failure/ Comments	Associated Fracture	Associated Injury	Wound Culture
24	Yes	9	3	Reverse cross finger flap, STSG	Pedicled		Open PIP		
21	Yes	19	3	Posterior interosseus artery flap, STSG	Pedicled	Partial flap loss	Open metacarpals Open phalanges		
23	Yes	59	6	Posterior interosseus artery flap, STSG	Pedicled	Partial flap loss	Open metacarpals		
23	Yes	59	6	Reverse cross finger flap	Pedicled		Open p1 phalanx		

IED = improvised explosive device, PIP = proximal interphalangeal, STSG = split-thickness skin graft.

colonization, massive soft tissue devitalization, and multiple concurrent injuries, early wound closure or flap reconstruction is avoided.

- In most instances, definitive wound coverage with a pedicled or free flap is performed prior to or at the time of the definitive bony fixation of fractures. Our preference is to avoid early internal fixation. In the upper extremity only, we prefer internal fixation at the time of wound closure with a vascularized flap. The use of additional external fixation for supplemental fixation or limb immobilization is useful to facilitate soft tissue rest. Internal fixation prior to the date of definitive wound coverage is generally avoided to decrease the risk of hardware colonization with bacteria and the establishment of bacterial biofilm on the hardware.

Definitive Management

GENERAL PRINCIPLES OF UPPER EXTREMITY COVERAGE

The soft tissue reconstruction of the upper extremity is extremely challenging in large part due to the upper extremity's versatile premorbid role in providing delicate tactile input from the environment while also remaining durable, highly mobile, and capable of tremendous productivity. The soft tissue envelope surrounding the upper extremity is relatively unforgiving. There is minimal fat, muscle, and redundant skin, yet critical neurovascular and musculotendinous units lie in a subcutaneous position, highly vulnerable to injury as well as desiccation if left exposed. For these reasons, a highly thoughtful reconstructive effort is mandated in order to cover the critical structures and to provide for a functional range of motion, protective sensation, and an acceptable aesthetic outcome.[19]

ALTERNATIVE TO FLAP RECONSTRUCTION

It would be ideal if vascularized healthy tissue coverage could be replaced by a synthetic off-the-shelf substitute. While this is currently unlikely to happen in the near future, new artificial skin substitutes, originally developed for burn patients, have proven to aid in the reconstruction of combat-wounded patients. Integra Bilayer Matrix Wound Dressing (Integra LifeSciences, Plainsboro, NJ) has been the most frequently used and studied in the combat patient. Integra is a bilaminar product that contains bovine collagen and shark chondroitin in the inner layer and silicone in the outer layer. After being applied to a clean, healthy wound bed, tissue grows into the collagen side akin to normal dermis. Following the incorporation of the dermal analog approximately 2 to 3 weeks after placement in a wound, a split-thickness skin graft is performed.

Helgeson and colleagues[20] reported successful results in achieving soft tissue coverage over exposed tendon or bone in 83% of patients using this method in the treatment of combat casualties at an Echelon V military treatment facility. The authors concluded that, when successful, the use of Integra eliminated the need for more sophisticated flap coverage. While we believe that Integra has a unique role in the management of these large open wounds with exposed tendons and bones, we have not used and do not recommend its use in the setting of an open fracture. The biologic demands of fracture healing require importation of vascularized tissue over the fracture site to correct the hypoxic low vascularity environment of the soft tissue avulsed fracture site.

TIMING OF UPPER EXTREMITY FLAP COVERAGE

The timing of upper extremity flap coverage remains controversial. The civilian literature indicates that early wound coverage provides better outcomes.[21-23] Godina[22] popularized early wound coverage (<72 hours) and indicated that optimal results in terms of flap success and avoidance of infection were obtained when flap coverage was provided within 72 hours from the time of the injury. Other authors subsequently reported successful outcomes in the early period and thus established the safety and efficacy of performing definitive soft tissue reconstruction in the early setting.[24-26] Despite the low infection rate and the high flap success rates, the fix and flap idea has not become mainstream thinking in the orthopedic or plastic surgery fields.[27] Most surgeons in the civilian setting strive for wound coverage as early as possible and usually within 7 days from the time of injury.[23,27-29]

The circumstances of war and the type of injuries sustained in the combat population make it nearly impossible to provide soft tissue coverage within 7 days of the injury. In a review of our experience treating combat casualties, we found that patients averaged 6 debridements prior to definitive closure.[3,12,13] Aside from the medical evacuation, reasons for a delay in flap coverage in this population include the stabilization of multiple concurrent injuries including the lower extremities, the cranium, and the torso; the progressive muscle necrosis in these high-energy blast injuries; and the necessity of creating a wound that is healthy and clean in the face of severe contamination.[13]

Despite the delay in wound coverage, excellent results have been obtained in the subacute or late time settings in the treatment of combat casualties.[3,13,14] We reported a 96% flap success rate with an infection rate of 8%.[13] With close review of the civilian literature, additional support for the successful result of coverage within the subacute time frame is garnered. Yaremchuk and Gan[30] found no negative effects with soft tissue coverage at an average of 17 days in patients with severe open IIIB tibia fractures. More recently, in a review of delayed flap coverage of both upper and lower extremity open fractures, Steiert and colleagues[31] reported a low rate of flap failure (10%) despite coverage with an average delay of 28 days.

Regardless of the timing of flap coverage, we believe that the timing of definitive orthopedic fracture fixation should be strongly considered in relation to the timing of flap coverage. In our experience, we almost always performed open reduction and internal fixation of fractures at the time of flap coverage or even after a 1-week delay when treating with ringed external fixation. While there is not overwhelming evidence to support the benefit of such a protocol, we achieved a high rate of success (95% union) when treating IIIB open tibia fractures in this manner and have had equally good short-term and intermediate results in the upper extremity.[13,32] In summary, despite the necessary delay in treating combat casualties, safe soft tissue coverage to include free tissue transfer can be performed with excellent outcomes. We also strongly recommend that there be no delay in flap coverage following definitive orthopedic fracture treatment.

FLAP SELECTION PRINCIPLES

In 1993, Levin and colleagues[33,34] introduced the concept of the reconstructive ladder. Wound closure by secondary intention is at the lowest rung of the ladder with progressive rungs displaying increasingly more sophisticated closures until the pinnacle of free tissue transfer is reached. The ladder was introduced in an effort to guide the selection of wound closure, and its creators indicated that a surgeon may go from one level to another and in many instances may simultaneously employ different aspects of the ladder.[33] When dealing with combat casualties with multiple extremity trauma and multiple organ system injuries, it is imperative to use the reconstructive ladder as a guide to provide the simplest and least morbid wound coverage.

The following factors play a critical role in the proper selection of flap coverage[24,35]:

- Patient factors (systemic illness, head trauma)
- Donor site availability (amputation of extremity)
- Genesis of the defect
- Location/size/depth of the defect
- Exposed structures
- Degree of contamination
- Quality of the surrounding tissues

In the combat-wounded setting, the availability of donor sites along with donor site morbidity considerations frequently play a pivotal role in flap selection. The high rate of concurrent injury and amputation may prevent traditional flap choices such as free fibula flaps or latissimus flaps from being viable options. Additionally, patients with severe systemic compromise and/or severe head trauma may not be ideal candidates for free tissue transfer procedures. In the upper extremity, there are a number of local pedicled flaps available for soft tissue coverage that will frequently suffice in the absence of very large tissue defects. In situations where appropriate local flaps are not available, distant pedicled flaps or free tissue transfer become necessary. In the civilian treatment of wounds requiring soft tissue flap coverage, there has been a trend toward performing more frequent free tissue transfer. The benefits of free tissue transfer include the possibility of a larger volume of durable, well-vascularized tissue without local tissue sacrifice from an already injured extremity, a one-stage coverage procedure, as well as the ability to perform the earliest range of motion. Despite this, there are circumstances frequently occurring in the combat wounded that lead toward the performance of less sophisticated local or distant pedicled flaps.[36-38] These pedicled flaps were used selectively when free flap donor sites were not available (eg, lower extremity amputations or blast injury) or when the overall patient condition required shorter operative times. The most significant advantage of the distant pedicled flap in the treatment of war wounds is that the vascular supply is obtained outside the often large zones of injury.

CRITICAL POINTS FOR OPTIMAL SUCCESS WITH FREE TISSUE TRANSFER

Patient and wound selection for free tissue transfer are the paramount factors for success. Often, a frank objective analysis of the wound and overall patient factors by a team of orthopedic and plastic surgeons will lead toward or against limb salvage. It is critical for optimal success in these situations to not perform free tissue transfer against one's better judgment when the limb is a better candidate for early amputation. In our experience, we performed few free muscle transfers to the upper extremity for soft tissue reconstruction. In the relatively few situations that a patient presented with an upper extremity that necessitated bulk muscle free tissue transfer for coverage of a wound, it was determined by a multidisciplinary team of orthopedic and plastic surgeons to be better served by early amputation unless extraordinary circumstances such as multiple limb amputations in a single patient were present. For this same reason, we did not often use vein grafts in free tissue transfer as the wounds that would have required them were frequently better candidates for amputation. In our free tissue transfers to the upper extremity, we used mainly fasciocutaneous flaps with long vascular pedicles in an effort to maximize vascular anastamoses outside the zone of injury. Liberal use of anticoagulation when not contraindicated with intravenous heparin (ptt goal 50 to 60) was used due to the wide zone of injury and multiple-level extremity injury often seen in the combat-injured patient.

ALGORITHM FOR UPPER EXTREMITY RECONSTRUCTION

While it is outside the scope of this chapter to discuss in detail all of the options for soft tissue coverage of the upper extremity, the following highlights our treatment algorithm and the flaps that we have used most frequently for wound coverage (Figure 18-1).

PEDICLED LATISSIMUS FLAP

The latissimus flap was most frequently used as a pedicled flap to provide coverage to the arm and proximal forearm, most frequently associated with open humerus and elbow fractures and associated triceps mechanism injury (Figure 18-2). While the latissimus is frequently taken as a free tissue transfer to provide bulk muscle coverage, in no instance was it used as a free tissue transfer in our cohort of upper extremity patients. The vascular pedicle for the latissimus flap is the thoracodorsal artery and its venae comitantes and the pedicle can be as long as 12 cm in length. The utility of this pedicled transfer lies in the fact that it is an expendable muscle and has the capability of reaching approximately 5 to 8 cm distal to the tip of the olecranon. It is the largest available muscle flap and is long, thin, and pliable. The average diameter of the thoracodorsal artery is 2.5 mm, and that of the venae comitantes is 3.0 mm.[39] While the latissimus flap may also be harvested as a myocutaneous flap, in most instances we have elected to take the flap as muscle only and then skin graft over the flap. The muscle-only variant facilitated flap inset and created a less bulky upper arm. The distal flap inset included appropriate tensioning to the ulnar or antebrachial fascia. In this configuration as a pedicled unipolar muscle transfer, the pedicled latissimus flap

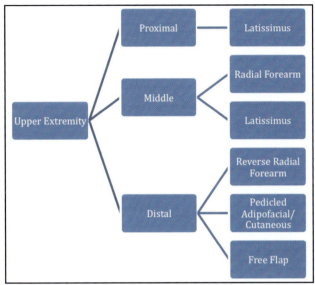

Figure 18-1. Reconstruction algorithm. Flap choices based on location of injury on the upper extremity.

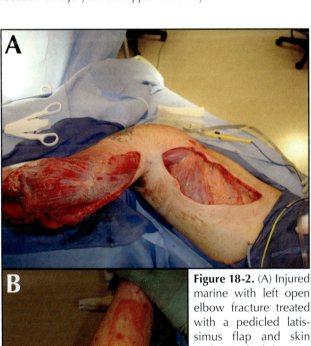

Figure 18-2. (A) Injured marine with left open elbow fracture treated with a pedicled latissimus flap and skin graft. (B) The left upper extremity 1 month status post inset and final skin graft.

served to both cover the exposed fracture and hardware as well as to reconstruct the damaged triceps extensor mechanism and serve as an in-phase functional muscle/tendon transfer for triceps function. While preoperative angiography is imperative prior to a free latissimus transfer, it is not as important with the pedicled transfer but should be performed if there is concern for a pedicle injury due to fragmentation. The most frequent complication following a pedicled latissimus transfer is a donor site seroma formation. For this reason, a surgical drain is usually used until drainage ceases.

Free Latissimus Flap

The free latissimus muscle flap was used very sparingly in upper extremity wound coverage. In most cases where bulk muscle transfer was required, the upper extremity was left with so few functional muscle tendon units that local reconstruction or delayed transfers were not possible. The free muscle flap was used in the devastating situation of the 3-limb amputation patient with only one arm remaining. This fortunately rare condition justifies the heroic salvage of the remaining limb to be used as an assist limb for transfers.

The details of flap elevation are described in the pedicled latissimus flap section. The recipient site preparation is extremely important in these technically demanding salvage procedures. The most common site of inset of the flap is the forearm and hand. This requires preparation of adequate inflow and outflow targets at the below-elbow level. The cephalic vein and antecubital veins are usually available for venous anastomosis at the elbow level. The brachial artery below the elbow is the most useful site for arterial anastomosis with an end-to-side configuration. The distal forearm and hand are often supplied by only one end arterial vessel, and preserving antegrade blood flow to the distal upper extremity is essential.

Radial Forearm Flap

Around the elbow and the proximal forearm, the workhorse radial forearm flap has been extensively used for coverage in civilian trauma.[40] The radial forearm flap is usually raised as a fasciocutaneous flap based upon the reliable arterial supply of the septocutaneous perforator branches of the radial artery. It was originally described as a free flap but has subsequently been used as a proximally based pedicled flap supplied by antegrade blood flow through the radial artery for coverage of defects around the elbow or the proximal forearm.[41,42] In the combat wounded, one of the most common contraindications to the use of the radial forearm flap has been significant trauma to

the soft tissue envelope of the forearm and/or injury to the radial artery or the venous system of the forearm or hand. We have used the radial forearm flap as a free tissue transfer from the contralateral upper extremity or as a flow through flap; however, we have seldom used it as a pedicled flap due to the frequent contraindications mentioned above.

Reverse Radial Forearm Flap

We have used the reverse radial forearm flap for dorsal hand coverage in the combat wounded. The reverse radial forearm flap provides ideal coverage for the dorsal hand due to its thin, supple nature (Figure 18-3).[41] The blood flow to the flap requires retrograde blood flow from the ulnar artery through the deep palmar arch, and it is imperative to ensure that the deep palmar arch is patent prior to performing this surgery. While a preoperative Allen's test will provide this information, it is wise in the combat wounded to perform preoperative angiography. One of the benefits of the reverse radial forearm flap is that it can still provide flap coverage in an upper extremity that has sustained trauma or undergone ligation of the radial artery proximal to the wrist, a situation that is not uncommon in the combat-wounded patient with severe upper extremity trauma.

Pedicled Adipofascial/ Cutaneous Flap

The family of distant pedicled adipofascial/cutaneous flaps includes distant pedicled flaps from the groin, trunk, or arm. We have used them routinely in the coverage of forearm and hand wounds in the combat injured and believe their role in the soft tissue coverage of distal upper extremity wounds is invaluable. These transfers were traditionally the mainstay of dorsal hand reconstruction; however, they have largely been replaced by local pedicled flaps or free tissue transfer (Figure 18-4).[21] The significant negatives of these distant pedicled flaps include the necessary 2-staged procedure as well as the prolonged period of immobilization and hand dependency.[21] In addition to the possibility of shoulder and elbow stiffness from the prolonged immobilization, the patient must endure the unnatural annoyance of having his or her hand attached to his or her body.[43]

Despite these negatives of the groin flap and other distant pedicled flaps, they will likely always have their place in the field of hand reconstruction and assuredly will continue to play a role in the reconstruction of combat-wounded patients.[19] The pedicled groin flap remains a useful and reliable technique in the properly selected patient. The groin flap has a relatively constant anatomy, and the dissection is

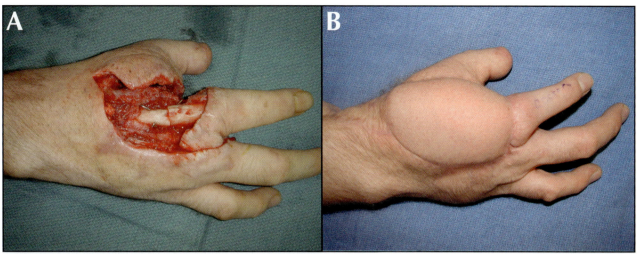

Figure 18-3. (A) Injured marine with right upper extremity dorsal hand injury after IED blast injury with exposed middle finger metacarpal arthrodesis. (B) The right hand 4 months after healed reconstruction with reverse radial forearm flap.

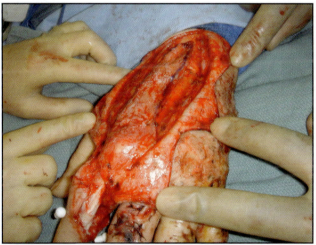

Figure 18-4. Injured marine with open left index finger fracture treated with pedicled adipofascial turnover flap and skin graft.

straightforward and requires minimal advanced training. One of the most significant advantages of the distant pedicled flap in the treatment of war wounds is that the vascular supply is more easily obtained outside the often large zone of injury. We have used single and multiple distant pedicled flaps successfully when traditional free flap reconstruction was contraindicated (eg, unable to anticoagulate) or not possible due to collateral damage or amputation (Figure 18-5).[36]

When performing distant pedicled flaps to the abdomen or groin, we have found that the use of an external fixator to immobilize the extremity to the pelvis is a useful adjunct.[36] First described by Drabyn et al in 1982,[44] this technique helps prevent skin maceration and pressure necrosis over the iliac crest, which can accompany the groin flap. The war-injured patients' care is frequently complicated by multiple other extremity injuries, traumatic brain injury, fre-

quent trips to the operating room with associated anesthesia, and intermittent postoperative delirium. We believe that external fixators provide rigid immobilization while avoiding the complications from poor hygiene, pressure necrosis, and flap separation.[44]

FREE ANTEROLATERAL THIGH FLAP

The anterolateral thigh flap is a versatile free flap capable of being harvested as a cutaneous, fasciocutaneous, or a musculocutaneous flap with the vastus lateralis. Most commonly, the anterolateral thigh flap is harvested as a fasciocutaneous flap based upon the perforator originating from the descending branch or transverse branch of the lateral femoral circumflex artery.[45] The often-encountered musculocutaneous variant of the anterolateral thigh flap can add additional time for flap harvest due to the technical demands of muscle perforator dissection into the skin paddle. The incorporation of a large segment of vastus lateralis with the skin paddle is usually not needed for upper extremity reconstruction. In our experience, the upper extremity reconstruction defect did not require significant dead space obliteration. The advantages of the anterolateral thigh flap include the potential large size of the flap (up to 35 x 25 cm)[46,47]; the ability to use a 2-team approach for harvest; the ability to obtain a long vascular pedicle up to 20 cm with the flap, thus often allowing for anastamosis outside the zone of injury; and relatively little donor site morbidity if minimal muscle harvest is performed.[39,46-48] Despite inconsistent thigh perforator anatomy, these advantages coupled with improved sensation and gliding surface make the anterolateral thigh flap our free flap of choice for reconstruction for distal upper extremity coverage (Figure 18-6).

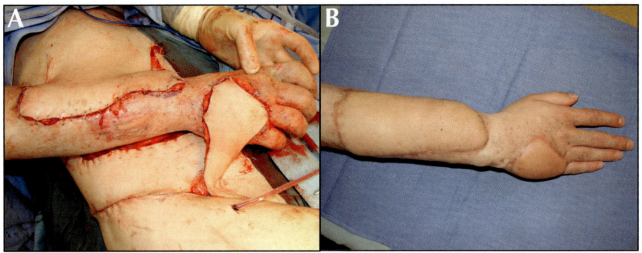

Figure 18-5. (A) Injured marine with right upper extremity open fractures treated with double pedicled flaps (abdominal and groin). (B) The right upper extremity 3 months after division and set of multiple pedicled flaps.

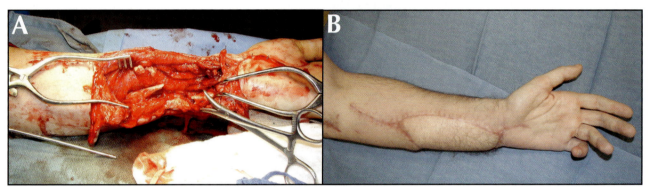

Figure 18-6. (A) Injured marine with left upper extremity open ulna fracture treated with an anterolateral thigh free flap. (B) The left upper extremity 6 months after injury and a flap revision.

In the preoperative planning for this flap, it is imperative that the inflow vessels be identified. For the combat-injured patient, this usually means that angiography of the upper extremity to receive the flap should be performed. In addition to verifying the inflow vessels, the patency of the palmar arch should be established if the arterial anastamosis is planned to be performed in an end-to-end fashion. Flap monitoring is imperative postoperatively. To facilitate close monitoring, we recommend 24 hours in an intensive care or step-down unit where adequate time and attention can be devoted to the flap.

Outcomes

In our previously reported experience with 32 upper extremity flap soft tissue reconstructions over a 30-month period, we found a flap success rate of 96%. Early infection (within 6 weeks of flap reconstruction) occurred in 2 patients (7%).[13] Three late cases of osteomyelitis (6 weeks to 528 days) occurred in 3 additional patients (11.5%). These infections were managed with surgical debridement and antibiotic therapy. All infections were successfully treated with retention of the limb. Total flap loss occurred in one patient. Three partial flap failures manifested as tip loss in 3 separate patients. The patient with total flap loss was reconstructed using a latissimus muscle flap. Flap failure was due to venous congestion secondary to axilla blast injury. Patients with partial flap loss were salvaged with negative pressure wound therapy, flap debridement, and re-advancement. The relationship between the timing of reconstruction and flap survival rate was not significant. Flap procedures were performed in the subacute period. Further stratification showed the timing of when the flap procedures occurred: early (5 to 21 days; n = 13, 50%), intermediate (within 21 days and 6 weeks; n = 7, 27%), and late (>6 weeks; n = 6, 23%). The average fracture time to union was 128 days, with a 96% union rate. The one patient with the nonunion went on to develop a nonpainful pseudarthrosis (distal ulna) and did not desire any further treatment. One patient elected early small finger amputation after partial flap loss, and one patient elected middle finger amputation 1 year after reconstruction due to finger stiffness. All patients underwent rehabilitation as indicated and prosthetic fitting when necessary (see Tables 18-1 through 18-3).

Our flap complication rate was very low with this severely injured cohort of combat patients. We strongly believe that the complication rates in these patients can be minimized with the combination of discriminating and precise patient selection as well as adherence to classic flap and microsurgical principles. It is imperative to closely look at the breakdown of our upper extremity flaps.

While excellent results have been obtained with the use of free tissue transfer, the majority of our patients' upper extremity wounds were successfully covered with pedicled flaps. Our review of soft tissue coverage in the upper extremity revealed that 81% of wounds were covered with pedicled flaps and the remaining 19% with free tissue transfer.[13] We had 100% success in the free flap cohort of patients. The high success rate overall and specifically with free tissue transfers highlights our critical selection bias in the performance of flap reconstruction. In further analysis of the free flaps performed, there were few free muscle flaps used in the coverage of upper extremity wounds in our patients for the reasons previously discussed.

Conclusion

Providing wound coverage to a combat-injured limb that would otherwise go on to amputation is a very rewarding yet humbling experience. It is imperative to recognize the unique nature of combat wounds and the differences in management of these wounds from civilian trauma. In the majority of instances in the upper extremity, pedicled flaps will provide reliable and durable soft tissue coverage when free tissue donor sites or patient characteristics prohibit free tissue transfer. When free tissue transfer is indicated, it can be provided successfully with stringent patient selection. With these principles in mind, success in the face of the demanding and unique challenges presented by modern battlefield injuries can be obtained.

References

1. Helling TS, McNabney WK. The role of amputation in the management of battlefield casualties: a history of two millennia. *J Trauma*. 2000;49(5):930-939.
2. Mabry RL, Holcomb JB, Baker AM, et al. United States Army Rangers in Somalia: an analysis of combat casualties on an urban battlefield. *J Trauma*. 2000;49(3):515-528; discussion 528-529.
3. Geiger S, McCormick F, Chou R, Wandel AG. War wounds: lessons learned from Operation Iraqi Freedom. *Plast Reconstr Surg*. 2008;122(1):146-153.
4. Nikolic D, Jovanovic Z, Popovic Z, Vulovic R, Mladenovic M. Primary surgical treatment of war injuries of major joints of the limbs. *Injury*. 1999;30(2):129-134.
5. Owens BD, Kragh JF Jr, Macaitis J, Svoboda SJ, Wenke JC. Characterization of extremity wounds in Operation Iraqi Freedom and Operation Enduring Freedom. *J Orthop Trauma*. 2007;21(4):254-257.
6. Dougherty PJ. Long-term follow-up study of bilateral above-the-knee amputees from the Vietnam War. *J Bone Joint Surg Am*. 1999;81(10):1384-1390.
7. Dougherty PJ. Transtibial amputees from the Vietnam War. Twenty-eight-year follow-up. *J Bone Joint Surg Am*. 2001;83-A(3):383-389.
8. Potter BK, Scoville CR. Amputation is not isolated: an overview of the US Army Amputee Patient Care Program and associated amputee injuries. *J Am Acad Orthop Surg*. 2006;14(10 Spec No.):S188-S190.
9. Stansbury LG, Lalliss SJ, Branstetter JG, Bagg MR, Holcomb JB. Amputations in U.S. military personnel in the current conflicts in Afghanistan and Iraq. *J Orthop Trauma*. 2008;22(1):43-46.
10. Stansbury LG, Branstetter JG, Lalliss SJ. Amputation in military trauma surgery. *J Trauma*. 2007;63(4):940-944.
11. Kumar AR. Standard wound coverage techniques for extremity war injury. *J Am Acad Orthop Surg*. 2006;14(10 Spec No.):S62-S65.
12. Kumar AR, Grewal NS, Chung TL, Bradley JP. Lessons from operation Iraqi freedom: successful subacute reconstruction of complex lower extremity battle injuries. *Plast Reconstr Surg*. 2009;123(1):218-229.
13. Kumar AR, Grewal NS, Chung TL, Bradley JP. Lessons from the modern battlefield: successful upper extremity injury reconstruction in the subacute period. *J Trauma*. 2009;67(4):752-757.
14. Chattar-Cora D, Perez-Nieves R, McKinlay A, Kunasz M, Delaney R, Lyons R. Operation Iraqi Freedom: a report on a series of soldiers treated with free tissue transfer by a plastic surgery service. *Ann Plast Surg*. 2007;58(2):200-206.
15. Graham B, Adkins P, Tsai TM, Firrell J, Breidenbach WC. Major replantation versus revision amputation and prosthetic fitting in the upper extremity: a late functional outcomes study. *J Hand Surg Am*. 1998;23(5):783-791.
16. Pollak AN. Use of negative pressure wound therapy with reticulated open cell foam for lower extremity trauma. *J Orthop Trauma*. 2008;22(10 Suppl):S142-S145.
17. Morykwas MJ, Argenta LC, Shelton-Brown EI, McGuirt W. Vacuum-assisted closure: a new method for wound control and treatment: animal studies and basic foundation. *Ann Plast Surg*. 1997;38(6):553-562.
18. Pollak AN, Powell ET, Fang R, Cooper EO, Ficke JR, Flaherty SF. Use of negative pressure wound therapy during aeromedical evacuation of patients with combat related blast injuries. *J Surg Orthop Adv*. 2010;19(1):44-48.
19. Friedrich JB, Katolik LI, Vedder NB. Soft tissue reconstruction of the hand. *J Hand Surg Am*. 2009;34(6):1148-1155.
20. Helgeson MD, Potter BK, Evans KN, Shawen SB. Bioartificial dermal substitute: a preliminary report on its use for the management of complex combat-related soft tissue wounds. *J Orthop Trauma*. 2007;21(6):394-399.
21. Page R, Chang J. Reconstruction of hand soft-tissue defects: alternatives to the radial forearm fasciocutaneous flap. *J Hand Surg Am*. 2006;31(5):847-856.
22. Godina M. Early microsurgical reconstruction of complex trauma of the extremities. *Plast Reconstr Surg*. 1986;78(3):285-292.
23. Byrd HS, Spicer TE, Cierney GR. Management of open tibial fractures. *Plast Reconstr Surg*. 1985;76(5):719-730.

24. Lister G, Scheker L. Emergency free flaps to the upper extremity. *J Hand Surg Am*. 1988;13(1):22-28.

25. Ninkovic M, Deetjen H, Ohler K, Anderl H. Emergency free tissue transfer for severe upper extremity injuries. *J Hand Surg Br*. 1995;20(1):53-58.

26. Chen SH, Wei FC, Chen HC, Chuang CC, Noordhoff MS. Emergency free-flap transfer for reconstruction of acute complex extremity wounds. *Plast Reconstr Surg*. 1992;89(5):882-888; discussion 889-890.

27. Levin LS. Early versus delayed closure of open fractures. *Injury*. 2007;38(8):896-899.

28. Ostermann PA, Henry SL, Seligson D. Timing of wound closure in severe compound fractures. *Orthopedics*. 1994;17(5):397-399.

29. Bhattacharyya T, Mehta P, Smith M, Pomahac B. Routine use of wound vacuum-assisted closure does not allow coverage delay for open tibia fractures. *Plast Reconstr Surg*. 2008;121(4):1263-1266.

30. Yaremchuk MJ, Gan BS. Soft tissue management of open tibia fractures. *Acta Orthop Belg*. 1996;62(Suppl):1188-1192.

31. Steiert AE, Gohritz A, Schreiber TC, Krettek C, Vogt PM. Delayed flap coverage of open extremity fractures after previous vacuum-assisted closure (VAC) therapy—worse or worth? *J Plast Reconstr Aesthet Surg*. 2009;62(5):675-683.

32. Keeling JJ, Gwinn DE, Tintle SM, Andersen RC, McGuigan FX. Short-term outcomes of severe open wartime tibial fractures treated with ring external fixation. *J Bone Joint Surg Am*. 2008;90(12):2643-2651.

33. Levin LS. The reconstructive ladder. An orthoplastic approach. *Orthop Clin North Am*. 1993;24(3):393-409.

34. Levin LS, Condit DP. Combined injuries—soft tissue management. *Clin Orthop Relat Res*. 1996;(327):172-181.

35. Wolf JM, Athwal GS, Shin AY, Dennison DG. Acute trauma to the upper extremity: what to do and when to do it. *J Bone Joint Surg Am*. 2009;91(5):1240-1252.

36. Tintle SM, Wilson K, McKay PL, Andersen RC, Kumar AR. Simultaneous pedicled flaps for coverage of complex blast injuries to the forearm and hand (with supplemental external fixation to the iliac crest for immobilization). *J Hand Surg Eur Vol*. 2010;35(1):9-15.

37. Lohman RF, Nabawi AS, Reece GP, Pollock RE, Evans GR. Soft tissue sarcoma of the upper extremity: a 5-year experience at two institutions emphasizing the role of soft tissue flap reconstruction. *Cancer*. 2002;94(8):2256-2264.

38. Hanumadass M, Kagan R, Matsuda T. Early coverage of deep hand burns with groin flaps. *J Trauma*. 1987;27(2):109-114.

39. Moran SL, Cooney WP. *Master Techniques in Orthopaedic Surgery: Soft Tissue Surgery*. Baltimore, MD: Lippincott Williams & Wilkins; 2008.

40. Orgill DP, Pribaz JJ, Morris DJ. Local fasciocutaneous flaps for olecranon coverage. *Ann Plast Surg*. 1994;32(1):27-31.

41. Jones NF, Jarrahy R, Kaufman MR. Pedicled and free radial forearm flaps for reconstruction of the elbow, wrist, and hand. *Plast Reconstr Surg*. 2008;121(3):887-898.

42. Song R, Gao Y, Song Y, Yu Y, Song Y. The forearm flap. *Clin Plast Surg*. 1982;9(1):21-26.

43. Gupta A, Shatford RA, Wolff TW, Tsai TM, Scheker LR, Levin LS. Treatment of the severely injured upper extremity. *Instr Course Lect*. 2000;49:377-396.

44. Drabyn GA, Porterfield HW, Mohler LR, Nappi JF. Wrist-iliac crest fixation for groin flap-thumb immobilization. *Plast Reconstr Surg*. 1982;70(1):98-99.

45. Song YG, Chen GZ, Song YL. The free thigh flap: a new free flap concept based on the septocutaneous artery. *Br J Plast Surg*. 1984;37(2):149-159.

46. Hsu CC, Lin YT, Lin CH, Lin CH, Wei FC. Immediate emergency free anterolateral thigh flap transfer for the mutilated upper extremity. *Plast Reconstr Surg*. 2009;123(6):1739-1747.

47. Koshima I. Free anterolateral thigh flap for reconstruction of head and neck defects following cancer ablation. *Plast Reconstr Surg*. 2000;105(7):2358-2360.

48. Park JE, Rodriguez ED, Bluebond-Langer R, et al. The anterolateral thigh flap is highly effective for reconstruction of complex lower extremity trauma. *J Trauma*. 2007;62(1):162-165.

Chapter 19

COMPLEX RECONSTRUCTIVE CHALLENGES IN HAND AND FOREARM WOUNDS

LTC(P) Martin F. Baechler, MD; LT Scott Tintle, MD;
COL Chester C. Buckenmaier III, MD; and MAJ Matthew L. Drake, MD

Compared to other types of injury, combat wounds sustained in modern warfare are more devastating in many ways. They result from the delivery of extremely high levels of energy to tissues, are highly contaminated, and occur very far from definitive care facilities. Although some civilian trauma techniques can be extrapolated to combat casualty care, war trauma remains unique and often necessitates novel approaches.

Epidemiology

The signature combat wound of the current US military conflicts is that caused by blast and fragmentation.[1,2] Projectile, thermal, and blast mechanisms combine to create diffuse, heterogeneous, extensive, and numerous wounds. It is common to have all tissue components of a limb affected. Not only are tissue planes dissected by the force of the blast, commonly there is projectile penetration across tissue planes far distant from the obvious wound, creating a large zone of injury with critical implications to reconstructive decision making.

With respect to tissue loss, one can imagine a wound resulting from modern warfare as being caused by the bite of a large animal (Figure 19-1). Indeed, the "shark bites" of modern warfare commonly have substantial volumes of segmental tissue loss. The combinations of tissue loss and the resulting dysfunction are infinitely variable and are not necessarily proportional. That is

to say, if vital structures are spared, an extremity with a large amount of tissue loss can function relatively well; whereas, if vital structures are affected, even minimal tissue injury can cause severe dysfunction. Therefore, each patient requires a unique reconstruction plan built upon fundamental principles.

Management in Theater

NUTRITION

Nutrition is to the trauma patient as ammunition is to the soldier; as the soldier needs more ammunition to wage a bigger fight, the patient needs more nutrition to heal a larger wound burden. However, despite their generally young and healthy physical condition, combat casualties are prone to nutritional deficiency. The process of casualty evacuation from a war zone is intense, occasionally demanding compromise between the nutrition and transportation needs of the casualty. Multiple surgical episodes, sometimes daily or every other day for extended periods, are common in the early stages of care. Each episode of anesthesia necessitates a period of antecedent and subsequent fasting. Prolonged mechanical ventilation and abdominal injuries are frequently concomitant with extremity injuries and impair nutrition, despite use of tube feeding and parenteral nutrition.[3,4] Nutrition must be emphasized and optimized at the earliest possible point in the patient's care.

Owens BD, Belmont PJ Jr, eds. *Combat Orthopedic Surgery:*
Lessons Learned in Iraq and Afghanistan (pp 169-180)
© 2011 SLACK Incorporated

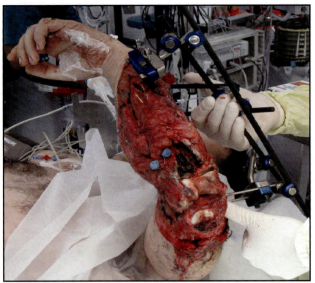

Figure 19-1. This is an example of a severe combat wound. Multiple specialized tissues are significantly injured or lost.

DEBRIDEMENT

The treatment of combat casualty wounds begins first and foremost with properly performed wound debridement. Insufficient debridement of a wound increases the risk of complications such as infection and exuberant scar formation. On the other hand, excessive debridement sacrifices vital structures that may heal and function satisfactorily given time. Thus, aggressive debridement of injured tissue and the selective preservation of vital structures are on opposite ends of a continuum. The dilemma of the surgeon is to strike the optimal balance between the two. Perhaps the best teachers of the skill are experience and mentoring; the relative lack of glamour in wound debridement should not cause the delegation of this surgical procedure for combat wounds to less experienced surgeons.

Generally, civilian trauma causes wounds that require only one or a few debridement procedures to render them clean and viable for reconstructive procedures. In contrast, combat wounds are prone to devolve in the short term and require an increased number of debridement procedures, somewhat analogous to burn wounds and frostbite.[5] Indeed, a combat wound that is aggressively debrided, even by a seasoned military surgeon, may appear alarmingly suboptimal several days later. When treating combat wounds sustained as a result of modern warfare, the surgeon must be patient and prepared for an increased number of debridement procedures.

Contrary to some surgeons' training, we commonly use a tourniquet during the debridement of combat wounds, even though the use of a tourniquet may affect the surgeon's ability to evaluate tissue

perfusion. Visualization of vital structures is vastly improved by a bloodless field. Also, it minimizes the transfusion requirement in patients undergoing multiple debridement procedures. At the conclusion of each debridement procedure, the tourniquet is released, vascularity of tissue is assessed, and further debridement of nonviable tissue is performed as needed.[6,7]

Pulsatile lavage may be useful in initial debridement procedures to remove large particulate debris and foreign matter. However, we believe the repetitive use of pulsatile lavage is of limited value. In fact, pulsatile lavage may cause cumulative surface trauma, dissect tissue planes unnecessarily, and lead to a paradoxical rebound in the bacterial count of the wound. Furthermore, irrigation with normal saline is preferred; additives such as bacitracin, Castile soap, and benzalkonium chloride, while reducing the bacterial load better than saline initially, result in a significant rebound in the bacterial count.[8] Low-pressure gravity flow irrigation of appropriate volumes of normal saline is recommended.

SUBATMOSPHERIC WOUND DRESSING

The interim treatment of war wounds about the hand and forearm with subatmospheric wound dressing (SAWD) has many benefits.[9] A main feature of SAWD is the regular removal of wound exudate, including metalloproteinases, which inhibit wound healing.[10] Without evacuation, excess wound exudate may cause tissue maceration and bacteria proliferation. Simultaneously, SAWD prevents wound desiccation by serving as a vapor barrier. Another significant benefit of SAWD is the elimination of bulky, odorous gauze dressings and the markedly decreased frequency of dressing changes, improving morale for the patient and caretakers alike. The low-profile dressing permits the patient to see and more readily move the extremity, affording the patient a better understanding of the nature of the injury and promoting participation in the recovery process. SAWD is an extremely effective anti-shear bolster dressing when applied over split-thickness skin grafts and engineered wound resurfacing products.

However, the merits of SAWD should not be overstated. SAWD will not clean, debride, or sterilize a wound and may actually cause an increase in bacterial load compared to gauze dressing.[11,12] Contraindications to the use of SAWD include an actively infected wound and the presence in the wound of exposed blood vessel or nerve. A SAWD that loses its negative pressure creates a partially closed system conducive to bacterial overgrowth; this condition must be immediately remediated. Lastly, SAWD promotes granulation tissue, which may be undesirable in many circumstances, as will be discussed.

EXTERNAL FIXATION

Immobilization of the injured extremity is an extremely important first aid principle. Patient comfort is significantly improved by immobilization. Splinting of bone and soft tissues promotes perfusion, reduces infection rates, blunts the inflammatory cascade in multitrauma patients, and facilitates hemodynamic stability by promoting clot formation at the fracture site.[13-17] Though a simple splint is an effective means of extremity immobilization, it is vastly inferior to external fixation in several ways when treating combat wounds caused by modern warfare. Patient transport is greatly facilitated by external fixation compared to simple splinting, which is extremely pertinent given that the combat casualty is subjected to transcontinental transport with multiple stops and transfers en route to a definitive care facility. Furthermore, external fixation provides relatively easy access to wounds for ongoing care both in the operating room and at the bedside.

In most cases, the application of an external fixator is not technically challenging, yet there are important principles that must be applied in order to maximize its effectiveness, avoid complications, and set the stage for future reconstruction. By nature of their communication with the environment, external fixation pins can introduce bacteria deep into an extremity. For this reason, when possible, external fixation pins should not be placed through fracture hematoma, open wounds, or areas of bone where a plate will later be placed. In some areas, such as the subcutaneous border of the ulna, pins may be placed through very small incisions with minimal concern for injury to vital deep structures. In other areas, the surgeon must be certain to avoid vital deep structures by making a surgical approach of adequate size to visualize the bone directly. In this situation, careful retraction and the use of drill sleeves should be used to avoid wrapping vital structures around the spinning drill bit. The notable and most frequently injured nerves are the superficial radial nerve and the lateral antebrachial cutaneous nerve, which are at risk throughout the length of the radius and the index metacarpal, and the radial nerve, which is at risk at the mid-lateral humerus.[18-20]

With threaded pins that require predrilling, the surgeon must ensure that the drill bit used is sharp before each use. With self-drilling, self-tapping, threaded pins, each pin should be new and as sharp as specified by its design. We prefer self-drilling, self-tapping, threaded pins over pins that require predrilling. However, in dense cortical bone, predrilling with a perfectly sharp drill bit may reduce heat generation and result in improved holding power, even when using self-drilling, self-tapping, threaded pins.

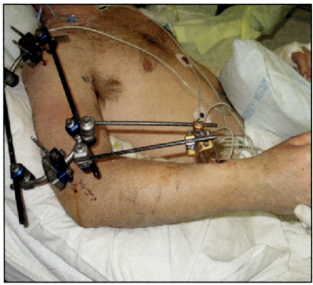

Figure 19-2. The external fixator spans midshaft humerus and proximal forearm fractures. Note the distal external fixator pins placed into the radius. This arrangement simultaneously splints elbow motion and forearm rotation. All pins were placed by directly visualizing bone to avoid injury to the radial nerve and the superficial branch of the radial nerve.

Additionally, placement with a powered drill is preferred over hand-powered insertion for several reasons. Clearly, time is saved with motor-powered insertion of self-drilling, self-tapping, threaded pins, while the heat produced by insertion is similar between motor-powered and hand-powered techniques.[21] Wobble is generally increased with hand-powered insertion, which can cause increased bone removal from the near-cortex hole and decrease pin stability.[22] When the external fixator is planned as the definitive fixation, the surgeon should consider using hydroxyapatite-coated pins, as they are more durable over time with respect to pull-out strength.[23-25]

When stabilizing the forearm, rather than simply spanning the radius or the ulna only, the surgeon should consider including both bones in the construct. By placing threaded pins proximally in the ulna and distally in the radius, for example, the forearm can be stabilized with a relatively simple construct that will simultaneously splint the fracture and soft tissues, maintain forearm length, and control forearm rotation. Alternatively, by placing pins proximally in the ulna and distally in the index metacarpal, the forearm and wrist are simultaneously splinted. When an unstable elbow is spanned, we recommend placing pins proximally in the lateral humerus and distally in the mid- or distal radius (Figure 19-2). This construct will simultaneously splint the elbow and control forearm rotation, immobilizing the extremity more effectively and completely compared to a spanning external fixator with pins in the humerus and ulna only.

Spanning external fixation also proves very useful in severe peri-articular wrist injuries and severe open carpal fractures with significant bone loss. In these cases, external fixator pins can be placed proximally in the radius or ulna and distally into a remaining metacarpal. The external fixator splints the joints and maintains length until conditions are optimized for bone reconstruction.

Contracture of the first web space is a common cause of compromised function of the hand in the combat casualty. While a simple web space splint may be effective, it is often inadequate due to poor patient compliance, concomitant hand injury, or wound issues. External fixation is effective in preventing a first web space contracture in the presence of a severe injury involving the hand (Figure 19-3).[26]

With the general acceptance of external fixation as a means of skeletal stabilization, along with improved external fixator design, its use in the hand has expanded. The ability to stabilize metacarpal or phalangeal fractures while minimizing further soft tissue dissection makes the use of the external fixator in the hand attractive. Sophisticated mini-external fixator designs for the hand now allow for independent and flexible pin and bar placement, minimal soft tissue damage, and a relatively stable construct.[27] In most series reported, mini-external fixators have been used in the setting of open, unstable, or comminuted fractures; severe soft tissue damage; or heavily contaminated fractures with substantial amounts of bone loss.[28-30]

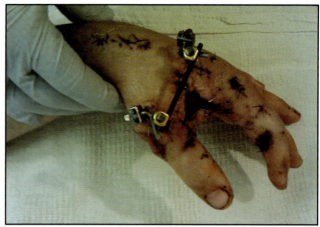

Figure 19-3. To minimize a first web space contracture, an external fixator is placed spanning the thumb and index metacarpals.

Definitive Management

Wound Closure

Upper extremity combat wounds of relatively low complexity may be satisfactorily treated using simple techniques, such as delayed primary closure, healing by secondary intention, early skin grafting over a suitably vascular bed, or delayed skin grafting on a bed of granulation tissue. Complex wounds with exposed fracture, joint, nerve, tendon, and bone often require advanced techniques to achieve wound healing, such as rotational, pedicled, or free flap coverage.

Often, wounds fall between these extremes. The surgeon must consider the future reconstructive and rehabilitative needs of the injured extremity in the earliest stages of wound management. For example, an injured extremity that would heal with simple skin grafting, or even direct closure, but with an associated complex deep wound may be better treated with composite flap coverage in order to set the stage for future reconstruction of specialized deep tissues. Reconstruction of structures deep to a heavily scarred or skin grafted area is technically difficult and

prone to poor wound healing and excessive scaring. Additionally, avoidance of linear scar contracture is another factor to consider when considering wound coverage options. Pliable skin with adequate excursion is necessary over a joint to allow normal joint mobility. Contracted scar tissue and grafted skin over and near a joint will tether its motion and should be prevented if possible.

In general, a wound should be definitively managed as soon as it is ready. Some authors have recommended that flap coverage occur within 72 hours of injury in order to avoid wound-healing complications and maximize eventual function.[31] Other authors have reported delayed reconstruction without apparent degradation of results.[32-34] Prospective studies on this issue are not available.

Based on their experience, the surgeons at Walter Reed Army Medical Center believe that treating combat wounds with zealous effort at immediate reconstruction of nerve, tendon, ligament, joint, and bone is fraught with pitfalls and complications. As discussed, prior to definitive wound coverage, the combat wound must undergo sufficient debridement to render it suitable for reconstruction. Furthermore, the patient must be physiologically stable, nutritionally optimized, and no longer require intensive interventions. When free-tissue transfer is to be employed, frequent trips to the imaging suite or operating room, as is commonly the case with the multiply injured war casualty, is undesirable, as this increases the risk of compromising the flap. Intensive support with vasopressors, which constrict blood vessels, precludes free-tissue transfer while they are being used. Concomitant injury may preclude some flaps, making selection of a donor site very challenging. Some patients require multiple free-tissue transfers for separate wounds, further complicating the situation. Close, frequent, efficient, and in-depth communication across surgical and medical specialties is critical to optimal care of the multiply injured war casualty, particularly in institutions with high volumes of such patients.

SYNTHETIC DERMAL REPLACEMENT

The array of engineered resurfacing products for the management of wounds has expanded in recent years. We have had a favorable experience with Integra Dermal Regeneration Template (Integra LifeSciences, Plainsboro, NJ), which is a bilayer dermal replacement system.[35,36] It is stored at room temperature, and application involves simply trimming the product to fit the dimensions of the wound to be covered, followed by stapling or suturing it to the wound edges. The dermal replacement layer consists of a porous matrix of cross-linked bovine tendon collagen fibers and a glycosaminoglycan (chondroitin-6-sulfate). It serves as a matrix for the infiltration of fibroblasts, macrophages, lymphocytes, and capillaries. The epidermal replacement layer is temporary and consists of a semi-porous silicone that serves as a vapor barrier. Once the dermal replacement layer has adequately vascularized, the silicone layer is removed, and a split-thickness skin graft is placed.

While the indications for use of this product are still in evolution, a number of short- and long-term benefits of the product are notable.[37] Upon initial application of the product, SAWD can be employed as an anti-shear bolster directly over the silicone layer. The vapor barrier function of the silicone layer is extremely effective in keeping the wound moist. It also allows relatively painless and easy bedside care as it does not adhere to gauze dressings. In fact, after 5 to 7 days, the initial SAWD typically can be removed at the bedside. Shaving the skin surrounding the wound at the time of SAWD application facilitates its bedside removal or exchange on the awake patient. The amount of drainage from the wound at this point is usually minimal. Adherence of the product to the wound bed and progressive vascularization are assessed, and areas of nonadherence and exudate accumulation are treated with selective debridement. Integra may be reapplied to these areas. Serial applications can be used to build up additional thickness of replacement dermis over critical structures or to improve the contour of the wound. We have found that a previously applied, adherent, and vascularized layer of Integra will readily accept additional layers of the product. A mature layer of Integra contains hues of yellow, orange, and red and is smooth as it follows the contour of the wound bed. Of note, the cellular and vascular infiltration of the Integra matrix does not appear to be the same as typical granulation tissue. Indeed, Integra seems to preclude the formation of granulation tissue on the wound bed. Perhaps

this is the mechanism by which the product appears to minimize contracture of the wound. After 14 to 21 days, the site is surgically prepped directly over the silicone layer. The silicone is then removed, and a split-thickness skin graft is applied. Again, as an anti-shear bolster, SAWD is used over the skin grafted area. The surgeon can expect uniformly successful skin graft results when conditions are optimized.

A mature wound that has been treated with Integra prior to skin grafting is more pliable and supple. The replacement dermis appears to develop some degree of differential excursion relative to the tissue underneath, improving wear characteristics and extremity function. Minimal or no wound contraction occurs, which is an important distinction compared to traditional split-thickness skin grafts. Selectively, when other means of wound coverage are not feasible, Integra can be placed over avascular structures, such as over tendon-lacking paratenon and bone-lacking periosteum. The dermal replacement matrix will allow cellular and vascular infiltration at the periphery of the Integra where it overlaps vascular tissue. The vascular infiltration will then continue throughout the Integra layer to eventually form a complete bed suitable for skin grafting. When used for this purpose, multiple applications of Integra may be necessary. The use of synthetic dermal replacement products directly over open fractures is not recommended.

Surgical Technique

INTERNAL FIXATION

Internal fixation of forearm and hand fractures resulting from modern warfare is often best managed with the traditional techniques of compression, neutralization, or bridge plating. The configuration of the construct and the timing of surgery are dictated by the specific fracture pattern, the particulars of the wound, and individual patient parameters.

The introduction of screws that lock into a plate at a fixed-angle is clearly a step forward in fracture care, particularly in peri-articular applications.[38] However, this technological advance should be considered by the surgeon merely as an adjunct to the basic principles of compression plating. Indeed, in many cases, the added rigidity afforded by locking plates may only be of theoretical benefit, as standard compression plating may be adequate. Furthermore, if the technique is applied incorrectly, a fracture may inadvertently be locked in distraction, or the stability afforded by the friction of a plate screwed tightly to a bone may be forfeited.[39] In the end, a hybrid of compression plating and locking screws, correctly applied, will capitalize on the benefits of each technique.[40]

Fractures resulting from modern warfare are frequently unsuited for internal fixation with plates and screws. Applying internal fixation may unacceptably complicate the wound by necessitating dissection of tissues that are already compromised. Furthermore, the mere presence of a plate may increase the burden of wound coverage if local soft tissue is inadequate to cover it. On the other hand, placing implants in the intramedullary position avoids additional soft tissue dissection. Unlocked intramedullary nailing of radius and ulna fractures in adults was described decades ago using smooth, noncontoured implants.[41] This technique has been used with success in open forearm fractures resulting from combat (Figure 19-4). More recently, intramedullary implants that are contoured and that can be interlocked with screws have been developed and appear to be effective, with reported union rates of 100%.[42-44]

In some cases of severe injury to the carpus and hand, to include severe fractures to the distal radius, neither standard internal fixation nor external fixation techniques may be suitable. For instance, the fracture pattern may defy the capabilities of the best surgeon armed with the latest plates. Or, a rather lengthy interval of time may separate injury from definitive surgery, making temporary external fixation undesirable. In such cases, the carpus can be temporarily spanned with an internal bridging plate from the radius to a metacarpal, or even to a phalanx, until the time is right for definitive fixation.[45,46]

Some hand fractures resulting from modern warfare can be managed nonoperatively; however, those with peri-articular involvement, metaphyseal comminution, segmental bone loss, or displacement may benefit from internal fixation. The goal is to restore anatomy while respecting the soft tissues, allowing early motion of the digits when possible. Hand stiffness is a very common complication of hand fractures, regardless of the method of treatment. Even with the theoretical advantage of early motion afforded by internal fixation of hand fracture, hand stiffness is still an issue.[47] Newer locking plate designs are now available for use in the hand; however, clinical data guiding their use are not yet available in peer-reviewed literature.

SEGMENTAL BONE LOSS

In our experience, segmental bone loss of the upper extremity is relatively common in wounds resulting from modern warfare. Bone grafting is rarely performed in the acute period due to concerns for infection and excessive inflammation, which may result in graft resorption. Options for reconstructing segmental bone loss include autograft bone, allograft bone, and bone graft substitutes, such as calcium sulfate and

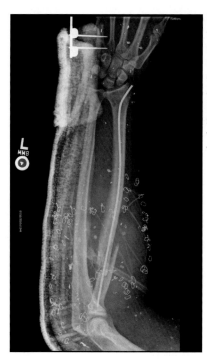

Figure 19-4. A titanium flexible nail is used to stabilize this proximal radius fracture. In this case, there was a large associated wound. The intramedullary implant stabilizes the bone without adding to the wound burden.

calcium phosphate. In order to maximize union and graft incorporation, it has been the practice at Walter Reed Army Medical Center to reconstruct segmental defects with autograft bone rather than allograft bone, whenever possible.

The decision to use cortical or cancellous autograft, or even both, is largely based on the particulars of the defect to be managed. If a diaphysis is being reconstructed, then a cortical graft may best reconstruct the defect. If the void is located in a metaphyseal region, cancellous bone may be more suitable. Small segmental bone loss (less than 4 cm) can generally be managed with autograft bone. Enough material for a 4-cm defect can predictably be obtained from one iliac crest.[48] Larger defects may require more elaborate reconstructive techniques, such as vascularized bone grafting.

We have had success with the recently described technique of induced membranes.[49,50] This technique involves placing a polymethylmethacrylate (PMMA) temporary spacer into a segmental bone defect. Its presence induces the formation of membranes rich in capillaries and various growth factors around the PMMA implant. Additionally, antibiotic-impregnated PMMA has been shown in lab animals to reduce infection rates.[51-53] After a period of 6 to 12 weeks, the PMMA spacer is removed, and cancellous autografting is performed. It is believed that the induced membrane reduces resorption of the autograft bone and secretes factors that promote remodeling and incorporation. This technique has been shown to be successful in healing defects up to 25 cm.[54]

For grafting of larger bone defects (larger than 4 cm), the ability to achieve a stable union is markedly enhanced by the technique of vascularized bone grafting. A free vascularized osteoseptocutaneus fibula is the workhorse for reconstructing large segmental long-bone defects (Figure 19-5).[55,56] This predictable flap is based on the peroneal artery, which has 2 venae comitantes and resides in the deep posterior compartment of the leg between the flexor hallucis longus and tibialis posterior muscles. Even if not needed for wound management, we regularly raise the fibula with a skin paddle, which serves well as a monitor of flap viability. The vascular pedicle length can be less than 3 cm, depending on the length of fibula harvested, and the average vessel diameter is 1.2 mm. While up to 26 cm of the fibula can be harvested, it is recommended to leave 8 to 10 cm distally to maintain ankle stability by ensuring preservation of the distal tibia-fibula ligaments. Proximally, the peroneal nerve must be carefully protected during the harvest. The patient and therapist must be instructed to stretch the great toe postoperatively to avoid the common complication of flexor hallucis longus contracture.[57]

Another promising technique is the free medial femoral condyle bone graft.[58] This flap has a variable arterial anatomy, with the most common variant being the descending genicular artery with a pedicle length of 13.7 cm and a diameter of 1.5 mm.[59] The flap can be raised as a thin corticoperiosteal sleeve, which is pliable compared to the rigid structure of the free fibula, or as a plug of corticocancellous bone. Recent investigators have published successful cases using this graft for difficult nonunions with bone loss in the humerus, radius, clavicle, ulna, and scaphoid.[60-62]

Though loss of forearm rotation significantly degrades function, creation of a one-bone forearm is reluctantly elected when reconstruction options are limited. Occasionally, a stable one-bone forearm can be created simply by allowing synostosis to occur while the forearm is immobilized in the selected position of rotation. Alternatively, the residual distal radius can simply be mounted on the residual proximal ulnar shaft and stabilized with a plate (Figure 19-6).[63] For reconstruction of segmental bone loss of the phalanges and metacarpals, salvage can be achieved using autograft bone blocks from the iliac crest.[64]

SEGMENTAL MUSCLE AND TENDON LOSS

Though the risk of tendon scarring and the need for eventual tenolysis is very high, direct tendon repair should be performed when possible in order to avoid the need for tendon grafting. When direct tendon repair is not possible, tendon reconstruction can be performed via grafting or tendon transfer, but usually must be delayed until inflammation is mini-

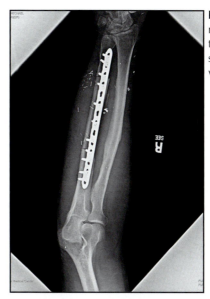

Figure 19-5. The segmental loss of bone of the ulna was reconstructed with a free vascularized fibula.

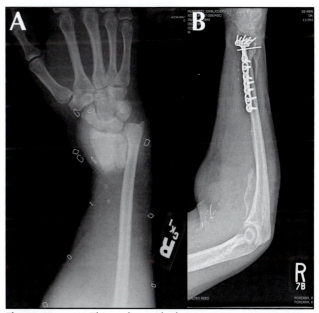

Figure 19-6. (A) This radiograph demonstrates a massive segmental bone loss of the radius. (B) The "one-bone" forearm is created by mounting the radius distally to the ulna proximally.

mal in order to minimize the formation of adhesions. However, the surgeon may consider placing silicone rods to create a favorable tunnel for future tendon grafting. As discussed, this is in contrast to the treatment of wounds caused by lower energy mechanisms wherein immediate and extensive reconstruction may be successful. Another consideration in the treatment of combat wounds is that the polytraumatized patient may have additional injuries competing for reconstruction and rehabilitation priority. Therefore, when considering the timing of tendon reconstruction, the ability of a patient to participate in postoperative tendon rehabilitation must be considered.

With extensive segmental muscle or tendon loss, anatomic reconstruction of the muscle-tendon unit simply may not be possible. In this situation, tendon transfers, tenodesis, and/or arthrodesis may be indicated. For example, if the long extensors of the wrist and hand are severely injured, tendon transfers typically used for radial nerve palsy can be considered.[65] However, satisfactory motor units may not be available for transfer. In this situation, the tenodesis effect may be employed, in which a joint is moved by the action of a motor unit on an adjacent joint. For example, if active wrist motion is preserved but active metacarpophalangeal joint extension is lost, the residual extensor digitorum comminus tendons may be surgically tethered proximal to the wrist, which would result in metacarpophalangeal joint extension when the wrist is actively flexed.[66,67] Wrist arthrodesis may be considered in certain cases where insufficient motor control of the wrist is present to use the tenodesis effect. This may free up any available wrist motors for transfer to the digits, but at the obvious cost of wrist motion.

Outcomes

Amputation Versus Limb Salvage

The dilemma of early amputation versus limb salvage involves multiple factors that can be extremely difficult to weigh, measure, and compare. Ultimately, the most prudent strategy requires careful reconciliation of expectation and feasibility. The reconstructive plan must be based on reasonable and achievable goals mutually derived by the surgical team and the patient. It must always be stressed that the reconstructive process does not end with the mere healing of a wound. Indeed, the surgeon must counsel the patient that wound healing is but one small component of the reconstruction process. Multiple procedures may be required before the patient reaches maximum function.

Despite all modern advances in design and materials, the prehensile function of the human hand is only marginally replicated by current prosthetic technology. For this reason, a "bad hand" may be more functional than the best prosthesis. However, late amputation after a prolonged effort at salvage, compared to early amputation, exacts a measurable financial cost to the health care system and an immeasurable personal cost to the patient. Simply, a patient may have been better off in the end with an early amputation. Unfortunately, there is no "crystal ball" for the surgeon or the patient to see the future and to know whether limb salvage or limb amputa-

tion would be the best option. Valid outcome predictors for severe trauma to the upper extremity have not been fully elucidated and are of limited value to the surgeon in counseling the individual patient on the decision for amputation versus limb salvage.[68] Furthermore, severity scores for the severely injured upper extremity are based on civilian trauma and may not be valid when applied to modern-day combat wounds.[69]

Therapy

An ever-present menace in hand surgery is the decided tendency for the hand to stiffen and to stiffen in the position of nonfunction.
—Sterling Bunnell

Therapy is one of the most important determinants of final outcomes in civilian mangled upper extremity injuries.[70] As the propensity for poor function due to scarring is proportionate to the amount of energy absorbed by the tissues, these observations apply with particular poignancy to injuries resulting from modern warfare. Due to systemic injury involving more than just limbs, wounded combatants are frequently subjected to prolonged periods of sedation and intensive care, resulting in the delay and detraction of therapy. Furthermore, multiple extremities are commonly involved, which can result in the dilution of attention being given to each injury.

While the therapist's role alone is critical, a close relationship among the patient, the therapist, and the reconstructive surgeon promotes success. The inflammation and propensity for scarring that accompanies severe injury can make casualties of adjacent and even noncontiguous tissues. In the early phases of rehabilitation of combat casualty wounds, the therapist attempts to minimize edema and prevent the stiffness and fibrosis of the upper extremity by performing passive range of motion of all noninjured joints. Active range of motion supplements this passive range of motion when possible. In this period, the surgical team assists the therapist by performing atraumatic passive range of motion of all uninjured upper extremity joints during episodes of anesthesia. Specialized custom splints are often created to facilitate immobilization in the most favorable position, depending upon the specific injury. As the patient progresses through the acute phase, therapy takes on an increasing role. Patients meet with their therapist often twice daily and engage in both active and passive motion protocols. In addition, custom dynamic splints are often created to facilitate rest in the position of function as well as to promote early tendon gliding and joint range of motion.

Complications

SCAR TISSUE

The formation of granulation tissue is the natural response of an open wound and is fundamental to the healing process in many ways. Granulation tissue is vascular and thus promotes healing and control of infection. It contracts, making a wound smaller. It proliferates in wounds and thus surrounds and protects exposed vital structures. The appearance of granulation tissue signals that a wound is no longer devolving and is capable of healing. On the local level, it signals that debridement has been sufficient to remove nonviable tissue and that infection is not present. On the systemic level, it signals that the patient's nutrition and physiology are at least minimally adequate.

Yet, the destiny of granulation tissue is to mature into bland cicatrix. Scar tissue simply cannot replace the highly specific function of specialized tissue such as bone, cartilage, ligament, tendon, muscle, nerve, or skin. Furthermore, scar adheres, binding together structures that are designed to excurse. The reconstructive surgeon cannot altogether avoid the formation of scar tissue, but its tendency to form and its ultimate impact can be minimized through adequate debridement, early definitive wound closure or coverage, appropriate staging of multiple reconstructive surgeries, and early aggressive rehabilitative therapy. We routinely debride some or all granulation tissue from a wound bed at the time of definitive wound closure.

PAIN MANAGEMENT

Pain management is a key element in complex reconstruction of the upper extremity that traditionally has been underemphasized. Until recently, pain has been seen merely as a symptom of the inciting disease process or trauma that, while unfortunate, had little to no impact on a patient's ultimate recovery. However, current evidence suggests that insufficient perioperative pain management may delay a patient's recovery and result in increased morbidity.[71] Evidence also indicates that inadequately treated perioperative pain can lead to chronic pain conditions.[72-74] More recently, early administration of morphine following traumatic injury was correlated with a reduction in the incidence of post-traumatic stress disorder, which suggests inadequate pain management has both physiologic and psychologic sequelae.[75]

In addition to the long-term morbidity associated with poorly managed pain, the surgeon must also recognize the broader, immediate negative impact of pain on patient recovery. Acute pain is associated with a variety of endocrine, metabolic, and inflammatory responses that adversely impact the patient's recuperation following acute trauma or surgery. Poorly managed pain, either during operative procedures or in the immediate postoperative period, leads to autonomic hyperactivity and a catecholamine surge that results in increased heart rate, blood pressure, peripheral vascular resistance, and myocardial oxygen consumption.[76] Pain often limits patient mobility and promotes muscle atrophy, thereby impeding rehabilitation efforts of the injured extremity. Immune function has also been shown to be adversely impacted by pain, which can be particularly undesirable in wounds prone to infection, such as open fractures and other contaminated traumatic wounds.[77] An effective pain management strategy must be an integral component to any rehabilitation plan.

Since the German pharmacist Friedrick Serturner isolated the substance from opium in 1805, morphine has been the gold-standard analgesic following acute trauma and surgery.[78] Indeed, the pre-eminence and success of opioid medications in the management of traumatic and surgical pain is indisputable. However, exclusive use of opioids for pain management is associated with significant side effects that are undesirable, if not deadly.[79] For example, there is growing evidence that opioids are immunosuppressive and may be dangerous in immunocompromised populations.[80]

As with all aspects of health care delivery, the management of pain exposes the patient to risk. These risks can be significantly mitigated when an organized acute pain medicine service is included as a component of a patient's reconstruction and rehabilitation milieu. An acute pain medicine service consists of physicians (usually anesthesiologists) and nurses specifically trained in the management of traumatic and surgical pain for a period that extends well beyond a patient's traumatic episode and/or surgical procedure(s). These providers should be integral members of the patient's rehabilitative team and should evaluate and treat patients on a daily basis from a pain perspective. An acute pain medicine service can provide the added benefit of being another physician-led team that can alert the surgeon of any difficulties or issues with their patients.

Acute pain medicine specialists are also knowledgeable in advanced regional anesthesia techniques, to include the continuous peripheral nerve block. First described by Halsted in 1884 when he used cocaine to anesthetize exposed roots of the brachial plexus, regional blocks using various local anesthetics have become increasingly used in upper extremity surgery.[81] Improvements in nerve localization with peripheral nerve stimulation and, more recently, ultrasound technology have revolutionized the practice of regional anesthesia by enabling the rapid and predictable placement of continuous infusion catheters adjacent to proximal extremity nerves.[82,83] Continuous peripheral nerve block has the added advantage of providing limb-specific analgesia. Redosing the indwelling catheter with local anesthetic is simple, thereby increasing the level of analgesia during dressing changes, therapy sessions, or repeat operations over days to weeks.[84] The safety of continuous peripheral nerve block in trauma patients has been confirmed in a variety of clinical situations, and these catheter infusions are being employed with some frequency in wounded warriors from the present conflicts in Iraq and Afghanistan.[85-87]

Multimodal analgesia refers to the concept of using multiple analgesics with different mechanisms of action that act synergistically to result in improved overall pain control while attempting to minimize the unwanted side effects of each individual medication by using less of each.[88]As part of a multimodal analgesic plan that includes systemic nonopioid pain medications (such as acetaminophen, nonsteroidal anti-inflammatory drugs, antidepressants, membrane stabilizers, and ketamine, among others) and regional anesthesia, opioid medications can be relegated to a secondary or even a tertiary pain management role.

In conclusion, we believe that the most efficient and effective method of managing acute traumatic and surgical pain is through the incorporation of an acute pain medicine service into the broader reconstruction and rehabilitation team. The adoption of the pain management principles outlined here will contribute to improved outcomes of patients undergoing complex reconstruction of the upper extremity.

References

1. Owens BD, Kragh JF Jr, Macaitis J, Svoboda SJ, Wenke JC. Characterization of extremity wounds in Operation Iraqi Freedom and Operation Enduring Freedom. *J Orthop Trauma.* 2007;21(4):254-257.
2. Owens BD, Kragh JF Jr, Wenke JC, Macaitis J, Wade CE, Holcomb JB. Combat wounds in Operation Iraqi Freedom and Operation Enduring Freedom. *J Trauma.* 2008;64(2): 295-299.
3. Fang R, Pruitt VM, Dorlac GR, et al. Critical care at Landstuhl Regional Medical Center. *Crit Care Med.* 2008;36(7 Suppl): S383-S387.
4. McCarthy MS, Fabling J, Martindale R, Meyer SA. Nutrition support of the traumatically injured warfighter. *Crit Care Nurs Clin North Am.* 2008;20(1):59-65, vi-vii.
5. Golant A, Nord RM, Paksima N, Posner MA. Cold exposure injuries to the extremities. *J Am Acad Orthop Surg.* 2008;16(12):704-715.
6. O'Mara MS, Goel A, Recio P, et al. The use of tourniquets in the excision of unexsanguinated extremity burn wounds. *Burns.* 2002;28(7):684-687.
7. Smoot EC. Modified use of extremity tourniquets for burn wound debridement. *J Burn Care Rehabil.* 1996;17(4):334-337.
8. Owens BD, White DW, Wenke JC. Comparison of irrigation solutions and devices in a contaminated musculoskeletal wound survival model. *J Bone Joint Surg Am.* 2009;91(1):92-98.
9. Geiger S, McCormick F, Chou R, Wandel AG. War wounds: lessons learned from Operation Iraqi Freedom. *Plast Reconstr Surg.* 2008;122(1):146-153.
10. Greene AK, Puder M, Roy R, et al. Microdeformational wound therapy: effects on angiogenesis and matrix metalloproteinases in chronic wounds of 3 debilitated patients. *Ann Plast Surg.* 2006;56(4):418-422.
11. Moues CM, Vos MC, van den Bemd GJ, Stijnen T, Hovius SE. Bacterial load in relation to vacuum-assisted closure wound therapy: a prospective randomized trial. *Wound Repair Regen.* 2004;12(1):11-17.
12. Weed T, Ratliff C, Drake DB. Quantifying bacterial bioburden during negative pressure wound therapy: does the wound VAC enhance bacterial clearance? *Ann Plast Surg.* 2004;52(3):276-279; discussion 279-280.
13. Zalavras CG, Patzakis MJ. Open fractures: evaluation and management. *J Am Acad Orthop Surg.* 2003;11(3):212-219.
14. Worlock P, Slack R, Harvey L, Mawhinney R. The prevention of infection in open fractures: an experimental study of the effect of fracture stability. *Injury.* 1994;25(1):31-38.
15. Jacob E, Erpelding JM, Murphy KP. A retrospective analysis of open fractures sustained by U.S. military personnel during Operation Just Cause. *Mil Med.* 1992;157(10):552-556.
16. Brundage SI, McGhan R, Jurkovich GJ, Mack CD, Maier RV. Timing of femur fracture fixation: effect on outcome in patients with thoracic and head injuries. *J Trauma.* 2002;52(2):299-307.
17. Pape HC, Hildebrand F, Pertschy S, et al. Changes in the management of femoral shaft fractures in polytrauma patients: from early total care to damage control orthopedic surgery. *J Trauma.* 2002;53(3):452-461; discussion 461-462.
18. Clement H, Pichler W, Tesch NP, Heidari N, Grechenig W. Anatomical basis of the risk of radial nerve injury related to the technique of external fixation applied to the distal humerus. *Surg Radiol Anat.* 2010;32(3):221-224.
19. Emami A, Mjoberg B. A safer pin position for external fixation of distal radial fractures. *Injury.* 2000;31(9):749-750.
20. Seitz WH Jr, Froimson AI, Leb RB. Reduction of treatment-related complications in the external fixation of complex distal radius fractures. *Orthop Rev.* 1991;20(2):169-177.
21. Wikenheiser MA, Markel MD, Lewallen DG, Chao EY. Thermal response and torque resistance of five cortical half-pins under simulated insertion technique. *J Orthop Res.* 1995;13(4):615-619.
22. Seitz WH Jr, Froimson AI, Brooks DB, Postak P, Polando G, Greenwald AS. External fixator pin insertion techniques: biomechanical analysis and clinical relevance. *J Hand Surg Am.* 1991;16(3):560-563.
23. Saithna A. The influence of hydroxyapatite coating of external fixator pins on pin loosening and pin track infection: a systematic review. *Injury.* 2010;41(2):128-132.
24. Moroni A, Cadossi M, Romagnoli M, Faldini C, Giannini S. A biomechanical and histological analysis of standard versus hydroxyapatite-coated pins for external fixation. *J Biomed Mater Res B Appl Biomater.* 2008;86B(2):417-421.
25. Moroni A, Pegreffi F, Cadossi M, Hoang-Kim A, Lio V, Giannini S. Hydroxyapatite-coated external fixation pins. *Expert Rev Med Devices.* 2005;2(4):465-471.
26. Acarturk TO, Ashok K, Lee WP. The use of external skeletal fixation to facilitate the surgical release of wrist flexion and thumb web space contractures. *J Hand Surg Am.* 2006;31(10):1619-1625.
27. Dailiana Z, Agorastakis D, Varitimidis S, Bargiotas K, Roidis N, Malizos KN. Use of a mini-external fixator for the treatment of hand fractures. *J Hand Surg Am.* 2009;34(4):630-636.

Complex Reconstructive Challenges in Hand and Forearm Wounds 179

28. Pennig D, Gausepohl T, Mader K, Wulke A. The use of minimally invasive fixation in fractures of the hand—the minifixator concept. *Injury.* 2000;31(Suppl):1102-1112.

29. Ugwonali OF, Jupiter JB. Mini external fixation in the hand. *Tech Hand Up Extrem Surg.* 2006;10(3):187-196.

30. Drenth DJ, Klasen HJ. External fixation for phalangeal and metacarpal fractures. *J Bone Joint Surg Br.* 1998;80(2):227-230.

31. Godina M. Early microsurgical reconstruction of complex trauma of the extremities. *Plast Reconstr Surg.* 1986;78(3):285-292.

32. Kumar AR, Grewal NS, Chung TL, Bradley JP. Lessons from the modern battlefield: successful upper extremity injury reconstruction in the subacute period. *J Trauma.* 2009;67(4):752-757.

33. Kumar AR, Grewal NS, Chung TL, Bradley JP. Lessons from operation Iraqi freedom: successful subacute reconstruction of complex lower extremity battle injuries. *Plast Reconstr Surg.* 2009;123(1):218-229.

34. Steiert AE, Gohritz A, Schreiber TC, Krettek C, Vogt PM. Delayed flap coverage of open extremity fractures after previous vacuum-assisted closure (VAC) therapy—worse or worth? *J Plast Reconstr Aesthet Surg.* 2009;62(5):675-683.

35. Helgeson MD, Potter BK, Evans KN, Shawen SB. Bioartificial dermal substitute: a preliminary report on its use for the management of complex combat-related soft tissue wounds. *J Orthop Trauma.* 2007;21(6):394-399.

36. Baechler MF, Groth AT, Nesti LJ, Martin BD. Soft tissue management of war wounds to the foot and ankle. *Foot Ankle Clin.* 2010;15(1):113-138.

37. Jeng JC, Fidler PE, Sokolich JC, et al. Seven years' experience with Integra as a reconstructive tool. *J Burn Care Res.* 2007;28(1):120-126.

38. Smith WR, Ziran BH, Anglen JO, Stahel PF. Locking plates: tips and tricks. *Instr Course Lect.* 2008;57:25-36.

39. Tan SL, Balogh ZJ. Indications and limitations of locked plating. *Injury.* 2009;40(7):683-691.

40. Haidukewych GJ, Ricci W. Locked plating in orthopaedic trauma: a clinical update. *J Am Acad Orthop Surg.* 2008;16(6):347-355.

41. Christensen NO. Kuntscher intramedullary reaming and nail fixation for nonunion of the forearm. *Clin Orthop Relat Res.* 1976;116:215-221.

42. Ozkaya U, Kilic A, Ozdogan U, Beng K, Kabukcuoglu Y. Comparison between locked intramedullary nailing and plate osteosynthesis in the management of adult forearm fractures. *Acta Orthop Traumatol Turc.* 2009;43(1):14-20.

43. Lee YH, Lee SK, Chung MS, Baek GH, Gong HS, Kim KH. Interlocking contoured intramedullary nail fixation for selected diaphyseal fractures of the forearm in adults. *J Bone Joint Surg Am.* 2008;90(9):1891-1898.

44. Visna P, Beitl E, Pilny J, et al. Interlocking nailing of forearm fractures. *Acta Chir Belg.* 2008;108(3):333-338.

45. Hanel DP, Lu TS, Weil WM. Bridge plating of distal radius fractures: the Harborview method. *Clin Orthop Relat Res.* 2006;44:591-599.

46. Nourissat G, Mudgal CS, Ring D. Bridge plating of the wrist for temporary stabilization of concomitant radiocarpal, intercarpal, and carpometacarpal injuries: a report of two cases. *J Orthop Trauma.* 2008;22(5):368-371.

47. Nalbantoglu U, Gereli A, Ucar BY, Kocaoglu B, Dogan T. Treatment of metacarpal fractures with open reduction and low-profile plate and screw fixation. *Acta Orthop Traumatol Turc.* 2008;42(5):303-309.

48. Green SA. Skeletal defects. A comparison of bone grafting and bone transport for segmental skeletal defects. *Clin Orthop Relat Res.* 1994;301:111-117.

49. Woon CY, Chong KW, Wong MK. Induced membranes—a staged technique of bone-grafting for segmental bone loss: a report of two cases and a literature review. *J Bone Joint Surg Am.* 2010;92(1):196-201.

50. Masquelet AC, Begue T. The concept of induced membrane for reconstruction of long bone defects. *Orthop Clin North Am.* 2010;41(1):27-37.

51. Beardmore AA, Brooks DE, Wenke JC, Thomas DB. Effectiveness of local antibiotic delivery with an osteoinductive and osteoconductive bone-graft substitute. *J Bone Joint Surg Am.* 2005;87(1):107-112.

52. Thomas DB, Brooks DE, Bice TG, DeJong ES, Lonergan KT, Wenke JC. Tobramycin-impregnated calcium sulfate prevents infection in contaminated wounds. *Clin Orthop Relat Res.* 2005;441:366-371.

53. Zalavras CG, Patzakis MJ, Holtom P. Local antibiotic therapy in the treatment of open fractures and osteomyelitis. *Clin Orthop Relat Res.* 2004;427:86-93.

54. Pelissier P, Masquelet AC, Bareille R, Pelissier SM, Amedee J. Induced membranes secrete growth factors including vascular and osteoinductive factors and could stimulate bone regeneration. *J Orthop Res.* 2004;22(1):73-79.

55. Adani R, Delcroix L, Innocenti M, et al. Reconstruction of large posttraumatic skeletal defects of the forearm by vascularized free fibular graft. *Microsurgery.* 2004;24(6):423-429.

56. Jupiter JB, Gerhard HJ, Guerrero J, Nunley JA, Levin LS. Treatment of segmental defects of the radius with use of the vascularized osteoseptocutaneous fibular autogenous graft. *J Bone Joint Surg Am.* 1997;79(4):542-550.

57. Strauch B, Yu H-L. *Atlas of Microvascular Surgery: Anatomy and Operative Approaches.* New York, NY: Thieme; 2006.

58. Sakai K, Doi K, Kawai S. Free vascularized thin corticoperiosteal graft. *Plast Reconstr Surg.* 1991;87(2):290-298.

59. Yamamoto H, Jones DB, Moran SL, Bishop AT, Shin AY. The arterial anatomy of the medial femoral condyle and its clinical implications. *J Hand Surg Eur.* 2010;35(7):569-574.

60. Del Pinal F, Garcia-Bernal FJ, Regalado J, Ayala H, Cagigal L, Studer A. Vascularised corticoperiosteal grafts from the medial femoral condyle for difficult non-unions of the upper limb. *J Hand Surg Eur Vol.* 2007;32(2):135-142.

61. Jones DB Jr, Burger H, Bishop AT, Shin AY. Treatment of scaphoid waist nonunions with an avascular proximal pole and carpal collapse. A comparison of two vascularized bone grafts. *J Bone Joint Surg Am.* 2008;90(12):2616-2625.

62. Jones DB Jr, Moran SL, Bishop AT, Shin AY. Free-vascularized medial femoral condyle bone transfer in the treatment of scaphoid nonunions. *Plast Reconstr Surg.* 2010;125(4):1176-1184.

63. Allende C, Allende BT. Posttraumatic one-bone forearm reconstruction. A report of seven cases. *J Bone Joint Surg Am.* 2004;86-A(2):364-369.

64. Bruner JM. Use of single iliac-bone graft to replace multiple metacarpal loss in dorsal injuries of the hand. *J Bone Joint Surg Am.* 1957;39-A(1):43-52.

65. Ropars M, Dreano T, Siret P, Belot N, Langlais F. Long-term results of tendon transfers in radial and posterior interosseous nerve paralysis. *J Hand Surg Br.* 2006;31(5):502-506.

66. Goubier JN, Teboul F. Management of hand palsies in isolated C7 to T1 or C8, T1 root avulsions. *Tech Hand Up Extrem Surg.* 2008;12(3):156-160.

67. Revol MP, Servant JM. Classification of the main tenodesis techniques used in hand surgery. *Plast Reconstr Surg.* 1987;79(2):237-242.

68. Saxena P, Cutler L, Feldberg L. Assessment of the severity of hand injuries using "hand injury severity score," and its correlation with the functional outcome. *Injury.* 2004;35(5):511-516.

69. Brown KV, Ramasamy A, McLeod J, Stapley S, Clasper JC. Predicting the need for early amputation in ballistic mangled extremity injuries. *J Trauma.* 2009;66(4 Suppl):S93-S97; discussion S97-S98.

70. Gupta A, Shatford RA, Wolff TW, Tsai TM, Scheker LR, Levin LS. Treatment of the severely injured upper extremity. *Instr Course Lect.* 2000;49:377-396.

71. Joshi GP, Ogunnaike BO. Consequences of inadequate post-operative pain relief and chronic persistent postoperative pain. *Anesthesiol Clin North America*. 2005;23(1):21-36.

72. Katz J, Jackson M, Kavanagh BP, Sandler AN. Acute pain after thoracic surgery predicts long-term post-thoracotomy pain. *Clin J Pain*. 1996;12(1):50-55.

73. Perkins FM, Kehlet H. Chronic pain as an outcome of surgery. A review of predictive factors. *Anesthesiology*. 2000;93(4):1123-1133.

74. Kehlet H, Jensen TS, Woolf CJ. Persistent postsurgical pain: risk factors and prevention. *Lancet*. 2006;367(9522):1618-1625.

75. O'Donnell ML, Creamer M, Holmes AC, et al. Posttraumatic stress disorder after injury: does admission to intensive care unit increase risk? *J Trauma*. 2010;69(3):627-632.

76. Liu SS, Block BM, Wu CL. Effects of perioperative central neuraxial analgesia on outcome after coronary artery bypass surgery: a meta-analysis. *Anesthesiology*. 2004;101(1):153-161.

77. Starkweather AR, Witek-Janusek L, Nockels RP, Peterson J, Mathews HL. Immune function, pain, and psychological stress in patients undergoing spinal surgery. *Spine (Phila Pa 1976)*. 2006;31(18):E641-E647.

78. Hamilton GR, Baskett TF. In the arms of Morpheus the development of morphine for postoperative pain relief. *Can J Anaesth*. 2000;47(4):367-374.

79. Taylor S, Voytovich AE, Kozol RA. Has the pendulum swung too far in postoperative pain control? *Am J Surg*. 2003;186(5):472-475.

80. Sacerdote P. Opioid-induced immunosuppression. *Curr Opin Support Palliat Care*. 2008;2(1):14-18.

81. Winnie AP. *Plexus Anesthesia*. Vol 1. Philadelphia, PA: WB Saunders; 1993:42-45.

82. Franco CD, Vieira ZE. 1,001 subclavian perivascular brachial plexus blocks: success with a nerve stimulator. *Reg Anesth Pain Med*. 2000;25(1):41-46.

83. Ootaki C, Hayashi H, Amano M. Ultrasound-guided infraclavicular brachial plexus block: an alternative technique to anatomical landmark-guided approaches. *Reg Anesth Pain Med*. 2000;25(6):600-604.

84. Stojadinovic A, Auton A, Peoples GE, et al. Responding to challenges in modern combat casualty care: innovative use of advanced regional anesthesia. *Pain Med*. 2006;7(4):330-338.

85. Buckenmaier CC 3rd, Rupprecht C, McKnight G, et al. Pain following battlefield injury and evacuation: a survey of 110 casualties from the wars in Iraq and Afghanistan. *Pain Med*. 2009;10(8):1487-1496.

86. Buckenmaier CC 3rd, Croll SM, Shields CH, et al. Advanced regional anesthesia morbidity and mortality grading system: regional anesthesia outcomes reporting (ROAR). *Pain Med*. 2009;10(6):1115-1122.

87. Buckenmaier CC 3rd, Shields CH, Auton AA, et al. Continuous peripheral nerve block in combat casualties receiving low-molecular weight heparin. *Br J Anaesth*. 2006;97(6):874-877.

88. Jin F, Chung F. Multimodal analgesia for postoperative pain control. *J Clin Anesth*. 2001;13(7):524-539.

Chapter

20

COMPLEX ELBOW AND SHOULDER INJURIES

Capt Robert McGill, MD and Col Damian Rispoli, MD

Devastating injuries about the elbow and shoulder are significant problems that confront the deployed orthopedic surgeon. In war injury registries from these latest conflicts, injuries involving the upper extremities account for 20% to 54.7% of combat injuries.[1-3] The deployed orthopedic surgeon, therefore, has a high likelihood of encountering complex elbow and shoulder trauma. A solid understanding of anatomy and biomechanics coupled with knowledge of the techniques of debridement and temporary and definitive fixation are necessary for optimal patient outcomes. The ongoing conflicts in Operation Iraqi Freedom/Operation Enduring Freedom (OIF/OEF) can provide valuable lessons for future management of these complex injuries.

Elbow

To understand and effectively treat complex elbow injuries, an understanding of normal elbow anatomy and biomechanics is paramount. The elbow articulation consists of 3 bony structures—the distal humerus, the proximal radius, and proximal ulna. The humerus has 2 distinct articular surfaces. The trochlea is a bilobed hyperbolic surface covered with articular cartilage through an arc of about 300 degrees, with the medial structure larger and more distal than the lateral.[4] The trochlea articulates with the radial notch of the proximal ulna. The capitellar portion of the distal humerus is a spheroidal surface covered in articular cartilage. The aptly named trochleocapitellar groove separates the trochlea and capitella, and the rim of the

radial head articulates with this groove throughout the arc of motion.

The orientation of the distal humerus dictates the position of the hand in space and the ability of the individual to fully manipulate his or her environment. In the lateral plane, the articular surface is flexed roughly 30 degrees in respect to the long axis of the humerus. Axially, the distal humerus is internally rotated about 6 degrees with respect to a line bisecting the midpoint of the epicondyles. Lastly, in the anterior-posterior plane, the articular portion of the distal humerus assumes an approximate 6 to 8 degrees valgus tilt.[4] The articular surface itself is supported similar to an arch between the medial and lateral columns. The central clearing between the columns and proximal to the articular surface allows for a full, unimpeded range of motion.

The congruity of the ulnohumeral and radiocapitellar articulations provides the osseous contribution to elbow stability. The proximal ulna articular portion consists of a greater sigmoid surface, terminating anteriorly in the coronoid process and posteriorly in the olecranon, and a lesser sigmoid notch that articulates with the radial head. The lesser notch sits lateral to the coronoid and proximal to the ulnohumeral articular surface.

The radial head is ellipsoid with roughly 240 degrees of articular cartilage that comes in contact with the ulna. There is a "safe zone" of about 110 degrees that is nonarticular and therefore amenable for open reduction/internal fixation (ORIF).[5] With the forearm in neutral rotation, the safe zone extends 65 degrees anterior and 45 degrees posterior to a line directly lateral on the radial head (Figure 20-1).

Owens BD, Belmont PJ Jr, eds. *Combat Orthopedic Surgery: Lessons Learned in Iraq and Afghanistan* (pp 181-190)
© 2011 SLACK Incorporated

Figure 20-1. Nonarticulating portion of the radial head. The 110-degree nonarticulating portion of the radial head is centered straight laterally with the hand in 10 degrees of supination.

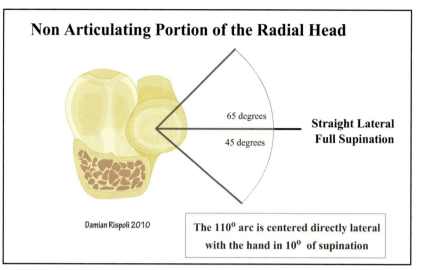

Non Articulating Portion of the Radial Head

65 degrees

45 degrees

Straight Lateral
Full Supination

Damian Rispoli 2010

The 110° arc is centered directly lateral with the hand in 10° of supination

In addition to the bony articulations, ligamentous restraints are key to the biomechanical stability of the elbow joint. Thickenings in the medial and lateral capsule comprise the collateral ligaments. The medial collateral ligament complex consists of anterior, posterior, and transverse components. The anterior component, which arises from the antero-inferior surface of the medial epicondyle and inserts near the coronoid at the sublime tubercle, is the most important portion of the medial collateral ligament complex with regard to valgus stability. At 90 degrees of flexion, the anterior bundle of the medial collateral ligament provides roughly 54% of valgus stability. Incidentally, due to its insertional proximity to the coronoid, valgus stability can be significantly impacted by even a minimally displaced coronoid fracture.[6] The anterior band can be divided even further into an anterior subportion and posterior subportion. The anterior subportion is a primary valgus restraint in angles of flexion of 90 degrees and less, while the posterior subportion is a co-primary valgus restraint (with the anterior subportion) at 120 degrees of flexion.[7]

The lateral collateral ligament complex consists of several, less well-defined components. Generally, the complex forms a "Y" shape, made up of the radial collateral ligament, the lateral ulnar collateral ligament, the annular ligament, and a variable accessory lateral collateral ligament. Of these, the lateral ulnar collateral ligament, which originates on the lateral epicondyle and inserts on the crista supinatoris, is the primary lateral stabilizer to varus stress.[4]

The combination of bony and ligamentous elbow constraints can be further divided into primary and secondary static constraints, with muscle forces acting as dynamic protection to all constraints. O'Driscoll and colleagues showed that the stabilizers can be likened to fortress defenses—primary stabilizers forming the outer wall and secondary static stabilizers

constituting the inner wall (Figure 20-2).[8] The primary static constraints to elbow instability are the lateral ulnar collateral ligament, ulnohumeral articulation, and the anterior band of the medial collateral ligament; the secondary constraints are the radial head, common flexor-pronator tendon, and common extensor tendon.

In addition to fractures through the bony components of the elbow, the articular surfaces can be damaged by dislocation without bony injury. This can result in either posterolateral rotatory instability (more common) or posteromedial instability and can greatly compromise function and lead to early joint degeneration. Emiko Hori developed the concept of progressive soft tissue damage about the elbow during subluxation and dislocation by a posterolateral rotatory mechanism; the "Circle of Hori" posits that soft tissue injury about the elbow progresses in 3 stages with the final stage leading to dislocation.[9] In the first stage, the lateral ulnar collateral ligament is disrupted. In the second stage, other anterior and posterior structures of the capsule are ruptured, but the medial collateral ligament complex is spared. In the final stage, the medial collateral ligament complex is disrupted either partially (only involving the posterior band) or completely (both the anterior and posterior). The resulting dislocation can be deceivingly unstable, with continued subluxation and even dislocation events after a careful reduction has been performed (Figure 20-3).

Complex war injuries to the elbow pose some unique challenges that are not necessarily present in civilian centers. The injuries show increased energy delivered to tissues. Explosive devices such as improvised explosive devices (IEDs) and high-energy projectile weapons (M-16, AK-47) impart significant energy to the soft tissues and bone. In addition, explosive device injuries are highly variable, especially

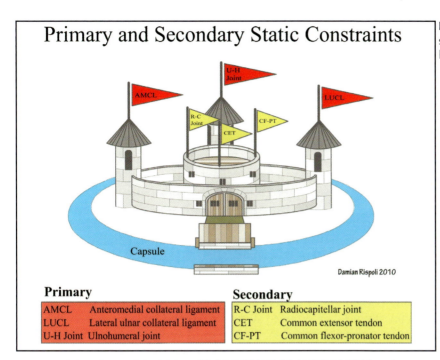

Figure 20-2. The primary and secondary static stabilizers of the elbow are shown likened to fortress defenses.

Primary and Secondary Static Constraints

Damian Rispoli 2010

Primary

AMCL	Anteromedial collateral ligament
LUCL	Lateral ulnar collateral ligament
U-H Joint	Ulnohumeral joint

Secondary

R-C Joint	Radiocapitellar joint
CET	Common extensor tendon
CF-PT	Common flexor-pronator tendon

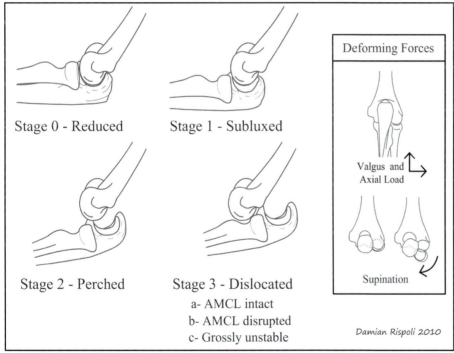

Stage 0 - Reduced

Stage 1 - Subluxed

Stage 2 - Perched

Stage 3 - Dislocated
   a- AMCL intact
   b- AMCL disrupted
   c- Grossly unstable

Deforming Forces

Valgus and Axial Load

Supination

Damian Rispoli 2010

Figure 20-3. Posterolateral rotatory mechanism of elbow dislocation. The 3 stages of posterolateral rotatory elbow instability follow the "Circle of Hori." The sentinel structure that is injured is the lateral ulnar collateral ligament, followed by the anterior and posterior capsules, and lastly by the failure of the anteromedial collateral ligament.

about the elbow, with varying degrees of soft tissue and bony loss. Explosive devices, especially, have wounding patterns that vary due to the composition of shrapnel. In recent modern combat, roughly 70% to 80% of extremity injury is due to explosive devices,[10] and roughly a quarter of injuries were associated with an injury to a major nerve or vessel. The body armor worn by US Forces protects the vital core, but the extremities remain at risk.

The surgical goals in complex combat elbow injuries are 3-fold. First, the soft tissues must be managed to allow for soft tissue coverage. Second, the repair or reconstruction must be useful. And, last, it must be durable. Lack of adherence to any of these basic goals will likely lead to poor results for the patient and frustration for the treating surgeon. To achieve these goals, a staged surgical plan is needed. In theater, the combat surgical team should provide stability for transport, adequate debridement, and pre-emptive actions to prevent tissue compromise during the evacuation chain. The actions may range from prophylactic fasciotomy, provisional fixation (external or internal), or delay in evacuation until a stable soft tissue envelope is achieved and the benefits of evacuation outweigh the risks. Literature clearly defining the timing of these actions or their efficacy does not currently exist.

Expeditious damage control surgery to control hemorrhage and limit contamination is the first step in management of a mangled elbow. The key at this stage is an adequate debridement. An adequate debridement includes removal of all necrotic and nonrecoverable tissue. Experience offers the only true guidance in this area, as contemporary concepts of color, capacity to bleed, and contractility as measures of muscular tissue viability have never been experimentally proven. Severely contused and ecchymotic muscle has the capacity to recover or worsen, probably as a function of blast or spallation energy imparted. The only true imperative is to save as much bone and soft tissue as possible without compromising patient survival. At the initial surgery, the surgeon should continually look toward the future by making choices that will help in re-explorations and the definitive repair. Irrigation is important with adequate debridement. A high volume (at least 6 L) of pulse lavaged normal saline has been shown to significantly reduce bacterial load in a wound model.[11] A trend has been observed toward the avoidance of pulsatile lavage as studies have noted translocation of bacteria deeper into the tissues[11] and surgeons anecdotally noted less soft tissue damage with low-pressure lavage. Digital massage of the tissue may be of benefit to dislodge more foreign matter, although this technique is not experimentally proven.

The surgical exposure needs to be adequate, and the 3-dimensional anatomy needs to be delineated. Unlike civilian projectile injuries, war-time injuries have an increased incidence of neurovascular injury. While adequate exposure and debridement are paramount, one should never forget that additional surgical trauma within tissue planes further compromises blood supply—an example of which is the vascular supply that pierces the fascia to supply the subcutaneous tissues and the skin. Structures that may be normally sacrificed in elective surgery can be the difference between being able to cover a wound with local tissue or the need for regional flaps or free tissue transfer. Long-bone injuries of the humerus, ulna, and radius should be stabilized, and length should be restored to the extent possible using internal fixation, external fixation, or any combination thereof. External fixation is normally placed from the lateral humerus to the ulna. Ulnar pins can be placed percutaneously. Humeral pins are best placed with direct visualization of the distal humeral shaft to ensure the radial nerve is protected. Initial reticence to use internal fixation has not been borne out by the current conflicts.[12] Selective revascularization should be performed in concert with a vascular-capable surgeon as indicated by the pre- and intraoperative presentation. The wound should be closed as soon as it is clean and stable. If wound closure is not possible at the initial surgical intervention, then management with dry dressing or negative pressure wound therapy should be considered. Regardless of the method of temporary wound coverage, care should be taken to manage the soft tissue with an eye to ultimately cover the deep tissues with a durable surface. Some level of traction to the skin will aid ultimately in coverage—especially in the upper extremity. If deep drainage is necessary, the drains can be brought through the negative pressure wound therapy sponge, and both the sponge and drain will be under suction (Figure 20-4).

The second stage of the surgical plan is outside of the operating room, where rewarming, resuscitation, and correction of coagulation can take place. This is an effort to avoid the "second hit" of a surgery in rapid succession.[13,14] The third and final stage is surgical re-exploration and definitive repair.

In the second "surgical look," it is important to again reassess the debridement. If the wound bed is clean and appropriate, the repair or reconstructive process can begin. Articular surfaces of the humerus, ulna, and radius can be reconstructed, and simple nerve injuries can be addressed. The chance of primary nerve repair success is low; however, it may make the later repair easier. Continued progression to final closure should be sought and plans for flap coverage of skin grafting made. With regard to skin closure, the soft tissue envelope of the upper extremity is usually fairly forgiving, and large defects in a quiescent wound may be primarily closed. Every attempt should be made to get muscular coverage over articular, neurovascular, and bony structures. Muscle, tendons with paratenon, fascia, and fat are amenable to split-thickness skin grafting or closure by secondary intention.

Special attention should be taken when dealing with injured skin tissue. Multiple operative procedures are often needed in these combat injured, and the effectiveness of these procedures is contingent upon a well-managed soft tissue envelope. Appropriate skin closure techniques can include local coverage, rotational flaps/skin, and fascia shifts/tissue expansion techniques such as pie crusting.[15] In the senior author's experience, a "Jacob's ladder" technique over a negative pressure wound therapy sponge provides some level of tension to assist in future skin closure.

A set of reconstructive options is useful for definitive treatment of the war-time mangled elbow. The first option is restoration of the normal bony and ligamentous anatomy. If possible, an elbow ORIF with or without ligament reconstruction would give the patient the best chance for functional limb salvage.

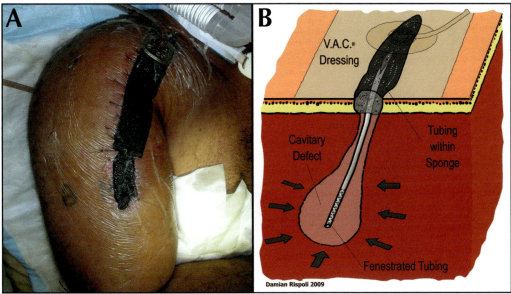

Figure 20-4. Technique of utilization of active suction for deep cavitary wounds. (A) The final negative pressure wound therapy construct. (B) Schematic of the negative pressure wound therapy construct.

A stable stiff elbow tends to be more functional than an unstable elbow, and open and arthroscopic options exist to release the stiff elbow. While restoration of the normal bony anatomy does not prevent all cartilage damage, the failure to restore bony anatomy predisposes the elbow to rapid degeneration, especially in the setting of persistent instability. With loss of osteochondral bone, an attempt should be made to restore ulnohumeral articulation with the use of structural osseous or osteochondral grafts.

Restoration of the articular surface should be the goal of ORIF. Columnar bone loss can be treated by primary shortening. Shortening of up to 2 cm has no effect on triceps strength.[16] We use the elbow in an internally rotated position, placing the ulnar collateral ligament complex in tension and placing compression across the anterior medial coronoid/anterior medial trochlea. Theoretically, restoration of the lateral ulnar collateral ligament and the anteromedial coronoid/trochlea should give the elbow a modicum of stability.

Traditional nonlocked and locked plating can be used to reconstruct bony abnormalities. Buttress plating can be effective along the medial aspect of the olecranon with highly comminuted fractures. Fine-threaded K-wires and headless screws can also be used to obtain solid fixation of articular fragments (Figure 20-5). The bridge plating method is also deserving of special consideration. By effective bridge plating, near-normal length can be achieved even with significant bone loss. Anatomic contouring of plates in and around the elbow can greatly aid restoration of normal architecture. A variety of plate benders can aid in fine tuning the plates to the individual patients. Utilization of a normal contralateral side to prebend the plates has been beneficial. Articulated external fixators can be used to provide stability and protect articular repair.

In the setting of an arthritic joint in a young patient or in a severely damaged articular surface, the next option is resurfacing arthroplasty. This includes interpositional arthroplasty, hemi-arthroplasty (both radiocapitellar and ulnohumeral), and total elbow arthroplasty. Interpositional arthroplasty has been advocated by some for treatment of articular degeneration in the younger, more active patient.[17] Reliable pain relief has been found to be unpredictable. Partial joint replacement can be considered in the elbow that is stable or can be rendered stable. Anecdotally, total elbow arthroplasty can be considered, but early failure will be the norm in active individuals.

The last option available is an elbow arthrodesis, which can be an effective procedure in war-time limb salvage. Reconstruction of bony defects can be obtained by structural bone graft, bone transport, or primary shortening. Traditionally, the optimal position of fusion depends on gender and the patient's occupation. However, with injuries in OIF/OEF, there may be significant bone loss and other factors that contribute to the final position of fusion. If possible, for a dominant arm with good shoulder and wrist range of motion, the fusion should be set at around 90 degrees. At this position, the hand can reach the mouth with compensatory shoulder, wrist, and neck motion.[18,19]

Heterotopic ossification is common in OIF/OEF injuries given the high rate of head injury and burns. Prophylactic treatment in the acute phase is not indicated given the risks associated with current modalities, specifically nonsteroidal anti-inflammatory drugs and radiation therapy.

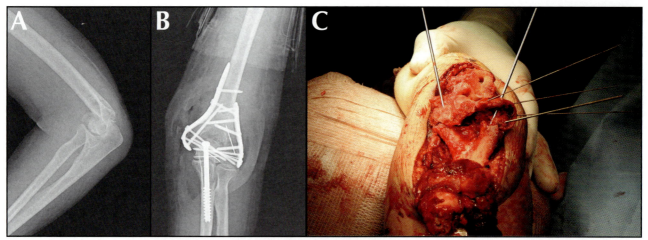

Figure 20-5. Fine-threaded Kirschner wires used to reconstruct a low intra-articular distal humerus fracture. (A) Preoperative radiograph. (B) Postoperative radiograph. (C) Fine-threaded Kirschner wires shown reconstructing the comminuted articular surface and parallel plating. Bone grafting using local bone graft was used to graft the articular defect.

Illustrative Case Examples

BRIDGE PLATING FOR HIGHLY COMMINUTED PROXIMAL ULNA

A 33-year-old male local national sustained a high-velocity gunshot wound to the proximal forearm. There was massive soft tissue injury, and radiographics revealed a severely comminuted proximal ulna fracture with significant bone loss. After physiologic stabilization, the patient was taken to the operating room for irrigation and debridement of the wound and primary bridge plating with a 4.5-mm locking plate (Figure 20-6).

HIGHLY COMMINUTED INTRA-ARTICULAR DISTAL HUMERUS FRACTURE

A 32-year-old male local national was seen immediately after an IED detonated near him. Among other injuries, this patient sustained a massively open, comminuted left elbow fracture. After appropriate resuscitation, the patient was taken to the operating room for management of his elbow injury. The wound was thoroughly debrided of all devitalized tissue and copiously irrigated, and then a spanning elbow external fixator was placed. One additional irrigation and debridement yielded a clean wound, and definitive fixation was performed. An initial screw construct was used to re-approximate the distal humerus intra-articular surface, and a 3.5-mm locking plate was used for ulnar fixation. The external fixator was left on. At the third irrigation and debridement, a more definitive distal humerus fixation was obtained with parallel plating. At this time, the external fixator was removed (Figure 20-7).

Shoulder

As with elbow injuries, the successful treatment of devastating shoulder injuries relies on a solid understanding of the relevant shoulder biomechanics. The bony shoulder consists of the proximal humerus and its articulation with the scapula. The proximal humerus comprises the humeral head, neck, and greater and lesser tuberosities. The humeral head is an ellipsoid surface covered in hyaline cartilage. The neck, or anatomic neck, is the transition zone from cartilage to capsular and tendinous insertions. The lesser tuberosity is the site of insertion for the subscapularis tendon, while the greater tuberosity is the site of insertion of the supraspinatus, infraspinatus, and teres minor tendons.

The morphology of the proximal humerus varies with respect to a person's overall size.[20] In one 3-dimensional study of the proximal humerus, head retroversion, inclination, radius of curvature, thickness, and head-center offset were measured in 30 pairs of proximal humeri. Average medial head center offset was 7 mm (4 to 12 mm) and posterior head center offset was 2 mm (-1 to 8 mm). Average head retroversion was 19 degrees (9 to 31 degrees) and head inclination was 41 degrees (34 to 47 degrees). Average head radius of curvature was 23 mm (17 to 28 mm) and average head cartilage thickness was 19 mm (15 to 24 mm).[20] With such a broad range of values, it is very important to individualize the reconstructive proximal humerus anatomy. Restoring the correct proximal humerus anatomy is very important for reconstituting range of motion, normal biomechanics, and kinematics.

The interturbercular groove, or bicipital groove, is an excellent bony landmark in the proximal humerus. The long head of the biceps tendon

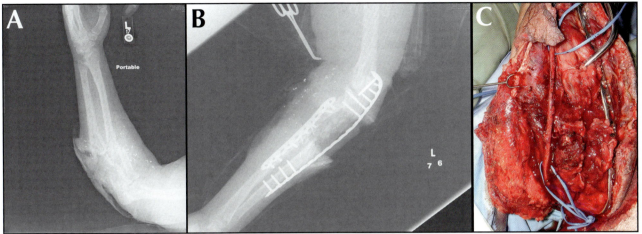

Figure 20-6. (A) Preoperative and (B) postoperative radiographs are shown. (C) Ulnar nerve exploration is shown at the second look irrigation and debridement.

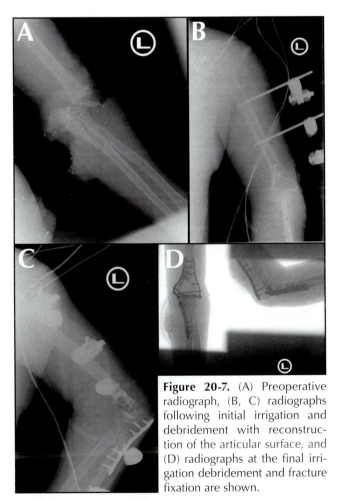

Figure 20-7. (A) Preoperative radiograph, (B, C) radiographs following initial irrigation and debridement with reconstruction of the articular surface, and (D) radiographs at the final irrigation debridement and fracture fixation are shown.

transverses this groove, covered by the variably strong transverse humeral ligament. The groove, too, has variable anatomy. The superior aspect of the interturbercular groove functions as a conduit for the ascending branch of the anterior humeral circumflex artery and arcuate artery, which provides the majority of blood supply for the humeral head.[21-24] Preservation

and/or restoration of this relationship in the complex shoulder injury is felt to be important for preventing humeral head collapse secondary to avascular necrosis. The presence and preservation of medial and posteromedial capsular vessels is also critical to preventing or limiting avascular necrosis.

As with complex war-time elbow trauma, complex shoulder injury should be approached in a logical, stepwise manner. Appropriate life-saving measures should first be applied to a combat casualty; then, attention can be turned to the mangled extremity. As with elbow injuries, a 3-fold scheme of recoverable tissue, useful repair/reconstruction, and durable construct should be followed. Multiple trips to the operating room are often needed to ensure an adequately debrided wound and to prepare for eventual closure. Meticulous tissue handling is paramount due to the devastating nature of infection in the shoulder region.

Unique to complex shoulder injury is the presence of the rotator cuff complex. Often, with high-energy injury, the rotator cuff tendons will be retracted, likely with variably sized fragments of their bony humeral insertions. It is important, if possible, to regain tension on the rotator cuff with temporary fixation. Healing of the tuberosity fragments to the remaining shaft is paramount for adequate shoulder function. This will facilitate improved shoulder mechanics after the definitive procedure. The use of muscular transfers may be beneficial for late reconstruction of deficient rotator cuff musculature, but outcomes generally lag behind that of the native rotator cuff.

The reconstructive options for the shoulder in or after sustaining injury in a war-time environment consist of ORIF, shoulder arthrodesis, replacement, and resection arthroplasty. Unlike elbow injury, there are exceedingly few indications for external fixation about the shoulder. External fixation may be an option to span the glenohumeral joint from the clavicle and/ or scapular spine to the humeral diaphysis. Currently, there are no case reports on the use of this type of fixation for acute trauma, although it has been used for shoulder fusion. The senior author has not found the need to use external fixation of the glenohumeral joint in theater or for late reconstruction.

Anatomic restoration of the glenohumeral articular surface and the restoration of normal anatomic alignment is the ultimate goal of ORIF. Conventional locked plating can be used in concert with articular restoration to reduce even comminuted humeral head fractures to the humeral shaft. Late arthrosis can be treated with resurfacing or replacement arthroplasty, whereas nonunion or loss of the tuberosities is an exceedingly difficult problem to treat.[25-28] Bridge plating is a viable option to bridge diaphyseal or meta-diaphyseal humerus fractures. With a properly contoured plate, the entire length of the humerus can be plated, with long areas of comminution avoided while still maintaining anatomic humeral alignment.

Shoulder arthrodesis is a viable late reconstructive option when managing complex shoulder injury, especially those with concurrent traumatic, complete brachial plexus injury. To ultimately have a good functional outcome, the scapula-stabilizing musculature must be functioning to some extent. Therefore, a contraindication to shoulder arthrodesis is paralysis of the trapezius, levator scapulae, serratus anterior, latissimus dorsi, and rhomboid musculature.[29] There is no true consensus on optimal arthrodesis position; however, any position that will allow the patient to reach his or her mouth, front, and back pockets is generally acceptable. Roughly, these goals can be reached with an arthrodesis of 10 to 15 degrees of forward flexion and abduction and 45 degrees of internal rotation. There are many techniques for glenohumeral arthrodesis. Each method falls into 2 main types (extra-articular and intra-articular) or a combination of both. Generally, a combination of both types will lead to the best eventual results.[30] In OIF/OEF causalties with high-energy injury mechanisms, the remaining humeral head articular surface is decorticated, along with the glenoid surface, and the 2 are positioned to maximize bony contact. The intra-articular surfaces are rigidly fixed, and then the remaining extra-articular surfaces, like the acromion, are brought into contact with the humeral head.

In the face of severe proximal humeral comminution, another option is resection arthroplasty. The nonviable proximal humerus is resected, and the resulting soft tissues are managed until the wounds are able to be closed. The resection arthroplasty is performed with the ultimate goal of proximal humeral hemi-arthroplasty on arrival to a tertiary care facility, either in the United States or Germany.

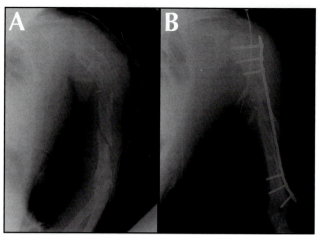

Figure 20-8. (A) Pre- and (B) postoperative radiographs are shown.

Illustrative Case Examples

OPEN REDUCTION/INTERNAL FIXATION HUMERUS WITH BRIDGE PLATING

A 28-year-old male US servicemember was involved in an explosion from a roadside IED, sustaining multiple injuries to include a segmental and comminuted left humerus fracture. The fracture extended into the proximal humeral metaphysis and distally to the distal third of the humerus above the condylar flare. The patient was stabilized from his acute injuries and was able to go to the operating room for definitive fixation at our Echelon III facility. A long bridge plating construct was selected due to the massive proximal comminution and high-energy mechanism. The plate was contoured to rest on the lateral humeral surface. The radial nerve was identified, retracted, and protected at the distal lateral incision allowing for safe plate fixation. Good screw purchase was obtained in the humeral head and again distally in the distal third of the diaphysis and in the distal metaphysis (Figure 20-8).

RESECTION ARTHROPLASTY

A 32-year-old male local national was struck in the right shoulder with a through-and-through high-velocity bullet, causing a massively comminuted proximal humerus and scapula fracture with associated near-complete loss of the humeral head. The patient was stabilized in the field and was brought to our Echelon III facility at Balad Air Base. The patient was taken to the operating room, and the wound was explored. The ruptured long head of the biceps tendon was located in the wound, along with the remaining supraspinatus, infraspinatus, and subscapularis tendons. After

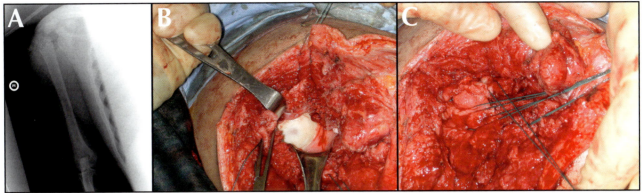

Figure 20-9. (A) Preoperative radiograph. (B) Exposed glenoid articular surface following adequate debridement. Note the volumetric loss of the anterior and lateral deltoid. (C) Rotator cuff tendons being imbricated over the top of the proximal humeral metadiaphysis. (Case performed by the senior author and Greg Osgood, MD.)

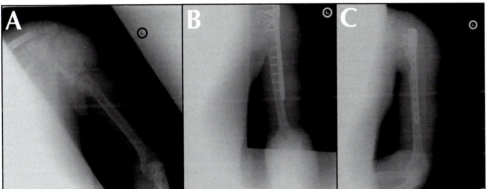

Figure 20-10. (A) Pre- and (B, C) postoperative radiographs shown.

adequate debridement of devitalized tissues and irrigation, the rotator cuff tendons were sutured together over the proximal humeral defect. This was likely the definitive procedure for this patient (Figure 20-9).

INTRA-ARTICULAR PROXIMAL HUMERUS

A 22-year-old male local national sustained a high-velocity gunshot wound to the right shoulder. Imaging revealed a severely comminuted interarticular proximal humerus fracture. The patient was stabilized in our Echelon III trauma room and was taken to the operating room for wound exploration. After determining that the tissues were appropriate for definitive fixation, the fracture was reduced (ensuring accurate positioning of the tuberosities) and a proximal humerus locking plate was used to stabilize the fracture. Ultimately, this patient will likely need a resurfacing procedure, but the results of that procedure will likely be rewarding if the tuberosities heal adequately to the shaft and the wound remains infection free (Figure 20-10).

References

1. Owens BD, Kragh JF Jr, Wenke JC, Macaitis J, Wade CE, Holcomb JB. Combat wounds in Operation Iraqi Freedom and Operation Enduring Freedom. *J Trauma.* 2008;64:295-299.
2. Geiger S. War wounds: lessons learned from Operation Iraqi Freedom. *Plast Reconstr Surg.* 2008;122:146.
3. Dougherty AL, Mohrle CR, Galarneau MR, Woodruff SI, Dye JL, Quinn KH. Battlefield extremity injuries in Operation Iraqi Freedom. *Injury.* 2009;40:772-777.
4. Morrey B, ed. *The Elbow and Its Disorders.* 4th ed. Philadelphia, PA: Saunders Elsevier; 2009.
5. Smith G. Radial head and neck fractures: anatomic guidelines for proper placement of internal fixation. *J Shoulder Elbow Surg.* 1996;5(2 Pt 1):113-117.
6. Sanchez-Sotelo J, O'Driscoll SW, Morrey BF. Medial oblique compression fracture of the coronoid process of the ulna. *J Shoulder Elbow Surg.* 2005;14(1):60-64.
7. Floris S, Olsen BS, Dalstra M, Sojbjerg JO, Sneppen O. The medial collateral ligament of the elbow joint: anatomy and kinematics. *J Shoulder Elbow Surg.* 1998;7(4):345-351.
8. O'Driscoll S, Jupiter JB, King GJW, Hotchkiss RN, Morrey BF. The unstable elbow. *J Bone Joint Surg.* 2000;82A:724.
9. O'Driscoll SW, Morrey BF, Korinek S, An KN. Elbow subluxation and dislocation. A spectrum of instability. *Clin Orthop Relat Res.* 1992;280:186-197.
10. Covey D. Musculoskeletal war wounds during Operation BRAVA in Sri Lanka. *Mil Med.* 2004;169(1):61-64.
11. Svoboda S. Comparison of bulb syringe and pulsed lavage irrigation with use of a bioluminescent musculoskeletal wound model. *J Bone Joint Surg Am.* 2006;88(10):2167-2174.

12. Keeney, et al. Surgical procedures performed at a combat hospital. Poster presentation, SOMOS 2009.
13. Tschoeke S, Hellmuth M, Hostmann A, Ertel W, Oberholzer A. The early second hit in trauma management augments the pro-inflammatory immune response to multiple injuries. *J Trauma.* 2007;62(6):1396-1403.
14. Schroeder J, Weiss YG, Mosheiff R. The current state in the evaluation and treatment of ARDS and SIRS. *Injury.* 2009;40 (Suppl 4):S82-S89.
15. Dunbar RP, Taitsman LA, Sangeorzan BJ, Hansen ST Jr. Technique tip: use of "pie crusting" of the dorsal skin in severe foot injury. *Foot Ankle Int.* 2007;28(7):851-853.
16. Hughes RE, Schneeberger AG, An KN, Morrey BF, O'Driscoll SW. Reduction of triceps muscle force after shortening of the distal humerus: a computational model. *J Shoulder Elbow Surg.* 1997;6(5):444-448.
17. Cheng SL, Morrey BF. Treatment of the mobile, painful, arthritic elbow by distraction interposition arthroplasty. *J Bone Joint Surg Br.* 2000;82(2):233-238.
18. Koch M. Arthrodesis of the elbow. *Clin Orthop Relat Res.* 1967;50.
19. McAuliffe J, Burkhalter WE, Ouellette EA, Carneiro RS. Compression plate arthrodesis of the elbow. *J Bone Joint Surg Br.* 1992;74(2):300-304.
20. Robertson DD, Yuan J, Bigliani LU, Flatow EL, Yamaguchi K. Three dimensional analysis of the proximal part of the humerus: relevance to arthroplasty. *J Bone Joint Surg.* 2000;82A(11):1594-1602.
21. Brooks C, Revell WJ, Heatley FW. Vascularity of the humeral head after proximal humeral fractures. *J Bone Joint Surg Br.* 1993;75(1):132-136.
22. Meyer C, Alt V, Hassanin H, et al. The arteries of the humeral head and their relevance in fracture treatment. *Surg Radiol Anat.* 2005;27(3):232-237.
23. Laing P. The arterial supply of the adult humerus. *J Bone Joint Surg Am.* 1956;38-A(5):1105-1116.
24. Duparc F, Muller JM, Freger P. Arterial blood supply of the proximal humeral epiphysis. *Surg Radiol Anat.* 2001;23(3):185-190.
25. Mansat P, Guity MR, Bellumore Y, Mansat M. Shoulder arthroplasty for late sequelae of proximal humeral fractures. *J Shoulder Elbow Surg.* 2004;13(3):305-312.
26. Boileau P, Chuinard C, Le Huec JC, Walch G, Trajani C. Proximal humerus fracture sequelae: impact of a new radiographic classification of arthroplasty. *Clin Orthop Relat Res.* 2006;422: 121-130.
27. Boileau P, Trojani C, Walch G, Krishnan SG, Romeo A, Sinnerton R. Shoulder arthroplasty for the treatment of the sequelae of fractures of the proximal humerus. *J Shoulder Elbow Surg.* 2001;10(4):299-308.
28. Boileau P, Krishnan SG, Tinsi L, Walch G, Coste JS, Mole D. Tuberosity malposition and migration: reasons for poor outcomes after hemiarthroplasty for displaced fractures of the proximal humerus. *J Shoulder Elbow Surg.* 2002;11(5):401-412.
29. Clare D, Wirth MA, Groh GI, Rockwood CA Jr. Shoulder arthrodesis. *J Bone and Joint Surgery.* 2001;83-A:693-600.
30. Gonzalez-Diaz R, Rodriguez-Merchan EC, Gilbert MS. The role of shoulder fusion in the era of arthroplasty. *Int Orthop.* 1997;21(3):204-209.

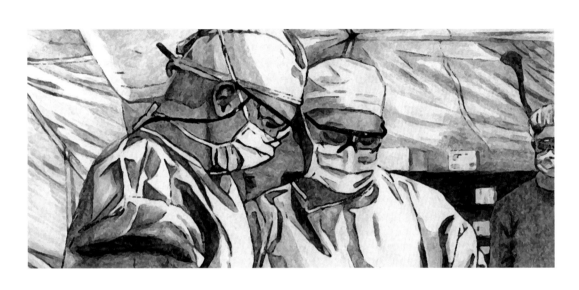

SECTION IV
LOWER EXTREMITY

Chapter 21

LOWER EXTREMITY LIMB SALVAGE

CPT Michael J. Beltran, MD; LTC(P) Romney C. Andersen, MD; and LTC Joseph R. Hsu, MD

The conflicts in Iraq and Afghanistan have exposed the devastating nature of modern combat warfare, with severe extremity trauma becoming the hallmark injury. As demonstrated by Owens and colleagues, injuries to the extremities represent more than half of all injuries sustained in the present conflicts, with a substantial number of these being open lower extremity fractures.[1,2] Injuries to the extremities have been shown to require the greatest amount of resources and lead to more disability than other combat injuries.[3] In previous military conflicts, severe fractures of the leg and hindfoot associated with bone and/or soft issue loss were often managed with amputation because the modern techniques of microvascular free flap coverage, advanced bone and soft tissue reconstruction, and distraction histiogenesis had not yet seen widespread use. Orthopedic surgeons deployed to combat zones today are increasingly tasked with the critical job of preserving limbs and avoiding amputation whenever possible, leaving definitive management and decisions regarding amputation versus limb salvage to experienced limb salvage surgeons at the definitive medical treatment facility in consultation with the patient.

The term *limb salvage* refers to the use of reconstructive surgery to preserve an extremity with a limb-threatening injury. Fractures of the tibia sustained in combat pose a major treatment dilemma for the orthopedic surgeon. Because the anteromedial surface of the tibia is subcutaneous along its entire surface, it is easily prone to injury, and the majority of these fractures are open and frequently complicated by bone and/or soft tissue loss.[2,4,5] The high-energy nature of tibial injuries also predisposes fractures to significant periosteal stripping, leaving large areas of bone devitalized, contaminated, or avascular. Salvage of limb-threatening tibia fractures sustained in combat is challenging and often requires a multidisciplinary approach, including surgical management by limb salvage orthopedic and plastic surgeons, aggressive physical therapy, and psychological and social support networks.

Epidemiology

Tibia fractures represent 48% of lower extremity fractures sustained in current military conflicts, and the vast majority of these are open injuries.[2] Combat-related tibia fractures are typically secondary to either single projectile penetrating injury from high-velocity gunshot wounds or multiple projectile penetrating injury from blast mechanisms.[2,4,5] Blunt trauma also is seen in theater, although with much less frequency. Blast trauma in particular is responsible for nearly 78% of all injuries sustained in Iraq and Afghanistan.[1] In comparison, civilian literature indicates that the majority of tibia fractures are the result of falls and motor vehicle collisions.[6] This difference in mechanism is critical in explaining the severe nature of combat-related tibia fractures and the frequent presentation with bone and soft tissue loss. Civilian blunt trauma open fractures generally occur from an inside-out mechanism, in which a force placed on the bone causes a fracture and the sharp end of the bone then penetrates out of the skin, exposing the

Owens BD, Belmont PJ Jr, eds. *Combat Orthopedic Surgery:*
Lessons Learned in Iraq and Afghanistan (pp 193-204)
© 2011 SLACK Incorporated

bone to bacteria. Deep contamination occurs when the bone is drawn back into the wound. Open fractures occurring from blast injuries occur from an outside-in mechanism, in which the blast causes deep penetration of foreign matter deep into the extremities' soft tissue envelope and bone. Blast mechanisms also behave similar to shotgun blasts, in which multiple small fragments create a wide zone of injury. Although each fragment travels at low velocity, coupled together, they impart a much higher total kinetic energy to the bone and soft tissue envelope.[7,8]

Management in Theater

DECISION MAKING REGARDING AMPUTATION VERSUS LIMB SALVAGE

The initial decision to amputate or salvage a mangled extremity in theater is a multidisciplinary team decision and should not be based on the opinion of a single surgeon. Rather, input from both trauma and vascular surgeons should be sought in conjunction with orthopedic expertise regarding the decision process. Orthopedic surgeons have a strong tendency to base decisions regarding amputation on anatomical considerations as opposed to the combat casualty's physiologic condition.[9] A recent survey found that orthopedic surgeons cited tibial nerve continuity and soft tissue coverage as the 2 most important determinants of a need for amputation. Injury Severity Score was not cited as a determining factor by orthopedists, although it was cited as most important by general surgeons.[9] In the acute setting, physiology should play a more critical role in determining whether to amputate or make an attempt at limb salvage. There is at least one case report of overaggressive limb salvage surgery resulting in the death of the patient.[10] Early management must focus on saving the life of the patient at the expense of the limb if necessary.

Patient resuscitation is a prerequisite for attempts at limb salvage in theater. Because the majority of wounds are to the extremities, control of hemorrhage is the most critical aspect of care prior to evacuation. Tourniquets, in particular, have led to a significant decrease in mortality through control of hemorrhage.[11] Tourniquets may be removed early if a patient is hemodynamically stable and anatomic control of bleeding is possible; otherwise, they should remain inflated until the patient reaches the operating room. Other modern modalities, including hemostatic chitosan dressings, are also available for control of extremity bleeding and are particularly effective for control of hemorrhage from cavitary wounds.[12,13] Patient resuscitation once evacuated to Echelon II or III continues with the aggres-

sive use of blood products, including whole blood and fresh frozen plasma.[14,15] Use of 1:1 transfusion ratios of packed red blood cells and fresh frozen plasma has been recommended.[16] Termed *damage control resuscitation*, this approach to patient resuscitation has led to a decrease in mortality among combat casualties during modern conflicts.[17] During resuscitation, tourniquets are left inflated until an adequate response is obtained based on multiple parameters, including base deficit, pH, blood pressure, international normalized ratio (INR), and body temperature. Once adequately resuscitated, direct control of bleeding and management of bone and soft tissue injury may commence. Prolonged muscle ischemia while tourniquets are inflated can lead to fatal reperfusion injury once deflated if proper measures are not taken, and this again requires a team approach between orthopedists, trauma surgeons, and anesthesiologists. Premedication with both insulin and calcium are necessary to prevent cardiopulmonary collapse from rapid increases in blood potassium levels, and aggressive alkalinization and urinary diuresis are needed to prevent renal failure. Failure of resuscitation, in the setting of progressive decompensation, is an indication to proceed with emergent amputation of injured hemorrhagic limbs to preserve a patient's life.

Multiple scoring systems have been devised in an attempt to determine which patients might benefit from acute amputation. These include the mangled extremity scoring system (MESS); predictive salvage index; limb salvage index; nerve injury, ischemia, soft tissue injury, skeletal injury, shock, age of patient score; and Hannover fracture scale, among others. Traditionally, the MESS score has been most frequently used, with a score of 7 or more predictive of the need for amputation.[18] Although a recent report validated the predictive value of the MESS for combat injuries, multiple other reports have found these systems, including the MESS, to be nonprognostic in large series of patients.[19-22]

Previous reports and opinions, most notably by Hansen in 1987, identified a higher rate of complications and lower functional results in patients managed with attempts at limb salvage versus acute amputation, giving credence to the notion that limb salvage left patients "demoralized, divorced, or destitute."[23-26] These reports seemed to indicate that attempts at limb salvage were inferior to acute amputation, with patients less likely to return to work and many ultimately requiring delayed amputation.[24-26] These assumptions were challenged by the Lower Extremity Assessment Project (LEAP) study, a large prospective, observational study of 545 patients comparing limb salvage versus amputation for limb-threatening lower extremity injuries. No difference was found between the 2 groups with regard to disability at 1, 2, or 7 years, and no difference was identified with regard to return-to-work rates.[27,28] Furthermore, a cost analysis study determined that the lifetime cost of a prosthesis was more than 3 times that of care rendered during limb salvage, with the lifetime costs associated with amputation exceeding $500,000.[29] The LEAP study also identified the limited utility of plantar sensation as a prognostic tool for amputation. Of salvage patients with initially absent plantar sensation, 55% had normal sensation at 2 years, with only a single patient having complete absence of sensation.[30] No difference was found in return-to-work rates between those patients with an initially insensate foot managed with either salvage or amputation.[30]

ORTHOPEDIC MANAGEMENT IN THEATER

Once the casualty is adequately resuscitated and all life-threatening injuries safely managed, the most forward-treating orthopedic surgeon may begin the most important aspect of open tibia fracture care, which consists of aggressive initial wound debridement and fracture stabilization. Antibiotic prophylaxis with a first-generation cephalosporin is recommended in the setting of all open fractures and should be given as soon as possible after injury. Little empiric evidence currently exists to recommend prophylactic gram-negative coverage with an aminoglycoside, and their initial use in theater should be discouraged.[31] The first debridement is the most critical and must be adequate. Surgeons are often tentative to remove potentially necrotic bone at the initial debridement given the implications for future reconstruction, but this remains a critical aspect of an adequate debridement and was shown by Edwards to lead to a lower incidence of deep infection.[32] Furthermore, studies from the civilian literature have demonstrated that continued trips to the operating room for multiple debridements may be associated with higher rates of nosocomial infection.[33-36] Once adequately debrided, the wound should be irrigated copiously to aid in removal of any additional gross or microscopic contamination. The amount of irrigation possible is dictated by level of care and assets available, but generally type III open tibia fractures should be irrigated with a minimum of 9 L of saline or other potable fluid.[31]

Skeletal fracture stabilization follows debridement. Fracture stabilization reduces bleeding, pain, and further injury to the soft tissue envelope. External fixation is preferred to provide more rigid stabilization during frequent transports and is generally available as far forward as the forward surgical team, which is an Echelon II level of care.[37] Possley and colleagues recently demonstrated that external fixator placement in theater is safe with an acceptable rate of complications.[38] Two half pins proximal and distal to

the fracture should be placed. Ideally, the pins should be placed near and far from the fracture in either fragment. Accurate pin placement may be difficult, however, if fluoroscopic imaging is unavailable.[39] Distal fractures involving the plafond or hindfoot should have the ankle spanned using a transfixion pin through the calcaneus. Although pins into the first metatarsal have been advocated to prevent equinus contracture, this has not been proven, and foot dorsiflexion has been shown to increase leg compartment pressures.[40] Bony contact remains the most important aspect of skeletal stabilization with external fixation. When faced with acute bone loss, increased stability may be gained by placement of a multiplanar frame or double stacking of bars; alternatively, a small amount of shortening may be accepted in an attempt to gain bony contact. A sterile dressing should be applied to the open soft tissue wound prior to recovery or transport.

As patients continue evacuation to higher echelons of care, repeat debridement at 24- to 48-hour intervals may be necessary until a clean wound bed is created and is amenable to definitive fracture management. Final evacuation to an Echelon V treatment facility within the United States for definitive fracture management typically occurs within 3 to 5 days of injury. This timeframe is critical; under ideal circumstances, soft tissue coverage is completed within 7 days of injury.[41] It is postulated that wounds are initially contaminated with bacteria but that after a short period of time wounds become colonized, leaving them more prone to infection. Although the results of subacute flap coverage in the civilian literature have been poor, a few recent series of combat limb salvage patients have demonstrated low flap infection rates and a high incidence of successful reconstruction, particularly with rotational flap coverage.[42-44] Once transport to a US facility is completed, planning for definitive management may commence (Figure 21-1).

Definitive Management

Definitive management of tibia fractures with loss of bone, soft tissue, or both begins with a careful and deliberate preoperative plan. The vascular status to the extremity must be known and well documented. Single-vessel vasculature can be a contraindication to microvascular free flap coverage due to microvascular steal syndrome and resultant risk for catastrophic limb compromise.[45,46] Microvascular free flap coverage also requires the expertise of an experienced flap surgeon, which may not be available. Despite results from the civilian literature indicating that rotational flap coverage may be contraindicated in tibia fractures

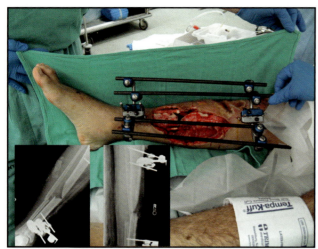

Figure 21-1. A 21-year-old active duty servicemember sustained a limb-threatening type IIIB right tibia fracture after blast injury with a large area of composite bone and soft tissue loss. The patient also sustained an ipsilateral femoral shaft fracture and comminuted open distal humerus fracture. The patient refused free flap coverage and desired limb salvage.

with severe bony injury,[47] this has not been found with respect to combat wounds.[4,42-44] Rotational coverage of proximal soft tissue defects has traditionally been accomplished with use of a gastrocnemius flap. Either the medial or lateral head may be rotated to fill the soft tissue defect, and this is determined by location of the soft tissue defect and local injury to the flap muscle in question. The medial head is preferable and has a greater excursion, as the fibula need not be circumvented. Soft tissue defects of the middle third of the tibia may be adequately covered with use of a hemisoleus flap, and again the adequacy is determined by local soft tissue injury and location of the defect. Wounds of the distal third of the tibia have traditionally been covered using a free flap; however, in certain circumstances, a reverse fasciocutaneus flap based on the sural artery may be employed.[48] When rotational flap coverage is contraindicated or a wound is too large, free flap coverage should be used if possible.

There are a number of situations in which soft tissue coverage is not possible with either a rotational flap or microvascular free tissue transfer. As alluded to above, contraindications to free flap coverage include single-vessel limbs and inexperience or unavailability of a qualified flap surgeon. Severe local damage to the vascular pedicle may also make rotational coverage impossible. In this setting, soft tissue closure may successfully be accomplished using the Ilizarov method. Ringed fixators are a powerful tool with which to manage both bone and soft tissue loss. Circular fixation has been used previously to close soft tissue defects via distraction histiogenesis,[49-51] but we have found that perhaps their most powerful use is through

acute shortening with or without angulation to close large soft tissue defects primarily. Because wounds benefit from closure as soon as possible to reduce the incidence of infection, this technique allows primary closure, with correction of bony deformity possible after a latency period allows the soft tissue defect to heal. Multiple authors have had success using this technique for soft tissue closure.[52-56] This soft tissue can subsequently be lengthened under the tension-stress effect described by Ilizarov.[57,58] All types of soft tissue can successfully be lengthened using this technique, including skin, muscle, nerves, and blood vessels.[49-51,57,58] New software-driven ringed fixators, including the Taylor Spatial Frame (Smith and Nephew, Memphis, TN), represent a powerful tool with which to generate and then later correct these intended deformities. Rings may be applied without the need for individualized preoperative planning or intraoperative frame construction. Once applied, a deformity may be induced with the soft tissue defect lying within the concavity of the deformity, allowing primary wound closure and obviating the need for coverage. This technique has been shown to be effective in circumstances where free flap coverage is not possible.[54,55] For large defects otherwise requiring free flap coverage, acute shortening and angulation may be combined with rotational flap coverage.[55] The limb is shortened and angulated as much as safely possible with the rotated muscle flap used to cover the remainder of the defect.

Management of bone loss is complex, and complications are frequent.[59-64] A myriad number of options exist to the limb salvage surgeon with regard to bone loss, among them acute shortening, cancellous autografting, vascularized free fibular transfer, and bone transport using distraction osteogenesis. Each technique has its own merits and weaknesses discussed below.

ACUTE SHORTENING

Primary acute shortening is a particularly effective strategy when faced with small bony defects of less than 3 cm (Figure 21-2).[63,65] It allows primary bony apposition and is most useful when it aids in primary soft tissue closure. Fracture stabilization can be accomplished with internal fixation using either a plate or an intramedullary nail. Alternatively, definitive management with external fixation may also be employed, particularly if one wishes to correct the induced limb length discrepancy via bifocal transport. Because primary bony apposition can be obtained, immediate fracture healing may commence, potentially obviating the need for staged bone grafting at a later date. Shortening of the tibia is made easier when fibula comminution is present; otherwise, a fibular

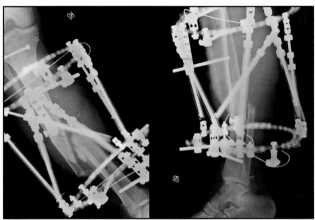

Figure 21-2. Radiographs after shortening and angulation with rotational gastrocnemius flap coverage. The limb was safely shortened 8 cm without complication. The soft tissue envelope was allowed to heal completely over 3 weeks prior to gradual deformity correction.

osteotomy should be performed to prevent angular deformity at the fracture site. Major drawbacks to acute shortening include creating a limb length discrepancy and soft tissue redundancy at the level of the closed wound, which may cause soft tissue swelling and may be cosmetically unappealing to the patient.

CANCELLOUS AUTOGRAFT

Cancellous autografting is an effective treatment modality to fill large diaphyseal bone defects. Autogenous cancellous graft material is highly osteogenic and osteoinductive, up-regulating multiple growth factors necessary for fracture healing and providing an osteoconductive scaffold for vascular and bony ingrowth.[66] The adult male pelvis possesses enough graft material to fill a 15-cm tibial defect, although this amount of bone should rarely ever be harvested.[67] It is also estimated that a tibial defect of 4 cm can be filled using the bone harvested from each posterior iliac crest.[67,68] Although the iliac crest has traditionally been the most common site for cancellous bone harvest, newer intramedullary harvest techniques (Reamer-Irrigator-Aspirator, Synthes, Paoli, PA) are now being employed and appear to offer an alternative graft source with abundant osteobiologic factors.[69,70]

Timing of autogenous bone grafting is a critical factor in determining the most appropriate treatment option for a tibia fracture with segmental bone loss and is dependent on the condition of the soft tissue envelope. It is recommended that bone grafting be delayed until after skeletal stabilization of open tibia fractures because the avascular graft material represents a potential nidus for infection.[71,72] A period of 2 weeks appears adequate to allow necessary wound healing and revascularization of tissues with mar-

ginal viability after local soft tissue coverage.[72] When free tissue transfer has been performed, a 6-week latency period is recommended.[71] This period allows the flap to epithelialize, which decreases bacterial contamination of the wound bed and allows healing of the flap to the surrounding native tissue.[71] A recent large series of combat-related tibia fractures managed with staged bone grafting demonstrated a union rate of 92% and a deep infection rate of only 8%, giving credence to this technique for war-time injuries.[4]

Definitive fracture stabilization is preferably performed after soft tissue reconstruction when the soft tissue envelope has begun to heal, usually around 2 weeks after coverage, and can be safely accomplished with use of either a bridge plate, intramedullary nail, or ringed fixator.[4] Proper restoration of axial length and rotation is difficult when segmental bone loss is present, but is critical and should not be overlooked. When faced with a large anteromedial soft tissue defect, minimally invasive percutaneous plate osteosynthesis techniques can be used to place an anterolateral bridge plate, avoiding the open soft tissue wound. Management of the bone void during the graft latency period can be accomplished with use of antibiotic beads or a spacer. Antibiotic spacers, in addition to their high local drug concentrations, maintain the wound bed and prevent accumulation of both scar tissue and hematoma through the formation of an induced membrane.[73] Induced membranes are highly vascular and have been shown to secrete multiple growth factors thought to stimulate bone production and prevent graft resorption. Pelissier and colleagues have demonstrated improved graft consolidation through these induced membranes.[74,75]

Multiple approaches can be used for delayed grafting of tibial bone defects. Harmon first described the use of a posterolateral approach in 1945.[76] Because most open wounds are located anteromedially, Harmon advocated this approach to avoid the compromised open soft tissues. The graft is placed along the interosseous membrane to affect a long synostosis of the tibia to the fibula, thereby spanning the defect. Harmon's technique is particularly risky when the remaining blood supply is from the peroneal artery and should not be used in proximal tibia fractures due to the close proximity to the neurovascular bundle. Other approaches that are commonly used in the setting of free flap coverage include anterolateral and posteromedial approaches. The flap can safely be raised from the side opposite the anastomosed vascular pedicle, allowing direct graft placement into the defect. During this direct access to the defect, all avascular scar tissue should be debrided and the medullary canal recanalized to aid in restoring blood supply. The graft can be firmly packed into the defect and contoured more accurately using this technique.

The major utility of autogenous grafting is in avoiding the need for prolonged frame time in an external fixator and in the relative simplicity of the technique. Graft consolidation is less reliable in larger defects, however.[77,78] This leaves the graft prone to delayed union, nonunion, or refracture. In addition, donor site morbidity remains a concern. Pain at the harvest site is common in addition to cosmetic concerns and nerve parasthesias over the buttock or lateral thigh.[79] Weight bearing should be limited until radiographic evidence of consolidation occurs, and continued radiographic surveillance is necessary after consolidation, as progressive deformity is possible even after apparent graft consolidation.[77]

FREE VASCULARIZED FIBULA TRANSFER

Transfer of a pedicled portion of the fibula represents an appealing technique in the management of tibial bone defects. Because the autogenous fibula relies on a vascular pedicle, immediate vascular inflow is accomplished, leading to a more predictable union than with cancellous grafting. Union rates approaching 90% have been reported in post-traumatic reconstruction.[80]

Free vascularized fibula transfer was first described as a microsurgical technique by Taylor and colleagues in the late 1970s.[81] Like all microvascular free tissue transfers, it requires the expertise of a microvascular surgeon. It is contraindicated in the setting of a single-vessel limb. The technique involves transfer of free vascularized fibula graft from the contralateral limb, which requires that the donor limb be uninjured. The entire length of the fibula can be safely harvested, taking care to leave the distal 5 cm to avoid problems with ankle stability and the proximal 7 cm to avoid injury to the peroneal nerve.[82] The graft ideally is 4 cm longer than the defect in question to allow 2 cm of overlap at either end available for stable fixation. Alternatively, ipsilateral pedicled fibular transfer has been described but is highly dependent on local injury characteristics.[83,84]

Union is more predictable with use of a vascularized fibula transfer when compared to cancellous autografting. Average union times in large series range from 3 to 6 months, although adequate graft hypertrophy takes approximately 2 years.[82,85,86] Failure to hypertrophy leads to graft fracture in 25% of cases. Watson and colleagues determined that fibular transfer was less efficacious in acute tibia fractures with bone loss when compared to other etiologies and recommended other techniques such as bone transport or cancellous grafting.[65] In addition to fracture through the graft and failure to hypertrophy, multiple other complications are inherent when using this technique. In a series of nearly 250 vascularized fibula grafts, Vail and Urbaniak identified a 19% incidence of donor site morbidity, including both objective and subjective motor and sensory loss, thromboembolism, and wound cellulitis.[86] The inherent advantages of the technique, immediate restoration of skeletal continuity, and preserved vascular inflow to the graft must be weighed against the potential significant complications.

DISTRACTION OSTEOGENESIS

Distraction osteogenesis, initially developed by G.A. Ilizarov in Russia to treat the war wound sequelae of World War II, represents an effective treatment strategy with a proven track record, particularly in the setting of large segmental bone defects that might otherwise be poorly treated with either cancellous or fibular autograft alone.[87] Using a ringed fixator, distraction osteogenesis may be performed using the monofocal bone transport technique originally described and disseminated by Ilizarov, or with more advanced techniques, including shortening and angulation, bifocal or trifocal transport, distraction over a nail, or hemifibular transport.[52,53,84,88,89] As described earlier, ringed fixators also represent a powerful tool with which to manage soft tissue defects. Frequently, both bone and soft tissue loss can be safely managed with the use of a ringed fixator alone.[52-56]

The decision to use a specific technique is dependent on the condition of the soft tissue envelope. When bone loss is not accompanied by a soft tissue defect, or when free flap coverage is used, simple monofocal bone transport techniques can be safely used to regenerate lost bone. The technique is not as technically demanding as bifocal transport, but does require additional surgical procedures, namely to remove antibiotic beads used to fill the dead space void during transport. Multiple authors have shown increased union rates when the docking site is bone grafted.[61,62,64] Bone transport requires a corticotomy, and this should be performed through an area of adequate soft tissue either proximally or distally to encourage healthy regenerate growth and consolidation. Whenever possible, the transport segment should be "pulled" by the transport ring to maintain better segment control. An intact fibula also helps to align the segment during transport. After a latency period, distraction may commence at the rate of 1 mm per day divided into 0.25-mm increments, although this rate should be adjusted based on the quality of regenerate bone one is expected to produce. Rate variability is also recommended to improve regenerate quality. Distraction is continued until the antibiotic bead spacer is sufficiently compressed, at which point the beads may be removed and bone grafting with or without osteobiologic adjuvants performed.

Distraction continues until bony contact is made, at which point compression can be performed until radiographic consolidation occurs.

Bifocal and trifocal transport techniques should be employed for defects larger than 6 or 7 cm. Because multiple segments of activity are involved, these techniques are technically more demanding and have a higher incidence of complications.[59,61-64,89-91] However, the techniques substantially decrease frame time because fracture shortening and compression can be carried out concurrently with lengthening performed along a different segment. Distraction should be performed wherever the soft tissue envelope is most healthy and amenable to successful regenerate development. The technique is particularly effective when a soft tissue defect is present, because lengthening can be performed distant from the zone of injury while either primary or gradual shortening is carried out at the level of the bone and soft tissue defect. Some authors recommend gradual shortening for defects greater than 4 cm due to concern for vascular compromise,[90] but others have not experienced those problems and have acutely shortened fractures up to 8 cm without complications.[54,55] Intraoperative Doppler examination is mandatory to assess the vascular status before, during, and after acute shortening. Any change in triphasic flow warrants a reduction in the amount of shortening. When gradual shortening is required, it can safely be done at the rate of 0.5 mm per day until docking is encountered. The fracture site should undergo compression until consolidation occurs. This typically occurs well before regenerate consolidation. If necessary, delayed bone grafting can be used to stimulate union. Regenerate maturation may also be expedited by the use of ultrasound therapy.[92]

Acute shortening and angulation represents another useful treatment strategy when faced with combined bone and soft tissue loss.[55,56] Acute shortening without angulation is effective; however, the technique is more likely to lead to soft tissue bunching or invagination than with fracture angulation, in which the soft tissues on the convex side are on tension. Acute shortening and angulation allows the soft tissue defect to be closed primarily and may allow bony apposition, although the primary concern with this technique is primary closure of the soft tissue envelope. A latency period is required to allow the soft tissue envelope to heal prior to distraction histiogenesis. Using a software-driven ringed fixator, the deformity may gradually be corrected while safely stretching the healing soft tissue defect at a rate of 1 mm per day.[55] Once alignment and rotation have been restored, the fracture may be actively compressed to stimulate union. Bifocal frames are commonly used to preserve limb length through distraction at a distant site. Bone grafting is frequently required at the fracture, particularly when good bony apposition cannot be obtained. Multiple authors have demonstrated good outcomes using this composite histiogenesis technique to manage combined bone and soft tissue defects.[52-56]

Surgical Technique

The authors prefer to manage combat casualty tibia fractures associated with bone and soft tissue defects with the use of ringed fixators according to the principles of Ilizarov. Smaller defects can be successfully managed with bone grafting alone, but in our experience the vast majority of tibia fractures sustained in modern combat environments involve greater amounts of bone and soft tissue loss. The technique of distraction histiogenesis to manage composite bone and soft tissue loss is described as follows.

TECHNIQUE

The patient is placed supine on a radiolucent or split leg table, which affords complete fluoroscopic visualization of the entire length of the tibia in both the anterior-posterior and lateral projections. A tourniquet is not used as it predisposes the bone to thermal injury during wire and half pin placement. Antibiotic prophylaxis with a first-generation cephalosporin should be initiated within 1 hour of surgery to reduce the risk of perioperative wound infection. Any necessary wound debridement or antibiotic bead placement is done before placement of the frame. If a rotational flap is to be used in conjunction with acute angulation, it should be mobilized prior to frame placement as well. We prefer to use a Taylor Spatial Frame for management of the fracture segment due to the improved control it affords; a simple Ilizarov frame with telescoping rods is all that is required for distraction osteogenesis at another bone segment. Because the Taylor Spatial Frame (Smith & Nephew, Memphis, TN) is software driven, no individualized preoperative frame planning is required, and intraoperative frame construction is not necessary. Rings are applied using the Rings First Method, in which the rings are first applied orthogonal to the proximal and distal fracture segments using a combination of half pins and thin wires. We recommend the use of hydroxyapatite-coated titanium half pins, due to the improved bone-pin interface obtained, which theoretically reduces pin sepsis and loosening.[93,94] Fast-fix struts are applied, and, with the construct unlocked, an induced deformity is created with the soft tissue defect within the concavity of the deformity. Doppler ultrasound is used before, during, and after shortening and angulation to detect any potential vascular compromise. Once the wound margins are approximated, the struts are locked, and primary closure of the soft tissue envelope can be performed. Sterile dressings and compressive foam bolsters should be applied to the pin sites to reduce pin tract complications during the first few postoperative weeks. Once the soft tissue wound has healed, typically within 2 or 3 weeks, frame care can commence with routine daily showering using soap and warm water. Wound healing also means that angular correction can commence. The Taylor Spatial Frame is designed to be used with its own software package. Using the "Total Residual Program," a correction can be performed based on good orthogonal radiographs of the deformity. The center of the deformity is defined as the "Structure at Risk," which is corrected at the rate of 1 mm per day until alignment and rotation are corrected. If fracture angulation is used, the structure at risk should be the concave wound skin edge. Repeat total residual programs can be run at scheduled office visits, and no frame adjustments are required. Based on the type of fracture and defect size, staged bone grafting or gradual shortening and compression may be used to obtain fracture union. When grafting is required, we will frequently augment healing with the use of recombinant bone morphogenic proteins. If limb lengthening is planned, a corticotomy distant from the fracture is performed through a healthy soft tissue envelope either proximal or distal. A metaphyseal corticotomy should be used whenever possible.[95] Distraction is performed at a rate of 1 mm day unless there is concern for healthy regenerate, in which case a slower rate of distraction is used until viable regenerate is visualized on plain films. Once length has been restored, the consolidation phase can begin. This period typically is 2 to 3 times as long as the distraction phase and represents the majority of the time the patient spends in the frame. Once mature regenerate appears on plain films, or if maturation appears to be delayed, frame dynamization can be used. The absence of pain is a strong indicator that maturation has occurred and frame removal can be performed. In instances of frame fatigue, the fixator can be removed prematurely, but regenerate and fracture stability must be ensured with another means of fixation. We prefer to apply a percutaneous plate in this circumstance because it can be applied without exposing the regenerate and does not rely on medullary continuity for successful placement. Intramedullary nailing, if undertaken, should be delayed until the pin sites have healed in order to reduce the likelihood of infection (Figure 21-3).

Outcomes

Little has been published regarding the use of distraction histiogenesis techniques for the management of combat-related tibia fractures associated with composite bone and soft tissue loss, although the results thus far are encouraging.[54,55] Large series of civilian patients managed with the techniques have been published with predictably good results. In general, union rates greater than 90% have been reported,[63,64,89] but expectations must be tempered by the high incidence of complications related to long periods of time in a ringed fixator.[62-64,67,68,89] The benefits of avoiding free tissue transfer must also be weighed when determining success with distraction histiogenesis. In both series by Beltran and Hsu, all patient wounds healed without the need for free tissue transfer.[54,55] Nho and colleagues,[52] as well as Gulsen and Ozkan,[56] have also demonstrated similar results. Free tissue transfer is a major reconstructive undertaking, and free flap complications and/or failure have been reported in more than 20% of patients in some series.[47,96,97]

Other recent reports from the conflicts in Iraq and Afghanistan have demonstrated good outcomes with limb salvage techniques, particularly when using circular fixation with or without soft tissue reconstruction.[4,42-44] Keeling and colleagues reported on 38 type III open tibia fractures managed with a ringed fixator-driven protocol.[4] Nearly half of these patients required soft tissue reconstruction with either rotational or free flap coverage. The deep infection rate was 8%, with all infections successfully managed without need for frame removal. Furthermore, only one patient ultimately required an amputation on a delayed basis.[4] Tintle et al[42] and Kumar and colleagues[43] have written extensively regarding soft tissue reconstruction of war wounds from Iraq and Afghanistan. In one report, only 1 of 46 flaps had total failure; in another, the infection rate was only 13% with flap failure reported in 2.8% of cases.[42,43]

Complications

Complications related to distraction osteogenesis techniques are common and generally fall into 3 categories: frame-related complications, problems with regenerate maturation, or problems related to healing of the docking site. Complication rates are highly variable in the literature but generally range from 33% to 60% if pin tract infections are excluded.[61-64,89] The majority of complications associated with distraction osteogenesis using ringed fixators fall into the category of frame complications, with pin tract sepsis and loosening by far the most common.[59,61-64,89,91] Newer tech-

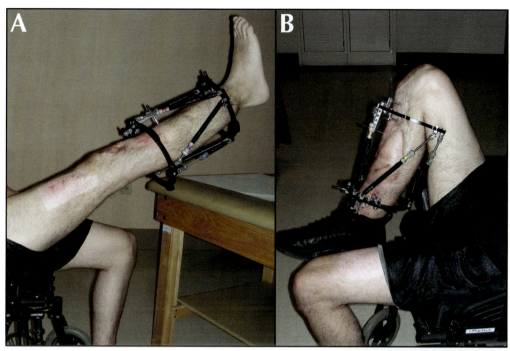

Figure 21-3. After 1 year in a circular external fixator, the fracture healed with restoration of limb length and mechanical axis. The knee regained a full range of motion. The patient has since returned to recreational activities and recently completed 2 marathons.

niques focused on use of more half pins and fewer soft tissue transfixing wires, use of hydroxyapatite-coated pins, and use of more biologically friendly materials such as titanium alloys have eased the burden placed on the soft tissue envelope and may lead to improved results.[93,94] Other frame-related complications encountered, although less frequently, include pin site pain, complex regional pain syndrome, frame failure or breakage, premature consolidation, and the potential for unintentional joint distraction or subluxation.[55]

Docking site nonunion occurs less frequently than pin tract sepsis but remains a concern as it delays frame removal and requires additional surgical procedures to facilitate fracture healing. As previously mentioned, during bone transport, the docking site can be bone grafted to reduce the incidence of nonunion and minimize frame times. When compressive techniques are employed and good bony apposition possible, one may potentially avoid the need for this secondary surgery; giving a fracture time to heal is warranted in this situation due to the powerful ability compression has to facilitate union. Results are also encouraging when using orthobiologics, namely recombinant bone morphogenic proteins.[55,64,91]

Although less common, problems related to regenerate maturation are more difficult to treat than docking site nonunions due to their propensity for collapse and resultant chronic deformity. It is imperative that frame removal not occur until regenerate maturation is complete unless regenerate stabilization occurs with additional fixation strategies. Computed tomography should be used in any instance where regenerate maturation is suspect on plain radiographs. Regenerate

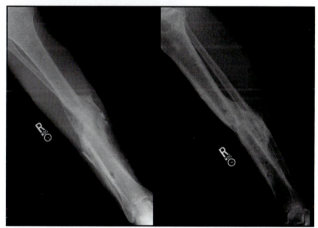

Figure 21-4. Final radiographs at 18 months after injury with continued fracture remodeling.

maturation may be speeded by the use of ultrasound therapy,[92] and this is routinely recommended. Proper distraction technique should also be employed, as healthy regenerate benefits from a variable rate of distraction. Although outcome studies are currently lacking, it appears newer techniques using orthobiologics and/or direct autogenous bone grafting may be beneficial in facilitating regenerate maturation (Figure 21-4).

Conclusion

Limb salvage of combat-related tibia fractures complicated by composite bone and soft tissue loss is technically challenging. Multiple options exist to manage these complex injuries, which can lead to predictably good results with regard to bony union, soft tissue closure, and return to functional activities. Amputation, the workhorse approach to these injuries in previous military conflicts, has been replaced by new, advanced surgical techniques and a multidisciplinary approach to patient management. Because of these strategies, soldiers sustaining these injuries are returning to duty and redeploying, ideas once thought to be impossible.

References

1. Owens BD, Kragh JF Jr, Wenke JC, Macaitis J, Wade CE, Holcomb JB. Combat wounds in Operation Iraqi Freedom and Operation Enduring Freedom. *J Trauma*. 2008;64:295-299.

2. Owens BD, Kragh JF Jr, Macaitis J, Svoboda SJ, Wenke JC. Characterization of extremity wounds in Operation Iraqi Freedom and Operation Enduring Freedom. *J Orthop Trauma*. 2007;21:254-257.

3. Masini BD, Waterman SM, Wenke JC, Owens BD, Hsu JR, Ficke JR. Resource utilization and disability outcome assessment of combat casualties from Operation Iraqi Freedom and Operation Enduring Freedom. *J Orthop Trauma*. 2009;23:261-266.

4. Keeling JJ, Gwinn DE, Tintle SM, Andersen RC, McGuigan FX. Short-term outcomes of severe open wartime tibial fractures treated with ring external fixation. *J Bone Joint Surg Am*. 2008;90:2643-2651.

5. Beltran MJ, et al. *Peripheral nerve recovery following type III combat-related open tibia fractures*. Presented at the 51st Annual Meeting of the Society of Military Orthopaedic Surgeons (SOMOS), December 14-18, 2009, Honolulu, HI.

6. Court-Brown CM, McBirnie J. The epidemiology of tibial fractures. *J Bone Joint Surg Br*. 1995;77:417-421.

7. Bartlett CS. Clinical update: gunshot wound ballistics. *Clin Orthop Relat Res*. 2003;408:28-57.

8. Deitch EA, Grimes WR. Experience with 112 shotgun wounds of the extremities. *J Trauma*. 1984;24:600-603.

9. MacKenzie EJ, Bosse MJ, Kellam JF, et al. Factors influencing the decision to amputate or reconstruct after high-energy lower extremity trauma. *J Trauma*. 2002;52:641-649.

10. Nessen SC, Lounsbury DE, Hetz SP, eds. *War Surgery in Afghanistan and Iraq: A Series of Cases 2003-2007*. Washington, DC: Office of the Surgeon General, Borden Institute; 2008:31-32.

11. Kragh JF Jr, Walters TJ, Baer DG, et al. Survival with emergency tourniquet use to stop bleeding in major limb trauma. *Ann Surg*. 2009;249:1-7.

12. Hsu JR. *"Reverse Roll" technique for chitosan hemostatic dressing in cavitary wounds*. Presented at the 48th annual meeting of the Society of Military Orthopaedic Surgeons (SOMOS), Honolulu, HI, 2006.

13. Wedmore I, McManus JG, Pusateri AE, Holcomb JB. A special report on the chitosan-based hemostatic dressing: experience in current combat operations. *J Trauma*. 2006;60:655-658.

14. Repine TB, Perkins JG, Kauvar DS, Blackborne L. The use of fresh whole blood in massive transfusion. *J Trauma*. 2006;60:S59-S69.

15. Spinella PC, Perkins JG, Grathwohl KW, Beekley AC, Holcomb JB. Warm fresh whole blood is independently associated with improved survival for patients with combat-related traumatic injuries. *J Trauma*. 2009;66:S69-S76.

16. Borgman MA, Spinella PC, Perkins JG, et al. The ratio of blood products transfused affects mortality in patients receiving massive transfusions at a combat support hospital. *J Trauma*. 2007;63:805-813.

17. Holcomb JB, Jenkins D, Rhee P, et al. Damage control resuscitation: directly addressing the early coagulopathy of trauma. *J Trauma*. 2007;62:307-310.

18. Johansen K, Daines M, Howey T, Helfet D, Hansen ST Jr. Objective criteria accurately predict amputation following lower extremity trauma. *J Trauma*. 1990;30:568-572.

19. Rush RM Jr, Kjorstad R, Starnes BW, Arrington E, Devine JD, Andersen CA. Application of the Mangled Extremity Severity Score in a combat setting. *Mil Med*. 2007;172:777-781.

20. Bonanni F, Rhodes M, Lucke MF. The futility of predictive scoring of mangled lower extremities. *J Trauma*. 2006;61:8-12.

21. Bosse MJ, MacKenzie EJ, Kellam JF, et al. A prospective evaluation of the clinical utility of the lower extremity injury severity scores. *J Bone Joint Surg Am*. 2001;83A:3-14.

22. Brown KV, Ramasamy A, McLeod J, Stapley S, Clasper JC. Predicting the need for early amputation in ballistic mangled extremity injuries. *J Trauma*. 2009;66(4 Suppl):S93-S97.

23. Hansen ST. The type-IIIC tibial fracture. Salvage or amputation. *J Bone Joint Surg Am*. 1987;69:799-800.

24. Purry NA, Hannon MA. How successful is below-knee amputation for injury? *Injury*. 1989;20:32-36.

25. Georgiadis GM, Behrens FF, Joyce MJ, Earle AS, Simmons AL. Open tibial fractures with severe soft-tissue loss. Limb salvage compared with below-the-knee amputation. *J Bone Joint Surg Am*. 1993;75:1431-1441.

26. Fairhurst MJ. The function of below-knee amputee versus the patient with salvaged grade III tibial fracture. *Clin Orthop Relat Res*. 1994;301:227-232.

27. Bosse MJ, MacKenzie EJ, Kellam JF, et al. An analysis of outcomes of reconstruction or amputation of leg-threatening injuries. *N Engl J Med*. 2002;347:1924-1931.

28. MacKenzie EJ, Bosse MJ, Pollak AN, et al. Long-term persistence of disability following severe lower-limb trauma. Results of a seven-year follow-up. *J Bone Joint Surg Am*. 2005;87:1801-1809.

29. MacKenzie EJ, Jones AS, Bosse MJ, et al. Health-care costs associated with amputation or reconstruction of a limb-threatening injury. *J Bone Joint Surg Am*. 2007;89:1685-1692.

30. Bosse MJ, McCarthy ML, Jones AL, et al. The insensate foot following severe lower extremity trauma: an indication for amputation? *J Bone Joint Surg Am*. 2005;87:2601-2608.

31. Murray CK, Hsu JR, Solomkin JS, et al. Prevention and management of infections associated with combat-related extremity injuries. *J Trauma*. 2008;64:S239-S251.

32. Edwards CC, Simmons SC, Browner BD, Weigel MA. Severe open tibial fractures. Results treating 202 injuries with external fixation. *Clin Orthop Relat Res*. 1988;230:98-115.

33. Templeman DC, Gulli B, Tsukayama DT, Gustilo RB. Update on the management of open fractures of the tibial shaft. *Clin Orthop Relat Res*. 1998;350:18-25.

34. Patzakis MJ, Harvey JP, Ivler D. The role of antibiotics in the management of open fractures. *J Bone Joint Surg Am*. 1974;56-A:532-541.

35. Benson DR, Riggins RS, Lawrence RM, Hoeprich PD, Huston AC, Harrison JA. Treatment of open fractures: a prospective study. *J Trauma*. 1983;23(1):25-30.

36. Delong WG Jr, Born CT, Wei SY, Petrik ME, Ponzio R, Schwab CW. Aggressive treatment of 119 open fracture wounds. *J Trauma*. 1999;46:1049-1054.

37. Szul AC, Davis LB, Walter Reed Army Medical Center Borden Institute, eds. *Emergency War Surgery*. 3rd US rev. Washington, DC: Walter Reed Army Medical Center Borden Institute; 2004.

38. Possley DR, Burns TC, Stinner DJ, et al. Temporary external fixation is safe in a combat environment. *J Trauma*. 2010;69(Suppl 1):S135-S139.

39. Topp R, Hayda R, Benedetti G, Twitero T, Carmack DB. The incidence of neurovascular injury during external fixator placement without radiographic assistance for lower extremity diaphyseal fractures: a cadaveric study. *J Trauma.* 2003;55:955-958.

40. Weiner G, Styf J, Nakhostine M, Gershuni DH. Effect of ankle position and a plaster cast on intramuscular pressure in the human leg. *J Bone Joint Surg Am.* 1994;76:1476-1481.

41. Cierny G 3rd, Byrd HS, Jones RE. Primary versus delayed soft tissue coverage for severe open tibial fractures. A comparison of results. *Clin Orthop Relat Res.* 1983;178:54-63.

42. Tintle SN, Gwin DE, Andersen RC, Kumar AR. Soft tissue coverage of combat wounds. *J Surg Orthop Adv.* 2010;19:29-34.

43. Kumar AR, Grewal NS, Chung TL, Bradley JP. Lessons from operation Iraqi freedom: successful subacute reconstruction of complex lower extremity battle injuries. *Plast Reconstr Surg.* 2009;123:218-229.

44. Burns TC, Stinner DJ, Possley DR, et al. Does the zone of injury in combat-related type III open tibia fractures preclude use of local soft tissue coverage? *J Orthop Trauma.* 2010 [Epub ahead of print].

45. Tosenovsky P, Zalesak B, Janousek L, Koznar B. Microvascular steal syndrome in the pedal bypass and free muscle transfer. *Eur J Vasc Endovasc Surg.* 2003;26(5):562-564.

46. Sonntag BV, Murphy RX Jr, Chernofsky MA, Chowdary RP. Microvascular steal phenomenon in lower extremity reconstruction. *Ann Plast Surg.* 1995;34:336-339.

47. Pollak AN, McCarthy ML, Burgess AR. Short-term wound complications after application of flaps for coverage of traumatic soft-tissue defects about the tibia. The Lower Extremity Assessment Project (LEAP) Study Group. *J Bone Joint Surg Am.* 2000;82-A:1681-1691.

48. Orr J, Kirk KL, Antunez V, Ficke J. Reverse sural artery flap for reconstruction of blast injuries of the foot and ankle. *Foot Ankle Int.* 2010;31:59-64.

49. Kocialkowski A, Marsh DR, Shackley DC. Closure of the skin defect overlying infected non-union by skin traction. *Br J Plast Surg.* 1998;51:307-310.

50. Lenoble E, Lewertowski JM, Goutallier D. Reconstruction of compound tibial and soft tissue loss using a traction histiogenesis technique. *J Trauma.* 1995;39:356-360.

51. Lerner A, Ullmann Y, Stein H, Peled IJ. Using the Ilizarov external fixation device for skin expansion. *Ann Plast Surg.* 2000;45:535-537.

52. Nho SJ, Helfet DL, Rozbruch SR. Temporary intentional leg shortening and deformation to facilitate wound closure using the Ilizarov/Taylor Spatial Frame. *J Orthop Trauma.* 2006;20:419-424.

53. Rozbruch SR, Weitzman AM, Watson TJ, Freudigman P, Katz HV, Ilizarov S. Simultaneous treatment of tibial bone and soft-tissue defects with the Ilizarov Method. *J Orthop Trauma.* 2006;20:197-205.

54. Hsu JR, Beltran MJ. Shortening and angulation for soft-tissue reconstruction of extremity wounds in a combat support hospital. *Mil Med.* 2009;174:838-842.

55. Beltran MJ, Ochoa LM, Graves RM, Hsu JR. Composite bone and soft tissue loss treated with distraction histiogenesis. *J Surg Orthop Adv.* 2010;19:23-28.

56. Gulsen M, Ozkan C. Angular shortening and delayed gradual distraction for the treatment of asymmetrical bone and soft tissue defects of tibia: a case series. *J Trauma.* 2009;66:E61-E66.

57. Ilizarov GA. The tension-stress effect on the genesis and growth of tissues. Part I: the influence of stability on fixation and soft-tissue preservation. *Clin Orthop Relat Res.* 1989;238:249-281.

58. Ilizarov GA. The tension-stress effect on the genesis and growth of tissues. Part II: the influence of the rate and frequency of distraction. *Clin Orthop Relat Res.* 1989;239:263-285.

59. Prokuski L, Marsh JL. Segmental bone deficiency after acute trauma: the role of bone transport. *Orthop Clin North Am.* 1994;25:753-763.

60. Watson JT, Anders M, Moed BR. Management strategies for bone loss in tibial shaft fractures. *Clin Orthop Relat Res.* 1995;315:138-152.

61. Cierny G, Zorn KL. Segmental tibial defects, comparing conventional and Ilizarov methodologies. *Clin Orthop Relat Res.* 1994;301:118-133.

62. Cattaneo R, Catagni M, Johnson E. The treatment of infected nonunions and segmental defects of the tibia by the methods of Ilizarov. *Clin Orthop Relat Res.* 1992;280:143-152.

63. Mahaluxmivala J, Nadarajah R, Allen PW, Hill RA. Ilizarov external fixator: acute shortening and lengthening versus bone transport in the management of tibial non-unions. *Injury.* 2005;36(5):662-668.

64. Paley D, Maar DC. Ilizarov bone transport treatment for tibial defects. *J Orthop Trauma.* 2000;14:76-85.

65. Watson JT. Treatment of tibial fractures with bone loss. *Tech Orthop.* 1996;11:132-143.

66. Stevenson S. Biology of bone grafts. *Orthop Clin North Am.* 1999;30:543-552.

67. Green SA. Skeletal defects: a comparison of bone grafting and bone transport for segmental skeletal defects. *Clin Orthop Relat Res.* 1994;301:111-117.

68. Green SA, Jackson JM, Wall DM, Marinow H, Ishkanian J. Management of segmental defects by the Ilizarov intercalary bone transport method. *Clin Orthop Relat Res* 1992;280:136-142.

69. Porter RM, Liu F, Pilapil C, et al. Osteogenic potential of reamer irrigator aspirator (RIA) aspirate collected from patients undergoing hip arthroplasty. *J Orthop Res.* 2009;27:42-49.

70. Kobbe P, Tarkin IS, Frink M, Pape HC. Voluminous bone graft harvesting of the femoral marrow cavity for autologous transplantation. An indication for the "Reamer-Irrigator-Aspirator" technique. *Unfallchirurg.* 2008;111:469-472.

71. Fischer MD, Gustilo RB, Varecka TF. The timing of flap coverage, bone-grafting, and intramedullary nailing in patients who have a fracture of the tibial shaft with extensive soft-tissue injury. *J Bone Joint Surg Am.* 1991;73-A:1316-1322.

72. Blick SS, Brumback RJ, Lakatos R, Poka A, Burgess AR. Early prophylactic bone grafting of high-energy tibial fractures. *Clin Orthop Relat Res.* 1989;240:21-41.

73. Masquelet AC, Begue T. The concept of induced membrane for reconstruction of long bone defects. *Orthop Clin North Am.* 2010;41:27-37.

74. Pelissier P, Masquelet AC, Bareille R, Pelissier SM, Amedee J. Induced membranes secrete growth factors including vascular and osteoinductive factors and could stimulate bone regeneration. *J Orthop Res.* 2004;22(1):73-79.

75. Pelissier P, Martin D, Baudet J, Lepreux S, Masquelet AC. Behaviour of cancellous bone graft placed in induced membranes. *Br J Plast Surg.* 2002;55(7):596-598.

76. Harmon PH. A simplified surgical approach to the posterior tibia for bone-grafting and fibular transference. *J Bone Joint Surg Am.* 1945;27:496-498.

77. Hertel L, Gerber A, Schlegel U, Cordey J, Ruegsegger P, Rahn BA. Cancellous bone graft for skeletal reconstruction. Muscular versus periosteal bed—preliminary results. *Injury.* 1994;25:S59-S70.

78. Weiland AJ, Phillips TW, Randolph MA. Bone graft: a radiological, histological, and biomechanical model comparing autografts, allografts, and free vascularized bone grafts. *Plast Reconstr Surg.* 1984;74:368-379.

79. Younger EM, Chapman MW. Morbidity at bone graft donor sites. *J Orthop Trauma.* 1989;3:192-195.

80. Weiland AJ, Moore JR, Daniel RK. The efficacy of free tissue transfer in the treatment of osteomyelitis. *J Bone Joint Surg Am.* 1984;66:181-193.

81. Taylor GI, Miller GD, Ham FJ. The free vascularized bone graft: a clinical extension of microvascular techniques. *Plast Reconstr Surg.* 1975;55:533-544.

82. DeCoster TA, Gehlert RJ, Mikola EA, Pirela-Cruz MA. Management of posttraumatic segmental bone defects. *J Am Acad Orthop Surg.* 2004;12:28-38.

83. Khan MZ, Downing, ND, Henry AP. Tibial reconstruction by ipsilateral vascularized fibular transfer. *Injury.* 1996;27:651-654.

84. Catagni MA, Camagni M, Combi A, Ottaviani G. Medial fibula transport with the Ilizarov frame to treat massive tibial bone loss. *Clin Orthop Relat Res.* 2006;448:208-216.

85. Weiland AJ. Current concepts review: vascularized free bone transplants. *J Bone Joint Surg Am.* 1981;63:166-169.

86. Vail TP, Urbaniak JR. Donor-site morbidity with use of vascularized autogenous fibular grafts. *J Bone Joint Surg Am.* 1996;78:204-211.

87. Rozbruch SR, Ilizarov S, eds. *Limb Lengthening and Reconstructive Surgery.* New York, NY: Informa Healthcare; 2007.

88. Raschke MJ, Mann JW, Oedekoven G, Claudi BF. Segmental transport after unreamed intramedullary nailing: preliminary report of a "monorail" system. *Clin Orthop Relat Res.* 1992;282:233-240.

89. Sen C, Kocaoglu M, Eralp L, Gulsen M, Cinar M. Bifocal compression distraction in the acute treatment of grade III open tibia fractures with bone and soft tissue loss: a report of 24 cases. *J Orthop Trauma.* 2004;18:150-157.

90. Watson JT. Distraction osteogenesis. *J Am Acad Orthop Surg.* 2006;14:S168-S174.

91. Paley D, Catagni MA, Argnani F, Villa A, Benedetti GB, Cattaneo R. Ilizarov treatment of tibial nonunions with bone loss. *Clin Orthop Relat Res.* 1989;2241:146-165.

92. Gold SM, Wasserman R. Preliminary results of tibial bone transports with pulsed low intensity ultrasound (Exogen). *J Orthop Trauma.* 2005;19:10-16.

93. Moroni A, Vannini F, Mosca M, Giannini S. State of the art review: techniques to avoid pin loosening and infection in external fixation. *J Orthop Trauma.* 2002;16:189-195.

94. Moroni A, Heikkila J, Magyar G, Toksvig-Larsen S, Giannini S. Fixation strength and pin tract infection of hydroxyapatite-coated tapered pins. *Clin Orthop Relat Res.* 2001;388:209-217.

95. Frierson M, Ibrahim K, Boles M, Bote H, Ganey T. Distraction osteogenesis: a comparison of corticotomy techniques. *Clin Orthop Relat Res.* 1994;301:19-24.

96. Gonzalez MH, Tarandy DI, Troy D, Phillips D, Weinzweig N. Free tissue coverage of chronic traumatic wounds of the lower leg. *Plast Reconstr Surg.* 2002;109:592-600.

97. Redett RJ, Robertson BC, Chang B, Girotto J, Vaughan T. Limb salvage of lower-extremity wounds using free gracilis reconstruction. *Plast Reconstr Surg.* 2000;106:1507-1513.

Chapter **22**

COMBAT-RELATED LOWER EXTREMITY AMPUTATIONS

MAJ Benjamin K. Potter, MD; LT Scott Tintle, MD; and
LCDR Jonathan Agner Forsberg, MD

The oldest known archeological evidence of an extremity amputation was found in modern-day Iraq and is more than 45,000 years old.[1] Since that time, the technical performance of extremity amputations as well as the indications for amputation have dramatically changed. With war remaining a nearly constant occurrence and weaponry having become progressively more destructive, there is an increasing prevalence of combat-related amputees worldwide. For thousands of years, the sacrifices of the combat wounded and the innovation and efforts of their surgeons have improved and advanced medicine and surgery. With regard to extremity amputations, the influence of Hippocrates and Celsus propagated the most significant changes in ancient amputation techniques, including the use of vessel ligation and wound compression to achieve hemostasis.[1] Their contributions developed into what we would recognize today as a nearly modern amputation technique.

A paradigm shift during the Napoleonic era, led by military surgeons George Guthrie and Dominique Jean Larrey, was equally important to combat surgery.[1] The two developed a system in which trained personnel received and evacuated the wounded. This represented a fundamental (and revolutionary) shift toward the performance of early, life-saving battlefield amputations of severely injured extremities and likely contributed to fewer battlefield fatalities than would have been expected otherwise. Prior to their influence, severely injured extremities were frequently symptomatically treated, and delayed amputations were performed 2 to 3 weeks after the initial injuries if the patient survived.[1]

With rapidly developing weapons, the American Civil War saw the first dramatic increase in the rate of amputations as a result of the French minie ball, which created extensive bone and soft tissue damage upon impact.[1] Since then, the development and progression of battlefield medicine; limb salvage capabilities; and the fields of orthopedic, plastic, and vascular surgery have generally led to decreased amputation rates as a result of combat injury. The Vietnam War is the exception, with a relative increase in the percentage of amputations due to increasingly destructive high-velocity firearms, landmines, and booby-traps[2,3] that led to more severe extremity injuries. Additionally, the introduction of body armor, an improved medical evacuation system, and the forward movement of medical capabilities and personnel led to an increased survival of American warriors, which likely contributed to the increase in the amputation incidence.[4]

Amputation rates of the current US conflicts in the Middle East have changed minimally since the Vietnam War.[4,5] The overall amputation rate remains elevated from prior wars and continues to underscore the increased destructiveness of modern weaponry and explosives as well as the increased survivability of combat injuries due to the aforementioned changes and resources. The robust amputee population from the recent conflicts highlights the fact that, despite the advancement of battlefield medicine and limb salvage surgery, amputation remains an important and all-too-often necessary facet of battlefield medicine.[4]

Owens BD, Belmont PJ Jr, eds. *Combat Orthopedic Surgery:
Lessons Learned in Iraq and Afghanistan (pp 205-220)*
© 2011 SLACK Incorporated

Epidemiology

In a review by Owens and colleagues[6] in 2007, 82% of combat casualties from the current conflicts were found to have sustained extremity injuries. Traumatic and trauma-related battlefield amputations from these conflicts comprise approximately 2.3% of all battlefield injuries, 5.4% of serious injuries, and 7.4% of major limb injuries.[4,7] As previously mentioned, these rates are consistent with the Vietnam War, yet would likely be markedly higher were it not for the improved medical evacuation and far-forward deployment of advanced medical resources, which have evolved in parallel with the advent of the devastating, and ubiquitous, improvised explosive device (IED).[4,5]

Despite the Lower Extremity Assessment Project (LEAP) study reviewing the economic impact of severe lower extremity trauma in the civilian population, this topic has been largely unstudied in the military population.[8] In a review by Masini and colleagues,[9] the initial inpatient utilization of resources for US combat-wounded patients from the recent conflicts was investigated, and the authors found that combat-related extremity injuries require the greatest use of resources in the initial post-injury period, cause the greatest number of disabled military servicemembers, and have the greatest projected disability benefit costs. The authors commented that the numbers they derived were likely conservative due to the fact that the study did not include outpatient visits, prosthesis costs, or rehabilitation expenditures that will inevitably and dramatically exceed initial inpatient resource use.[9]

In spite of the advancement in prosthetics, rehabilitation, and the re-establishment of regional amputation centers at strategic military treatment facilities, the return to active duty following amputation was recently shown to be only 16.5%.[10] Additionally, officers and senior enlisted returned to duty at significantly higher rates of 35.3% and 25.5%, respectively, versus the junior enlisted rate of 7.0%. Multiple extremity amputees had a return to active duty rate of only 3%.[10] It is worth noting, however, that active duty retention likely depends as much on the patient's wishes and willingness or ability to reclassify to a different military occupational specialty, when necessary, as it does on specific injuries or amputations.

Management in Theater

TOURNIQUET USE

The development of a practical, one-handed, and intuitive field tourniquet with universal training and distribution was a significant advance in modern battlefield medicine. This is a dramatic improvement from the tourniquet's historical (and largely anecdotal) application as a last resort following the onset of shock. An educational campaign directed toward not only battlefield medical personnel but toward all military servicemembers has focused on the benefit of early application in the setting of a severely injured extremity. Widespread use of the battlefield tourniquet has since shown consistent benefit in controlling life-threatening hemorrhage following major extremity trauma.[11,12]

LIMB SALVAGE VERSUS AMPUTATION

The goals of limb salvage are to provide a functional limb with reasonable sensation and practical mobility. Predicting which limbs will ultimately possess this capacity is difficult. In the combat-wounded patient, the salvage of life is the utmost priority, and patient stability is the most critical variable when choosing to pursue initial limb salvage versus amputation. The mechanisms of injury, commonly blasts and high-energy projectiles, produce severe extremity and systemic trauma and often also include thoraco-abdominal and head trauma. The result is a severely wounded patient for whom the salvage of life may preclude heroic early limb salvage efforts. In these instances, stopping the hemorrhage to save the patient's life often makes an emergent amputation the only option afforded to the combat surgeon (Figure 22-1).

The absolute indications for major extremity amputation remain a mangled extremity with a patient in extremis or an unrepairable vascular injury with a warm ischemia time of greater than 6 hours. There are numerous relative indications, and frequently the combination of a few of these relative indications should and will lead to early amputation.[13] While vascular injury was historically a major indication for amputation, reperfusion by a general or vascular surgeon can frequently be accomplished in a far-forward setting. Likewise, the absence of plantar sensation, historically a relative indication for amputation, is no longer used in the absence of documented tibial nerve transection or loss.[14] Massive loss of bone, also an historical relative indication for amputation, can now be temporarily stabilized using external fixation and reconstructed using advanced reconstruction techniques including free vascularized bone grafting or a bone-transport procedure.[15,16]

The severity of soft tissue injury thus appears to be the best predictor of long-term function, as we currently have no good solution for massive volumetric muscle loss. The loss of muscle in multiple compartments carries a poor prognosis and often results in delayed amputation when initial limb salvage is attempted. Despite the battlefield indications for amputation,

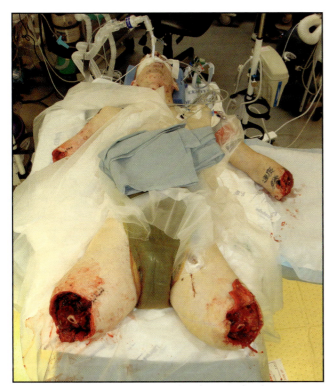

Figure 22-1. Clinical photograph of a quadruple amputee. The patient sustained severe injuries to all 4 extremities as well as an open carotid laceration. In addition to the relative indication of near-traumatic amputations, immediate definitive amputation of all limbs was required in order to control hemorrhage and save the patient's life.

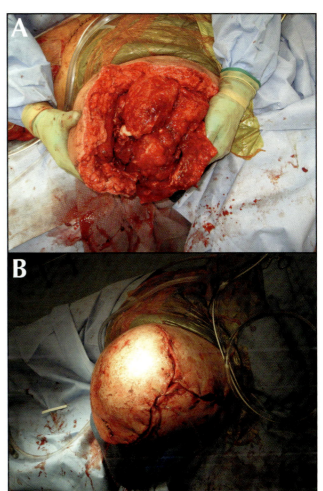

Figure 22-2. Intraoperative clinical photographs of a transfemoral amputation. Despite the irregular appearance of the fasciocutaneous flaps (A), early salvage of this viable tissue permitted maintenance of critical residual limb length and delayed primary closure (B) at a functional level at the time of definitive revision.

the limb should be spared whenever practicable, and conditions for subsequent reassessment and informed discussion should be established. It is imperative that discussion regarding the severity of an extremity injury begins with the patient as soon as he or she is capable. Discussions with the patient by treating surgeons should be predicated on the following important concept: while the preservation of a questionably salvageable limb for the benefit of facilitating the definitive amputation can substantially improve the ability to preserve limb length as well as the quality of soft tissue coverage, it can also prove psychologically damaging to a patient who has become convinced that sensate and functional extremity salvage is practicable because of the persistence of his or her "intact" limb up to that point. Early, frank discussions with patients and family about the anticipated practicality and outcomes of definitive limb salvage versus amputation are therefore a necessity.

EARLY SURGICAL GOALS

In addition to salvage of life, the initial goals when treating severe extremity injuries are the expeditious control of hemorrhage, debridement of the contaminated wounds, and preservation of as much

salvageable tissue as possible. All devitalized muscle, skin, and bone must be removed during both the initial and each ensuing debridement. Conversely, any viable muscle, bone, and fasciocutaneous tissue should be maintained for possible use in the definitive reconstruction as "flaps of opportunity" (Figure 22-2). At this time, there is no indication to perform a "guillotine" amputation. It is an antiquated technique that then requires additional and substantial bone shortening to allow for adequate soft tissue coverage of the residual limb (Figure 22-3).

An extremely important principle in the management of combat amputations is that the wounds should remain open until thorough, serial, and adequate debridement occurs and the wound remains stable.[17] Negative pressure wound therapy allows for safe wound containment in the care of combat amputations while allowing the wound to remain

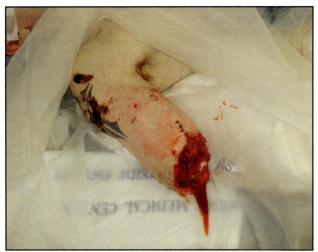

Figure 22-3. Clinical photograph of a guillotine transhumeral amputation. This antiquated technique is highlighted only to be condemned; guillotine amputations compromise subsequent reconstructive efforts and require substantial shortening for definitive coverage and closure. Furthermore, there is no evidence that guillotine amputations decrease blood loss or improve patient survival over the preferred, modern technique of open, length-preserving amputation.

open for serial assessment and debridement. While the role of negative pressure wound therapy throughout the medical evacuation chain continues to evolve, its use at definitive treatment centers is well-established. The wound vacuum-assisted closure has been suggested to decrease edema and facilitate wound closure by applying macrostrain to soft tissues, stimulating fibroblast proliferation, removing destructive proteinases from the wound, facilitating bacterial clearance from the wound, and limiting cross contamination from the patient's environment.[18,19] These benefits, especially when espoused with the use of vessel loops in a so-called Jacob's ladder or shoelace manner, have likely contributed to the salvage of amputation length similar to the highly touted skin traction techniques that were practiced in Vietnam and previous conflicts.[20]

In addition to the use of negative pressure wound therapy, antibiotic-impregnated polymethylmethacrylate beads have also been frequently used in the early and provisional management of lower extremity amputations. While difficult to study in humans due to host and wound variability, animal data have demonstrated efficacy of local antibiotic beads within wounds to prevent infection.[21] While so-called bead pouches and the temporary closure of residual limbs over antibiotic beads have been used, antibiotic beads are also frequently used in conjunction with negative pressure wound therapy, but the efficacy of this regimen remains unproven to date.

Definitive Management

LEVEL SELECTION

Amputation length in combat trauma is often predetermined based upon the location of the worst soft tissue injury. Energy considerations are of utmost importance, as increasing oxygen is required with each progressively more proximal amputation level.[22-25] This is a major reason why a longer residual limb is usually associated with better functional outcomes. One distinct exception to this occurs in the setting of severe foot and ankle injuries. Although early salvage of hindfoot or Symes amputations is indicated, the authors prefer to recommend a transtibial amputation to our patients. The transtibial level allows for optimal prosthetic fit and a more robust soft tissue envelope and frequently allows previously high-functioning people to return to their pre-amputation activities.

One additional situation with regard to level selection warrants special mention. Through-the-knee amputations were originally a popular level of amputation prior to the introduction of anesthesia. The lack of bone cuts made the procedure quick and hemodynamically attractive, as there was minimal blood loss. Early in the development of this level of amputation, a posterior fasciocutaneous flap was used, providing little to no padding over the distal femoral condyles as it was felt that this was a "weight bearing" amputation level.[1] Because of this poor soft tissue coverage, however, the through-the-knee amputation quickly fell out of favor due to patient rejection of prostheses.[1] The more recent introduction of a long posterior myofasciocutaneous flap that padded the distal femoral condyles has increased the popularity of this level.[26-28] However, the role of knee disarticulation remains somewhat limited in trauma due to the fact that a high transtibial amputation can often be performed when there is viable gastrocnemius available for coverage; it is a relatively rare situation that there is adequate gastrocnemius available for the long posterior myofasciocutaneous flap but complete loss of the proximal tibia. The LEAP study did not show much success with its 17 knee disarticulations. These patients did very poorly, but it was noted that at least 12 of them had no gastrocnemius available for distal bone coverage, and it was reported that definitive closure of this level occurred much later than those for transtibial or transfemoral amputations, further suggesting that marginal soft tissues were used for coverage.[8] This is likely a major reason for the poor outcomes associated with this level in that study. Transfemoral amputation may have been more appropriate due to the lack of adequate myofasciocutaneous coverage in those instances.[1,25]

AMPUTATION CLOSURE AND WOUND COVERAGE

Atypical flap coverage is very common in combat-related amputations, and closure usually occurs within the zone of injury. While the LEAP study suggested that there is not a higher rate of complications in their civilian patients treated with atypical flap coverage, we have noted both a higher rate of wound problems and an increased rate of heterotopic ossification (HO) with atypical flap coverage within the zone of injury.[8,29,30] Despite the increased complication and HO rates, closure within the zone of injury is often indicated to salvage residual limb length or functional joint levels. In certain situations, such as when attempting to salvage the knee joint (Figure 22-4), the use of split-thickness skin grafting and even free tissue transfer may be warranted in order to maintain length. However, the performance of such heroic length- or level-saving procedures will often result in an increased rate of wound complications, delayed prosthetic fitting, and frequent late revision surgery.[31-44] Nonetheless, the authors believe that such measures are warranted in select cases.

Likewise, the use of turn-up techniques can also be useful in the preservation of amputation length in the combat wounded. The tibial turn-up technique has been described to salvage transtibial-level amputations as well as to increase the length of transfemoral amputees.[45-48] We have used both techniques with good early results (Figure 22-5). The premise of this operation is to use the healthy distal portion of tibia with sound posterior skin and soft tissues to replace the more proximal tibial bone and anterior soft tissue loss. Prerequisite to performing this vascularized rotational flap is a healthy, patent posterior tibial artery from which the bone and posterior soft tissues are supplied.

SOFT TISSUE MANAGEMENT

Muscle

The proper management of the residual muscle is critical to the outcome of a combat-related amputation. Myofascial and myoplasty techniques are frequently performed in dysvascular and even civilian trauma amputee populations, and most extremity surgeons are familiar with these techniques.[8,49,50] It is important to note that though they are useful supplemental techniques in the combat amputee, neither should be performed in isolation. Rather, myodesis is the preferred technique of soft tissue stabilization following trauma-related amputation.[51,52] Myodesis is performed by suturing the muscular fascia to the distal end of the bone via drill holes or by direct suturing to the periosteum.

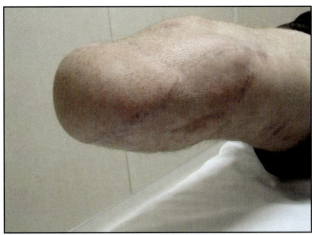

Figure 22-4. Clinical photograph of a proximal transtibial amputation in which a free latissimus dorsi myofasciocutaneous flap and subsequent split-thickness skin grafting were used to salvage a functional and uninjured knee joint.

Myofascial and myoplasty techniques are then performed to supplement the myodesis to improve the contour of the distal residual limb. While no definitive evidence exists to support myodesis over the other techniques, our institutional experience with scores of lower extremity amputees presenting with findings of myodesis or myoplasty failure (a painful residual limb and an unstabilized or retracted muscle mass and poor distal bone coverage) highlights the importance of a well-performed myodesis (Figure 22-6). Tenodesis is also an acceptable form of muscle stabilization at appropriate amputation levels.

Nerve

Symptomatic neuromata accompany 0% to 25% of major limb amputations and are a frequent indication for revision surgery.[53-55] Noxious stimuli such as stretching and pressure near the amputation closure or the distal end of the limb may lead to pain, resulting in limited prosthesis wear and ambulation. Multiple techniques have been suggested for dealing with the nerves at the time of amputation.[55-59] None has proven superior to a carefully performed traction neurectomy and burying the cut nerve ends deep in the proximal soft tissues. The traction neurectomy places the severed nerve and resulting neuroma away from the scarring, ligated blood vessels, and distal end of the residual limb. It is recommended for all named and other grossly visible nerves of the lower extremity at the various amputation levels. The anecdotal experience of the authors has found this step to be one frequently overlooked by surgeons performing an amputation. When performing a traction neurectomy of the sciatic nerve proximally in high transfemoral amputations, the nerve may be ligated prior to transection to avoid bleeding from the substantive vaso nervosum.

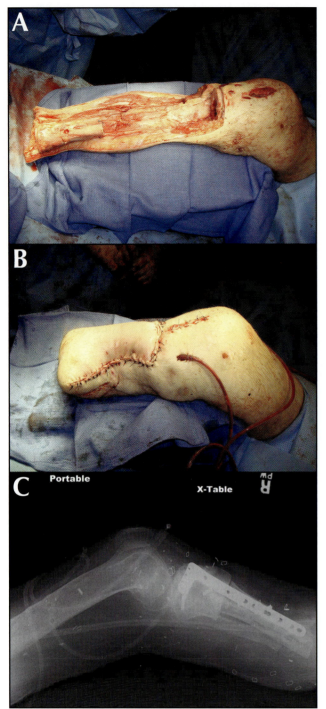

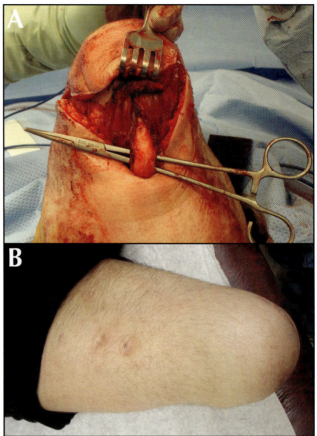

Figure 22-6. Clinical photographs of transfemoral amputations demonstrating (A) a conical residual limb resulting from inadequate supplementary myoplasty of the hamstrings to the quadriceps apron, permitting retraction of the soft tissues over time, and (B) a more desirable, cylindrical and rounded, residual limb with robust soft tissue coverage following hamstring myodesis and quadriceps myoplasty. In the first patient, the sciatic nerve (running over the tonsil hemostat) has unfortunately been left long, and the resulting neuroma, in addition to the poor soft tissue coverage, caused distal symptoms during prosthesis wear for ambulation.

Figure 22-5. Intraoperative clinical photographs demonstrating the soft tissue dissection with maintenance of distal posterior myofasciocutaneous and osseous blood supply (A) and definitive closure (B) of a tibial turn-up plasty to salvage a transtibial amputation level in a patient with an infected non-union of the proximal tibia with segmental bone loss. (C) Postoperative lateral radiograph from the same case. The patient ambulated without difficulty in a prosthesis at 12 weeks postoperatively, after allowing for initial bone healing. In addition to protection of the distal soft tissue and osseous blood supply, the procedure requires anticipation of difficult proximal soft tissue closure and a greater-than-intuitive intercalary soft tissue gap to accommodate the 180-degree rotation of the distal bone.

Postoperative Care

Vigilance in the early postoperative period is indicated based on the high rate of early wound infections and wound healing complications that occur after the performance of combat-related amputations within the zones of injury.[30] Frequently used postoperative bandage techniques following amputation are soft and rigid dressings and the immediate postoperative prosthesis (IPOP).[60-66] Each technique has advantages and disadvantages, but none has proven superior in the avoidance of complications or improving outcomes. The principles behind each technique, however, are to provide gentle, balanced compression to the residual limb in order to control swelling, decrease pain, and attempt to stabilize limb volume.

Rigid dressings and the IPOP have frequently been used following transtibial and more distal amputations. The benefit of the rigid dressing lies in its ability to control edema, prevent joint contractures, and improve pain control. Despite multiple studies showing trends toward improved wound healing and improved pain control with a rigid dressing, we caution its use in the combat amputee.[60-66] The authors advocate, instead, soft bandages in most instances due to the ease of wound inspection, the improved ability to mobilize patients early, and the decreased risk of pressure ulceration, particularly over the patella. It is the opinion of the authors that rigid dressings are hazardous in the setting of combat amputees rendered insensate by regional anesthesia. Nevertheless, certain situations may require the use of rigid dressings in the form of splinting material, for instance, on the residual limb. This technique should be employed with extreme caution. Despite traditional teaching, rigid dressings are frequently not necessary, even at the transtibial level, as the limb can be adequately and safely splinted in extension through the generous use of soft cast padding. Additionally, knee contractures are rarely problematic in our patient population who are routinely treated with early physical therapy and mobilization.

The IPOP was proposed shortly after World War I and has been intermittently used, advocated, and modified following all wars up until the current conflicts.[67-70] The benefits of IPOP have been demonstrated mainly in a nontrauma population and largely include improved psychological outlook, less perceived loss of function, shorter hospital stays, and a faster time to initial prosthesis fitting.[61,65,71,72] In the combat amputees who are almost invariably receiving treatment at a national amputee center, the psychological benefits would likely prove less evident; our patients have immediate peer support and exposure to high-performance amputees from the time of admission to one of these centers. Additionally, the high risk of early wound breakdown and infection, coupled with concomitant injuries that frequently preclude early ambulation with a prosthesis, make the IPOP unwarranted in the combat population in most instances.

Surgical Technique

A detailed discussion of every operative step for each amputation level is beyond the scope of this chapter, and frequently atypical closures or coverage are required in the combat-related amputation setting. The following sections highlight important considerations and pitfalls in the performance of definitive amputation, revision amputations, and closure at specific amputation levels.

LISFRANC/CHOPART AMPUTATIONS

These levels are often given little consideration in the young active combat amputee due to frequent injury to or loss of plantar tissues, difficult prosthetic fitting, and difficulty in returning to athletic and running activities. There are 2 proposed benefits that warrant consideration in a patient satisfied with a more sedentary lifestyle or with excellent soft tissue coverage. Patients are frequently capable of weight bearing on these levels without the use of a prosthesis, and these levels have the optimal cosmetic appearance.[1] However, the negatives of these levels deter their performance in the combat-wounded population. Prosthetic fitting can be difficult with these distal level amputations and, more importantly, the powerful plantarflexors of the foot often overpower the weaker remaining extensors and contort the foot into a poorly functioning equinovarus deformity.[73]

In attempts to prevent these equinovarus deformities, significant (but often humbling) efforts are warranted. Multiple procedures to include percutaneous heel cord lengthening, cast immobilization in dorsiflexion, external fixation in dorsiflexion, tenomyoplastic procedures, and even fusion of the midtarsal joints to prevent this deformity have been proposed.[74-77] In our limited experience with these levels, the combat-wounded amputee is seldom satisfied with his or her functional result, but good results are occasionally achieved for patients in whom both aggressive tendon balancing and early therapy are successful.

SYMES

The Symes ankle disarticulation, originally described by James Symes in 1843, has been met with varying levels of acceptance around the world.[78] It has been very popular in Europe and Canada but less well accepted in the United States. The significant advantage of this amputation level is the potential to bear weight on the residual limb in the absence of a prosthesis.[79] Despite this highly touted benefit, multiple studies have demonstrated that 30% to 50% of amputees are not capable of bearing full weight through their residual limb without a prosthesis.[60,79] This level of amputation may be useful in the elderly diabetic population due to the decreased energy required for ambulation; however, its role in the combat-wounded patient should be limited. The improved cosmesis, the numerous prosthetic options, and the functional outcomes of transtibial amputees make a transtibial amputation more desirable for most combat-wounded warriors.[2,80,81]

Prerequisites to the performance of the Symes level of amputation include a patent posterior tibial artery and an intact, robust heel pad, which ultimately forms the padding for the residual limb.[82,83] Technically, the malleoli should be narrowed modestly in a fashion that still allows for the benefits of a supramalleolar fit of a prosthesis but also minimizes the extruding bony prominences to prevent painful bursal formation or skin breakdown.[84,85] The final priority is the maintenance of the mobile but secure heel pad beneath the tibia. The heel pad is pulled, and often migrates, posteriorly by the force of the triceps surae. Tenodesis of the Achilles tendon to the distal tibia to maintain the heel pad directly in line with the tibia is therefore imperative when performing this amputation.[86]

Transtibial Amputation

This is the most common level of amputation following combat trauma. It is the least debilitating of the major amputation levels and requires less energy for ambulation than more proximal levels.[87,88] Prosthesis use at this level is maximized. A study by Purry and Hannon[81] reported that 84% of their patients wore a prosthesis for more than 13 hours a day. Seventy-two percent of their patients could walk farther than a mile, and 84% considered themselves only minimally disabled. In a 2001 study of Vietnam War amputees with 28 years of follow-up, Dougherty[2] reported that isolated transtibial amputees without other injuries had SF-36 scores similar to population controls without an amputation. A study of Iranian veterans by Taghipour[80] in 2009 reported slightly contrasting results in that the SF-36 scores of their transtibial amputees were significantly lower than a control group; however, the SF-36 scores still remained significantly higher than those of transfemoral amputees.

The standard Burgess technique for amputation at this level is frequently performed in the primary setting. General guidelines for optimal residual limb length include 2.5 cm of bone for every 30 cm of a patient's height. This usually translates to between 12.5 and 17.5 cm of residual tibia as measured from the medial tibial plateau, although we recommend adding 1 to 2 cm to this calculation for patients in whom robust and healthy soft tissue coverage permits.[89] The fibula should be transected about 1 to 2 cm proximal to the tibial osteotomy to ensure that the fibula does not become prominent and painful with prosthetic wear. Important considerations include beveling the anterior tibia and posterolateral fibula to prevent a sharp edge that may prove painful in the future and careful traction neurectomies of the saphenous, sural, superficial and deep peroneal, and tibial nerves. This step is not particularly difficult or time consuming, and it may prevent significant long-term pain and revision surgery in the future. Locating

the sural nerve proximally between the 2 heads of the gastrocnemius via an anterior approach through the wound will allow the sural nerve end to retract out of the distal subcutaneous tissue that will drape over the distal end of the residual limb while maintaining the vascularity of the posterior skin flap (Figure 22-7). Despite the LEAP study finding that only 22.8% of transtibial amputees had a myodesis performed, the authors emphatically stress the importance of performing this critical step at this and all levels of amputation in the combat-wounded amputee.[8]

DISTAL TIBIOFIBULAR SYNOSTOSIS

The creation of a synostosis between the distal tibia and the fibula following transtibial amputation was first proposed by Bier in 1892 but subsequently popularized by von Ertl.[1] Ertl and his proponents describe that his modification allowed for a more normal, end-bearing residual limb.[90] In the many years since its description, multiple modifications to the original technique have been suggested, and it has been the subject of many heated debates both within and outside of the literature.[91,92] In 2006, Pinzur and colleagues[93] indicated that patient-perceived outcomes may be improved by performing the distal tibiofibular synostosis. However, he was unable to reproduce these results in a similar study using the prior data from Brazil and his own patients in the United States.[94] While evidence suggests that it can safely be performed in the young patient population without significant untoward events, the indications for and benefits of performing this procedure remain controversial.[30] To date, there is no definitive evidence demonstrating improved patient outcomes after the performance of a bone bridging amputation, and there are unique complications seen in the follow-up of these patients. We have performed multiple revision surgeries for nonunions and for prominent hardware or suture that were used for fixation of the bone strut. Nonetheless, this surgery is still performed in carefully selected patients by ourselves and other surgeons at our institution after detailed preoperative counseling, and we will perform this as a revision surgery when a patient strongly desires it or when late symptomatic fibular instability occurs. We recommend using #5 nonabsorbable suture or the Tightrope suture bridge device (Arthrex Inc, Naples, FL) for bone bridge fixation as it is stable but pliable and may be less prone to implant failure or late implant-related symptoms. We routinely remove the silicone-coated Fiberwire suture from the Tightrope suture washers and replace it with #5 braided nylon suture due to concerns about host reactions to silicone.[95] However, good results have also been achieved with screw fixation (Figure 22-8).

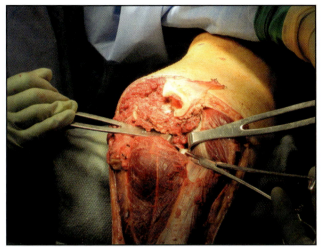

Figure 22-7. Intraoperative clinical photograph of the sural nerve identified and isolated proximally, without devascularization or stripping of the posterior fasciocutaneous flap, by limited splitting of the soleus median and the raphe between the medial and lateral heads of the gastrocnemius via an anterior approach. This technique leaves the posterior soft tissues intact and vascularized, but allows transection of the sural nerve proximal to the weight-bearing distal residual limb and prevents symptoms due to the inevitable sural neuroma. Identifying the nerve distally and providing traction with a hemostat is useful for localizing the nerve superficial or deep (depending on the patient and the level of amputation) to the fascia of the posterior triceps surae.

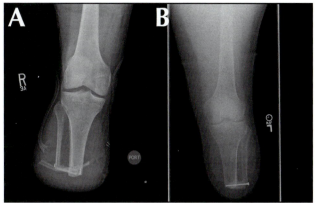

Figure 22-8. Postoperative anterior-posterior radiographs of transtibial amputations performed with a so-called modified Ertl, distal tibiofibular bridge synostosis technique stabilized with (A) a Tightrope suture bridge and (B) screw fixation.

Knee Disarticulation

As previously mentioned, the LEAP study has recently cast a negative light on through-the-knee amputations. Their patients with through-the-knee amputations had the lowest walking speed and lowest self-reported outcome scores.[8] Despite these findings, other studies in nontrauma populations have reported better walking stability, a decreased metabolic cost of ambulation, and higher scores on the physical component of the SF-36 as compared to transfemoral amputees.[25,80,96] Additionally, the longer lever arm allows for better sitting balance, and the improved biomechanics as a result of the maintained adductor insertional footprint and the improved proprioception of this level have led to improved outcomes and popularity at this level in nontrauma populations.[97] When a knee disarticulation with gastrocnemius coverage and a tenodesis of the patellar tendon can be performed with subsequent gastrocnemius to extensor retinaculum myoplasty, we recommend this level over a more proximal transfemoral amputation. Even greater consideration to knee disarticulation is warranted in the patient with a contralateral knee disarticulation or transfemoral amputation, as many of the drawbacks of this level, relative knee level asymmetry and space for prosthetic components, are obviated by the absence of the other knee.

When performing a through-the-knee amputation, careful ligation of the popliteal artery must be performed distal to the sural artery take-off to preserve the blood supply to the gastrocnemius. If debridement of the gastrocnemius is necessary, the sural artery pedicle must also be protected as it enters each head of the gastrocnemius 1 to 2 cm from their origin. The leg is sharply removed through the knee, and the patellar tendon is sharply dissected off of the tibial tubercle in order to maintain tendon length for tenodesis to the cruciate remnants, which should likewise be released from the tibial side. The patella may then be removed at the surgeon's discretion in attempts at preventing patellofemoral pain, although we do not do this routinely in the absence of overt chondral injury or other indication. Modest trimming of the medial and lateral condyles is sometimes performed to decrease their bulk. More significant trimming, including posterior condylectomy, can be performed when necessary depending on the length of the posterior myofasciocutaneous flap for coverage.

Transfemoral Amputations

Transfemoral amputations require significantly more energy for ambulation than more distal amputations. This is due to a shorter lever arm as well as the loss of an increasing number of muscle insertions as the level of amputation is made more proximally. Unfortunately, this amputation is all too frequently performed without consideration for the resulting biomechanical changes of the residual limb. The LEAP study demonstrated that only 53.3% of transfemoral amputations performed for trauma underwent adductor myodesis.[8] Gottschalk and Stills[98] demonstrated that the loss of the adductor magnus insertion that occurs from a transfemoral amputation leads to an overall loss of 70% of the adductor moment on the femur. The result is an unopposed pull of the hip abductors leading to an abduction deformity and a lateral drift of the femur within the soft tissue envelope. This abducted position also renders the abductors ineffective in maintaining normal pelvic tilt and leads to an abductor lurch during swing phase, further increasing energy consumption. Gottschalk's work, along with other studies, demonstrated the importance of performing an adductor myodesis during a transfemoral amputation, and this has dramatically improved modern transfemoral amputee function.[99-101]

After the adductor magnus tendon is identified and tagged, the distal 9 to 12 cm of the femur is removed in order to ensure robust distal soft tissue padding to leave room for prosthetic components and maintenance of equal knee levels. All of the nerves, to include both divisions of the sciatic nerve (at distal levels), the saphenous and terminal femoral and obturator nerves, and the posterior and lateral femoral cutaneous nerves, need to be identified and traction neurectomies performed. Double ligation of the vessels using suture ligatures on the femoral artery, and the adductor magnus myodesis to the lateral cortex should be performed, when possible, with the residual limb maximally adducted and slightly extended. The adductor magnus may be further stabilized with medial suture to avoid posterior subluxation and loss of muscle tension. Following this, we advocate semimembranosis myodesis to prevent a flexion deformity and to further stabilize the subsequent hamstring-quadriceps myoplasty. Secondary myoplasty of additional muscle groups (eg, the sartorius, gracilis, semitendinosis, and biceps femoris) may be performed deep to the quadriceps apron in an effort to prevent soft tissue retraction and the resulting conical residual limb shape. The quadriceps apron is then pulled distally over the end of the residual limb, and a myoplasty is performed, providing robust musculotendinous padding over the residual limb.

Hip Disarticulation

Hip disarticulations are amputations of last resort that are usually performed in an attempt to stop life-threatening hemorrhage. Historically, these amputees have functioned poorly and have often been bound to wheelchairs. Recently, however, through the use of modern suction-fit, microprocessor-assisted prostheses, remarkable function has been recovered by some patients following hip disarticulation. A high transfemoral amputation proximal to the lesser trochanter will function as a hip disarticulation, and consideration toward a hip fusion should be given. The flap for closure is electively based upon the gluteal musculature posterolaterally. In the trauma setting, any available flap, and sometimes even rotational rectus flaps, may be needed for soft tissue coverage. The femoral, sciatic, and obturator nerves must be identified and transected or ligated as they exit the true pelvis as far proximal as possible to avoid symptomatic neuroma formation.[1] Suture ligatures should be used to ligate the common femoral artery and vein, and careful dissection around the sciatic notch must be performed to avoid injury to the gluteal vessels supplying blood to the posterolateral flap. Postoperatively, incisional and flap complications are common; thus, it is imperative to monitor the wound carefully. It is also helpful to avoid direct pressure to the flap by requiring the patient to lie on the unaffected side during the early postoperative phase.

FUNCTIONAL OUTCOMES

Pierce and colleagues[53] discovered that 51% of their trauma-related amputees experienced anatomic or physical problems related to their amputation. Smith and colleagues[102] further debunked the myth that lower extremity trauma-related amputees routinely do well when they reported that isolated transtibial amputees scored significantly lower than age-matched controls on the SF-36 in physical functioning and role limitations due to physical health problems. Most recently, the LEAP study confirmed that severe disability was common following above-ankle amputations for trauma and continues to heighten awareness that trauma-related amputations are not the panacea for severe lower extremity injuries.[8]

The long-term functional outcomes of combat-injured amputees were reviewed by Dougherty in 2001.[2,3,103] His review of Vietnam veterans is likely the best outcome data available for extrapolation to the present-day combat amputee. His cohort of transtibial amputees sustained their injuries as a result of landmine or booby-trap at least 65% of the time.[2] In his review of isolated transtibial amputees, he described 2 groups of patients. The first group sustained only an isolated amputation, whereas the second group sustained a transtibial amputation and an additional major injury to include a major long-bone fracture; burns covering more than 20% of the body; or a wound to the chest, abdomen, face, or head. After an average of 28 years, 72 patients were available for follow-up. An interview as well as the SF-36 questionnaire was administered to all amputees. In the isolated transtibial amputee group, the average scaled SF-36 scores were similar to age- and gender-matched controls. The group 2 patients with at least one other major injury had significantly lower SF-36 scores ($P<0.001$). In addition, significantly more patients in group 2 required psychological counseling or support ($P<0.001$).

In a similar fashion, Dougherty[3,103] reviewed the outcomes of unilateral and bilateral transfemoral amputees from the Vietnam War. Forty-six patients with unilateral transfemoral amputations were available for follow-up; 63% of these amputations were the result of landmines or booby-traps, and 61% sustained at least one other major injury. The SF-36 scores obtained from this group were significantly lower than an age- and gender-matched control group (*P*<0.01). SF-36 scores were also significantly lower than the transtibial amputation group in the physical function (*P*<0.001) and general health subcategories (*P*<0.007). In the bilateral transfemoral amputation group, SF-36 scores were expectedly lower than a control group with regard to physical function, but other subcategories of the SF-36 as well as interview data obtained regarding education, employment, marriage, family life, prosthetic use, and psychological care indicated that, despite the portrayal by the popular media that a bilateral amputee is condemned to live with severe physical and emotional difficulties, these patients "led relatively normal and productive lives within the context of their physical limitations."[3,103]

Long-term follow-up studies from civilian amputee populations have, however, demonstrated that trauma-related amputees suffer from significant long-term residual limb, phantom, back, and joint pain.[104-107] Low back pain is the most significant chronic disabling pain experienced by amputees. Smith and colleagues[107] reported that 71% of their patients experienced significant back pain following a unilateral amputation. The study subjects indicated that the back pain was significantly more bothersome than any other pain experienced. The frequency of back pain was also significantly more common in transfemoral amputees.

Despite the chronic pain symptoms experienced by amputees, the most concerning issue relating to the long-term health of the amputee population was described by Robbins and colleagues.[104] The authors performed a systematic review of the long-term health outcomes associated with war-related amputations and demonstrated that amputees were at a significantly higher risk of developing cardiovascular disease and cardiovascular mortality when compared to a control group of matched patients.

Another area in which the outcome of trauma-related amputations should be evaluated is in the ability of these patients to return to productive vocational lives following their amputations. The majority of trauma-related amputees are able to return to work; however, they frequently require a change in their occupation following injury.[108] In a recent review by Stinner and colleagues[10] of 395 major limb amputations sustained during combat from the recent conflicts, 65 patients (16.5%) returned to duty following rehabilitation.

Despite this relatively low overall rate of return to duty, it is significantly higher than the 2.3% return to duty reported after amputations performed during the 1980s.

PSYCHOSOCIAL IMPACT OF AMPUTATION

In the LEAP study, 42% to 48% of patients screened positive for a psychological disorder between 3 and 24 months after their injury.[109] The LEAP study group thus has heightened the awareness of the psychosocial disability that lower extremity amputees, and limb salvage patients, endure.[8] In an attempt to address all the components of an amputee's rehabilitation, including the psychological needs, the US military has established Amputee Care Programs during the current conflicts as well as during and after all previous conflicts beginning with World War I. These programs have historically served to standardize patient care as well as pool the resources and expertise in the care of the military amputees.[1,3] The current program recognizes the complex recovery of the war-injured patients and has taken steps to provide optimal support in all areas relating to recovery to meet foreseeable physical, emotional, and psychological needs.[4]

Unique Complications

Recently, the LEAP study group reported short-term complications seen following trauma-related lower extremity amputations.[54] Despite these reports, there is a relative paucity of literature addressing the surgical complications in the short- and long-term follow-up of trauma-related amputations, in general, and of combat-related amputations in particular. In the review by the LEAP study group, more than 85% of patients who had a trauma-related amputation had a significant complication within 6 months of amputation. Nearly half of these patients had either a wound infection or wound necrosis. The most common non-wound–related complications included symptomatic neuromas and phantom and residual limb pain.[54]

Less frequently reported short- and intermediate-term complications that have contributed substantively to our current operative caseload include bone spurs, heterotopic ossification, symptomatic neuromas, and myodesis failures.[29] Anecdotally, we believe that the long-term follow-up of combat-related amputees throughout and after their initial rehabilitation will identify a large number of patients with these conditions, which limit their prosthesis wear and functional outcomes. Following surgical treatment and/or revision amputation, dramatic pain relief and increased prosthesis wear are common.

HETEROTOPIC OSSIFICATION

HO frequently forms in the residual limbs of amputees and is a well-known cause of limited prosthesis use.[29,110] Potter and colleagues[29] indicated that at least 36% of all combat-related amputees from the recent conflicts have radiographic evidence of HO in their residual limbs. When only limbs with adequate radiographs are evaluated, the prevalence jumps to 63%. Despite the selection bias that is seen with this figure, the true prevalence likely lies somewhere between the two and likely approaches 50% of all amputees. As such, HO remains a significant problem among combat amputees. Potter and colleagues[29] advocated an exhaustive nonoperative treatment regimen for these patients prior to proceeding to surgical intervention.[111] Nonoperative treatments for symptomatic HO include rest; nonsteroidal anti-inflammatory medications; evaluation for other causes of residual limb pain; and serial prosthetic alignment and socket, suspension, and liner modifications. With these treatments, the authors concluded that only 7% of all amputees required surgical excision of HO and that exhaustive nonoperative methods were warranted prior to excision because the surgical removal of HO is fraught with wound- and infection-related complications.[29]

The relatively high incidence of postoperative wound and infectious complications following combat-related amputations can likely be attributed to compromised soft tissue envelopes, latent chronic infections and deep tissue colonization, and the frequently culture-positive nature of excised HO specimens. For these reasons, tissue from resected HO should be sent for culture, and, in an effort to minimize these complications, wounds should be thoroughly irrigated following excision, meticulous hemostasis obtained, and closure should be performed over surgical drains.

SYMPTOMATIC NEUROMATA

As previously mentioned in the technique section, symptomatic neuromas remain a common reason for surgical revision in the intermediate postoperative period and frequently limit prosthesis wear. Symptomatic neuroma formation has been reported in the 2% to 30% range, but in our opinion is likely near the higher end of this spectrum.[112,113] A significant number of these patients can, however, be managed nonoperatively through the use of neuroleptic medications, prosthesis and socket adjustments, local anesthetic patches, and even Botox (onabotulinumtoxinA) injections or percutaneous proximal neural ablation. When surgical intervention is necessary, the first treatment is effective in improving patient symptoms in approximately 65% of patients. When a second surgery for a neuroma is required, the success rate falls to

13%.[114] The commonly used method for addressing a symptomatic neuroma is to perform a traction neurectomy proximal to the symptomatic area as previously discussed. Ensuring that the nerve is nestled deep to the muscle is necessary to prevent symptomatic recurrence. One must avoid avulsing the nerve prior to sharp division, however, as this may lead to an increase in postoperative neuropathic pain or a more distal and potentially symptomatic neuroma.

MYODESIS FAILURE

There is very little mention of this complication in the civilian literature, and this is not surprising considering the large number of patients treated with trauma-related amputations who have not undergone a primary myodesis. In elderly or sedentary patients, the lack of myodesis performance is less likely to become a problem, but in the young, active combat amputee population, the lack of a myodesis can result in decreased function. In the LEAP study, only 21% of transtibial and 63% of transfemoral amputees underwent a primary myodesis.[8] We advocate myodesis for all amputations, when practicable, but myodesis failure remains a relatively common indication for revision surgery. The loss of the myodesis results in 2 significant problems. The first is the lack of residual limb padding and coverage, and the second is the loss of active muscle tension and control of the distal residual limb necessary for most efficient control. This can lead to poor prosthetic fit, pain, and decreased ambulation status and function for these patients.

Once the identification of myodesis failure has been made, there is little that nonoperative management can provide. While prosthetic adjustments can be made to accommodate poor distal coverage, no muscle strength or control will be regained without surgical intervention. Revision adductor myodesis at the transfemoral level as well as revision gastrocnemius myodesis at the transtibial level are challenging procedures and often require shortening of the residual limb to achieve adequate myodesis. Despite the difficulty of these procedures, they are usually warranted to improve overall function for the amputee.

Conclusion

Although both operative and nonoperative complications remain common in the combat-amputee population, adherence to the key surgical and anatomic principles described in this chapter can optimize combat-related amputee functional outcomes. When major complications do occur, diligent and conscientious treatment can salvage good outcomes in most instances. As such, the treatment of combat-related lower extremity amputations is a rewarding experience, and we continue to be amazed by the resilience and determination of our wounded warrior patients.

References

1. Smith DG, Michael JW, Bowker JH, eds. *Atlas of Amputations and Limb Deficiencies*. 3rd ed. Rosemont, IL: American Academy of Orthopaedic Surgeons; 2004.
2. Dougherty PJ. Transtibial amputees from the Vietnam War. Twenty-eight-year follow-up. *J Bone Joint Surg Am*. 2001;83-A(3):383-389.
3. Dougherty PJ. Long-term follow-up study of bilateral above-the-knee amputees from the Vietnam War. *J Bone Joint Surg Am*. 1999;81(10):1384-1390.
4. Potter BK, Scoville CR. Amputation is not isolated: an overview of the US Army Amputee Patient Care Program and associated amputee injuries. *J Am Acad Orthop Surg*. 2006;14(10 Spec No.):S188-S190.
5. Stansbury LG, Branstetter JG, Lalliss SJ. Amputation in military trauma surgery. *J Trauma*. 2007;63(4):940-944.
6. Owens BD, Kragh JF Jr, Macaitis J, Svoboda SJ, Wenke JC. Characterization of extremity wounds in Operation Iraqi Freedom and Operation Enduring Freedom. *J Orthop Trauma*. 2007;21(4):254-257.
7. Stansbury LG, Lalliss SJ, Branstetter JG, Bagg MR, Holcomb JB. Amputations in U.S. military personnel in the current conflicts in Afghanistan and Iraq. *J Orthop Trauma*. 2008;22(1):43-46.
8. MacKenzie EJ, Bosse MJ, Castillo RC, et al. Functional outcomes following trauma-related lower-extremity amputation. *J Bone Joint Surg Am*. 2004;86-A(8):1636-1645.
9. Masini BD, Waterman SM, Wenke JC, Owens BD, Hsu JR, Ficke JR. Resource utilization and disability outcome assessment of combat casualties from Operation Iraqi Freedom and Operation Enduring Freedom. *J Orthop Trauma*. 2009;23(4):261-266.
10. Stinner DJ, Burns TC, Kirk KL, Ficke JR. Return to duty rate of amputee soldiers in the current conflicts in Afghanistan and Iraq. *J Trauma*. 2010;68(6):1476-1479.
11. Kragh JF Jr, Littrel ML, Jones JA, et al. Battle casualty survival with emergency tourniquet use to stop limb bleeding. *J Emerg Med*. 2009; Epub ahead of print.
12. Kragh JF Jr, Walters TJ, Baer DG, et al. Survival with emergency tourniquet use to stop bleeding in major limb trauma. *Ann Surg*. 2009;249(1):1-7.
13. Lange RH, Bach AW, Hansen ST Jr, Johansen KH. Open tibial fractures with associated vascular injuries: prognosis for limb salvage. *J Trauma*. 1985;25(3):203-208.
14. Bosse MJ, McCarthy ML, Jones AL, et al. The insensate foot following severe lower extremity trauma: an indication for amputation? *J Bone Joint Surg Am*. 2005;87(12):2601-2608.
15. Noonan KJ, Leyes M, Forriol F, Canadell J. Distraction osteogenesis of the lower extremity with use of monolateral external fixation. A study of two hundred and sixty-one femora and tibiae. *J Bone Joint Surg Am*. 1998;80(6):793-806.
16. Han CS, Wood MB, Bishop AT, Cooney WP. Vascularized bone transfer. *J Bone Joint Surg Am*. 1992;74(10):1441-1449.
17. Szul AC, Davis LB, Walter Reed Army Medical Center Borden Institute, eds. *Emergency War Surgery*. 3rd US rev. Washington, DC: Walter Reed Army Medical Center Borden Institute; 2004.
18. Pollak AN. Use of negative pressure wound therapy with reticulated open cell foam for lower extremity trauma. *J Orthop Trauma*. 2008;22(10 Suppl):S142-S145.
19. Morykwas MJ, Argenta LC, Shelton-Brown EI, McGuirt W. Vacuum-assisted closure: a new method for wound control and treatment: animal studies and basic foundation. *Ann Plast Surg*. 1997;38(6):553-562.
20. Harris I. Gradual closure of fasciotomy wounds using a vessel loop shoelace. *Injury*. 1993;24(8):565-566.
21. Seligson D, Mehta S, Voos K, Henry SL, Johnson JR. The use of antibiotic-impregnated polymethylmethacrylate beads to prevent the evolution of localized infection. *J Orthop Trauma*. 1992;6(4):401-406.
22. Waters RL, Hislop HJ, Perry J, Antonelli D. Energetics: application to the study and management of locomotor disabilities. Energy cost of normal and pathologic gait. *Orthop Clin North Am*. 1978;9(2):351-356.
23. Waters RL, Lunsford BR, Perry J, Byrd R. Energy-speed relationship of walking: standard tables. *J Orthop Res*. 1988;6(2):215-222.
24. Waters RL, Perry J, Antonelli D, Hislop H. Energy cost of walking of amputees: the influence of level of amputation. *J Bone Joint Surg Am*. 1976;58(1):42-46.
25. Pinzur MS, Gold J, Schwartz D, Gross N. Energy demands for walking in dysvascular amputees as related to the level of amputation. *Orthopedics*. 1992;15(9):1033-1036; discussion 1036-1037.
26. Pinzur MS, Bowker JH. Knee disarticulation. *Clin Orthop Relat Res*. 1993;61:23-28.
27. Bowker JH, San Giovanni TP, Pinzur MS. North American experience with knee disarticulation with use of a posterior myofasciocutaneous flap. Healing rate and functional results in seventy-seven patients. *J Bone Joint Surg Am*. 2000;82-A(11):1571-1574.
28. Klaes W, Eigler FW. A new technique of transgenicular amputation. *Chirurg*. 1985;56(11):735-740.
29. Potter BK, Burns TC, Lacap AP, Granville RR, Gajewski DA. Heterotopic ossification following traumatic and combat-related amputations. Prevalence, risk factors, and preliminary results of excision. *J Bone Joint Surg Am*. 2007;89(3):476-486.
30. Gwinn DE, Keeling J, Froehner JW, McGuigan FX, Andersen R. Perioperative differences between bone bridging and non-bone bridging transtibial amputations for wartime lower extremity trauma. *Foot Ankle Int*. 2008;29(8):787-793.
31. Gallico GG, Ehrlichman RJ, Jupiter J, May JW Jr. Free flaps to preserve below-knee amputation stumps: long-term evaluation. *Plast Reconstr Surg*. 1987;79(6):871-878.
32. Ghali S, Harris PA, Khan U, Pearse M, Nanchahal J. Leg length preservation with pedicled fillet of foot flaps after traumatic amputations. *Plast Reconstr Surg*. 2005;115(2):498-505.
33. Gumley GJ, MacLeod AM, Thistlethwaite S, Ryan AR. Total cutaneous harvesting from an amputated foot—two free flaps used for acute reconstruction. *Br J Plast Surg*. 1987;40(3):313-316.
34. Henman PD, Jain AS. Skin grafting an amputation stump: considerations for the choice of donor site. *Br J Plast Surg*. 2000;53(4):357.
35. Kasabian AK, Colen SR, Shaw WW, Pachter HL. The role of microvascular free flaps in salvaging below-knee amputation stumps: a review of 22 cases. *J Trauma*. 1991;31(4):495-500; discussion: 500-501.
36. Kasabian AK, Glat PM, Eidelman Y, et al. Salvage of traumatic below-knee amputation stumps utilizing the filet of foot free flap: critical evaluation of six cases. *Plast Reconstr Surg*. 1995;96(5):1145-1153.
37. Kuntscher MV, Erdmann D, Homann HH, Steinau HU, Levin SL, Germann G. The concept of fillet flaps: classification, indications, and analysis of their clinical value. *Plast Reconstr Surg*. 2001;108(4):885-896.
38. Pelissier P, Pistre V, Casoli V, Martin D, Baudet J. Reconstruction of short lower leg stumps with the osteomusculocutaneous latissimus dorsi-rib flap. *Plast Reconstr Surg*. 2002;109(3):1013-1017.

39. Shenaq SM, Krouskop T, Stal S, Spira M. Salvage of amputation stumps by secondary reconstruction utilizing microsurgical free-tissue transfer. *Plast Reconstr Surg.* 1987;79(6):861-870.

40. Wood MR, Hunter GA, Millstein SG. The value of stump split skin grafting following amputation for trauma in adult upper and lower limb amputees. *Prosthet Orthot Int.* 1987;11(2):71-74.

41. Wieslander JB, Wendeberg B, Linge G, Buttazzoni G, Buttazzoni AM. Tissue expansion: a method to preserve bone length and joints following traumatic amputations of the leg—a follow-up of five legs amputated at different levels. *Plast Reconstr Surg.* 1996;97(5):1065-1071.

42. Rees RS, Nanney LB, Fleming P, Cary A. Tissue expansion: its role in traumatic below-knee amputations. *Plast Reconstr Surg.* 1986;77(1):133-137.

43. Jupiter JB, Tsai TM, Kleinert HE. Salvage replantation of lower limb amputations. *Plast Reconstr Surg.* 1982;69(1):1-8.

44. Dedmond BT, Davids JR. Function of skin grafts in children following acquired amputation of the lower extremity. *J Bone Joint Surg Am.* 2005;87(5):1054-1058.

45. Younge D, Dafniotis O. A composite bone flap to lengthen a below-knee amputation stump. *J Bone Joint Surg Br.* 1993;75(2):330-331.

46. Song EK, Moon ES, Rowe SM, Chung JY, Yoon TR. Below knee stump reconstruction by turn-up technique. Report of 2 cases. *Clin Orthop Relat Res.* 1994;307:229-234.

47. Morgan SJ, Newman J, Ozer K, Smith W, Gurunluoglu R. Salvage of a below-the-knee amputation level following a type-IIIB open tibial fracture. A case report. *J Bone Joint Surg Am.* 2007;89(12):2769-2778.

48. McDonald DJ, Scott SM, Eckardt JJ. Tibial turn-up for long distal femoral bone loss. *Clin Orthop Relat Res.* 2001;383:214-220.

49. Burgess EM, Romano RL, Zettl JH, Schrock RD Jr. Amputations of the leg for peripheral vascular insufficiency. *J Bone Joint Surg Am.* 1971;53(5):874-890.

50. Pedersen HE. The problem of the geriatric amputee. *Artif Limbs.* 1968;12(2)(Suppl):1-3.

51. Smith DG, Fergason JR. Transtibial amputations. *Clin Orthop Relat Res.* 1999;361:108-115.

52. Pinzur MS, Gottschalk F, Pinto MA, Smith DG. Controversies in lower extremity amputation. *Instr Course Lect.* 2008;57:663-672.

53. Pierce RO Jr, Kernek CB, Ambrose TA. The plight of the traumatic amputee. *Orthopedics.* 1993;16(7):793-797.

54. Harris AM, Althausen PL, Kellam J, Bosse MJ, Castillo R. Complications following limb-threatening lower extremity trauma. *J Orthop Trauma.* 2009;23(1):1-6.

55. Ducic I, Mesbahi AN, Attinger CE, Graw K. The role of peripheral nerve surgery in the treatment of chronic pain associated with amputation stumps. *Plast Reconstr Surg.* 2008;121(3):908-914; discussion 915-917.

56. Rahimi F, Muehleman C. Epineurial capping via Surgitron and the reduction of stump neuromas in the rat. *J Foot Surg.* 1992;31(2):124-128.

57. Whipple RR, Unsell RS. Treatment of painful neuromas. *Orthop Clin North Am.* 1988;19(1):175-185.

58. Swanson AB, Boeve NR, Lumsden RM. The prevention and treatment of amputation neuromata by silicone capping. *J Hand Surg Am.* 1977;2(1):70-78.

59. Martini A, Fromm B. A new operation for the prevention and treatment of amputation neuromas. *J Bone Joint Surg Br.* 1989;71(3):379-382.

60. Barber GG, McPhail NV, Scobie TK, Brennan MC, Ellis CC. A prospective study of lower limb amputations. *Can J Surg.* 1983;26(4):339-341.

61. Deutsch A, English RD, Vermeer TC, Murray PS, Condous M. Removable rigid dressings versus soft dressings: a randomized, controlled study with dysvascular, trans-tibial amputees. *Prosthet Orthot Int.* 2005;29(2):193-200.

62. Frogameni AD, Booth R, Mumaw LA, Cummings V. Comparison of soft dressing and rigid dressing in the healing of amputated limbs of rabbits. *Am J Phys Med Rehabil.* 1989;68(5):234-239.

63. Kane TJ, Pollak EW. The rigid versus soft postoperative dressing controversy: a controlled study in vascular below-knee amputees. *Am Surg.* 1980;46(4):244-247.

64. Nawijn SE, van der Linde H, Emmelot CH, Hofstad CJ. Stump management after trans-tibial amputation: a systematic review. *Prosthet Orthot Int.* 2005;29(1):13-26.

65. Smith DG, McFarland LV, Sangeorzan BJ, Reiber GE, Czerniecki JM. Postoperative dressing and management strategies for transtibial amputations: a critical review. *J Rehabil Res Dev.* 2003;40(3):213-224.

66. Mooney V, Harvey JP Jr, McBride E, Snelson R. Comparison of postoperative stump management: plaster vs. soft dressings. *J Bone Joint Surg Am.* 1971;53(2):241-249.

67. Wilson PD. Early weight-bearing in the treatment of amputations to the lower limbs. *J Bone Joint Surg Am.* 1922;4:224-227.

68. Berlemont M, Weber R. Temporary prosthetic fitting of lower limb amputees on the operating table. Technique and long-term results in 34 cases. *Acta Orthop Belg.* 1966;32(5):662-667.

69. Burgess EM, Romano RL. The management of lower extremity amputees using immediate postsurgical prostheses. *Clin Orthop Relat Res.* 1968;57:137-146.

70. Mooney V, Nickel VL, Snelson R. Fitting of temporary prosthetic limbs immediately after amputation. *Calif Med.* 1967;107(4):330-333.

71. Schon LC, Short KW, Soupiou O, Noll K, Rheinstein J. Benefits of early prosthetic management of transtibial amputees: a prospective clinical study of a prefabricated prosthesis. *Foot Ankle Int.* 2002;23(6):509-514.

72. Weinstein ES, Livingston S, Rubin JR. The immediate postoperative prosthesis (IPOP) in ischemia and septic amputations. *Am Surg.* 1988;54(6):386-389.

73. Greene WB, Cary JM. Partial foot amputations in children. A comparison of the several types with the Syme amputation. *J Bone Joint Surg Am.* 1982;64(3):438-443.

74. Marquardt E. Chopart exarticulation using tenomyoplasty. *Z Orthop Ihre Grenzgeb.* 1973;111(4):584-586.

75. Letts M, Pyper A. The modified Chopart's amputation. *Clin Orthop Relat Res.* 1990;256:44-49.

76. Persson BM, Soderberg B. Pantalar fusion for correction of painful equinus after traumatic Chopart's amputation—a report of 2 cases. *Acta Orthop Scand.* 1996;67(3):300-302.

77. DuParc J. *Surgical Techniques in Orthopaedics and Traumatology: v. 1-8.* St. Louis, MO: Elsevier Health Sciences; 2003.

78. Cottrell-Ikerd V, Ikerd F, Jenkins DW. The Syme's amputation: a correlation of surgical technique and prosthetic management with an historical perspective. *J Foot Ankle Surg.* 1994;33(4):355-364.

79. Gaine WJ, McCreath SW. Syme's amputation revisited: a review of 46 cases. *J Bone Joint Surg Br.* 1996;78(3):461-467.

80. Taghipour H, Moharamzad Y, Mafi AR, et al. Quality of life among veterans with war-related unilateral lower extremity amputation: a long-term survey in a prosthesis center in Iran. *J Orthop Trauma.* 2009;23(7):525-530.

81. Purry NA, Hannon MA. How successful is below-knee amputation for injury? *Injury.* 1989;20(1):32-36.

82. Harris RI. Syme's amputation: the technical details essential for success. *J Bone Joint Surg Br.* 1956;38-B(3):614-632.

83. Syme J. Amputation at the ankle joint. *London and Edinburgh Monthly Journal of Medical Sciences.* 1843;393.

84. Mazet RJ. Syme's amputation. A follow-up study of fifty-one adults and thirty-two children. *J Bone Joint Surg Am.* 1968;50(8):1549-1563.

85. Sarmiento A. A modified surgical-prosthetic approach to the Syme's amputation. A follow-up report. *Clin Orthop Relat Res*. 1972;85:11-15.

86. Smith DG, Sangeorzan BJ, Hansen ST Jr, Burgess EM. Achilles tendon tenodesis to prevent heel pad migration in the Syme's amputation. *Foot Ankle Int*. 1994;15(1):14-17.

87. Gonzalez EG, Corcoran PJ, Reyes RL. Energy expenditure in below-knee amputees: correlation with stump length. *Arch Phys Med Rehabil*. 1974;55(3):111-119.

88. Bard G, Ralston HJ. Measurement of energy expenditure during ambulation, with special reference to evaluation of assistive devices. *Arch Phys Med Rehabil*. 1959;40:415-420.

89. Canale ST, Beaty JH. *Campbell's Operative Orthopaedics*. 11th ed. St. Louis, MO: Mosby; 2007.

90. Ertl J. About amputation stumps. *Chirurgie*. 1949;20:212-218.

91. Anderson C, Unger D. Recent advances in lower-extremity amputations. *Current Opinion in Orthopaedics*. 2007;18(2):137-144.

92. Berlet GC, Pokabla C, Serynek P. An alternative technique for the Ertl osteomyoplasty. *Foot Ankle Int*. 2009;30(5):443-446.

93. Pinzur MS, Pinto MA, Saltzman M, Batista F, Gottschalk F, Juknelis D. Health-related quality of life in patients with transtibial amputation and reconstruction with bone bridging of the distal tibia and fibula. *Foot Ankle Int*. 2006;27(11):907-912.

94. Pinzur MS, Beck J, Himes R, Callaci J. Distal tibiofibular bone-bridging in transtibial amputation. *J Bone Joint Surg Am*. 2008;90(12):2682-2687.

95. Mack AW, Freedman BA, Shawen SB, Gajewski DA, Kalasinsky VF, Lewin-Smith, MR. Wound complications following the use of FiberWire in lower-extremity traumatic amputations. A case series. *J Bone Joint Surg Am*. 2009;91(3):680-685.

96. Pinzur MS, Smith D, Tornow D, Meade K, Patwardhan A. Gait analysis of dysvascular below-knee and contralateral through-knee bilateral amputees: a preliminary report. *Orthopedics*. 1993;16(8):875-879.

97. Baumgartner RF. Knee disarticulation versus above-knee amputation. *Prosthet Orthot Int*. 1979;3(1):15-19.

98. Gottschalk FA, Stills M. The biomechanics of trans-femoral amputation. *Prosthet Orthot Int*. 1994;18(1):12-17.

99. James U. Maximal isometric muscle strength in healthy active male unilateral above-knee amputees, with special regard to the hip joint. *Scand J Rehabil Med*. 1973;5(2):55-66.

100. Thiele B, James U, Stalberg E. Neurophysiological studies on muscle function in the stump of above-knee amputees. *Scand J Rehabil Med*. 1973;5(2):67-70.

101. Jaegers SM, Arendzen JH, de Jongh HJ. An electromyographic study of the hip muscles of transfemoral amputees in walking. *Clin Orthop Relat Res*. 1996;328:119-128.

102. Smith DG, Horn P, Malchow D, Boone DA, Reiber GE, Hansen ST Jr. Prosthetic history, prosthetic charges, and functional outcome of the isolated, traumatic below-knee amputee. *J Trauma*. 1995;38(1):44-47.

103. Dougherty PJ. Long-term follow-up of unilateral transfemoral amputees from the Vietnam war. *J Trauma*. 2003;54(4):718-723.

104. Robbins CB, Vreeman DJ, Sothmann MS, Wilson SL, Oldridge NB. A review of the long-term health outcomes associated with war-related amputation. *Mil Med*. 2009;174(6):588-592.

105. Ehde DM, Smith DG, Czerniecki JM, Campbell KM, Malchow DM, Robinson LR. Back pain as a secondary disability in persons with lower limb amputations. *Arch Phys Med Rehabil*. 2001;82(6):731-734.

106. Norvell DC, Czerniecki JM, Reiber GE, Maynard C, Pecoraro JA, Weiss NS. The prevalence of knee pain and symptomatic knee osteoarthritis among veteran traumatic amputees and nonamputees. *Arch Phys Med Rehabil*. 2005;86(3):487-493.

107. Smith DG, Ehde DM, Legro MW, Reiber GE, del Aguila M, Boone DA. Phantom limb, residual limb, and back pain after lower extremity amputations. *Clin Orthop Relat Res*. 1999;361:29-38.

108. Millstein S, Bain D, Hunter GA. A review of employment patterns of industrial amputees—factors influencing rehabilitation. *Prosthet Orthot Int*. 1985;9(2):69-78.

109. McCarthy ML, MacKenzie EJ, Edwin D, Bosse MJ, Castillo RC, Starr A. Psychological distress associated with severe lower-limb injury. *J Bone Joint Surg Am*. 2003;85-A(9):1689-1697.

110. Forsberg JA, Pepek JM, Wagner S, et al. Heterotopic ossification in high-energy wartime extremity injuries: prevalence and risk factors. *J Bone Joint Surg Am*. 2009;91(5):1084-1091.

111. Forsberg JA, Potter BK. Heterotopic ossification in wartime wounds. *J Surg Orthop Adv*. 2010;19(1):51-61.

112. Nashold BS Jr, Goldner JL, Mullen JB, Bright DS. Long-term pain control by direct peripheral-nerve stimulation. *J Bone Joint Surg Am*. 1982;64(1):1-10.

113. Nelson AW. The painful neuroma: the regenerating axon versus the epineural sheath. *J Surg Res*. 1977;23(3):215-221.

114. Tupper JW, Booth DM. Treatment of painful neuromas of sensory nerves in the hand: a comparison of traditional and newer methods. *J Hand Surg Am*. 1976;1(2):144-151.

Chapter *23*

PROSTHESES FOR
MAJOR EXTREMITY AMPUTATIONS

Zach Harvey, BS, CPO and MAJ Benjamin K. Potter, MD

odern medical advances in amputation surgery, rehabilitation, and prosthesis technology have afforded more servicemembers
sustaining limb loss as a result of battlefield conflict
the ability to regain greater function and indepen-
dence. As of January 2010, 953 US servicemembers
have sustained major limb loss during Operation Iraqi
Freedom and Operation Enduring Freedom (OIF/
OEF). In contrast, World War II resulted in approximately 15,000 amputations.[1] The infrastructure at that
time did not exist to handle such a high demand of
specialized patient care. Early dissatisfaction with the
availability of prosthesis technology and training in
an immature medical system led to the establishment
of 7 military treatment facility (MTF) amputee centers
throughout the country and a workforce of professionals centered on amputee care. As a result, the field of
prosthetics advanced with an increased understanding of gait and upper extremity biomechanics, socket
system innovation, and the development of new and
improved prosthetic components.[2] Today, comprehensive amputee care is conducted in three major MTFs in
the United States: Walter Reed Army Medical Center
(WRAMC) in Washington, DC; Brooke Army Medical
Center in San Antonio, TX; and the Naval Medical
Center in San Diego, CA.

A recent survey analyzing patient satisfaction at
WRAMC revealed an overall high level of satisfaction
among amputees, particularly regarding the therapy
received while in treatment.[3] This satisfaction was
attributed to the time commitment and availability of
therapists and the use of a progressive rehabilitation
model, starting with basic rehabilitation and progress-

ing toward more advanced, sports medicine-based
models of rehabilitation. Concurrent with overall
satisfaction rates for rehabilitation are the MTF standards of care for amputation procedures and prostheses, which require expedited prosthetic fittings and
maintaining a well-fitting socket at all times.[4,5]

While amputation surgery, rehabilitation techniques, and prosthetic technology have improved,
the full restoration of a functional equivalent to the
native human limb remains lacking, especially for
more proximal amputation levels. Lessons learned
from working with the challenging but gratifying
population of combat-injured amputees from OIF/
OEF must therefore continue to drive improvements
for current and future amputee rehabilitation. The
following is not intended as a comprehensive overview of all prosthetic options, but rather as a review
of current technology and practice based on the
WRAMC experience.

The Prosthetic Process

The prosthetist is responsible for helping formulate
the initial prosthetic prescription as well as facilitating an appropriate pace of advancement in prosthesis
rehabilitation. His or her experience working with
a variety of patients, technical knowledge of the latest industry products, and physical assessment of
the individual patient add valuable input into the
provision of the best prosthetic device or devices for
a particular patient. Prosthetics can be thought of as
an art, based on science. No two residual limbs are

- 221 -

Owens BD, Belmont PJ Jr, eds. *Combat Orthopedic Surgery:*
Lessons Learned in Iraq and Afghanistan (pp 221-236)
© 2011 SLACK Incorporated

exactly alike, yet many problems are common and can be solved using similar prosthetic and biomechanical principles. Selective loading of the residual limb skeletal anatomy, while maintaining total contact of soft tissue, requires a precise fit with low tolerance for error. Quantitative measurement tools to assess socket fit are lacking in clinical practice, although research has shown that peak pressures within a socket vary substantially with minimal alterations in socket design.[6] It is common, especially with more recent amputees, to frequently replace sockets as the shape and volume of the residual limbs change and to replace and change component types as activity levels, performance status, and patient needs evolve.

The prosthetic process generally starts with a functional assessment, patient and residual limb measurements, and a cast impression (Figure 23-1) or a digital scan of the residual limb that is used in computer-aided design/computer-aided manufacture. A plan is made for a follow-up patient visit, and the fabrication of the socket begins. A positive model of the limb is rectified, the prosthetist modifies the shape, and a provisional socket is created with an attachment plate secured to the distal end of the limb in a critical orientation. Appropriate components are selected and ordered based on information such as patient weight, activity level, skin tone, and measurements. Upon return of the patient, the fit of the socket is assessed and adjusted as necessary. Static and dynamic alignment is achieved, and adjustments to components are made physically to the device or via computer interfaces. The patient is educated, and a plan is made for another follow-up visit. Patient follow-up is critical, and positive molds of the limb are often saved in order to make alterations to a socket shape or to duplicate a socket for a different device. Alignment can be duplicated as well and can be transferred to additional sockets through the use of a specialized vertical alignment jig.

Lower Extremity Prostheses

MODERN-DAY PROSTHETIC ADVANCES AND HISTORY

As health care providers, it is important to provide reliable information to the patient early on in order to facilitate understanding and mental preparation for what lies ahead, while tempering early expectations appropriately. Even within the scope of the combat-injured amputee population, a great degree of variability exists from person to person; frequent setbacks are the rule for some, while recovery moves forward quickly for others. Such apparent hurdles and limitations may be attributed to external factors, such as the

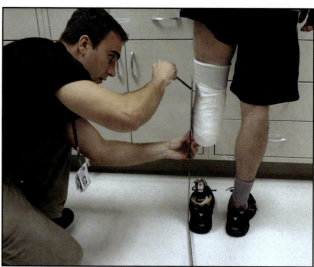

Figure 23-1. After careful assessment of the residual limb, the prosthetist takes a cast impression and measurements to begin formation of the prosthetic socket. Notation of knee joint alignment facilitates proper prosthetic foot placement in order to achieve optimal gait biomechanics.

fit and function of the prosthesis or associated injuries, as well as to internal factors, such as patient motivation, perhaps the most critical attribute leading to, or preventing, a successful recovery. The traumatic amputee is generally healthy prior to injury, and initial expectations are for a rapid recovery.[7] Unfortunately, complications and difficulties requiring revision surgery for traumatic amputations even in the civilian sector have been reported at a rate of greater than 30%.[7] Perhaps most disturbing is that the current literature suggests that a large percentage of these traumatic amputees become severely disabled.[7,8] In light of these data, it is reasonable to conclude that limb length should be preserved, but not at the expense of nonhealing or painful residual limb with poor soft tissue coverage. Dramatic outcomes are possible with proper amputation techniques and appropriate attention to avoiding well-documented technical errors[9] in combination with meticulous work by the auxiliary rehabilitation team. The recent experience with combat-injured amputees from OIF/OEF has produced a plethora of successful wounded warrior outcomes via use of prostheses. From the onset of OIF/OEF through 2008, 17% to 20% of patients who desired to were able to pass the requisite standard or modified physical fitness tests and remain on active duty.[10] Others may have retained the functional abilities of a soldier, but chose to retire from the military and reintegrate into civilian life.

Socket design, materials, and the application of techniques have evolved, and prosthetic manufacturers continue to develop new products; however, many of the options used today are not entirely, or even remotely, new. According to Bowker and Prithan:

The concept of ischial weight bearing in transfemoral sockets was introduced in 1790. The suction valve, now a preferred method of suspension, was invented in 1863. Total contact socket designs, hydraulic knee joints, and thermoset materials are now commonplace and were introduced following WWII around 1950. Heat adjustable thermoplastics, such as polypropylene and polyethylene, emerged in the 1960s. Endoskeletal components replaced exoskeletal systems for lower extremity devices as they became mass-produced by the 1970s. Gel liners, ischial containment sockets, compliant thermoplastics, computer-aided design/computer-aided manufacture, elevated vacuum suspension, microprocessor knee joints, and dynamic response feet, all commonly used today, were developed and refined in the 1980s and 1990s.[11]

STAGING OF CARE

The lower extremity prosthesis phases mirror the timelines of those for physical therapy. MTF phases of prosthetic care have been established as 1) pre-prosthetic phase, 2) interim prosthetic phase, 3) basic prosthetic phase, and 4) advanced prosthetic phase.[4] Some of the pre-prosthetic goals of physical therapy include wound healing, edema control, infection control, contracture prevention, and pain management. Ace bandages and shrinkers help prepare the shape and size of the residual limb for prosthetic fitting. A gel liner is generally applied when open wounds have healed, and initial fitting with the early postoperative prosthesis occurs when the patient is cleared by the orthopedic surgeon. The patient then enters the interim prosthetic phase of care. It should be noted that contralateral limb injuries may not necessitate the delay of initial fitting because physical therapy can still work on weight bearing using a tilt table, crutches, parallel bars, or a rolling stool (Figure 23-2).

The benefits of early fitting are well documented and include reduction in pain and edema, prevention of contractures, and increased residual limb viability. The first day using an early postoperative prosthesis is a tremendous benchmark in the recovery process for an individual who recently lost a limb. A patient may be placed on a conservative wear schedule with limited weight bearing as indicated, and regular skin checks are imperative at this stage, especially when there is a lack of protective sensation. Frequent follow-up care with the prosthetist at this stage may be necessary, and good communication between the physical therapist, treating physicians, and prosthetist is required as limb volume changes, wear time increases, and activity level progresses. During this phase of care, sockets are commonly replaced and are constructed out of highly adjustable but durable plastic.

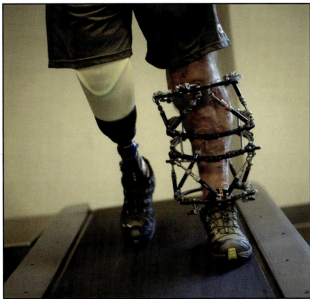

Figure 23-2. The decision to amputate versus salvage a limb is weighted with a multitude of considerations. Amputation is not the panacea of lower extremity injuries, but may be a better functional option than limb salvage in many instances, particularly when a transtibial amputation level is an option.

The basic phase of prosthetic care is entered as activity level increases and impact and load bearing through the prosthesis becomes greater. A foot offering greater dynamic response and rigidity may be used once this phase is reached. During the advanced phase of care, specialty prostheses for sports and recreation are made available, with requisite training for the successful utilization and integration of each new device. These prostheses should be constructed from definitive materials to prevent breakage. Prosthetist follow-up becomes less frequent as reintegration into active duty or civilian life is established. For those wounded warriors returning to duty, provision of versatile and low maintenance components along with back-up supplies and devices is advised.

PROSTHETIC OPTIONS BY LEVEL OF AMPUTATION

Partial Foot and Symes Amputations

Prosthetic options for partial foot amputations include low-profile and high-profile designs, depending on the level of support needed. Replacing part of a lost limb, a goal of prosthetics, and restoring functionality, a goal of orthotics, are the combined goal of the *prosthesis*, as it has been aptly termed, for these amputation levels. Although the length of the foot is decreased, peak magnitude of the forces, using gait analysis, are higher with a partial foot amputation.[12,13]

Thus, it is critical to consider principles of foot orthotics into a design that is cosmetically acceptable and comfortable to wear. Low-profile designs may use lightweight foam to prevent the shoe box from collapsing and carbon plates to provide rigidity throughout the terminal stance of the gait cycle. High-definition silicone restorations are an option for this type of amputation and may employ suction suspension or a zipper. High-profile designs may incorporate various types of ankle-foot orthoses, depending on the level of support needed.

The Symes amputation affords the ability to bear weight distally and allows some room for a low-profile prosthetic foot. Minimal clearance and foot options are a disadvantage to this amputation level, especially for a highly active individual. Socket designs must allow passage on the bulbous distal end through the socket and may incorporate a bivalve door or window. Other options include a foam inner liner or custom liner with buildups to create a "stovepipe" design, an expandable wall design, and sockets with localized elastic materials. Modern advances now allow running feet to be attached to the posterior aspect of a Symes socket.

Transtibial Amputation

The retention of the anatomic knee joint allows most transtibial amputees, regardless of age, the ability to achieve pre-amputation ambulatory level.[14] With a pain-free residual limb, well-fitted socket, a properly selected and aligned prosthetic foot, and good physical therapy training, nearly full symmetry can be expected in motivated patients when analyzed using observational gait analysis.

Because of the osseous anatomy of the transtibial residual limb, a soft interface is necessary in order to provide cushioning and shear absorption. Gel liners with sleeve suction, elevated vacuum, pin suspension, or seal-in suspension are common socket suspension systems. The evolution of current socket designs can be traced from the days when open-ended designs were the norm to the introduction of total contact designs, such as the patella tendon-bearing design, developed by Radcliffe in 1961, which advocated loading pressure-tolerant areas and relieving pressure-sensitive areas.[15] Total surface bearing theory subsequently sought to maximize contact surface area of the limb to distribute pressure and thus modified the shape of the unrectified cast less than that of the patella tendon-bearing design.[16] Hydrostatic socket theory employs a casting method under pressure, with little or no modification to the positive mold.[17] Regardless of the technique, or combination of techniques, used by the prosthetist, successful outcomes rely on careful analysis of the residual limb characteristics. Knee stability, strength, range of motion, Q-angle, and residual limb

length must be assessed, and each of these characteristics influence socket design, trim-lines, and alignment. Special consideration must be given to amputations using the modified Ertl distal bone-bridge procedure because osseous structure is often prominent distally and requires intimate contouring. Weight-bearing restrictions may prohibit early full ambulation if this surgical technique is used, although generally only for a few weeks. Solid radiographic healing is not required for community ambulation following transtibial amputation bone-bridge procedures.

For the unlimited community ambulator, one who walks on uneven terrain and at variable cadence, a dynamic response foot with spring-like properties is generally indicated. A number of different options are available if space underneath the socket permits; these include models with torsion adapters, vertical shock pylons, and multi-axial units. While greater length salvage, robust soft tissue coverage permitting, is generally preferable, at least 10 to 11 inches of ground clearance (from sound limb heel) is required to enable the direct utilization of all transtibial prosthesis options. Differences in properties of the feet are subtle but apparent, especially during certain activities. For example, a torsion adapter offers greater axial rotation during a golf swing. Foot efficiency depends simultaneously on foot design and gait style.[18] It can reasonably be concluded that new amputees tend to bear less weight through the prosthesis and are more comfortable using a foot with compliant, multi-axial characteristics.[19] Prosthetic goals should focus on minimizing component weight while facilitating a more normal and efficient gait.

Knee Disarticulation and Transfemoral Amputation

Knee disarticulation amputations with adequate soft tissue coverage generally tolerate distal weight bearing, and the sockets are generally more comfortable and less restrictive than transfemoral sockets that often must support weight through the pelvis. This type of socket design does not enclose the pelvic anatomy and allows full range of motion of the hip. If soft tissue coverage is lacking, a socket design incorporating the pelvic anatomy may be required. Cosmetically, the knee joint on a knee disarticulation prosthesis is lower than anatomic and protrudes slightly during sitting; however, low-profile couplings and polycentric knee joints are an option to minimize this effect. These knees provide a more proximal "virtual knee center" and allow shortening during swing phase of the gait cycle.[20] For the aforementioned reasons, preference should be given to the knee disarticulation amputation if a transtibial amputation is not an option only when distal soft tissue coverage is adequate. If soft tissue coverage is inadequate, a transfemoral amputation should be performed in most instances.

The femoral condyles and patella, when present, are easily palpable through the soft tissue. A soft interface can protect these prominences, which are susceptible to localized pressure and shear forces. If the femoral condyles are not reduced during amputation surgery, the residual limb has a deliberately bulbous shape. This improves suspension but can make socket design more difficult for the prosthetist, who must seek to maintain total contact but ensure ease of donning and doffing. Options in this case include sockets with flexible plastic and rigid frames, a removable "window," soft foam inserts, and custom gel liners. If the femoral condyles are reduced during surgery, a more cylindrical morphology results, yielding a comfortable, simple to use, "push-in" suction socket.

Many theories and principles of transfemoral sockets have evolved since the days of "plug-fit" socket designs prior to 1950. Since then, ischial weight-bearing quadrilateral sockets and narrower ischial containment sockets have been developed and widely used. Because the proximal thigh soft tissue is mobile, various socket shapes and contours are possible, the selection of which depends on the characteristics of the individual patient.[21,22] Hip rotation is somewhat restricted because of the need for high socket trim-lines. Positional rotators, which add about 2 cm in length, permit the ability to unlock and rotate the prosthesis, thereby facilitating changing a shoe, entering a car, or sitting cross-legged.

The distal femur and the ischial tuberosity of the pelvis are generally protected by soft tissue at the transfemoral amputation level, and, unless adherent scars or skin grafts are present, a soft interface may not be needed once limb volume stabilizes. With this system, the socket is worn directly against the skin and is held on by suction. Specialized gel liners can be used when suction is a primary means of suspension. These liners are called Seal-In liners (Össur, Aliso Viejo, CA) and incorporate a hypobaric seal that flattens as the limb is pushed into the suction socket. Gel liners with distal pin locks or lanyard suspension are especially beneficial for new amputees, in whom limb volume fluctuates, or when suction is not an option. Regardless of the type of interface, a flexible inner socket and rigid frame can be designed to balance support and comfort (Figure 23-3).[23] Nonessential parts of the rigid frame are cut away to allow flexibility along the brim of the socket, the posterior proximal aspect (for sitting), and over muscle bellies or problematic areas. Auxiliary suspension and support may be necessary in the form of a soft belt or hip joint and pelvic band, particularly in the case of very short transfemoral amputations.

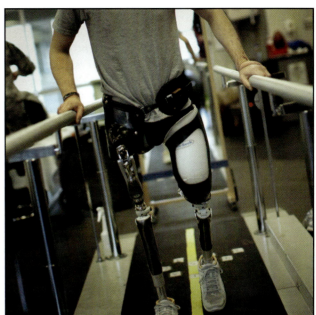

Figure 23-3. This creative hip disarticulation socket design incorporates custom gel shorts with integrated ratchet locks and straps, allowing a lower profile and potentially more comfortable design than traditional style sockets (Medical Center Orthotics and Prosthetics, Silver Spring, MD). Flexible inner liners and rigid frames allow comfort and flexibility on the left transfemoral socket. Shortening the prosthetic height is advantageous for balance and stability during early training.

Consensus has not been reached regarding specific techniques and philosophical approaches, even among the team of prosthetists at WRAMC, but successful transfemoral socket fittings are generally achieved by all. The Marlo Anatomical Socket (MAS) is a socket design with aggressive ischial ramus containment and low posterior trim-lines, below the gluteal fold. Perceived advantages of this design include decreased inhibition of hip extension and rotation range of motion and increased comfort during sitting. Standard ischial containment sockets are less aggressive medially and have higher posterior trim-lines. Perceived advantages of these designs include load sharing onto the gluteus maximus and arguably greater comfort along the medial aspect of the socket. Double-wall elevated vacuum sockets are more complicated to fabricate and don, but they have proven useful, especially for patients experiencing residual limb volume fluctuation. Although objective measures to evaluate transfemoral socket fit are currently undefined, patient acceptance of various socket designs often reveals the best fit for each individual.

Coronal plane biomechanics are slightly different between knee disarticulation and transfemoral prostheses. Due to the fact that most knee disarticulation sockets allow for distal weight bearing, the socket tends to rotate around this point of contact; in comparison, the transfemoral socket rotates around the ischium.[24] Therefore, one of the objectives with transfemoral sockets is to bring the position of the residual femur as close to anatomical alignment as possible. Research is inconclusive and controversial, but this may be accomplished through surgical technique[25] or socket design and alignment.[26]

Alignment in the sagittal plane is critical for optimum performance of the prosthetic knee joint. Because of the longer lever arm and better balanced hip musculature, a patient with a knee disarticulation amputation is less susceptible to development of a hip flexion contracture. Therefore, socket alignment is generally more upright in comparison to the transfemoral socket. With transfemoral amputees, initial flexion of the socket puts the gluteus maximus in a position of strength, and additional socket flexion is required if a hip flexion contracture is present.[27,28] If posterior offset of the knee joint in relation to the socket does not accompany added socket flexion, the knee may be prone to buckle inadvertently.

Prosthetic knee joint options can be described in terms of the number of mechanical axes—single axis or polycentric; the mechanism of control—hydraulic, pneumatic, or friction; or the existence of electronic circuitry—microprocessor or nonmicroprocessor. The goal of every prosthetic knee is to respond to the movements of the amputee, judiciously altering between stability and mobility. *Voluntary control* is a term used to describe the direct influence of the amputee on the movement of the prosthetic knee. As the center of mass moves posterior in relation to the mechanical knee joint axis, either mechanical stability warranted by resistance of the knee or voluntary control using hip extensor strength is necessitated in order to prevent the knee from buckling. Because the gluteus maximus is the primary hip extensor with knee disarticulation and transfemoral amputation levels, the control pattern to stabilize the prosthetic knee joint is indirect and therefore not intuitive. For this reason, physical therapy is imperative for new amputees, especially when lacking an anatomical knee joint, to relearn altered motor patterns to appropriately compensate and achieve the most normal gait pattern practicable.[29]

Jacquelin Perry defined the gait cycle into eight phases: Initial contact, loading response, mid-stance, terminal stance, pre-swing, initial swing, mid-swing, and terminal swing.[30] During initial contact/loading response of the gait cycle, certain prosthetic knees are designed to provide "stance flexion," which is a normal shock-absorbing feature of the intact biological limb. Stance phase vertical displacement of the trunk has been shown to be influenced by the stance flexion feature of a prosthetic knee.[31] Practical use of this feature is not universal for all amputees, especially those with longer, stronger residual limbs, because the feeling

that the knee is buckling is not desirable. When stance flexion is activated during mid to terminal stance phase, "extension dampening" is an adjustable feature for some prosthetic knees; this serves to function similar to the intact popliteal musculature. During pre-swing phase, the release criteria of the prosthetic knee are met in order to advance the prosthesis, swinging it forward. Release criteria parameters differ among knee joints and can be adjusted. Gait training during this phase of the gait cycle teaches the amputee to rotate the pelvis in coordination with activating the prosthetic knee to flex.[32] Swing phase adjustments on the prosthetic knee may limit the amount of heel rise during initial swing phase, the swing speed during mid-swing phase, and the amount of terminal impact dampening during terminal swing phase. For those amputees who walk at variable cadences, certain mechanical and microprocessor-controlled knees can be adjusted to synchronize how quickly the prosthesis swings into an extended position. These movements entail many variables to execute successfully, so it is advantageous, especially in the case of a new patient, for the physical therapist and prosthetist to work together. Voluntary control may increase as new walking patterns become reinforced and the hip musculature becomes stronger. Concomitant prosthetic adjustments may reduce provisional stability, affording freer mobility and perhaps greater energy efficiency.

Microprocessor knees (Figure 23-4), such as the C-Leg (Otto Bock, Minneapolis, MN), use algorithms and real-time data to adjust stance phase stability and to initiate and properly time the swing phase in order to prevent the user from having to "think" during ambulation.[32,33] A number of recent and ongoing studies have examined the C-Leg in comparison to a nonmicroprocessor single-axis hydraulic knee. Results indicate superiority of the C-Leg for most parameters, including energy efficiency,[34,35] stairs and hills,[36] self-selected walking speed,[37] gait kinematics,[38] fall risk,[39] maneuverability,[40] psychological adjustment,[41] quality of life,[42] activity level,[43] and patient satisfaction and preference over other knees.[36,40] A microprocessor knee may be especially advantageous when less voluntary control is possible. For highly active athletic individuals with long, strong, and flexible residual limbs, anecdotal reports suggest a preference for nonmicroprocessor knees for certain activities. This may be explained by the limited foot selection with the current C-Leg. An ongoing study at WRAMC is evaluating the efficacy of the C-Leg in comparison to a single-axis hydraulic nonmicroprocessor knee for initial fitting on unilateral transfemoral amputees.[44] Higher profile feet with more dynamic response and vertical shock-absorbing properties have adequate clearance distal to the knee joint with a nonmicroprocessor knee joint, which may partially explain user preference of

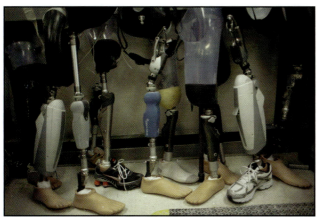

Figure 23-4. Research has demonstrated that microprocessor knee joints are advantageous in restoring complex algorithms of control for amputation levels proximal the knee joint. Some of the latest prosthetic knee joints incorporate more on-board sensors, power generation, and artificial technology (Otto Bock Healthcare, Minneapolis, MN; Össur, Aliso Viejo, CA).

nonmicroprocessor knees for highly active individuals. Other microprocessor knees are similar in build height to nonmicroprocessor knees and are preferred over other options by some users.

The properties of the prosthetic foot determine how ground reaction forces interact with the prosthetic knee joint. If the heel of the foot is too soft, less energy is allowed to transfer proximally to create a knee flexion moment during loading response; if too stiff, excessive knee flexion moment and instability may result. The roll-over characteristics of the foot during stance phase of gait may influence how long the foot stays plantargrade, the amount of energy return at terminal stance, and how quickly the knee will meet swing phase criteria. For this reason, the properties of the foot should complement the properties of the knee for safety and efficiency during walking.

Hip Disarticulation and Hemipelvectomy (Transpelvic) Amputations

It is not surprising that the loss of the entire limb results in energy demands almost two-fold that of able-bodied individuals.[45] It is also not surprising that high levels of prosthesis rejection and wheelchair-only ambulation were reported in 1983 for these amputation levels, citing prosthesis comfort as the biggest complaint.[46,47] Since then, improvements to materials and concepts have been developed and offer more options for greater comfort and mobility. However, the biomechanical principles of traditional Canadian hip disarticulation prostheses have not changed substantively since Radcliffe described them in 1957, and they are applicable to modern design.[48] Nonetheless,

in our experience, hip disarticulation amputees from the current conflicts without major contralateral limb injuries are universally capable of prolonged ambulation without the use of nonprosthetic assist devices; remarkably good function is therefore possible even at these very proximal amputation levels.

A well-fitting and suspended socket is critical because the trunk (in the case of the hemipelvectomy) and pelvis (in the case of the hip disarticulation) accept ground reaction forces during stance phase and power the forward progression of the prosthesis during swing phase of the gait cycle. The use of flexible inner liners with rigid frame sockets helps to provide support and maximize comfort. Interface options include knit body socks, Lycra-based garments, and gel liners. Suspension is traditionally obtained through an anatomical lock on the pelvis anatomy. Some creative designs incorporate straps attached to a gel liner that ratchet into a lock on the socket and afford a lower profile and potentially more comfortable, one-piece socket design with waist strap (see Figure 23-3).

The hip joint alignment is such that it positions the prosthetic knee joint in line with the center of mass. Adjustments can be made by the prosthetist to set resistance levels on the hip joint that are appropriate for maximum gait efficiency. The choice of prosthetic knee depends on the activity level of the patient and environmental barriers he or she may encounter. For these more proximal amputation levels, fluid-controlled knees and dynamic-response feet demonstrate improved results in gait biometrics and contribute to a faster cadence.[49,50] Good communication, patience, gait training, and persistent follow-up with the prosthetist are keys to successful ambulation with these amputation levels.

BILATERAL LOWER EXTREMITY PROSTHETIC CONSIDERATIONS

Gait analysis of bilateral transtibial amputations has revealed slower speeds, lower cadences, shorter step lengths, altered kinematics of the ankle and knee joints, reduced power generation, and increased compensatory hip hiking.[51-53] Shock absorption was described as a primary function of normal walking[54] and, without a compensatory sound side, is even more of a requirement with bilateral amputees (Figure 23-5). Prosthetic feet and specialized pylons have been shown to reduce forces transmitted to the body.[55]

Lowering the center of gravity through shortened prosthesis height (see Figure 23-3) lessens mechanical forces transmitted through the sockets, increases safety and stability, and increases energy efficiency; although many patients object to giving up height for long-term use, provisional prosthesis shortening can be a useful training modality.[56] A minimum of 18 inches

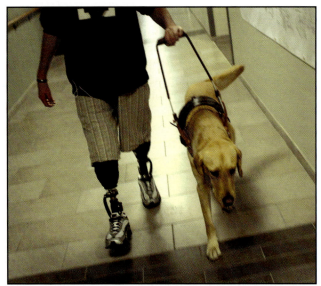

Figure 23-5. Bilateral lower extremity amputees often benefit from the use of vertical shock-absorbing feet or pylons to reduce the impact of ground reaction forces.

has been recommended to facilitate getting out of a chair.[57] "Stubbies" are designed without knee joints and are beneficial for bilateral transfemoral amputees during initial rehabilitation and for short-distance walking, such as around the house. Length is progressively added as patients gain balance and strength. Microprocessor knee joints are added later as goals and milestones are reached in physical therapy. Low back pain is extremely common following lower limb amputation,[58] and a careful assessment of hip flexion range of motion and degree of compensatory lumbar lordosis during standing can help the prosthetist decide the best prosthetic alignment as a basis for lumbar support.

LOWER EXTREMITY PROSTHETIC OPTIONS FOR SPORTS AND RECREATION

The benefits of exercise are well known, and combat-related lower limb amputees express a strong desire to participate in sports and recreational activities and not to be limited by the functional capacity of the prosthesis.[59] Removal of the prosthesis is the first option for participants of certain activities, such as swimming, skiing, or wheelchair sports. The general-use prosthesis is a second option, and, often, alteration to equipment and/or prosthetic alignment may be all that is required. However, this is not advisable for a number of reasons: 1) general-use prostheses sometimes include an optional cosmetic cover and skin that is subject to wear and tear with high activity; 2) functional performance may be compromised, and excessive forces may cause stress on prosthetic components and the body[59]; and 3) in the worst-case scenario, if a component breaks during high impact

and a back-up device is not available, an emergency situation may develop due to secondary injuries or immobility. Specialized lower extremity prostheses are a third option and can be created for nearly every sport. Some specialized prostheses used at WRAMC include those for running, cycling, rock climbing, hiking, water sports, winter sports, in-line skating, and golf.[60-62] Common component options to consider in the design of sport-specific prostheses include torsion adapters, vertical shock absorbers, multi-axial feet, adjustable ankles, knees with shock units, and quick-disconnect couplers. For amputation levels proximal to the knee joint, prosthetic knees with mountain biking shock units have proven useful in restoring quadriceps function during activities requiring an athletic stance (Symbiotech, McMinnville, OR; Left Side Inc, Snohomish, WA). Versatile, modular designs are advisable, whenever possible.

Prosthetic feet specific to running do not require a heel and are therefore made by simply gluing the sole of a shoe onto the "C- shaped" or "J-shaped" carbon fiber spring. Running comes after months of physical therapy and pre-running training drills, typically on a dynamic response foot. Transfemoral amputees have the option of using a straight pylon without a knee joint and circumducting the prosthesis, or using a mechanical hydraulic knee joint with a more natural-looking running gait. Specialized equipment, such as a suspended track system (Solo-Step, Sioux Falls, SD) and antigravity treadmill (Alter-G, Freemont, CA), can make the transition to running safer and help instill confidence in the patient. Per WRAMC protocol, the prescription of running leg(s) comes only after compliance in physical therapy is met and when bone density is proved adequate as determined by physician-reviewed DEXA (dual energy x-ray absorptiometry) scan.

LOWER EXTREMITY PROSTHETIC RESEARCH AND DEVELOPMENT

A formalized understanding of biomechanics principles originated following World War II, and gait labs emerged, which are currently instrumental in gathering data on kinetics, kinematics, energy consumption, virtual reality, and motion analysis for purposes of research and clinical evaluation. Research is sparse for the field of rehabilitation, despite a developing interest in evidence-based practice and outcome measures.[63,64] A recent symposium brought a diverse team of experts together to identify research needs, particularly of the combat amputee.[65] Experts agreed that more longitudinal studies, better outcome measures, development and funding for gait labs, and validation of new technology are needed in order to advance current practice.

Exciting advances are emerging in lower extremity prosthetics. Microprocessor knee technology is progressing with the use of more on-board sensors, better batteries, artificial intelligence, and powered actuators.[66] More versatile designs will facilitate mobility and increased functionality as the specific needs of the prosthetic knee change and different environmental barriers are encountered. The first ankle joint to employ an electrically powered actuator is already on the market (Össur), and future developments are in progress to restore active plantarflexion to the gait cycle. Current vacuum-assisted socket systems introduced by TEC Interface Systems (St. Cloud, MN) and Otto Bock currently help "solidify" the residual limb inside the socket. Variable socket technology may soon improve socket comfort, permitting adaptations to sweating and limb volume fluctuations throughout the day. Problems associated with poor socket fit become non-issues when osseointegration is successful. Since the inception by Branemark, a Swedish engineer, the majority of osseointegration procedures have been performed in Europe on patients with transfemoral amputations.[67,68] As complication rates associated with osseointegration decrease and device longevity improves, this technique may become a new standard of care.[69]

Upper Extremity Prostheses

MODERN-DAY PROSTHESIS ADVANCES AND HISTORY

Upper extremity technology in use today dates back to 1816, when the first body-powered device was created, and 1919, when myoelectric-controlled devices were incepted.[2] A breakdown of prosthetic options by level of amputation, and advantages and disadvantages of all of the different components and combinations of components is beyond the scope of this chapter. A general description of the current state of prosthetic technology and rehabilitation methods of the upper extremity amputee follows.

STAGING OF CARE

Reconstructing a damaged hand and fingers often leads to better functional outcomes than amputation and the use of a prosthesis.[70] Surgical protocols at WRAMC advise retention of the remaining digits if at least two are sensate and mobile.[5] Historically, prosthetic abandonment rates for unilateral upper extremity were high, especially for proximal levels of amputation.[71] A number of factors contribute to the overall success rate of prosthetic use, the importance of which cannot be underestimated. The use of a prosthesis is beneficial in preventing overuse injuries to the other hand and wrist,[72,73] in addition to maximizing ultimate patient function. It has been well documented that the likelihood of prosthetic wear increases when the elbow joint is retained. Early prosthetic fitting within the first 30 to 90 days has also been shown to improve success and acceptance rates.[74] Properly staging the introduction to different types of prosthetic devices in coordination with the rehabilitation team is the key to preventing patient frustration and integrating the prosthesis into his or her lifestyle. This is especially true with more complex cases, proximal amputations, and bilateral injuries.[75]

Treatment protocols for the staging of upper extremity prostheses have been published at WRAMC, dividing the process into 3 phases: the pre-prosthetic phase, the interim prosthetic phase, and the advanced prosthetic phase.[5] Pre-prosthetic training helps to develop strength, range of motion, myo-site development, and desensitization prior to the prosthesis being worn. After early prosthetic fitting, the interim stage of care begins. Therapy changes focus to training with the initial prosthesis. During this time, sockets are frequently replaced, and different types of prostheses and terminal devices are serially introduced. Months later, the first definitive devices are provided, and the advanced stage of care is entered. Therapy in this stage focuses on helping the patient to achieve long-term goals and use of the prosthesis for real-world activities.

The success of an upper extremity prosthesis starts with a pain-free residual limb and ends with a comfortable socket. Flexible plastics and rigid frames allow compliance and support in respective parts of the socket (Figure 23-6). It is not uncommon to have to adjust or replace sockets, especially in the beginning stages before limb volume has stabilized. Suspension may take place through a harness, a suction valve, a pin/lanyard lock, or anatomical compression. With a suction interface, the socket is worn directly against the skin. A gel liner interface is also a possibility and is a good option for weight-bearing activities. Comfortable suspension is paramount for the upper extremity amputee because, unlike the lower extremity amputee who experiences the weight of the prosthesis only when it is lifted off of the ground, the upper extremity device is nearly constantly suspended. Socket design can be self-suspending or may require a harness for support. Anatomically contoured transradial socket designs capture dynamic muscular hypertrophy, thus aiding in control and suspension of the prosthesis.[76] Transhumeral designs are cut low proximally, yet extend onto the chest and back in order to allow greater shoulder abduction range of motion and aid in rotational control. Designs for amputation levels about the shoulder incorporate

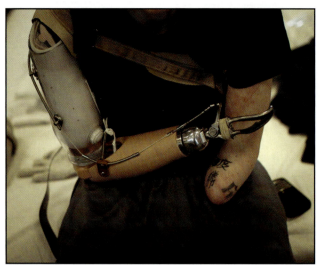

Figure 23-6. Bilateral upper extremity amputees rely a great deal on the prosthetic device functionality. Pictured is a body-powered elbow with a flexion wrist joint and voluntary opening hook. Advances in surgical technique and prosthetic technology for the upper extremity are emerging to improve current standards of care.

a lower profile, X-frame design.[77] These designs have replaced traditional designs as a standard of care at WRAMC.[5]

PROSTHETIC OPTIONS BY DEVICE TYPE

Prosthetic options available for some upper limb amputation levels can be categorized into 5 basic types: 1) passive prosthesis/cosmetic restoration, 2) body-powered prosthesis, 3) electric-powered prosthesis, 4) hybrid prosthesis, and 5) activity-specific prosthesis. Each prosthesis type has certain advantages and disadvantages, and no single device is superior in all circumstances.[5] When adequate clearance permits, in the case of transradial amputations, a quick-disconnect mechanism aids in this purpose, allowing terminal devices to be changed out as necessitated by activity. In the case of the wrist disarticulation amputation level, a quick-disconnect wrist joint adds undesirable length, and the exchange of terminal devices requires additional time and effort. However, the wrist disarticulation level of amputation is advantageous and is arguably more desirable than proximal amputation levels when full retention of wrist pronation and supination is possible.

Passive Prosthesis/ Cosmetic Restoration

Passive/cosmetic restorations do not allow active prehension, but the functionality of these devices cannot be overlooked. Several grasp patterns may still be possible, even though active prehension is not present.[78,79] Passive devices may be constructed out of robust, nonanthropomorphic materials and can serve as opposition posts for residual fingers. These may also be adapted for specific activities, including sports. High-definition silicone restorations look strikingly realistic and are available with fingers that can be passively positioned into place. For higher levels of amputation, silicone restorations are available with an endoskeletal locking elbow joint. The color of the device does not change like human skin, but a recent survey found that most upper extremity amputees were more concerned about shape than color.[80]

Body-Powered Prosthesis

The body-powered prosthesis uses excursion of the back and shoulders to power a cable-operated device (see Figure 23-6). These components are generally lighter and more durable than their motorized counterparts. Elbow joints can be flexed, locked, and unlocked using specific motions of the residual limb and/or back and contralateral shoulder. Terminal devices are available as voluntary opening or voluntary closing and are controlled by the harness through cable excursion. When a prosthetic elbow joint is included, the terminal device is operated sequentially after the elbow joint is locked into position. Other motions that can be operated by cable excursion or passively on certain devices include 1) wrist joint rotation and flexion and 2) shoulder joint rotation, flexion/extension, and abduction/adduction. Passive movement of the arm may require the use of the contralateral side for positioning, bumping the prosthesis against an object, or using momentum or gravity to assist. Some advantages of the body-powered device include the provision of proprioceptive feedback through tension on the cable and harness,[81] speed and accuracy of functional performance,[82-84] and relative durability and decreased expense to maintain.[5]

Electric-Powered Prosthesis

For the electric-powered prosthesis, current motorized components allow finger flexion/extension, terminal device open/close, wrist rotation, elbow flexion and extension, and locking. These motorized components are commonly controlled by myoelectrodes placed strategically over muscle bellies within the socket. Myoelectrodes pick up EMG currents that allow the operation of the hand, hook, wrist, or elbow. Intuitive control is easier when the residual muscle that previously performed a function is used. For example, with a transhumeral amputation, myoelectrodes may be placed in contact with the biceps and/or triceps, which in turn control an open/close function of the terminal device. This requires considerably more learning than when terminal device open/close function is controlled by the flexor/extensor muscles in the transradial or wrist disarticulation amputee. A number of other options are available in addition to or in place of myoelectrodes, including sensors that may be connected to the harness and controlled through slight excursion. In most cases, action speed of the device may be modulated proportional to the strength and accuracy/reproducibility of the signal input by the user. For more proximal amputation levels, a combination of control options and control schemes may be required for dedicated control of each movement.[85] Sensory feedback is primarily visual.[86,87] Some advantages of the electrically powered device include larger functional work envelope, reduced forces on the residual limb,[5] and high-performance anthropomorphic hand function.[5,88] Because the forces on the residual limb are thought to be lessened with an externally powered device in comparison to those generated by a body-powered device, externally powered prostheses for the initial prosthesis are the option of choice at WRAMC.

Hybrid Prosthesis

A hybrid prosthesis most commonly uses a body-powered elbow and an electrically powered terminal device, although an electrically powered elbow with a body-powered terminal device is an option. Advantageous to the hybrid design is that control can be "dedicated" more easily to each motion and the overall weight of the prosthesis is reduced. Dedicated control warranted by the hybrid prosthesis can sometimes permit simultaneous movement of the elbow and terminal device as a coordinated movement.

Activity-Specific Prosthesis

The complexity of the human hand is only marginally replicated with current technology.[89] The 2- or 3-point prehensile function of prosthetic hooks and hands is simply not adequate for optimal performance of certain activities and sports. There are a multitude of activity-specific terminal devices available that may be constructed as part of a separate prosthesis or may be quickly exchanged with a hook or hand in order to perform a specific activity.[90,91] Specialized devices may facilitate gripping onto a bicycle handle, golf club, dumbbell, or kayak paddle, for example, or may provide support for activities such as boxing, basketball, or gymnastics. Not only do these devices offer better function, they save wear and tear on the device and/or cosmetic glove used for everyday activities. A vast assortment of tools and eating utensils are available with the ability to be quickly exchanged in and out of the wrist joint. Our experience has found that, in most circumstances, however, it is more efficient and more convenient for the upper extremity amputee to adapt grasp patterns in order to eat and work with tools.

BILATERAL UPPER EXTREMITY PROSTHETIC CONSIDERATIONS

Bilateral amputees adapt quickly to using a prosthesis because use of an intact, physiologic arm is not an option. Because of the high reliance on the prosthesis, rapid training and prosthetic fitting gain increased importance. Harnessing and control options become quite complicated with more proximal levels of amputation, particularly because contralateral shoulder/thorax control is often not an option due to the prosthetic needs of the other residual limb. Wrist flexion units allow positioning of the terminal device along the midline of the body. Functional requirements are rated as most important for bilateral transhumeral patients in comparison to comfort being rated highest among those with unilateral amputations (see Figure 23-6).[91] Considering this, combining a body-powered device with hook terminal device on one side, and an electrically powered device on the other, has been advocated.[92]

UPPER EXTREMITY PROSTHETIC RESEARCH AND DEVELOPMENT

Better outcome measures assessing components and technology are needed for upper extremity prosthetics.[75] Once identified, such measures should be easy to apply universally so that multicenter reviews can capture the same information.[92] Prosthetic use research is also needed in order to determine predictors of abandonment rates based on level of amputation and dominant versus nondominant upper limb in order to further develop the prescription process.[75]

Compared to lower extremity patients, the number of upper extremity amputees is much lower. For this reason, advances in upper extremity technology have been slow to emerge. However, the recent OIF/OEF conflicts and improvements to body armor have resulted in a relatively large number of upper extremity amputations. In response, many organizations have undertaken efforts to drive improvements. Exciting advances are currently being developed, most of which are focused on improving the mechanism of prosthetic control and increasing the degrees of freedom provided by electrically powered prostheses. Three neural-machine interfaces are currently being investigated: brain-machine interfaces, peripheral nerve interfaces, and targeted muscle reinnervation.

While brain-machine interfaces are the most far-reaching technology being researched, they are potentially the most intuitive.[93-95] Peripheral nerve interfaces are the second closest means to direct thought-control prosthesis activation but have some obstacles to overcome before they are practical.[95,96] Targeted muscle reinnervation was developed by Kuiken and

Dumanian to enhance the current myoelectric prostheses and to make residual muscle(s) a better amplifier of neural signals. By surgical rewiring of branches of the brachial plexus, more intuitive control is ostensibly obtainable. To date, marked improvements of upper extremity prosthetic function have been achieved at WRAMC following targeted muscle reinnervation surgery and rehabilitation protocols.[97-99] Patient-specific advanced pattern recognition techniques may enhance the benefits of targeted muscle reinnervation even further.[77,99]

As less morbid regimens for the prevention of tissue rejection become available, composite tissue allotransplantation (eg, hand transplants) may become a more accepted and practical alternative to amputation and prosthetic use. As complication rates are gradually reduced, osseointegration may become a viable option to replace otherwise heavy and cumbersome prosthetic sockets.

Developments in mechatronics have taken place through 2 projects funded through the Defense Advanced Research Projects Agency. Although not yet commercially available, these devices are designed to provide increased degrees of freedom when compared to current prosthetic technology. In the future, smaller batteries, better actuators and transmissions, and improved sensors and controls will continue to improve electric-powered prosthetic technology.[79]

COMPLICATING FACTORS AFFECTING PROSTHESIS USE

Successful use of a prosthesis may become limited due to problems associated with pressure from the socket, which may or may not be complicated by medical conditions. A generally poor-fitting socket does not distribute pressure optimally throughout the surface area of the residual limb. If the socket continues to be worn, pain may be aggravated, and skin breakdown may occur. Discontinuing or limiting prosthesis use until the wound heals is prudent in this situation. Adjustments to the current socket may alleviate symptoms, or socket replacement may be necessary if the socket is not adjustable due to the material properties or the amount of alteration required. Some residual limb shapes are particularly challenging to fit due to shape, length, and anatomy. Comfort and control within the socket may be difficult to achieve and may require more test socket fittings than usual. Patience and persistence are the keys to success in working with these residual limb types. With new socket changes, it often takes time to tell how well the adjustments have worked. Considering the risk of developing musculoskeletal imbalances and pathologies,[100,101] periodic follow-up to check prosthesis height and alignment should be taken.

Pain-related issues are common and are best handled through good communication and a multidisciplinary approach because medication, injections, prosthetic adjustments, therapeutic treatment, surgery, and other treatment modalities can have combined effects in the pain subsiding or persisting. Hypersensitivity of the residual limb poses a much different problem than the lack of sensation, and both can add to the degree of complexity in managing a particular patient's care.

Common medical complications affecting successful wear of the prosthesis include infection, scar irritation, open wounds, heterotopic ossification, myodesis failure, neuromas, ingrown hairs, skin conditions, and symptomatic bursas. A multidisciplinary clinic is ideal for sorting out the cause of a problem and formulating a treatment plan. All too often, the prosthetist works hard to reduce pressure differently throughout the socket, only to discover that a medical problem was left undiagnosed or untreated.

Heterotopic ossification deserves special attention because it is extremely prevalent in amputation following injury in theater for OIF/OEF.[102] This ectopic bone formation presents challenges to the rehabilitation team because removal is not generally advisable until growth is complete and mature. Fitting a comfortable socket presents a challenge and may not be possible, especially when even the low amount of pressure from wearing a gel liner alone is painful. The use of radiographs and 3-D imaging models can be helpful for the prosthetist to understand the underlying topography. In the best of circumstances, the heterotopic ossification does not have to be removed, the range of motion of surrounding joint(s) is not restricted, and the asymptomatic heterotopic ossification can even assist in prosthesis load transmission and suspension.

Conclusion

The lessons learned from individuals sustaining limb loss in OIF/OEF have helped to improve and standardize modern methods of care, identify current and future gaps for research and development, and inspire motivation in providers. The capacity of the human spirit to recover from catastrophic injury and attain acceptance back to active duty or civilian life is rewarding for those who provide care to the heroes of our nation. Understanding the state of science with regard to prosthetic technology, as illustrated in this chapter, is important for the orthopedic surgeon making decisions about amputation surgery as well as for the physiatrist, physical therapist, or prosthetist subsequently caring for these wounded warriors. With diligent efforts by all parties, the functional and psychosocial outcomes of all servicemembers with limb loss can be maximized.

References

1. US military builds on rich history of amputee care. *Military In-Step.* http://www.amputee-coalition.org/military-instep/rich-history.html. Last updated 9/18/2008.
2. Bowker JH, Prithan CH. The history of amputation surgery and prosthetics. In: Smith DG, Michael JW, Bowker JH, eds. *Atlas of Amputations and Limb Deficiencies: Surgical, Prosthetic, and Rehabilitation Principles.* 3rd ed. Rosemont, IL: American Academy of Orthopedic Surgeons; 2004:11-14.
3. Pasquina PF, Tsao JW, Collins DM, et al. Quality of medical care provided to service members with combat-related limb amputations: report of patient satisfaction. *J Rehabil Res Dev.* 2008;45:953-960.
4. Kapp S, Miller JA. Lower limb prosthetics. In: Lenhart MK, Pasquina PF, Cooper RA, *Textbooks of military medicine: Care of the combat amputee.* Washington, DC: Office of the Surgeon General Department of the Army, United States of America; 2009:578.
5. Miguelez J, Conyers D, Lang M, Gulick K. Upper extremity prosthetics. In: Lenhart MK, Pasquina PF, Cooper RA, *Textbooks of military medicine: Care of the combat amputee.* Washington, DC: Office of the Surgeon General Department of the Army, United States of America; 2009:618-639.
6. Dumbleton T, Buis AWP, McFadyen A, et al. Dynamic interface pressure distributions of two transtibial prosthetic socket concepts. *J Rehabil Res Dev.* 2009;46:405-416.
7. Pierce ROJ, Kernek CB, Ambrose T. The plight of the traumatic amputee. *Orthopedics.* 1993;16:793-797.
8. Harris AM, Althausen PL, Kellam J, Bosse MJ, Castillo R. Complications following limb-threatening lower extremity trauma. *J Orthop Trauma.* 2009;23:1-6.
9. Smith DG. General principles of amputation surgery. In: Smith DG, Michael JW, Bowker JH, eds. *Atlas of Amputations and Limb Deficiencies: Surgical, Prosthetic, and Rehabilitation Principles.* 3rd ed. Rosemont, IL: American Academy of Orthopedic Surgeons; 2004:21-30.
10. US Army Military Amputee Care Data Base. Washington, DC: Walter Reed Army Medical Center.
11. Bowker JH, Prithan CH. The history of amputation surgery and prosthetics. In: Smith DG, Michael JW, Bowker JH, eds. *Atlas of Amputations and Limb Deficiencies: Surgical, Prosthetic, and Rehabilitation Principles.* 3rd ed. Rosemont, IL: American Academy of Orthopedic Surgeons; 2004:11-14.
12. Chrzan JS, Giurini JM, Hurchik JM. A biomechanical model for the trans-metatarsal amputation. *J Am Podiatr Med Assoc.* 1993;83:82-86.
13. Boyd LA, Rao SS, Burnfield JM, et al. Forefoot rocker mechanics in individuals with partial foot amputation. *Gait Posture.* 1999;9:144.
14. Pinzur MS, Gottschalk F, Smith DG, et al. Functional outcome of below-knee amputation in peripheral vascular insufficiency: a multicenter review. *Clin Orthop.* 1993;286:247-249.
15. Rosenkranz G. The patella-tendon-bearing prosthesis. *Artificial Limbs.* 1962;6:1-3.
16. Staats TB, Lundt J. The UCLA total surface bearing suction below knee prosthesis. *Clin Prosthet Orthot.* 1987;11:118-130.
17. Guh JC, Lee PV, Chong SY. Stump/socket pressure profiles of the pressure cast prosthetic socket. *Clin Biomech.* 2003;18:237-238.
18. Goujon H, Bonnet X, Sautreuil P, et al. A functional evaluation of prosthetic foot kinematics during lower-limb amputee gait. *Prosthet Orthot Int.* 2006;30:213-223.
19. Marinakis GNS. Interlimb symmetry of traumatic unilateral transtibial amputees wearing two different prosthetic feet in the early rehabilitation stage. *J Rehabil Res Dev.* 2004;41:581-590.
20. Van de Veen PG. *Above-Knee Prosthesis Technology.* The Netherlands: PG van de Veen Consultancy (Enschede); 2001.
21. Schuch CM. Modern above-knee fitting practice: a report on the ISPO workshop on above-knee fitting and alignment techniques. *Prosthet Orthot Int.* 1988;12:77-90.
22. Hoyt C, Littig D, Lundt J, Staats TB. *The UCLA CAT-CAM Above-Knee Prosthesis.* 3rd ed. Los Angeles, CA: UCLA Prosthetic Education and Research Program; 1987.
23. Kristinsson O. Flexible above-knee socket made from low density polyethylene suspended by a weight transmitting frame. *Orthot Prosthet.* 1983;37:25-27.
24. Hughes J. Biomechanics of the through-knee prosthesis. *Prosthet Orthot Int.* 1983;7:96-99.
25. Gottschalk FA, Kourosh S, Stills M, McClellan B, Roberts J. Does socket configuration influence the position of the femur in above-knee amputation? *J Prosthet Orthot.* 1990;2:94-102.
26. Pritham CH. Biomechanics and shape of the above-knee socket considered in light of the ischial containment concept. *Prosthet Orthot Int.* 1990;14:9-21.
27. Anderson MH, Sollars RE, eds. *Prosthetic Principles: Above Knee Amputations.* Springfield, IL: Charles C. Thomas Publishers; 1960:129-146.
28. Anderson MH, Sollars RE, eds. *Manual of Above Knee Prosthetics for Physicians and Therapists.* 2nd ed. Los Angeles, CA: UCLA School of Medicine, Prosthetics Education Program; 1957:86-111.
29. Gailey RS, Gailey AM. *Prosthetic Gait Training for Lower Limb Amputees.* Miami, FL: Advanced Rehabilitation Therapy Inc; 1989.
30. Perry J, ed. *Gait Analysis: Normal and Pathological Function.* Thorofare, NJ: SLACK Incorporated; 1992.
31. Gard SA, Childress DS. The influence of stance-phase knee flexion on the vertical displacement of the trunk during normal walking. *Arch Phys Med Rehabil.* 1999;80:26-32.
32. Williams RM, Turner AP, Orendurff M, et al. Does having a computerized prosthetic knee influence cognitive performance during amputee walking? *Arch Phys Med Rehabil.* 2006;87:989-994.
33. Hafner BJ, Willingham LL, Buell NC, Allyn KJ, Smith DG. Evaluation of function, performance, and preference as transfemoral amputees transition from mechanical to microprocessor control of the prosthetic knee. *Arch Phys Med Rehabil.* 2007;88(2):207-217.
34. Seymour R, Engbretson B, Kott K, et al. Comparison between the C-leg microprocessor-controlled prosthetic knee and non-microprocessor control prosthetic knees: a preliminary study of energy expenditure, obstacle course performance, and quality of life survey. *Prosthet Orthot Int.* 2007;31(1):51-61.
35. Schmalz T, Blumentritt S, Marx B. Biomechanical analysis of stair ambulation in lower limb amputees. *Gait and Posture.* 2007;25:267-278.
36. Kahle JT, Highsmith MJ, Hubbard SL. Comparison of non-microprocessor knee mechanism versus C-Leg on prosthesis evaluation questionnaire, stumbles, falls, walking tests, stair descent, and knee preference. *J Rehabil Res Dev.* 2008;45(1):1-14.
37. Segal AD, Orendurff MS, Klute GK, et al. Kinematic and kinetic comparisons of transfemoral amputee gait using C-leg and Mauch SNS prosthetic knees. *J Rehabil Res Dev.* 2006;43(7):857-870.
38. Johansson JL, Sherrill DM, Riley PO, Bonato P, Herr H. A clinical comparison of variable-damping and mechanically passive prosthetic knee devices. *Am J Phys Med Rehabil.* 2005;84:563-575.
39. Blumentritt S, Schmalz T, Jarasch R. Safety of C-leg: biomechanical tests. *J Prosthet Orthot.* 2009;21(1):2-17.
40. Berry D, Olson MD, Larntz K. perceived stability, function, and satisfaction among transfemoral amputees using microprocessor and nonmicroprocessor controlled prosthetic knees: a multicenter survey. *J Prosthet Orthot.* 2009;21:32-42.

41. Bunce DJ, Breakey JW. The impact of C-Leg on the physical and psychological adjustment to transfemoral amputation. *J Prosthet Orthot.* 2007;19(1):7-14.

42. Gerzeli S, Torbica A, Fattore G. Cost utility analysis of knee prosthesis with complete microprocessor control (C-leg) compared with mechanical technology in transfemoral amputees. *European Journal of Health Economics.* 2008. (e-publication ahead of print.)

43. Kaufman KR, Levine JA, Brey RH, McCrady SK, Padgett DJ, Joyner MJ. Energy expenditure and activity level of transfemoral amputees using passive mechanical and microprocessor-controlled prosthetic knees. *Arch Phys Med Rehabil.* 2008;89(7):1380-1385.

44. Harvey ZT. *Microprocessor vs. Hydraulic Controlled Prosthetic Knee in Early Stage Rehabilitation for Transfemoral Amputees: A Pilot Study.* Washington, DC: Walter Reed Army Medical Center; on-going.

45. Waters RL, Perry J, Antonelli D, Hislop H. Energy cost of walking of amputees: the influence of level of amputation. *J Bone Joint Surg Am.* 1976;58:42-46.

46. Shurr DG, Cook TM, Buckwalter JA, Cooper RR. Hip disarticulation: a prosthetic follow-up. *Orthot Prosthet.* 1983;37:50-57.

47. Steen Jensen J, Mandrup-Poulsen T. Success rate of prosthetic fitting after major amputations of the lower limb. *Prosthet Orthot Int.* 1983;7:119-121.

48. Radcliffe CW. The biomechanics of the Canadian-type hip-disarticulation prosthesis. *Artif Limbs.* 1957;4:29-38.

49. van der Waarde T, Michael J. Hip disarticulation and transpelvic amputation: Prosthetic management. In: Bowker JH, Michael JW, eds. *Atlas of Limb Prosthetics: Surgical, Prosthetic, and Rehabilitation Principles.* 2nd ed. Rosemont, IL: American Academy of Orthopedic Surgeons; 2002:539-552.

50. Michael J. Energy storing feet: a clinical comparison. *Clin Prosthet Orthot.* 1987;11:154-168.

51. Su PF, Gard SA, Lipschultz RD, Kuiken TA. Gait characteristics of persons with bilateral transtibial amputations. *J Rehabil Res Dev.* 2007;44:491-502.

52. Torburn L, Perry J, Ayyappa E, Shanfield SL. Below-knee amputee gait with dynamic elastic response prosthetic feet: a pilot study. *J Rehabil Res Dev.* 1990;27(4):369-384.

53. Prince F, Winter DA, Sjonnensen G, Powell C, Wheeldon RK. Mechanical efficiency during gait of adults with transtibial amputation: a pilot study comparing the SACH, Seattle, and Golden-Ankle prosthetic feet. *J Rehabil Res Dev.* 1998;35(2):177-185.

54. Perry J, ed. *Gait Analysis: Normal and Pathological Function.* Thorofare, NJ: SLACK Incorporated; 1992.

55. Gard SA, Konz RL. The influence of prosthetic shock absorbing pylons on transtibial amputee gait. *Gait Posture.* 2001;13:303.

56. McCollough NC III, Harris AR, Hampton FL. The bilateral lower-limb amputee. In: American Academy of Orthopaedic Surgeons. *Atlas of Limb Prosthetics: Surgical and Prosthetic Principles.* St. Louis, MO: CV Mosby; 1981:417-422.

57. Uellendahl JE. Bilateral lower limb prostheses. In: Smith DG, Michael JW, Bowker JH, eds. *Atlas of Amputations and Limb Deficiencies: Surgical, Prosthetic, and Rehabilitation Principles.* 3rd ed. Rosemont, IL: American Academy of Orthopedic Surgeons; 2004:623.

58. Smith DG, Ehde DM, Legro MW, Reiber GE, del Aguila M, Boone DA. Phantom limb, residual limb, and back pain after lower extremity amputations. *Clin Orthop Relat Res.* 1999;Apr(361):29-38.

59. Kegel B. Physical fitness: sports and recreation for those with lower limb amputation or impairment. *J Rehab Res Dev Clin Suppl.* 1985;1:1-125.

60. Harvey ZT. The desire to achieve. *O&P Edge.* www.oandp.com/articles/2008-03_04.asp. Accessed November 9, 2010.

61. Fergason JR, Boone DA. Prostheses for sports and recreation. In: Smith DG, Michael JW, Bowker JH, eds. *Atlas of Amputations and Limb Deficiencies: Surgical, Prosthetic, and Rehabilitation Principles.* 3rd ed. Rosemont, IL: American Academy of Orthopedic Surgeons; 2004:633-640.

62. Fergason JR, Harsch PD. Lower limb prosthetics for sports and recreation. *Textbooks of military medicine: Care of the combat amputee.* Washington, DC: Office of the Surgeon General Department of the Army, United States of America; 2009:581-595.

63. Geil MD. Assessing the state of clinically applicable research for evidence-based practice in prosthetics and orthotics. *J Rehabil Res Dev.* 2009;46:305-314.

64. Pasquina PF, Fitzpatrick KF. The Walter Reed experience: current issues in the care of the traumatic amputee. *J Prosthet Orthot.* 2006;18:119-122.

65. Collinger J, Grindle GG, Heiner C, et al. Road map for future amputee care research. *Textbooks of Military Medicine: Care of the Combat Amputee.* Washington, DC: Office of the Surgeon General Department of the Army, United States of America; 2009:731-739.

66. Martinez-Villalpando EC, Herr H. Agonist-antagonist active knee prosthesis: a preliminary study in level-ground walking. *J Rehabil Res Dev.* 2009;46:361-374.

67. Hagberg K, Branemark R. One hundred patients treated with osseointegrated transfemoral amputation prostheses—rehabilitation perspective. *J Rehabil Res Dev.* 2009;46:331-344.

68. Branemark R, Branemark PI, Rydevik BL, Myers RR. Osseointegration in skeletal reconstruction and rehabilitation: a review. *J Rehabil Res Dev.* 2001;38:175-191.

69. Sensinger J, Pasquina PF, Kuiken T. The future of artificial limbs. *Textbooks of Military Medicine: Care of the Combat Amputee.* Washington, DC: Office of the Surgeon General Department of the Army, United States of America; 2009:721-730.

70. Baccarani A, Follmar KE, De Santis G, et al. Free vascularized tissue transfer to preserve upper extremity amputation levels. *Plast Reconstr Surg.* 2007;120:971-981.

71. Pinzur MS, Angelats J, Light TR, Izuierdo R, Pluth T. Functional outcome following traumatic upper limb amputation and prosthetic limb fitting. *J Hand Surg Am.* 1994;19:836-839.

72. Reddy MP. Nerve entrapment syndromes in the upper extremity contralateral to amputation. *Arch Phys Med Rehabil.* 1984;65:24-26.

73. Jones LE, Davidson JH. Save that arm: a study of problems in the remaining arm of unilateral upper limb amputees. *Prosthet Orthot Int.* 1999;23:55-58.

74. Malone JM, Fleming LL, Roberson J, et al. Immediate, early, and late postsurgical management of upper-limb amputation. *J Rehabil Res Dev.* 1984;21:33-41.

75. Uellendahl JE. Bilateral upper limb prostheses. In: Smith DG, Michael JW, Bowker JH, eds. *Atlas of Amputations and Limb Deficiencies: Surgical, Prosthetic, and Rehabilitation Principles.* 3rd ed. Rosemont, IL: American Academy of Orthopedic Surgeons; 2004:313.

76. Miguelez JM, Lake C, Conyers D, Zenie J. The transradial anatomically contoured (TRAC) interface: design principles and methodology. *J Prosthet Orthot.* 2003;15:148-157.

77. Miguelez JM, Miguelez MD. The MicroFrame: the next generation of interface design for glenohumeral disarticulation and associated levels of limb deficiency. *J Prosthet Orthot.* 2003;15:66-71.

78. Roeschlein RA, Domholdt E. Factors related to successful upper extremity prosthetic use. *Prosthet Orthot Int.* 1989;13:14-18.

79. Muilengurg AL, LeBlanc MA. Body-powered upper-limb components. In: Atkins DJ, Meier RH III, eds. *Comprehensive Management of the Upper-Limb Amputee* (pp 28-38). New York, NY: Springer-Verlag; 1989.

80. Schultz AE, Baade SP, Kuiken TA. Expert opinions on success factors for upper-limb prostheses. *J Rehabil Res Dev.* 2007;44:483-490.

81. Heckathorne CW. Manipulation in unstructured environments: extended physiological proprioception, position control, and arm prostheses. *Proceedings of the International Conference on Rehabilitation Robotics.* 1990:25-40.

82. Billock JN. The Northwestern University supracondylar suspension technique for below-elbow amputations. *Orthot Prosthet.* 1972;26:16-23.

83. Kritter AE. Myoelectric prostheses. *J Bone Joint Surg Am.* 1985;67:654-657.

84. Northmore-Ball MD, Heger H, Hunter GA. The below-elbow myoelectric prosthesis: a comparison of the Otto Bock myoelectric prosthesis with the hook and functional hand. *J Bone Joint Surg Br.* 1980;62:363-367.

85. Uellendahl JE, Heckathorne CW. Creative prosthetic solutions for the person with bilateral upper extremity amputations. In: Atkins D, Meier R, eds. *Functional Restoration of Adults and Children With Upper Extremity Amputation.* New York, NY: Demos Medical Publishing; 2004:225-237.

86. Stein RB, Walley M. Functional comparison of upper extremity amputees using myoelectric and conventional prostheses. *Arch Phys Med Rehabil.* 1983;64:243-248.

87. Uellendahl JE. Upper extremity myoelectric prosthetics. *Phys Med Rehabil Clin N Am.* 2000;11:639-652.

88. Millstein SG, Heger H, Hunter GA. Prosthetic use in adult upper limb amputees: a comparison of the body powered and electrically powered prostheses. *Prosthet Orthot Int.* 1986;10:27-34.

89. Radocy R. Upper limb prosthetics for sports and recreation. *Textbooks of Military Medicine: Care of the Combat Amputee.* Washington, DC: Office of the Surgeon General, Department of the Army, United States of America; 2009:641-681.

90. Radocy R. Prosthetic adaptations in competitive sports and recreation. In: Smith DG, Michael JW, Bowker JH, eds. *Atlas of Amputations and Limb Deficiencies: Surgical, Prosthetic, and Rehabilitation Principles.* 3rd ed. Rosemont, IL: American Academy of Orthopedic Surgeons; 2004:327-337.

91. Heckathorne CW, Krick H, Uellendahl J, Wu Y, Childress DS. Achieving complementary manipulative function with bilateral hybrid upper-limb prostheses. *Arch Phys Med Rehabil.* 1990;71:773.

92. Miller LA, Swanson S. Summary and recommendations of the academy's state of the science conference on upper limb prosthetic outcome measures. *J Prosthet Orthot.* 2009;21:83-89.

93. Musallam S, Corneil BD, Greger B, Scherberger H, Andersen RA. Cognitive control signals for neural prosthetics. *Science.* 2004;305:258-262.

94. Hochberg LR, Serruya MD, Friehs GM, eds. Neuronal ensemble control of prosthetic devices by a human with tetraplegia. *Nature.* 2006;442:164-171.

95. Upshaw B, Sinkjaer T. Digital signal processing algorithms for the detection of afferent nerve activity recorded from cuff electrodes. *IEEE Trans Rehabil Eng.* 1998;6:172-181.

96. Childress D, Weir RF. Control of limb prostheses. In: Smith DG, Michael JW, Bowker JH, eds. *Atlas of Amputations and Limb Deficiencies: Surgical, Prosthetic, and Rehabilitation Principles.* 3rd ed. Rosemont, IL: American Academy of Orthopedic Surgeons; 2004:173-195.

97. Lipschutz RD, Miller LA, Stubblefield KA, Dumanian GA, Phillips ME, Kuiken TA. Transhumeral level fitting and outcomes following targeted hyper-reinnervation nerve transfer surgery. In: *Proceedings of the myoelectric control symposium.* Fredericton, New Brunswick, Canada: University of New Brunswick; 2005:2-5.

98. Stubblefield KA, Miller LA, Lipschutz RD, Kuiken TA. Occupational therapy protocol for amputees with targeted muscle reinnervation. *J Rehabil Res Dev.* 2009;46:481-488.

99. Kuiken TA, Dumanian GA, Lipschutz RD, Miller LA, Stubblefield KA. The use of targeted muscle reinnervation for improved myoelectric prosthesis control in a bilateral shoulder disarticulation amputee. *Prosthet Orthot Int.* 2004;28:245-253.

100. Robbins CB, Vreeman DJ, Sothmann MS, Wilson SL, Oldridge NB. A review of the long-term health outcomes associated with war-related amputation. *Mil Med.* 2009;174:588-592.

101. Gailey R, Allen K, Castles J, Kucharik J, Roeder M. Review of secondary physical conditions associated with lower-limb amputation and long-term prosthesis use. *J Rehabil Res Dev.* 2009;45:15-30.

102. Potter BK, Burns TC, Iacap AP, Granville RR, Gajewski DA. Heterotopic ossification following traumatic and combat-related amputations. Prevalence, risk factors, and preliminary results of excision. *J Bone Joint Surg Am.* 2007;89:476-478.

Chapter 24

LONG-BONE FRACTURE MANAGEMENT

MAJ Travis C. Burns, MD; CPT Daniel J. Stinner, MD; and LTC Joseph R. Hsu, MD

Extremity injuries are the most common injuries sustained in recent conflicts, and lower extremity fractures are the most common fractures treated by orthopedic surgeons.[1,2] A treatment algorithm is critical for the deployed orthopedic surgeon to ensure appropriate, timely decisions in mass casualty situations that tax resources and preclude consultation. In creating such an algorithm, the treating orthopedic surgeon must have knowledge of the available surgical set and prefabricated splint inventory, air evacuation procedures, and contact information for the next higher echelon of care.

Epidemiology

Eighty-two percent of injured US military personnel have sustained extremity injuries during the ongoing conflicts in Afghanistan and Iraq.[3] The majority of these combat-related injuries (78%) are secondary to explosions. In a recent review of battlefield injuries during the current conflicts, Owens and colleagues reported 915 fractures sustained by US military personnel, with 758 (82%) of those being open fractures, signifying the severe nature of these injuries.[2] In this review, the fractures were evenly distributed between the upper and lower extremities: 461 upper extremity fractures (50%) and 454 lower extremity fractures (50%). Not surprisingly, fractures of the tibia and fibula accounted for the majority of lower extremity fractures (48%). Just over a quarter of the lower extremity fractures were femur fractures (27%).[2] In another review of the injuries sustained by a single

US Army brigade combat team during Operation Iraqi Freedom, Belmont and colleagues also identified a high rate of lower extremity long-bone fractures sustained during combat, with fractures of the tibia, fibula, and femur accounting for nearly one-third of all fractures (31%).[4]

Management in Theater

GENERAL PRINCIPLES OF LONG-BONE MANAGEMENT

Damage control orthopedics is a philosophical departure from "early total care" and evolved from damage control surgery in the management of abdominal injuries. Abdominal damage control surgery involves early laparotomy for hemorrhage control, resuscitation in the intensive care unit, followed by a return to the operating room for definitive surgery. Damage control orthopedics largely refers to the use of temporary external fixation to stabilize extremity fractures to help mitigate the physiologic consequences of long-bone fractures.[5-8] Stabilization of long-bone fractures in polytrauma patients reduces both narcotic requirements and inflammatory mediators and results in improved ventilation.[8-10] Temporary external fixation provides patients the benefit of early fracture stabilization, while avoiding the physiologic "second hit" associated with early definitive fracture stabilization.[6] The concept of damage control surgery is especially useful in a combat theater of operations where early internal fixation is avoided secondary to

Owens BD, Belmont PJ Jr, eds. *Combat Orthopedic Surgery: Lessons Learned in Iraq and Afghanistan (pp 237-252)*
© 2011 SLACK Incorporated

resource limitations and significant contamination associated with combat injuries.[11] Damage control orthopedics in this scenario allows for both optimization of the patient's physiologic status and transport to a more appropriate tertiary care facility for definitive management.

In assessing patients for damage control algorithms, the civilian literature divides patients into categories based on overall status: stable, borderline, unstable, and in extremis.[12] Physiologically unstable patients and those in extremis are best treated with damage control surgical intervention and early external fixation of lower extremity long-bone fractures.[6,12,13] Borderline patients are those patients predisposed to deterioration, and while the definition varies between institutions, it often includes patients with thoracic or head injuries.[6,9,14] Borderline patients with tibia and femur fractures are also best treated with external fixation due to the physiologic benefits of stabilization and the difficulty of monitoring and treating patients during evacuation flights. Stable patients can be treated with external fixation or splinting based on injury characteristics and the surgeon's perceived utility of the treatment methods. In contrast to treatment of civilian injuries where the clinical decision rests between early total care and damage control orthopedics, in the combat setting, there are only 2 options for long-bone fracture treatment: external fixation or splint immobilization.

There are numerous benefits of fracture stabilization provided by external fixation besides the physiologic effects in severely injured patients. Stabilizing the fracture site reduces further trauma to the zone of injury, can protect a vascular repair, and may reduce hemorrhage by reducing displaced fracture surfaces. The reduced soft tissue injury afforded by external fixation may also reduce the risk of infection.[15,16] External fixation additionally provides easy access for wound monitoring and treatment, is less bulky than traction and splinting devices, and can be constructed to suspend the injured extremity to limit pressure on soft tissue.

Several studies evaluating safety of external fixation have demonstrated that lower extremity pin placement has a very low rate of neurologic or vascular injury.[17-19] In a cadaveric study evaluating lower extremity external fixator placement without fluoroscopic assistance, Topp and colleagues demonstrated a 2% risk of neurovascular injury.[20] Dwyer, after studying pin insertion in cadaver specimens, noted that vessels are usually pushed to the side as the pin penetrates the soft tissue.[21] This supports Burny's report of 1421 tibia fractures treated with an external fixation device without a neurovascular injury.[18]

External fixation has associated disadvantages.[22,23] Safe placement of the device requires technical expertise and knowledge of the anatomy. The minimal amount of equipment required may still be unavailable in austere combat environments. Damage to surrounding neurovascular structures is rare, but is of special concern in applying external fixation to the upper extremities. A communication track is created from the external environment to the bone, which introduces the risks of pin track osteomyelitis and joint sepsis if intracapsular pins are placed. A series of civilian tibia fractures reported a 78% incidence of pin track infections treated initially with external fixation.[24] Although frequently used in the combat environment, the effect of temporary external fixation on osseous union rate and deep infection rate is unknown.

Splinting is a rapid means of supporting an injured extremity that is low cost, requires minimal equipment and technical expertise, and does not require a sterile environment for application. It provides more soft tissue support than external fixation, does not introduce additional sources of infection, and preserves the maximum number of definitive treatment options for the receiving orthopedic surgeon.[25] Splints, however, may provide inadequate stability for unstable fracture patterns associated with combat injuries. More importantly, anatomic location of the fracture often determines a splint's utility. Splint application is useful for injuries more distal in the appendicular skeleton (eg, wrist, hand, ankle, foot), as immobilizing the joints above and below the fracture is more easily accomplished.

In addition, splints often lose stability with removal, which frequently necessitates fabrication of a new one. The extremity is often unstable during the repeat splinting, and the patient may require sedation for correct application. Splinting a long-bone fracture associated with a wound that will require repeat dressing changes and evaluation during the evacuation process may be less than ideal. Splint materials may also become saturated with wound drainage. Despite these limitations, splints or traction devices must be used in situations where external fixation is unavailable or not practicable.

FEMORAL FRACTURES

Femur fractures have historically been a devastating injury in combat casualties. Femur fractures were often associated with significant morbidity and mortality in early conflicts.[26] Devised in the late 1800s, the Thomas splint was a device that used traction to reduce and stabilize femur fractures. During World War I, physicians attributed a reduced mortality from femur fractures to the use of the Thomas splint.[27] The Thomas splint and several similar devices (eg, NATO splint, HARE traction) are still useful today in the temporary stabilization of lower extremity long-bone fractures.

During the same time the Thomas splint was developed, several surgeons described external fixation devices for fracture stabilization. Malgaigne first described the use of external fixation in 1847, but it did not gain much acceptance until it became more frequently used in combat operations during World War II.[28,29] The Hoffmann II External Fixation System and Sterile Field Kit (Stryker, Mahwah, NJ) was designed for military application and was largely based on Raoul Hoffmann's early designs.[30,31] The important characteristics of an external fixation system used in combat operations are a minimum amount of necessary equipment, sufficient rigidity for fracture stability during transport, and modular design that can be adjusted or modified at subsequent levels of care.

The Hoffmann II External Fixation System provides self-drilling, self-taping pins that allow placement of the external fixator and stabilization of the fracture without need for electrical power. The modular design combines clamps, side posts, and carbon fiber rods to connect the pins on either side of the fracture. The system allows for placement of unilateral frames that may be modified with additional components as fracture stability requires at higher levels of care when more resources and imaging are available.

Femur Fracture Treatment Options

External Fixation (Indications, Risks, Benefits)

In the conflicts in Iraq and Afghanistan, external fixation is a commonly used treatment for femur fractures.[32,33] The precise indications for external fixator application for combat-related femur fractures have not been defined.[25] Relative indications from the *Emergency War Surgery* manual include need for soft tissue wound access (eg, evaluation or treatment en route), vascular injury, femur fracture with abdominal injury, extensive burns on ipsilateral extremity necessitating soft tissue access, polytrauma patients, and fractures with significant comminution or bone loss (Table 24-1).[25]

Due to the average 6-day evacuation time from theater, the necessity of multiple litter transfers, and the benefits of patient comfort and fracture stabilization provided by external fixation, we recommend external fixation of all open, displaced, or unstable femur fractures when technically feasible.

The basic requirements for application of external fixation in theater are a thorough understanding of the anatomy and safe zones for pin placement, a modular external fixator equipment set, and a sterile operating room environment with appropriate support staff. The Hoffmann II External Fixator System and Sterile Field Kit can safely be applied without power or fluoroscop-

Table 24-1

Indications for External Fixation of Femur Fracture

Relative Indications

Segmental bone loss
Open fractures
Vascular injury
Polytrauma
Multiple long-bone fractures
Femur fracture in physiologically unstable
Need for soft tissue access
　　Extensive burns
　　Repeat debridements
　　Compartment monitoring

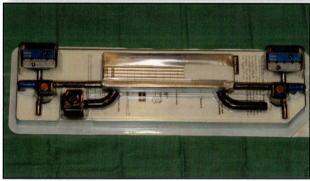

Figure 24-1. The Hoffmann II External Fixation System and Sterile Field Kit (Stryker, Mahwah, NJ) as shown in its off-the-shelf sterile peel pack was designed to allow temporary, rapid stabilization of long-bone fractures in the combat or austere environment.

ic imaging if unavailable (Figure 24-1).[20] A radiolucent bed is used when available; otherwise, the standard operating room table may be used. The entire limb is prepared for surgery in sterile fashion from the anterior superior iliac crest to the foot. Irrigation and debridement of the open wound should be completed to remove all contamination and devitalized tissue. If the wound is grossly contaminated, the extremity should be sterilely prepped a second time after debridement with an aseptic solution.

For a diaphyseal femur fracture, a padded "bump" should be applied under the fracture site for gross limb alignment. The pin entrance sites should be identified based on location of the fracture and the soft tissue wound and to avoid hip or knee intracapsular pin placement. The pins should be a minimum of 1 inch from the fracture site to avoid propagating the fracture and infecting the fracture hematoma.[25,34] For subtrochanteric and pertrochanteric proximal femur fractures with a very short proximal fracture segment, external fixator pins can be placed into the femoral

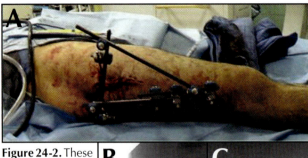

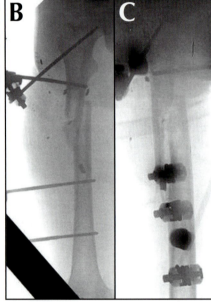

Figure 24-2. These figures demonstrate the application of an external fixator for a proximal femur fracture with proximal pin fixation in the femoral neck.

neck (Figure 24-2).[35-38] Pelvifemoral or hip-spanning external fixation is an alternative method of external fixation if proximal femoral bone stock is insufficient for pin fixation.[39] Both methods of proximal femur fracture stabilization with external fixation are more technically demanding than diaphyseal fixation, and the associated risks may outweigh the benefits depending on surgeon experience and available fluoroscopic imaging resources.

Soft Tissue Anatomy Considerations

The important structures surrounding the femur that may be injured during pin placement are the femoral vessels, femoral nerve, sciatic nerve, and hip and knee joints. The femoral nerve and superficial femoral artery enter the leg through the inguinal canal in the proximal anterior thigh and are covered by the sartorius muscle down the anterior medial thigh. The saphenous nerve joins the femoral vessels in the proximal thigh and courses through the adductor canal (Hunter's canal) to a more posterior location in the popliteal fossa. Hunter's canal can extend from the midpoint of the femur to the distal one-sixth.[40] Due to their fixed position adjacent to the bone, the femoral vessels are most at risk in Hunter's canal from overpenetrated pins through the medial cortex. The sciatic nerve remains posterior to the femur throughout its

course and is not in direct contact with the bone. The knee joint capsule extends anteriorly approximately 6.3 cm above the proximal pole of the patella. The capsule inserts approximately 1 cm proximal to the articular margins medially, laterally, and posteriorly.[40]

Safe Corridors for Femoral Pin Placement

Safe pin placement for femoral external fixation is laterally and anteriorly. The femoral vessels are at risk with medial pin placement, and their approximate position can be identified by a straight line from the most medial aspect of the medial femoral condyle and the anterior superior iliac spine.[41] The sciatic nerve lies directly posterior to the femoral shaft, and pins should not be placed in this region. Anterior pin placement is a safe alternative to lateral pin placement; however, some authors believe this can cause knee stiffness due to adhesions from rectus femoris pin penetration.[41] Also, anterior pins should be avoided in the distal femur due to the 6.3 cm proximal extension of the suprapatellar pouch.

Femoral External Fixation Technique[42]
Indications: Femur Fracture, Proximal Femur Fracture:
- Identify appropriate pin location, keeping in mind to place the pins adjacent to the fracture site a minimum of 1 inch from the fracture.
- A 1-cm longitudinal stab incision is made.
- Bluntly spread down to bone.
- Put a 5-mm half-pin down on the bone, and determine the midportion of the bone by moving the pin gently back and forth across the width of the femur. Assistant should provide stability and counter pressure.
- Two taps on the end of the pin with a mallet should provide an indent in the bone and allow you to start insertion. The pin can be placed by hand or with power.
- Insert the pin in the midportion of the bone through both the near and far cortex.
- Experience will enable the surgeon to detect an increase in the resistance, or a change in the pitch of the drill when using power, as the far cortex is encountered. If using power to insert the pins, it is recommended to change from power to hand insertion as the far cortex is encountered to control depth of placement.
- Two complete revolutions of the pin after initial contact with the far cortex will advance the 5-mm half pin far enough to allow for sufficient penetration.
- Place a multi-pin clamp over the inserted pin. Ideally, the pin should occupy one of the end positions for greater pin spread, increasing stability of the construct.

- Using the clamp as a guide, insert a second pin through the clamp. The second pin must be parallel to the first.
- Ensure that the multi-pin clamp is in line with the bone and that bi-cortical purchase is obtained with the second pin.
- A third pin may be inserted if needed for additional construct stability.
- Apply a second multi-pin clamp and pins in the same manner to the distal femoral fracture fragment. Pins should be placed parallel to the distal articular surface.
- Connect the 2 clamps with elbows, bar-to-bar clamps, and 2 longitudinal bars placed parallel to each other.
- Reduce the fracture with longitudinal traction. Manipulating the fracture fragments using the clamps may be helpful. Once adequate reduction is achieved, tighten all the connections. While maintenance of length is advantageous, precise reduction is not necessary.

Pin Placement in Femoral Neck
- Under fluoroscopic guidance, two parallel 5-mm pins are placed across the femoral neck into the femoral head.
- The start point on the lateral femur is at or above the level of the lesser trochanter.
- Pins are inserted to approximately 1 cm from the chondral surface.
- Care is taken to ensure appropriate pin placement in the femoral neck and head on fluoroscopic images or orthogonal radiographs to minimize the risks of joint sepsis from pin track infections.

Pin Placement in Iliac Wing
- A 3-cm incision is made over iliac crest 3-cm posterior to anterior superior iliac spine.
- Sharp dissection is carried down to the iliac crest.
- The periosteum is incised in-line with the iliac crest, and periosteum is elevated anteriorly and posteriorly.
- Starting at the junction of the medial one-third and the lateral two-thirds, 6-mm pins are placed in the cancellous bone between the inner and outer pelvis tables.
- Pins should be aimed toward the greater trochanter.
- Extra pins placed along the inner and outer tables can assist with trajectory.

Splint or Traction (Hip Spica, NATO, HARE, Thomas) (Indications, Risks, Benefits)

Splints support fractures by providing a rigid structure adjacent to a fracture, while traction devices reduce the fracture fragments indirectly via ligamentotaxis and provide stability through longitudinal traction. Due to the difficulty of immobilizing across the hip joint, splinting or traction provides significantly less stability than external fixation of femur fractures. Due to the need to cross the hip, splints are also more cumbersome and less comfortable during transport. As a result, we recommend splint or traction treatment of femur fractures in 3 general instances: external fixation is not possible, stable fracture patterns with patient comfortable in splint, and femoral neck fractures.

Splint Application Technique[42]
Technical considerations for splint application during air evacuation include the following:
- All circumferential casts must be bi-valved prior to air evacuation to minimize the risks of cast-induced compartment syndrome.
- All casts must fit the patient within the dimensions of the standard NATO litter (22" x 72" in Field Manual 8-10-6).[25]
- Hanging traction is not allowed during air evacuation for concern of patient injury during turbulence or flight maneuvering (Air Force Guide 41-307).
- Draw the fracture pattern, and note the dates of wounding and surgery, if performed, on the cast.

Hip Spica Transportation Cast[42]
Indications: Proximal Femur Fracture
- Patient is placed on fracture table.
- Stockinette is placed over abdomen, distal thigh of uninvolved side, and foot of the involved side.
- Felt padding is placed over sacrum and anterior superior iliac spine and other bony prominences.
- Towel is placed over abdomen to allow breathing space.
- Six-inch Webril or similar cotton batting is wrapped, 2 to 4 layers.
- Six-inch casting material is then rolled over the Webril from anterior superior iliac spine to the foot on the affected side and to the distal thigh on the unaffected side. Additional splints are applied over the posterior, lateral, or groin areas to reinforce the groin. Use a finishing roll after turning down the edges of the stockinette to give a neat appearance.
- An adequate perineal space must be left for hygiene.
- Use a 1/2" dowel or similar material to make anterior/posterior crossbars.
- Affected knee should be bent about 20 degrees.
- Space between feet must not exceed standard litter, although this makes perineal access difficult.

- Towel is removed, cast is bi-valved, and a circular area over the abdomen is cut out.

Traction Application Technique (HARE, NATO, SAGER, etc)

There are multiple off-the-shelf traction splints available for use, and the treating orthopedic surgeon should refer to the instructions for each specific device.

Indications: Femur Fracture, Tibia Fracture, Proximal Femur Fractures With Proximal Ischial Pad:

- Adjust splint length based on uninjured extremity.
- Open all strap attachments.
- While assistant pulls longitudinal traction on extremity, slide device under injured leg.
- Slide traction device from distal to proximal, and place proximal pad against ischial tuberosity. Apply ischial strap at hip.
- Attach ankle hitch and apply traction.
- Attach straps from distal to proximal. Place 2 straps above and 2 straps below fracture site for ideal placement. Do not place strap over fracture site.
- Reassess neurovascular status after application.

Abduction Pillow (Indications, Risks, Benefits)

Proximal femur fractures may have insufficient proximal femoral bone stock for external fixator pin placement. If a surgeon decides against hip-spanning external fixation, the patient may be given an abduction pillow for transport. Off-the-shelf pillows are available, but in the absence of a prefabricated device, a wedge-shaped structure can be created by taping pillows and/or blankets together. A 3-pillow configuration with 1 pillow perpendicular to the long axis of the bed and 2 pillows on top in line with the bed, using an Ace wrap to wrap around the pillows and/or patient's legs has been described.[43] The device should fit comfortably between the patient's legs, keeping the legs abducted approximately 30 degrees, while ensuring the patient fits within the borders of the NATO litter. This can be an effective temporizing measure while the patient is transported to a higher echelon of care.

Authors' Recommended Treatment Method in Theater (Echelon II and III Facilities)

Femoral Neck Fracture

The author recommends open reduction and internal fixation if the necessary surgical equipment,

implants, and radiologic imaging are available. If any of the above is not available, it is recommended to use an abduction pillow and aeromedically evacuate the combat casualty either emergently or urgently depending upon the operational scenario.

Pertrochanteric Femur Fracture

The author recommends using a HARE traction splint or other traction splint with medial ischial pad. In the case of a combat casualty with a severely comminuted pertrochanteric femur fracture or one with segmental bone loss, hip-spanning external fixation can be used if the necessary surgical equipment, implants, and radiologic imaging are available.

Diaphyseal Femur Fracture

The author recommends using lateral uniplanar external fixation.

Distal Femur Fracture

The author recommends using knee-spanning external fixation.

Femoral Fracture Soft Tissue Considerations

Compartment syndrome in the thigh after long-bone fracture is much less common than in the leg.[44] However, suspicion for thigh compartment syndrome should be raised in high-energy fractures, vascular injuries, and blunt trauma. Delayed treatment of compartment syndrome of the thigh is associated with significant morbidity including sensory deficits, motor weakness, muscle necrosis, and amputation.[45,46] The anterior compartment of the thigh is the most commonly affected compartment.[47] While compartment syndrome is a clinical diagnosis, the surgeon may have to rely on compartment measurements in obtunded patients. Due to the need for transport and inability to perform fasciotomies during flight, we recommend aggressive compartment releases when suspected clinically or when compartment pressures are either greater than 30 mm Hg or within 30 mm Hg of the diastolic blood pressure. Compartment measurements should be performed for the anterior, posterior, and adductor compartments. Compartment pressures can be measured with a Stryker Intracompartmental Pressure Monitor System (Stryker, Mahwah, NJ) or with an arterial line manometer. A side-port needle or slit catheter should be used as straight needles have been shown to overestimate pressure.[48] While a definitive time to irreversible damage after compartment syndrome has not been elucidated, compartments should be released in an emergent manner. It has been estimated that 37% of patients with acute compartment syndrome develop muscle necrosis within 3 hours of the injury.[49]

Fasciotomy Technique[46]

- The patient is placed in a supine position with a "bump" under the ipsilateral buttocks.

- The anterior and posterior compartments of the thigh can be accessed through a single lateral incision.

- The incision is made in line with the femoral shaft from the greater trochanter to the femoral condyle.

- Incise the fascia lata for the length of the incision to release the anterior compartment.

- Retract the vastus lateralis superiorly and medially to expose the lateral intermuscular septum.

- Incise along the lateral intermuscular septum for the complete length of the skin incision, releasing the posterior compartment. Incise the septum away from the bone to minimize disruptions of the perforating vessels.

- The adductor or medial compartment is rarely involved in thigh compartment syndrome. If the pressure is elevated preoperatively, a repeat measurement should be obtained after release of the anterior and posterior compartments.

- Medial compartment can be released with an anteromedial incision along the course of the saphenous vein. The sartorius is just posterior to the course of the saphenous vein. Release of the fascia overlying the sartorius is usually sufficient. For further release, identify the medial intermuscular septum anterior to the sartorius, and release this fascia for the length of the skin incision. Note the femoral vessels are just anterior to this septum.

Tibial Fractures

Open tibia fractures are the most common open long-bone fractures that orthopedic surgeons will treat in combat operations.[2,50] This is likely a combined result of proximity to the ground or the floor of the vehicle and a relatively small soft tissue envelope. The distal location on the limb, consistent anatomy, and subcutaneous location of the medial tibial cortex makes stabilization of tibia fractures possible with external fixation or splinting. The decision between the methods of treatment depends upon the soft tissue envelope, inherent stability of the fracture, and associated injuries.

Tibial Fracture Treatment Options

External Fixation (Indications, Risks, Benefits)

Due to the subcutaneous location of the tibia, external fixator pin placement is ideally suited for severe,

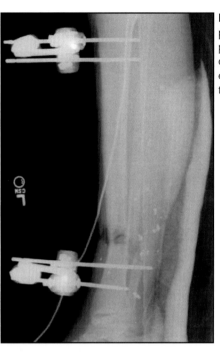

Figure 24-3. Overpenetration of the proximal pin in the distal clamp can easily be seen on this radiograph.

open tibia fractures. External fixation of severe open tibia fractures in combat casualties relies on applying pins and producing a construct that does not damage vital structures, provides access for secondary procedures, and fulfills mechanical demands of the patient and injuries.[51] This is achieved through bi-cortical pin placement within Behren's safe zones, while avoiding pin placement within the fracture hematoma and overpenetration of the pins (Figure 24-3).[51]

A review of external fixator placement for severe open tibia fractures in the conflicts in Iraq and Afghanistan revealed a very low rate of external fixator-related complications.[17] The authors noted that approximately 20% of devices could have had improved placement to reduce potential complications, mostly due to pin placement either too close to the fracture or joint capsule.

Soft Tissue Anatomy Considerations

The popliteal fossa is bound proximally by the biceps femoris and the semimembranosus and distally by the medial and lateral heads of the gastrocnemius. The major structures it contains are the popliteal vessels, tibial nerve, and peroneal nerve. The common peroneal nerve passes laterally in a subcutaneous location posterior to the head of the fibula. It is closely opposed to the periosteum of the fibula as it courses anteriorly around the fibular neck, where it divides into the superficial and deep peroneal nerves. The superficial peroneal nerve travels in the lateral compartment, and, while variable, it passes out of the fascia approximately 10 to 12 cm proximal to the tip of the lateral malleolus.

Figure 24-4. Intra-capsular pin placement, as seen in the distal tibial pin, should be avoided due to the potential development of septic arthritis.

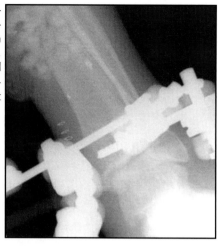

Safe Corridors for Tibial Pin Placement

Safe pin placement in the tibia is easier than in other long bones due to the subcutaneous location of the tibia. Pins can be placed from anterior or medial, while pins placed perpendicular to the anteromedial tibial cortex may be the easiest to place bi-cortically. The triangular cross-section of the tibia should be considered while determining pin trajectory to obtain bi-cortical purchase. Pin placement within 14 mm of the tibial plateau and 10 mm of the tibial plafond should be avoided to avoid intracapsular pin placement (Figure 24-4).[52,53]

Tibial Shaft External Fixation Technique[42]
Indications: Open or Unstable Diaphyseal Tibia Fracture

- The anteromedial surface is the safest way to introduce pins into the tibia. Palpate the antero-medial border of the tibia. Make a 1-cm longitudinal incision over the midportion of the surface.
- The pin closest to the fracture site should be a minimum of 1-inch outside the hematoma.
- Insert one pin into either the proximal or distal fragment, engaging both cortices. This pin should be placed perpendicular to the subcutaneous border of the tibia and centered across the width of the tibia.
- The proximal tibia should be palpated on the anteromedial surface, and the anterior and posterior border should be identified. Midway anterior/posterior, a 1-cm longitudinal stab incision should be made and a blunt soft tissue dissection made to bone.
- Using the multi-pin clamp as a guide, insert a second pin through the clamp. An assistant should hold the clamp and provide counterpressure. Ensure that the clamp is in line with the bone and that bi-cortical purchase is obtained with the second pin. Use the pin sites as far apart on the clamp as possible for biomechanical stability.

- Apply a second multi-pin clamp and 2 pins in the same manner to the other main fracture fragment. Connect the 2 clamps via two elbows, bar-bar clamps, and a carbon fiber rod.
- Comminuted fractures should be stabilized using a 2-bar construct, while a single bar is sufficient for stable fractures.

Knee-Spanning External Fixation Technique[42]
Indications: Proximal Tibia Fracture, Distal Femur Fracture, Unstable Knee After Dislocation (Especially Those With Vascular Repair in Popliteal Fossa)

- General reduction maneuver should be longitudinal traction with slight (10 to 15 degrees) flexion at the knee.
- Pins are placed anteromedially on the proximal tibia and anterolaterally on the distal femur. Pin placement should be outside of the zone of injury, a minimum of 1 inch from the fracture site, and outside of the knee joint. Lateral pins placed in the distal femur should be proximal to the intercondylar notch. Pins should not be within 14 mm of the proximal tibia articular surface due to the risk of intracapsular penetration.
- At the distal femur, a longitudinal stab incision is made over the anterolateral aspect of the bone, so that the pin may be inserted into the center of the bone at about a 45-degree angle from the horizontal. Depending on the fracture configuration, it may also be placed directly anteriorly, though it is generally better to avoid the quadriceps tendon.
- Blunt dissection is used to create a corridor to the bone. A single pin is inserted by hand through both cortices of the bone fragment.
- A multi-pin clamp is used as a guide for a second pin. The second pin must be parallel to the first and also bi-cortical—care should be taken to maintain pin alignment.
- The proximal tibia should be palpated on the anteromedial surface, and the anterior and posterior border should be identified. Midway anterior/posterior, a 1-cm longitudinal stab incision should be made and a blunt soft tissue dissection made to bone. A multi-pin clamp should be used as a guide to insert a second pin in the proximal tibia.
- The 2 pin clusters (femur and tibia) should be connected via 2 elbows, 2 bar-bar clamps, and a single bar. The knee should be aligned and/or fracture reduced with longitudinal traction and the bar clamps tightened. A second bar should be added in the manner described above with additional bar clamps from the elbows.

Ankle-Spanning External Fixation Technique[42]

Indications: Distal Tibia Fracture

- Pins should be inserted on the anteromedial surface of the tibia and the medial aspect of the calcaneus.

- Identify the posterior tibial artery and dorsalis pedis pulses.

- Palpate the anteromedial border of the tibia. Make a 1-cm longitudinal incision midway between the anterior and posterior border of the tibia. Insert the most distal pin on the tibia outside the zone of injury, a minimum of 1 inch from the fracture site.

- Using a multi-pin clamp as a guide, insert a second pin in the tibia more proximal to the first. The pin must be parallel and be aligned in the longitudinal axis to the first.

- Palpate the medial border of the calcaneus. Over the calcaneus, make a longitudinal incision, which should be a safe distance posterior and inferior to the neurovascular structures.

- Bluntly dissect down to the bone with a hemostat and insert the pin. A centrally threaded 5-mm pin can be used to construct an "A" frame. Insert the pin in the central portion of the calcaneus parallel with the distal tibia joint line, and advance to the lateral skin surface. Incise the skin where pin prominence is noted, and allow passage of the pin through the skin until the centrally threaded portion of the pin is in the calcaneus.

- Alternatively, a unilateral frame can be constructed with a medial pin (not centrally threaded) using the standard technique.

- Connect the 2 clamps via 2 elbows, 2 bar-bar clamps, and a single bar.

Extremity Splint

- Hold the knee flexed about 20 degrees.

- Apply Webril/cotton padding from the toes to the tibial tubercle (or to the groin if spanning knee with splint) with attention to bony prominences around malleoli, fibular head, and posterior heel.

- Place the L/U splint of 5″ plaster measured to appropriate length just below tibial tubercle.

- Do not fold over the proximal or distal portion of the cast to avoid iatrogenic thermal cast injuries.[54]

- Alternatively, 6-inch wide casting material can be rolled over this region, with a turn-down of the stockinette prior to the final layer.

- For above-knee splints, reinforce the knee to strengthen the cast. Make a supracondylar mold to provide stabilization.

- If a circumferential cast is placed, bivalve.

- Elevate the leg so the tibia is parallel to the litter or bed.

Authors' Recommended Treatment Method

Tibial Plateau Fracture

The author recommends in combat casualties with open or unstable tibial plateau fractures to use a knee-spanning external fixator. In the case of a combat casualty with a stable, closed tibial plateau fracture, a knee-spanning splint or a knee-immobilizing off-the-shelf brace can be used.

Diaphyseal Tibia Fracture

The author recommends in combat casualties with open or unstable diaphyseal tibial fractures to use external fixation. In the case of a combat casualty with a stable, closed diaphyseal tibial fracture, a knee-spanning splint can be used.

Distal Tibia or Pilon Fracture

The author recommends in combat casualties with open or unstable distal tibia or pilon fractures to use an ankle-spanning external fixator. In the case of a combat casualty with a stable, closed distal tibia or plafond fracture, an L/U splint can be used.

Tibial Fracture Soft Tissue Considerations

Compartment Syndrome

Compartment syndrome of the leg is associated with high-energy injury mechanisms common in combat operations. Delayed diagnosis or treatment of lower extremity compartment syndrome is associated with significant morbidity including muscle necrosis, neurologic injury, long-term dysfunction, and amputation.[44,48,55] A recent review of fasciotomies performed during Operation Iraqi Freedom and Operation Enduring Freedom reported that patients who received fasciotomies in theater, earlier in their clinical course, had lower rates of muscle excision, amputation, and mortality.[44] There is significant research attention evaluating the utility of continuous compartment pressure monitoring and noninvasive pressure monitoring, but these devices are currently not routinely available in the combat deployed setting.[56-58] Diagnosis of compartment syndrome remains a clinical diagnosis based on pain out of proportion or increasing narcotic requirements. In an obtunded patient, pressure monitoring can be performed for the anterior, lateral, deep posterior, and superficial posterior compartments as discussed above. Fasciotomies performed for combat injuries should be extensile in nature, and care should be taken to ensure release of all 4 leg compartments. The anterior compartment was the most commonly neglected compartment in a recent review of 643 combat-related fasciotomies.[44]

Fasciotomy 2-Incision Technique

- Incisions must extend the entire length of the calf to release all of the compressing fascia and skin.

- An approximately 15-cm lateral incision is made centered between the fibula and anterior tibial crest.

- The lateral intermuscular septum and superficial peroneal nerve are identified. The superficial peroneal nerve has a variable course and can pass through the fascia from 3 to 18 cm, most commonly 12 cm, proximal to the lateral maleolus.[8,59]

- A transverse incision is made over the fascia to allow clear identification of the intermuscular septum.

- Blunt-tipped scissors are used to initially spread above and below the fascia in both compartments.

- The anterior compartment is released with blunt-tipped scissors in line with longitudinal axis of the limb from Gerdy's tubercle to the extensor retinaculum. The lateral compartment is then released in similar fashion.

- A second incision of approximately 15 cm in length is made medially at least 2 cm posterior to the posterior palpable edge of the tibia. A medial incision posterior to the subcutaneous surface of the tibia is used to avoid exposure of the tibia when the tissues retract.

- The saphenous vein and nerve are retracted anteriorly.

- Once down to the fascia, undermine anteriorly to identify posterior tibial margin.

- Incise fascia just posterior to tibia through length of incision. Elevate the soleus from posterior tibia to expose fascia covering flexor digitorum longus and posterior tibialis.

- Incise this fascia through the length of the incision.

Definitive Management

FEMORAL FRACTURE DEFINITIVE TREATMENT

Recently, Department of Defense and civilian experts performed an evidence-based review of the pertinent literature on both combat-related and severe civilian open fractures.[11,60] The goal of this review was to provide evidence-based recommendations for management of combat-related injuries to include definitive fixation of femur and tibia fractures. This review along with subsequent publications in both the military and civilian literature are the basis for the recommendations in the definitive management of femur and tibia fractures.

Conversion of external fixation to intramedullary fixation should be performed with some caution, because increased infectious complications have been reported with conversion of femur external fixation to intramedullary nails after 14 days in some series.[61] An evidence-based review of the literature demonstrated that infection rates for conversion of external fixation to intramedullary nails in femurs was 3.6% (95% CI: 1.8% to 7.4%).[62]

Closed and open femur fractures in civilian series generally lend themselves to intramedullary nailing with union rates of 98% to 99% and infection rates around 1%.[63,64] There appears to be some benefit in reaming femur fractures, as some series have demonstrated decreasing rates of nonunion and implant failure with reaming.[65] Immediate reamed intramedullary nailing of open femur fractures demonstrates infection rates of 1.8% to 5%.[66-68] Application of the civilian data to battlefield injuries must be done on a case-by-case basis, because severe soft tissue injury may accompany fractures with an explosion mechanism of injury. Because most infections in open femur fractures occur in type III open injuries,[66,69] we may expect a greater proportion of infectious complications in the combat injured. Unfortunately, there are limited data from this conflict on femur fractures. In one civilian series, 11% of type IIIB open fractures became infected and accounted for all of the infections in the entire series. The multivariate analysis by Noumi and colleagues showed that age, time to debridement, and reaming did not affect rates of infectious complications. Only open fracture type correlated with infection, with Gustilo type III open femur fractures with the highest rate of infection.[69]

Definitive circular fixation plays a very limited role even in the treatment of combat femur fractures due to conflicting literature on their outcomes and rates of fixation-related complications.[70-72] It does, however, remain a treatment option for the unusual injury complicated by infection.[73]

The authors recommend timely conversion of external fixation to a locked, intramedullary nail. Reaming appears to be beneficial and safe in all but the most severe (IIIB and IIIC) open femur fractures.

TIBIAL FRACTURE DEFINITIVE TREATMENT

Temporary external fixation is commonly used in this conflict and appears to be safe.[17] It is rarely used for definitive management of combat-related tibia fractures. A recent evidence-based review of the literature demonstrated that plausible infection rates for conversion of external fixation to intramedullary nails in tibia fractures is 9% (95% CI: 7% to 12%). This review also found that limiting the duration of tibial external fixation to 28 days decreased the infection rate by 83% (95% CI: 62% to 93%).[62] A pin tract infection in the temporary fixator is a predictor of subsequent deep infection after conversion to a nail.[74]

Open reduction and internal plate fixation of open tibia shaft fractures has an unacceptably high rate of deep infection compared to external fixation (19% versus 3%).[75] Unfortunately, definitive management of open tibia fractures with unilateral external fixation has had some unfavorable results in the past. One series reported a 43% pin tract infection rate and malalignment greater than 5 degrees in 38% of the cases.[24] In contrast, some series demonstrate reasonable results with unilateral external fixation.[75,76]

While trends in the recent civilian trauma literature favor immediate nailing of open tibia fractures due to fewer re-operations and better alignment compared to external fixation,[77-83] some studies continue to demonstrate worrisome infection rates as high as 12.5% to 35% in type IIIB open injuries.[79,80,82,84] Older literature favored reaming, because it did not seem to increase the infection rate in open tibia fractures while providing the benefits of fewer nonunions and hardware failures.[65,77,78,80,83,85] The Study to Prospectively Evaluate Reamed Intramedullary Nails in Tibial Fractures (SPRINT) trial demonstrated benefits of reaming only in closed tibia fractures. There was no difference in "event" rate with open fractures.[86]

Type III open fractures of the tibia represent a larger proportion of tibia fractures in military conflicts than in civilian series. Most are due to blast injuries.[2,87] Favorable clinical results with severe open tibia fractures have been demonstrated with the use of circular external fixation.[88-92] A series of 24 patients with combat-related type III open tibia fractures were treated with circular (Ilizarov) external fixation. One patient had an amputation (4.2%), and one patient developed a deep infection (4.2%).[91] A recent series of combat injured from the current conflicts in Iraq and Afghanistan demonstrated a low infection rate and reasonable clinical outcomes with circular fixation[93] compared to other series of predominately internal fixation with higher infection rates.[17,94] Another series from these conflicts demonstrates the ability to reconstruct both the bone and soft tissue injury simultaneously using the Ilizarov method principles of distraction histiogenesis.[95]

Recommendations for definitive management of combat-related tibia fractures undoubtedly spark intense debate. Intramedullary nailing with or without reaming seems appropriate for closed fractures and open fractures with minimal soft tissue injury. For those fractures with larger soft tissue injury, we recommend the use of circular fixation due to the benefits of decreased infection rates and ability to use distraction histiogenesis.

Outcomes

FEMUR FRACTURES

There are limited prospective data on combat injuries and specifically combat-related femur fracture outcomes. Outcome and complication rates are derived from case series and extrapolation from civilian data.

Proximal Femur

A review of 17 combat-related high-energy open proximal femur fractures treated with hip-spanning external fixation revealed a 100% union rate at an average of 11.5 months.[96] The authors concluded that hip-spanning external fixation provides stable fixation and allows for soft tissue management when internal fixation is not possible. Internal fixation is not commonly performed in the combat environment predominately due to concerns of infections. A recent review of internal fixation in theater revealed that fractures of the proximal femur accounted for 28% of surgeries performed on US military servicemembers in the combat environment.[97] There were no postoperative infections in this cohort, and 93% (13 of 14) went on to union.

Proximal femur fractures, including femoral neck fractures, can be temporarily treated in traction or with an abduction pillow prior to definitive care. A prospective civilian trial of closed, displaced femoral neck fractures did not detect a difference in union rates or occurrence of avascular necrosis if surgical stabilization was delayed more than 48 hours.[98] A meta-analysis using 12 hours to define early or late surgery, similarly, did not identify differences in outcomes.[99]

Diaphyseal Femur

Historically, combat-related femoral shaft fractures were treated in traction or with use of the Thomas splint.[15,43,48] The "successful" use of the Thomas splint is well described during World War II,[48] but the drawbacks of keeping patients immobilized necessitated alternative treatment. During the Korean Conflict, balanced traction with delayed conversion to intramedullary nail fixation was becoming commonplace for the treatment of these injuries.[15] During the past 2 decades, a transition has been made to the treatment of unstable femur fractures with external fixation.[19,100]

Despite this, when in an environment with limited resources, Clasper and colleagues demonstrated satisfactory short-term outcomes to include wound healing and fracture union (92%) when treating ballistic femur fractures without internal or external fixation.[101] One report on 173 combat-related femur fractures treated with external fixation reported an average time of 128 days in an external fixator.[102]

In civilian trauma centers, temporary external fixation is frequently converted to internal fixation. Bhandari and colleagues performed an evidence-based review and determined that plausible infection rates for conversion of external fixators to intramedullary nails in femurs was 3.6% (95% CI: 1.8% to 7.4%).[103] A retrospective study of severely injured civilian trauma patients with 59 femur fractures reported outcomes and complications associated with initial external fixation and then conversion to intramedullary nail fixation.[104] The authors reported that 32% of the fractures were open, the external fixation was used on average for 7 days, there was a 97% union rate by 6 months, and there was a 1.7% infection rate. Despite this low risk of infection, caution must be exercised when extrapolating these data to combat-related injuries as the mechanisms of injury, initial operating room environment, and evacuation needs are vastly different.

There are few studies evaluating intramedullary nail fixation in an austere environment for patients without access to evacuation. A review of 23 femur fractures in host or third country nation patients treated with closed intramedullary nailing demonstrated a low infection rate and good results, but lacked adequate follow-up to make practice-changing conclusions.[105]

Distal Femur

Combat-related distal femur fractures are typically treated initially with knee-spanning external fixation, prior to conversion to definitive fixation. There are limited data describing outcomes of combat-related distal femur fractures. Zlowodzki and colleagues performed an evidence-based review of operative treatment of acute distal femur fractures and found that operative treatment, when compared to nonoperative management, results in a 32% reduction in the risk of poor results.[106] They also identified no differences between implants in nonunions, infections, fixation failures, and revision surgeries. Overall, they found a 2.7% risk of deep infection (CI: 2.0% to 3.5%), 6% nonunion rate (CI: 4.9% to 7.2%), and a high rate of secondary surgical procedures (16.8%) (CI: 15.1% to 18.6%).[106]

TIBIA FRACTURES

Severe open tibia fractures in combat are most commonly due to blast mechanisms, frequently require long evacuation times, and may have poor outcomes. In a study on war injuries, Lerner reported on 64 open fractures from projectiles.[91] The authors noted a 90% union rate at an average of 8 months after treating the patients initially with an external fixator and then converting them to Ilizarov or hybrid frames. A recent review of combat-related tibia fractures from the current conflicts in Iraq and Afghanistan treated with ringed external fixation revealed a time to healing of 7.2 months.[93] In our series of combat-related open tibia fractures, we retrospectively evaluated 213 consecutive type III open diaphyseal tibia fractures (unpublished data), and 80.3% of fractures united at an average of 9.2 months. There was a 27% deep infection rate, and 22% of patients ultimately required an amputation at 24 months of follow-up. In a large civilian series of 523 closed and open tibia fractures, Court-Brown reported an average time to union of 38.2 weeks.[107]

The outcomes, associated complications, and safety of short-term external fixator use in the treatment of combat-related open fractures is controversial. In a review of 15 external fixators applied to upper and lower extremities in a combat environment, one report noted an 86.7% device revision or removal rate secondary to instability, pin loosening, and pin track infections.[22] Due to the high early complication rate, the authors cautioned against universal acceptance of external fixation for combat injuries. This study is in contrast to an evaluation of 55 external fixators applied to US service-members during the conflicts in Iraq and Afghanistan.[17] The authors recorded no major complications from external fixator application, and 77% were applied "successfully" without potential complications. The study concluded that external fixation was effective in attaining the limited goals of safe, provisional stabilization for open tibia fractures in a combat environment.

Complications

FEMUR FRACTURES

Infection

Because there are few data describing outcomes of combat-related femur fractures, infection rates must be extrapolated from civilian data. Due to the significant soft tissue envelope and limited soft tissue stripping associated with femoral nailing, infection rates remain low in the civilian literature following internal fixation of both closed (1%) and open femur fractures (1.8% to 5%).[63,64,66,67,69] The majority of infections occur in Gustilo type III open femur fractures.[66,69] This was shown by Noumi and colleagues, who performed a multivariate analysis of factors contributing to deep infection in open femur fractures, concluding that only Gustilo type correlated with the occurrence of deep infection, with Gustilo type III open femur fractures with the highest rate of infection.[69]

Temporary external fixation of femur fractures is frequently used in the combat environment with delayed conversion to intramedullary nail fixation following medical evacuation. Infection rates following conversion of external fixation to intramedullary nails have been demonstrated to be higher when performed after 14 days in the civilian literature.[61] This finding was supported in an evidence-based review by Bhandari and colleagues, who demonstrated a plausible infection rate of 3.6% (95% CI: 1.8% to 7.4%) following conversion from temporary external fixation to intramedullary nails.[62]

Nonunion

Both closed and open femur fractures have a high rate of union in the civilian literature, with rates typically around 98% to 99% when treated with intramedullary nailing.[63,64] In a review of internal fixation performed in the combat environment with an average follow-up of 17 ± 2 months, 1 of 14 (7%) hip/proximal femur fractures resulted in nonunion.[97] Although limited by lack of follow-up, another review of 23 femoral shaft fractures in host or third country nation patients treated in the combat environment with intramedullary nailing reported no known cases of nonunion.[105]

TIBIA FRACTURES

Complications associated with open tibia fractures are related to the severity of the fracture and soft tissue injury.[108,109]

Infection

Civilian series have noted open tibia fracture infection rates of 5% to 65%.[24,100,110,111] Three recent studies on combat-related, open, lower extremity long-bone fractures from the recent conflicts in Iraq and Afghanistan reported deep infection rates ranging from 8% to 40%.[32,93] Studies have reported an increased infection rate with internal fixation after temporary external fixator stabilization. Has and colleagues reported an infection rate of 9.3% in long-bone fractures treated with external fixation and an infection rate of 42.8% for those that received a subsequent internal fixation procedure due to inadequate fracture healing.[112] A recent meta-analysis of sequential intramedullary nail fixation after external fixation of tibia fractures revealed a 90% union rate and a 9% infection rate.[110] There was evidence to support a lower infection rate if the duration of external fixator use was less than 28 days.

A recent study on combat-related open lower extremity fractures from these conflicts evaluated sequential conversion from temporary external fixa-

tion to an intramedullary nail. The authors reported a 40% infection rate and a 17% rate of osteomyelitis.[32] The pin track infection rate for tibial external fixation is thought to be lower than femoral or upper extremity external fixation as the half-pins are not required to pass through muscle prior to bone insertion.[24]

Nerve Injury

Previous reports have demonstrated that peripheral nerve injuries are involved in as many as 30% of combat-related extremity injuries.[113] This is substantially higher than the results of a recent cohort of 5000 civilian trauma patients, in which only 3% were found to sustain a peripheral nerve injury.[114] The Lower Extremity Assessment Project (LEAP) study group reported a high rate of sensory recovery in civilian patients with severe lower extremity injuries.[115] A recent series of combat-related open tibia fractures identified a 22% incidence of neurologic injury, with improvement seen in 50% of motor and 27% of sensory nerve deficits.[116]

Nonunion

Severe open tibia fractures have been shown in multiple studies to require a prolonged time to healing and to have high complication rates. A separate review of 42 open type III tibia fractures in civilian trauma patients revealed a 70% delayed union rate.[24]

Amputation

Similar to the infection rate and time to union, the ultimate amputation rate of open tibia fractures corresponds to the fracture severity and presence of arterial injury. An amputation rate of up to 25% for open tibia fractures has been reported in a civilian series assessing limb-threatening injuries.[117] The rate of amputation has been reported between 40% and 86% if the open fracture is associated with an arterial injury requiring repair.[19,108,111] We identified a 22% amputation rate for all type III open tibia fractures, but the rate was 72% for those with an arterial injury requiring repair (unpublished data). The majority of amputations occur in the acute setting after injury, emphasizing the need for expedient hemorrhage control, revascularization, and fracture stabilization.[118,119]

References

1. Lin DL, Kirk KL, Murphy KP, McHale KA, Doukas WC. Orthopedic injuries during Operation Enduring Freedom. *Mil Med.* 2004;169:807-809.
2. Owens BD, Kragh JF Jr, Macaitis J, Svoboda SJ, Wenke JC. Characterization of extremity wounds in Operation Iraqi Freedom and Operation Enduring Freedom. *J Orthop Trauma.* 2007;21:254-257.

3. Owens BD, Kragh JF Jr, Wenke JC, Macaitis J, Wade CE, Holcomb JB. Combat wounds in operation Iraqi Freedom and operation Enduring Freedom. *J Trauma.* 2008;64:295-299.
4. Belmont PJ Jr, Goodman GP, Zacchilli M, Posner M, Evans C, Owens BD. Incidence and epidemiology of combat injuries sustained during "the surge" portion of operation Iraqi Freedom by a U.S. Army brigade combat team. *J Trauma.* 2010;68:204-210.
5. Scalea TM, Boswell SA, Scott JD, Mitchell KA, Kramer ME, Pollak AN. External fixation as a bridge to intramedullary nailing for patients with multiple injuries and with femur fractures: damage control orthopedics. *J Trauma.* 2000;48:613-621; discussion 21-23.
6. Roberts CS, Pape HC, Jones AL, Malkani AL, Rodriguez JL, Giannoudis PV. Damage control orthopaedics: evolving concepts in the treatment of patients who have sustained orthopedic trauma. *Instr Course Lect.* 2005;54:447-462.
7. Renaldo N, Egol K. Damage-control orthopedics: evolution and practical applications. *Am J Ortho.* 2006;35:285-291; discussion 291.
8. Pape HC, Grimme K, Van Griensven M, et al. Impact of intramedullary instrumentation versus damage control for femoral fractures on immunoinflammatory parameters: prospective randomized analysis by the EPOFF Study Group. *J Trauma.* 2003;55:7-13.
9. McKee MD, Schemitsch EH, Vincent LO, Sullivan I, Yoo D. The effect of a femoral fracture on concomitant closed head injury in patients with multiple injuries. *J Trauma.* 1997;42:1041-1045.
10. Camuso MR. Far-forward fracture stabilization: external fixation versus splinting. *J Am Acad Orthop Surg.* 2006;14:S118-S123.
11. Murray CK, Hsu JR, Solomkin JS, et al. Prevention and management of infections associated with combat-related extremity injuries. *J Trauma.* 2008;64:S239-S251.
12. Pape HC, Hildebrand F, Pertschy S, et al. Changes in the management of femoral shaft fractures in polytrauma patients: from early total care to damage control orthopedic surgery. *J Trauma.* 2002;53:452-461; discussion 461-462.
13. Rixen D, Grass G, Sauerland S, et al. Evaluation of criteria for temporary external fixation in risk-adapted damage control orthopedic surgery of femur shaft fractures in multiple trauma patients: "evidence-based medicine" versus "reality" in the trauma registry of the German Trauma Society. *J Trauma.* 2005;59:1375-1394; discussion 1394-1395.
14. Pape HC, Giannoudis P, Krettek C. The timing of fracture treatment in polytrauma patients: relevance of damage control orthopedic surgery. *Am J Surg.* 2002;183:622-629.
15. Jacob E, Erpelding JM, Murphy KP. A retrospective analysis of open fractures sustained by U.S. military personnel during Operation Just Cause. *Mil Med.* 1992;157:552-556.
16. Worlock P, Slack R, Harvey L, Mawhinney R. The prevention of infection in open fractures: an experimental study of the effect of fracture stability. *Injury.* 1994;25:31-38.
17. Possley DR, Burns TC, Stinner DJ, et al. Temporary external fixation is safe in a combat environment. *J Trauma-Inj Infect Crit Care.* 2010;69:S135-S139.
18. Burny F. *Elastic External Fixation of Tibial Fractures: Study of 1421 Cases.* Baltimore, MD: Williams & Wilkins; 1979.
19. Edwards CC, Simmons SC, Browner BD, Weigel MC. Severe open tibial fractures. Results treating 202 injuries with external fixation. *Clin Orthop Relat Res.* 1988;May(230):98-115.
20. Topp R, Hayda R, Benedetti G, Twitero T, Carmack DB. The incidence of neurovascular injury during external fixator placement without radiographic assistance for lower extremity diaphyseal fractures: a cadaveric study. *J Trauma.* 2003;55:955-958; discussion 958.
21. Dwyer NS. Preliminary report upon a new fixation device for fractures of long bones. *Injury.* 1973;5:141-144.
22. Clasper JC, Phillips SL. Early failure of external fixation in the management of war injuries. *J R Army Med Corps.* 2005;151:81-86.
23. Coupland RM. War wounds of bones and external fixation. *Injury.* 1994;25:211-217.
24. Clifford RP, Lyons TJ, Webb JK. Complications of external fixation of open fractures of the tibia. *Injury.* 1987;18:174-176.
25. Szul A. Extremity fractures. In: Szul AC, Davis LB, Walter Reed Army Medical Center Borden Institute, eds. *Emergency War Surgery.* 3rd US rev. Washington, DC: Walter Reed Army Medical Center Borden Institute; 2004.
26. Kirkup J. Foundation lecture. Fracture care of friend and foe during World War I. *ANZ J Surg.* 2003;73:453-459.
27. Henry BJ, Vrahas MS. The Thomas splint. Questionable boast of an indispensable tool. *Am J Orthop.* 1996;25:602-604.
28. Malgaigne JF. *Traité des Fractures et des Luxations.* Paris, France; 1847.
29. Sisk TD. External fixation. Historic review, advantages, disadvantages, complications, and indications. *Clin Orthop Relat Res.* 1983;Nov(180):15-22.
30. Hoffmann R. Rotules à os pour la réduction dirigée non sanglante des fractures. *Congrès Français de Chirurg.* 1938:601-610.
31. Bosse MJ, Holmes C, Vossoughi J, Alter D. Comparison of the Howmedica and Synthes military external fixation frames. *J Orthop Trauma.* 1994;8:119-126.
32. Mody RM, Zapor M, Hartzell JD, et al. Infectious complications of damage control orthopedics in war trauma. *J Trauma-Inj Infect Crit Care.* 2009;67:758-761.
33. Camuso MR. Far-forward fracture stabilization: external fixation versus splinting. *J Am Acad Orthop Surg.* 2006;14:S118-S123.
34. Green SA. Complications of external fixation. *Instructional Course Lectures.* 1984;33:138-143.
35. Vossinakis IC, Badras LS. The external fixator compared with the sliding hip screw for pertrochanteric fractures of the femur. *J Bone Joint Surg Br.* 2002;84:23-29.
36. Alcivar E. A new method of external fixation for proximal fractures of the femur. *Injury.* 2001;32 Suppl 4:SD107-SD114.
37. Scott IH. Treatment of intertrochanteric fractures by skeletal pinning and external fixation. *Clin Orthop.* 1957;10:326-334.
38. Barros JW, Ferreira CD, Freitas AA, Farah S. External fixation of intertrochanteric fractures of the femur. *Int Orthop.* 1995;19:217-219.
39. Miric DM, Bumbasirevic MZ, Senohradski KK, Djordjevic ZP. Pelvifemoral external fixation for the treatment of open fractures of the proximal femur caused by firearms. *Acta Orthop Belg.* 2002;68:37-41.
40. Gianchino A. *Anatomic Considerations in the Placement of Percutaneous Pins.* Berlin, Germany: Springer-Verlag; 1982.
41. Sabharwal S, Kishan S, Behrens F. Principles of external fixation of the femur. *Am J Orthop.* 2005;34:218-223.
42. Szul AC, Davis LB, Walter Reed Army Medical Center Borden Institute, eds. *Emergency War Surgery.* 3rd US rev. Washington, DC: Walter Reed Army Medical Center Borden Institute; 2004.
43. Baker JF, Mulhall KJ. A simple substitute for when the abduction pillow is unavailable. *Injury.* 2010;41:425-426.
44. Ritenour AE, Dorlac WC, Fang R, et al. Complications after fasciotomy revision and delayed compartment release in combat patients. *J Trauma.* 2008;64:S153-S161; discussion S61-S62.
45. Mithoefer K, Lhowe DW, Vrahas MS, Altman DT, Erens V, Altman GT. Functional outcome after acute compartment syndrome of the thigh. *J Bone Joint Surg Am.* 2006;88:729-737.
46. Schwartz JT Jr, Brumback RJ, Lakatos R, Poka A, Bathon GH, Burgess AR. Acute compartment syndrome of the thigh. A spectrum of injury. *J Bone Joint Surg Am.* 1989;71:392-400.
47. Mithoefer K, Lhowe DW, Vrahas MS, Altman DT, Altman GT. Clinical spectrum of acute compartment syndrome of the thigh and its relation to associated injuries. *Clin Orthop Relat Res.* 2004;(425):223-229.
48. Boody AR, Wongworawat MD. Accuracy in the measurement of compartment pressures: a comparison of three commonly used devices. *J Bone Joint Surg Am.* 2005;87:2415-2422.

49. Vaillancourt C, Shrier I, Vandal A, et al. Acute compartment syndrome: How long before muscle necrosis occurs? *CJEM.* 2004;6:147-154.

50. Labeeu F, Pasuch M, Toussaint P, Van Erps S. External fixation in war traumatology: report from the Rwandese war (October 1, 1990 to August 1, 1993). *J Trauma.* 1996;40:S223-S227.

51. Behrens F, Searls K. External fixation of the tibia. Basic concepts and prospective evaluation. *J Bone Joint Surg Br.* 1986;68:246-254.

52. Hutson JJ Jr. The centered lateral fluoroscopic image of the knee: the key to safe tensioned wire placement in periarticular fractures of the proximal tibia. *J Orthop Trauma.* 2002;16:196-200.

53. Stavlas P, Polyzois D. Septic arthritis of the major joints of the lower limb after periarticular external fixation application: are conventional safe corridors enough to prevent it? *Injury.* 2005;36:239-247.

54. Halanski M, Noonan KJ. Cast and splint immobilization: complications. *J Am Acad Orthop Surg.* 2008;16:30-40.

55. Frink M, Klaus AK, Kuther G, et al. Long term results of compartment syndrome of the lower limb in polytraumatised patients. *Injury.* 2007;38:607-613.

56. Harris IA, Kadir A, Donald G. Continuous compartment pressure monitoring for tibia fractures: does it influence outcome? *J Trauma.* 2006;60:1330-1335; discussion 1335.

57. Katz LM, Nauriyal V, Nagaraj S, et al. Infrared imaging of trauma patients for detection of acute compartment syndrome of the leg. *Crit Care Med.* 2008;36:1756-1761.

58. Wiemann JM, Ueno T, Leek BT, Yost WT, Schwartz AK, Hargens AR. Noninvasive measurements of intramuscular pressure using pulsed phase-locked loop ultrasound for detecting compartment syndromes: a preliminary report. *J Orthop Trauma.* 2006;20:458-463.

59. Adkison DP, Bosse MJ, Gaccione DR, Gabriel KR. Anatomical variations in the course of the superficial peroneal nerve. *J Bone Joint Surg Am.* 1991;73:112-114.

60. Hospenthal DR, Murray CK, Andersen RC, et al. Guidelines for the prevention of infection after combat-related injuries. *J Trauma.* 2008;64:S211-S220.

61. Harwood PJ, Giannoudis PV, Probst C, et al. The risk of local infective complications after damage control procedures for femoral shaft fracture. *J Orthop Trauma.* 2006;20:181-189.

62. Bhandari M, Zlowodzki M, Tornetta P 3rd, et al. Intramedullary nailing following external fixation in femoral and tibial shaft fractures. *J Orthop Trauma.* 2005;19:140-144.

63. Wolinsky PR, McCarty E, Shyr Y, et al. Reamed intramedullary nailing of the femur: 551 cases. *J Trauma.* 1999;46:392-399.

64. Winquist RA, Hansen ST Jr, Clawson DK. Closed intramedullary nailing of femoral fractures. A report of five hundred and twenty cases. *J Bone Joint Surg.* 1984;66:529-539.

65. Bhandari M, Guyatt GH, Tong D, et al. Reamed versus non-reamed intramedullary nailing of lower extremity long bone fractures: a systematic overview and meta-analysis. *J Orthop Trauma.* 2000;14:2-9.

66. Brumback RJ, Ellison PS Jr, Poka A, et al. Intramedullary nailing of open fractures of the femoral shaft. *J Bone Joint Surg.* 1989;71:1324-1331.

67. Lhowe DW, Hansen ST. Immediate nailing of open fractures of the femoral shaft. *J Bone Joint Surg.* 1988;70:812-820.

68. O'Brien PJ, Meek RN, Powell JN, et al. Primary intramedullary nailing of open femoral shaft fractures. *J Trauma.* 1991;31:113-116.

69. Noumi T, Yokoyama K, Ohtsuka H, et al. Intramedullary nailing for open fractures of the femoral shaft: evaluation of contributing factors on deep infection and nonunion using multivariate analysis. *Injury.* 2005;36:1085-1093.

70. Pavolini B, Maritato M, Turelli L, et al. The Ilizarov fixator in trauma: a 10-year experience. *J Orthop Sci.* 2000;5:108-113.

71. Kumar P, Singh GK, Singh M, et al. Treatment of Gustilo grade III B supracondylar fractures of the femur with Ilizarov external fixation. *Acta Orthop Belg.* 2006;72:332-336.

72. Arazi M, Memik R, Ogun TC, et al. Ilizarov external fixation for severely comminuted supracondylar and intercondylar fractures of the distal femur. *J Bone Joint Surg Br.* 2001;83:663-667.

73. Hsu JR. Options and decision making in complex war trauma. Case presentations. In: Hayda RH, ed. Orthopedic Trauma Association 24th Annual Meeting. Denver, CO; 2008.

74. Maurer DJ, Merkow RL, Gustilo RB. Infection after intramedullary nailing of severe open tibial fractures initially treated with external fixation. *J Bone Joint Surg Am.* 1989;71:835-838.

75. Bach AW, Hansen ST Jr. Plates versus external fixation in severe open tibial shaft fractures. A randomized trial. *Clin Orthop Relat Res.* 1989:89-94.

76. Marsh JL, Nepola JV, Wuest TK, et al. Unilateral external fixation until healing with the dynamic axial fixator for severe open tibial fractures. *J Orthop Trauma.* 1991;5:341-348.

77. Bhandari M, Guyatt GH, Swiontkowski MF, et al. Treatment of open fractures of the shaft of the tibia. *J Bone Joint Surg.* 2001;83:62-68.

78. Finkemeier CG, Schmidt AH, Kyle RF, et al. A prospective, randomized study of intramedullary nails inserted with and without reaming for the treatment of open and closed fractures of the tibial shaft. *J Orthop Trauma.* 2000;14:187-193.

79. Keating JF, Blachut PA, O'Brien PJ, et al. Reamed nailing of Gustilo grade-IIIB tibial fractures. *J Bone Joint Surg.* 2000;82:1113-1116.

80. Keating JF, O'Brien PI, Blachut PA, et al. Reamed interlocking intramedullary nailing of open fractures of the tibia. *Clin Orthop Relat Res.* 1997;May(338):182-191.

81. Tornetta P 3rd, Bergman M, Watnik N, et al. Treatment of grade-IIIb open tibial fractures. A prospective randomised comparison of external fixation and non-reamed locked nailing. *J Bone Joint Surg.* 1994;76:13-19.

82. Tu YK, Lin CH, Su JI, et al. Unreamed interlocking nail versus external fixator for open type III tibia fractures. *J Trauma.* 1995;39:361-367.

83. Ziran BH, Darowish M, Klatt BA, et al. Intramedullary nailing in open tibia fractures: a comparison of two techniques. *Int Orthop.* 2004;28:235-238.

84. Court-Brown CM, Keating JF, McQueen MM. Infection after intramedullary nailing of the tibia. Incidence and protocol for management. *J Bone Joint Surg.* 1992;74:770-774.

85. Keating JF, O'Brien PJ, Blachut PA, et al. Locking intramedullary nailing with and without reaming for open fractures of the tibial shaft. A prospective, randomized study. *J Bone Joint Surg Am.* 1997;79:334-341.

86. Bhandari M, Guyatt G, Tornetta P 3rd, et al. Randomized trial of reamed and unreamed intramedullary nailing of tibial shaft fractures. *J Bone Joint Surg Am.* 2008;90:2567-2578.

87. Lacap A, Anderson RC. *Infection Rate With Intramdullary Nailing of Combat Related Tibia Fractures.* Washington, DC: Walter Reed Army Medical Center; 2007.

88. Ullmann Y, Fodor L, Ramon Y, et al. The revised "reconstructive ladder" and its applications for high-energy injuries to the extremities. *Ann Plastic Surg.* 2006;56:401-405.

89. Delimar D, Klobucar H, Jelic M, et al. Treatment of defect pseudoarthroses with bone segment transport. *Acta Chirurgiae Orthopaedicae et Traumatologiae Cechoslovaca.* 2001;68:109-111.

90. Korzinek K. War injuries to the bone and joint system: reconstructive surgery. *Arch Ortho Trauma Surg.* 1994;113:180-187.

91. Lerner A, Fodor L, Soudry M. Is staged external fixation a valuable strategy for war injuries to the limbs? *Clin Orthop Rel Res.* 2006;448:217-224.

92. Hutson JJ Jr, Dayicioglu D, Oeltjen JC, et al. The treatment of Gustilo grade IIIB tibia fractures with application of antibiotic spacer, flap, and sequential distraction osteogenesis. *Ann Plast Surg.* 2010;64:541-552.

93. Keeling JJ, Gwinn DE, Tintle SM, et al. Short-term outcomes of severe open wartime tibial fractures treated with ring external fixation. *J Bone Joint Surg Am.* 2008;90:2643-2651.

94. Johnson EN, Burns TC, Hayda RA, et al. Infectious complications of open type III tibial fractures among combat casualties. *Clin Infect Dis.* 2007;45:409-415.

95. Beltran MJ, Ochoa LM, Graves RM, et al. Composite bone and soft tissue loss treated with distraction histiogenesis. *J Surg Orthop Adv.* 2010;19:23-28.

96. Miric D, Bumbasirevic M, Radulovic N, Lesic A. [External fixation of war injuries of the proximal femur]. *Acta Chir Iugosl.* 2005;52:101-105.

97. Stinner DJ, Keeney JA, Hsu JR, et al. Outcomes of internal fixation in a combat environment. *J Surg Orthop Adv.* 2010;19:49-53.

98. Upadhyay A, Jain P, Mishra P, Maini L, Gautum VK, Dhaon BK. Delayed internal fixation of fractures of the neck of the femur in young adults. A prospective, randomised study comparing closed and open reduction. *J Bone Joint Surg.* 2004;86:1035-1040.

99. Damany DS, Parker MJ, Chojnowski A. Complications after intracapsular hip fractures in young adults. A meta-analysis of 18 published studies involving 564 fractures. *Injury.* 2005;36:131-141.

100. Koval KJ, Clapper MF, Brumback RJ, et al. Complications of reamed intramedullary nailing of the tibia. *J Orthop Trauma.* 1991;5:184-189.

101. Clasper JC, Rowley DI. Outcome, following significant delays in initial surgery, of ballistic femoral fractures managed without internal or external fixation. *J Bone Joint Surg Br.* 2009;91(1):97-101.

102. Oberli H, Frick T. [The open femoral fracture in war—173 external fixators applied to the femur (Afghanistan war)]. *Helv Chir Acta.* 1992;58:687-692.

103. Bhandari M, Guyatt GH, Tong D, Adili A, Shaughnessy SG. Reamed versus nonreamed intramedullary nailing of lower extremity long bone fractures: a systematic overview and meta-analysis. *J Orthop Trauma.* 2000;14:2-9.

104. Nowotarski PJ, Turen CH, Brumback RJ, Scarboro JM. Conversion of external fixation to intramedullary nailing for fractures of the shaft of the femur in multiply injured patients. *J Bone Joint Surg Am.* 2000;82:781-788.

105. Keeney JA, Ingari JV, Mentzer KD, Powell ET. Closed intramedullary nailing of femoral shaft fractures in an echelon III facility. *Mil Med.* 2009;174:124-128.

106. Zlowodzki M, Bhandari M, Marek DJ, Cole PA, Kregor PJ. Operative treatment of acute distal femur fractures: systematic review of 2 comparative studies and 45 case series (1989 to 2005). *J Orthop Trauma.* 2006;20(5):366-371.

107. Court-Brown CM, McQueen MM, Quaba AA, Christie J. Locked intramedullary nailing of open tibial fractures. *J Bone Joint Surg Br.* 1991;73:959-964.

108. Court-Brown CM, Wheelwright EF, Christie J, McQueen MM. External fixation for type III open tibial fractures. *J Bone Joint Surg Br.* 1990;72:801-804.

109. Khatod M, Botte MJ, Hoyt DB, Meyer RS, Smith JM, Akeson WH. Outcomes in open tibia fractures: relationship between delay in treatment and infection. *J Trauma.* 2003;55:949-954.

110. Bhandari M, Zlowodzki M, Tornetta P 3rd, et al. Intramedullary nailing following external fixation in femoral and tibial shaft fractures. *J Orthop Trauma.* 2005;19:140-144.

111. Gustilo RB, Mendoza RM, Williams DN. Problems in the management of type III (severe) open fractures: a new classification of type III open fractures. *J Trauma.* 1984;24:742-746.

112. Has B, Jovanovic S, Wertheimer B, Mikolasevic I, Grdic P. External fixation as a primary and definitive treatment of open limb fractures [see comment]. *Injury.* 1995;26:245-248.

113. Roganovic Z, Savic M, Minic L, et al. [Peripheral nerve injuries during the 1991-1993 war period]. *Vojnosanit Pregl.* 1995;52:455-460.

114. Noble J, Munro CA, Prasad VS, Midha R. Analysis of upper and lower extremity peripheral nerve injuries in a population of patients with multiple injuries. *J Trauma.* 1998;45:116-122.

115. Bosse MJ, McCarthy ML, Jones AL, et al. The insensate foot following severe lower extremity trauma: an indication for amputation? *J Bone Joint Surg.* 2005;87:2601-2608.

116. Beltran M, et al. Peripheral nerve recovery following combat-related type III open tibia fractures. Presented at Society of Military Orthopedic Surgeons 51st Annual Meeting. Honolulu, HI; 2009.

117. Bosse MJ, MacKenzie EJ, Kellam JF, et al. An analysis of outcomes of reconstruction or amputation after leg-threatening injuries. *N Engl J Med.* 2002;347:1924-1931.

118. Stinner DJ, Burns TC, Kirk KL, Ficke JR. Return to duty rate of amputee soldiers in the current conflicts in Afghanistan and Iraq. *J Trauma.* 2010;68:1476-1479.

119. Stansbury LG, Lalliss SJ, Branstetter JG, Bagg MR, Holcomb JB. Amputations in U.S. military personnel in the current conflicts in Afghanistan and Iraq. *J Orthop Trauma.* 2008;22:43-46.

Chapter 25

LOWER EXTREMITY COVERAGE: MANAGEMENT OF COMBAT-RELATED SOFT TISSUE INJURY OF THE LOWER EXTREMITY

CDR (Ret) Anand R. Kumar, MD; CAPT Alan A. Lim, MD; LT Scott Tintle, MD; and James P. Bradley, MD

The occurrence of extremity trauma has increased during recent military conflicts.[1-5] There has also been a rapid progression in the destructive power of combat weaponry since the Vietnam War, yet, as a result of the advancement of battlefield medicine, improved body armor, and progressive limb salvage capabilities, the extremity amputation rate has only minimally changed.[6,7] A significant development in limb salvage surgery has been the ability to provide safe, vascularized wound coverage in the form of rotational, pedicled, and free tissue transfer in the subacute or late time periods.[8-11] This capability has significantly contributed to maintaining the current extremity amputation rate.

Lower extremity combat injuries from the recent conflicts have presented a significant challenge to reconstructive surgeons. The blast mechanism frequently leaves a large zone of composite tissue loss, with the remaining tissue highly contaminated and its vascularity often impaired. These large zones of injury, coupled with the complex microflora seen in battlefield extremity wounds and concurrent injuries, make soft tissue reconstruction challenging and mandate a cooperative effort amongst trauma, orthopedic, and plastic surgeons in order to achieve optimal outcomes.

These injuries often require prolonged reconstruction over many months and multiple surgical interventions. For this reason, durable and well-vascular-

ized soft tissue coverage must be provided in order to allow for repeated surgeries. The ultimate goal of achieving an extremity with healed fractures, a functional range of motion, and protective sensation, capable of ambulation, must be equally embraced by all members of the reconstructive team. This chapter outlines the principles of management and describes a reconstruction algorithm for these complex lower extremity wounds based upon our experiences at an Echelon V treatment facility.

Epidemiology

A previously published review of our experience with lower extremity flap reconstruction revealed the following epidemiologic data. Patient age ranged from 19 to 37 years (mean age: 25). The injuries in order of incidence included improvised explosive devices (76%), assault rifle projectiles (11%), mortars (7%), and motor vehicle accidents (6%). Our patients all sustained type IIIB and IIIC fractures requiring soft tissue coverage. The resulting fractures included 22% thigh (femur/hip), 52% upper-middle leg (tibia/fibula), 22% lower leg (ankle/foot), and 4% sacral injuries. Twenty-six percent of the fractures were type IIIC and thus required vascular repair for limb salvage. The average time to flap reconstruction was 21 days (range: 7 to 82 days). Lower extremity reconstructive

Owens BD, Belmont PJ Jr, eds. *Combat Orthopedic Surgery: Lessons Learned in Iraq and Afghanistan* (pp 253-268)
© 2011 SLACK Incorporated

delays occurred with several patients who sustained multiple concurrent traumatic injuries including brain trauma and abdominal organ injuries. Our treatment approach included approximately 5 pre-reconstructive washouts (range: 2 to 13) per patient, and negative pressure wound therapy was used in 100% of the patients between debridements (Tables 25-1 through 25-3).

Management in Theater

While the specific early management of combat wounds has been previously discussed in the text, we will highlight the National Naval Medical Center limb salvage protocol:

- Combat-injured patients with open wounds are rapidly assessed and evacuated to local medical treatment facilities.

- The initial treatment at these facilities includes gross decontamination of foreign material and the debridement of nonviable tissue. Following adequate early debridement, a copious amount of irrigation is used.

- Vascular repair and fasciotomies are performed if necessary, and, if indicated, monopolar external fixation is applied.

- Wound debridement and irrigation are then performed every 48 to 72 hours following the initial debridement and stabilization until arrival in the United States.

- Upon arrival at the tertiary care center in the United States, trauma surgery, orthopedic surgery, and plastic surgery evaluate each of these patients.

- Broad-spectrum antibiotics are always started on these patients and are continued until all wounds are closed.

- Patients return to the operating room every 48 to 72 hours until definitive wound closure or coverage. Aggressive debridement is performed at every procedure. Due to the high rate of bacterial colonization, massive soft tissue devitalization, and multiple concurrent injuries, early wound closure or flap reconstruction is avoided. Early internal fixation is avoided in order to decrease the risk of bacterial colonization and adherence of bacterial biofilm to implanted hardware.

In most instances, definitive wound coverage with a pedicled or free flap is performed prior to or at the time of the definitive bony fixation of fractures. Very rarely does internal fixation occur prior to definitive wound coverage. Our preference for lower extremity fracture fixation is external fixation, flap coverage, and then conversion to multiplanar spatial frames 1 to 2 weeks after flap coverage. This is different than our upper extremity protocol where internal fixation when indicated was performed at the time of or immediately before flap coverage of the combat extremity wound.

In general, one of the most important points for Echelons II and III levels of care is that, regardless of proceeding with early limb salvage or amputation, all viable tissue should be spared. If proceeding with amputation, a guillotine amputation should almost never be performed. The atypical flaps that remain after a tissue-sparing amputation may lead to length preservation of an amputation or may even be used in a spare parts surgery to cover contralateral extremity wounds (Figure 25-1).

Definitive Management

SALVAGE VERSUS AMPUTATIONS

Amputation is often the only option in the treatment of severe lower extremity combat trauma. In other situations, however, the patient and the team of surgeons may choose amputation of a potentially salvageable extremity as the preferred reconstructive method.[6,12] While limb salvage versus amputation has been discussed in other chapters, it is critical that this decision involve the surgeon who will perform the definitive soft tissue coverage if limb salvage is chosen by the patient. This decision is likely one of the most important ones in terms of the overall outcome, and it should be a multidisciplinary decision among orthopedic and plastic surgeons with experience treating these combat injuries.

ALTERNATIVE TO FLAP RECONSTRUCTION

Artificial skin substitutes, originally developed for burn patients, have been proven to aid in the reconstruction of combat wounded patients. Integra Bilayer Matrix Wound Dressing (Integra LifeSciences, Plainsboro, NJ) has been the most frequently used and studied in combat casualties. Integra is a bi-laminar product that contains bovine collage and shark chondroitin in the inner layer and silicone in the outer layer. After being applied to a clean, healthy wound bed, tissue grows into the collagen side akin to normal dermis. Following the incorporation of the dermal analog approximately 2 to 3 weeks after placement in a wound, a split-thickness skin graft is performed (Figure 25-2).

Helgeson and colleagues[13] reported successful results in achieving soft tissue coverage over exposed tendon or bone in 83% of patients using this method

Table 25-1

Fasciocutaneous Flap Reconstruction

Age	IED Injury	Time to Flap (Days)	# Prior Washouts	Flap Type	Connection	Flap Failure/ Comments	Associated Fracture	Associated Injury	Wound Culture
21	Yes	23	6	Anterolateral thigh flap	Free		Open metatarsals Calcaneus		*Bacillus* spp.
23	No	41	13	Extended tensor fascia lata flap	Pedicled		Open femur Acetabular hip	EIA w/ Fem-Fem Bypass	*Acinetobactor calcoaceticus baumannii*
35	No	26	5	Retrograde sural artery flap	Pedicled	Elective amputation (tip loss, osseous nonunion)	Open ankle		
33	Yes	16	3	Dorsalis pedis rotation Local flap, STSG	Pedicled		Open cuboid		*Acinetobactor calcoaceticus baumannii*
25	Yes	18	6	Anterolateral thigh flap	Free	Total flap loss (elective BKA)	Open calcaneus		
20	Yes	20	4	Anterolateral thigh flap	Free		Open metatarsals		
21	Yes	23	8	Crossleg flap	Pedicled		Exposed Achilles		*Acinetobactor calcoaceticus baumannii*
19	No	22	5	Lateral arm flap	Free		Open metatarsal		*Acinetobactor calcoaceticus baumannii*
34	Yes	21	5	Anterolateral thigh flap	Free		Open IIIB tibia		
23	No	27	10	Extended tensor fascia lata flap	Pedicled		Open sacral	Hypogastric artery, pelvic nerves, sacral plexus	*Candida albicans*

BKA = below-knee amputation, IED = improvised explosive device, STSG = split-thickness skin graft.

Table 25-2

Musculocutaneous Flap Reconstruction

Age	IED Injury	Time to Flap (Days)	# Prior Washouts	Flap Type	Connection	Flap Failure/ Comments	Associated Fracture	Associated Injury	Wound Culture
22	Yes	12	5	Oblique rectus abdominus flap	Pedicled		Open femur		Acinetobacter calcoaceticus baumannii
20	Yes	19	6	Rectus abdominus flap	Free		Open IIIB tibia	Tibial nerve	Acinetobacter calcoaceticus baumannii
24	Yes	33	6	Medial gastrocnemius flap	Pedicled		Open femur Tibial plateau	Forward popliteal bypass	Enterobacter Klebsiella Acinetobactor
23	No	19	3	Soleus flap, STSG	Pedicled		Open IIIB tibia		
23	Yes	82	3	Lateral gastrocnemius flap	Pedicled		Open lateral tibia		Staphlococcus epidermidis
27	No	17	8	Gastrocnemius flap	Pedicled		Open tibia		
23	Yes	94	4	Local ankle flap x 2 STSG	Bipedicled		Open ankle		
22	No	13	3		Pedicled		Open femur	SFA vein interposition graft, exposed	
37	Yes	23	8	Serratus flap	Free		Open calcaneus		Enterococcus faecalis Aeromonas hydrophillia Pseudomonas aeruginosa
23	Yes	15	3	Oblique rectus abdominus flap, STSG	Pedicled		Open femur	Lateral femoral cutaneous nerve	Acinetobactor calcoaceticus baumannii
24	Yes	7	3	Soleus flap, STSG	Pedicled		Open IIIC tibia	Popliteal artery (vein graft)	Alternaria
23	Yes	8	2	Soleus flap	Pedicled	Partial flap loss	Open tibia		
23	Yes	20	5	Rectus abdominis flap	Free	Failed soleus flap	Open tibia		Staphlococcus haemolyticus Coagulase negative Staph
20	Yes	38	4	Soleus flap, STSG	Pedicled		Open tibia		Pseudomonas aeruginosa
25	Yes	16	6	Gastrocnemius flap, STSG	Pedicled		Open femur		
23	Yes	20	4	Gastrocnemius flap, STSG	Pedicled		Open tibia		Acinetobacter calcoaceticus baumannii Klebsiella pneumoniae Enterococcus faecalis
27	Yes	21	10	Gastrocnemius flap, STSG	Pedicled		Open femur	Sciatic nerve	Acinetobacter calcoaceticus baumannii

IED = improvised explosive device, SFA = superficial femoral artery/vein, STSG = split-thickness skin graft.

(continued)

Table 25-2 (continued)

Musculocutaneous Flap Reconstruction

Age	IED Injury	Time to Flap (Days)	# Prior Washouts	Flap Type	Connection	Flap Failure/ Comments	Associated Fracture	Associated Injury	Wound Culture
22	Yes	17	4	Latissimus flap, STSG	Free		Open tibia		Enterobacter cloacae
20	No	11	3	Soleus flap, STSG	Pedicled		Open tibia		
32	Yes	8	2	Gastrocnemius flap, STSG	Pedicled		Open knee, patellar loss		
32	Yes	10	3	Gastrocnemius flap, STSG	Pedicled		Open femur		
32	Yes	10	3	Lateral gastrocnemius flap	Pedicled		Open femur		
33	Yes	24	7	Rectus abdominus flap, STSG	Free		Open tibia		Acinetobacter calcoaceticus baumannii
24	Yes	11	3	Lateral gastrocnemius flap, STSG	Pedicled		Open tibia		
22	Yes	14	4	Peroneus brevis flap, STSG	Pedicled		Open tibia		
20	Yes	12	3	Medial gastrocnemius flap, STSG	Pedicled		Open fibula	Peroneal nerve (grafted)	Acinetobacter calcoaceticus baumannii
19	Yes	25	4	Gluteus maximus flap, STSG	Pedicled		Open sacral fractures		
25	Yes	19	3	Lateral gastrocnemius flap	Pedicled		Open tibia		
36	Yes	19	3	Lateral gastrocnemius flap, STSG	Pedicled		Open femur		
24	Yes	14	4	Medial gastrocnemius flap, STSG	Pedicled		Open tibia		
22	Yes	12	3	Medial gastrocnemius flap, STSG	Pedicled		Open tibia		Acinetobacter calcoaceticus baumannii
27	Yes	12	3	Lateral gastrocnemius flap, STSG	Pedicled		Open tibia Open femur		
23	No	15	3	Soleus flap, STSG	Pedicled		Open tibia	Deep peroneal nerve	
21	No	11	3		Pedicled	Nosocomial subflap infection	Open fibula		Nosocomial Staph aureus Acinetobacter calcoaceticus baumannii

IED = improvised explosive device, STSG = split-thickness skin graft.

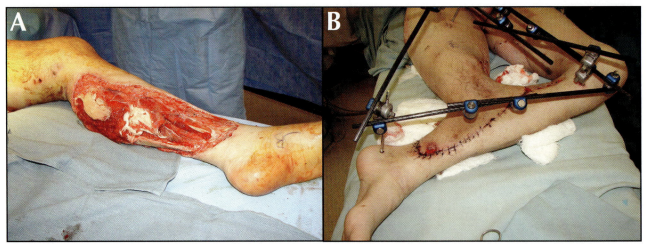

Figure 25-1. (A) Injured Marine with degloved left leg with exposed Achilles tendon after severe blast injury. (B) Left leg wound reconstructed with cross leg fillet flap with supplemental external fixation.

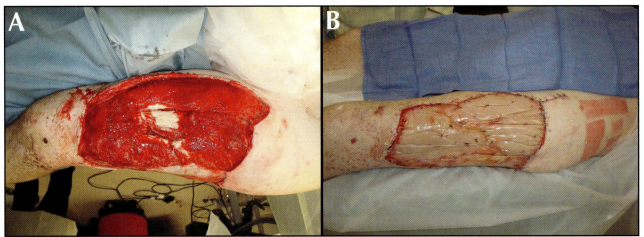

Figure 25-2. (A) Injured marine with left lateral thigh wound with exposed muscle and tendon and no underlying fracture. (B) The left lateral thigh wound after 2.5 weeks demonstrating sufficient revascularization of the dermal template. Note the paradoxical white appearance. The template appears red when initially placed on the wound bed.

at an Echelon V military treatment facility in combat patients. The authors concluded that when successful, the use of the Integra eliminated the need for more sophisticated flap coverage. While we do believe that Integra has a unique role in the management of these large open wounds, we have not and do not recommend its use in the setting of an open fracture. The use of Integra in the lower extremity is also limited to wounds where bacterial colonization has been adequately controlled and active infection is not present. The unique wound with exposed tendon or exposed nonfractured bone is an ideal candidate for Integra in our opinion.

TIMING OF LOWER EXTREMITY FLAP COVERAGE

In 1986, Marco Godina[14] published his landmark paper that challenged the standard of care on the tim-

ing of flap reconstruction, yet controversy continues to this day. Godina's paper reviewed his team's experience with the performance of 532 microsurgical reconstructions involving 134 open fractures. The results of his work revealed that early flap coverage within 3 days from the time of injury had a significantly higher rate of success with the lowest rate of infection as compared to more delayed coverage (P<0.0005). They also found that the rate of total flap necrosis and postoperative wound infections rose to between 20% and 30% when flap coverage was provided outside the 72-hour interval from injury.[14]

Byrd and colleagues,[15] as well as others, have also documented the necessity of radical wound debridement and early (<5 days) vascularized soft tissue coverage of grade III extremity injuries.[16-23] Despite these studies, early flap coverage is not frequently performed at Echelon V military facilities treating combat casualties for a number of reasons.[3,9-11] The

Table 25-3

Adipofascial Flap Reconstruction

Age	IED Injury	Time to Flap (Days)	# Prior Washouts	Flap Type	Connection	Flap Failure/ Comments	Associated Fracture	Associated Injury	Wound Culture
22	No	20	4	Local flap	Pedicled	Elective BKA	Open IIIB tibia/fibula	Popliteal artery	
22	Yes	15	3	Supramalleolar flap, STSG	Pedicled	Partial flap loss	Open calcaneus		Nosocomial *Enterococcus faecium* Coagulase negative *Staph* Yeast

BKA = below-knee amputation, IED = improvised explosive device, STSG = split-thickness skin graft.

large amount of soft tissue contamination, the delayed appearance of progressive muscle necrosis, multiple concomitant injuries, and the delayed presentation due to medical evacuation make it nearly impossible to perform coverage within the early time period.

This delay, however, has not unfavorably affected outcomes.[9-11] Provided that one adheres to the established principles of creating a clean wound bed and using healthy vascularized coverage, then infection and flap failure can be minimized and good results obtained. In our experience, even in the presence of heavy wound colonization, we have achieved low flap failure rates and acceptable postoperative infection rates. There is also supporting civilian literature that indicates that good results can be obtained during the subacute and late time periods. Yaremchuk and colleagues[24] found no untoward effects with soft tissue coverage at an average of 17 days in patients with severe open IIIB tibia fractures. Ironically, he reported this in 1986, the same year as Marco Godina's paper. More recently, in a review of delayed flap coverage of both upper and lower extremity open fractures, Steiert and colleagues found a low rate of both infection (0.0%) and flap failure (2.6%) when coverage was performed in the subacute time period (mean: 28 days).[25]

Steiert and colleagues[25] highlighted the advances in wound care over the past 20 years and specifically discussed the use of the wound vacuum-assisted closure device as a significant contributor to the overall success of flap coverage in this subacute time period. In contrast to his results, however, a recent review of type IIIB open tibia fractures at a Level I trauma center within the United States revealed an overall infection rate of 36% when flap coverage was provided in the first 7 days after injury.[26] When delayed coverage was provided outside of the first 7 days, the infection rate soared to 57%. The treatment protocol at this trauma center included wound vacuum-assisted closure application to open wounds following initial debridement and stabilization and then repeat irrigation and debridement procedures in the operating room every 48 hours until definitive soft tissue coverage.[26] What was not clear from this study, however, was the method of definitive fracture fixation nor the timing of such treatment in relation to definitive wound coverage. The high rate of early infection in the group that underwent flap coverage within 7 days (36%) raises concern about the overall treatment protocol.

We believe that the successful coverage of open fracture wounds in the lower extremity is possible within the subacute and late time frame for a number of reasons. The timing delay ensures that patients' overall condition and nutrition is optimized. It ensures that more urgent surgeries such as thoraco-abdominal, spinal, or cranial surgeries are performed

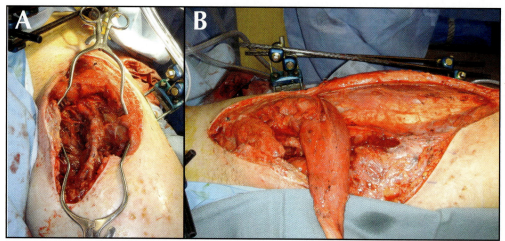

Figure 25-3. (A) Injured Marine with left open femur fracture and exposed vascular bypass graft. (B) The left rectus femoris muscle flap prior to inset.

and that these systems have stabilized prior to flap reconstruction. In addition, the delay allows for the appreciation and subsequent debridement of all necrotic tissue in the evolving combat wound prior to flap reconstruction.

Regardless of these benefits, we strongly believe that the greatest contribution to the success of this limb salvage protocol was the orthoplastic approach to the treatment of these injuries. Daily consultation between the orthopedic surgeon and plastic surgeon was imperative. Both surgeons were present in the operating room for a majority of the debridements. All fracture stabilization and soft tissue procedures were thoroughly timed and planned by both the plastic and orthopedic surgeons with the best overall outcome in mind, as opposed to the usual interest in selective flap success or fracture union.

FLAP SELECTION PRINCIPLES

In 1993, Levin and colleagues[27,28] introduced the concept of the reconstructive ladder. Wound closure by secondary intention is at the lowest rung of the ladder with progressive rungs displaying increasingly more sophisticated closures until the pinnacle of free tissue transfer is reached. The ladder was introduced in an effort to guide the selection of wound closure, and its creators indicated that a surgeon may go from one level to another and in many instances may simultaneously employ different aspects of the ladder.[27] When treating combat casualties with multiple organ system injuries, it is imperative to use the reconstructive ladder as a guide to provide the simplest and least morbid wound coverage.

The following factors play a critical role in the proper selection of flap coverage[29,30]:
- Patient factors (systemic illness, head trauma)
- Donor site availability (amputation of extremity)

- Genesis of the defect
- Location/size/depth of the defect
- Exposed structures
- Degree of contamination
- Quality of the surrounding tissues

In combat-wounded servicemembers, the availability of donor sites along with donor site morbidity considerations play a pivotal role in flap selection. The high rate of concurrent injury and amputation may make traditional flap choices such as free fibula flaps or latissimus flaps nonviable options. In addition, patients with severe systemic compromise and/or severe head trauma may not be ideal candidates for free tissue transfer procedures. In the lower extremity, there are a number of local pedicled flaps available for soft tissue coverage that will frequently provide the necessary coverage. In situations where appropriate local flaps are not available, free tissue transfer usually becomes necessary.

While it is outside the scope of this chapter to discuss in detail all of the options for soft tissue coverage of the lower extremity, the following highlights our treatment algorithm and a few of the flaps that we have used most frequently for wound coverage. The optimal flap used for lower extremity wound reconstruction should be made by analyzing all the anatomic, functional, and aesthetic reconstructive requirements. In our experience, proximal hip wounds are best treated with rectus abdominus flaps or rectus femoris flaps (Figure 25-3). The sacrum, an extremely challenging location, can best be treated with the extended fascia lata flap, local gluteus muscle flaps if not significantly injured, and/or free latissimus flaps. Upper one-third and middle one-third leg wounds are best treated with gastrocnemius and soleus flaps, respectively, and rarely with free tissue transfer. Distal

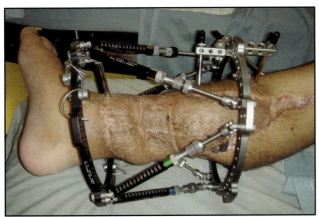

Figure 25-4. Distal tibia fracture and soft tissue defect reconstructed using a free rectus flap and skin graft. Two weeks after free flap reconstruction the monoplanar frame is then converted to a multiplanar weight-sharing frame after soft tissue reconstruction viability is ensured.

lower extremity wounds were best treated with local pedicled flaps or free tissue transfer.

EXTENDED TENSOR FASCIA LATA FLAP

The tensor fascia lata (TFL) flap, first introduced in 1978, was originally used as both a free flap and a pedicled flap for coverage of wounds around the hip and the abdominal wall.[31-33] It is most frequently used as a transposition flap.[33] This is a musculocutaneous flap, and its blood supply is derived from the lateral femoral circumflex artery, which originates from the profunda femoris artery. The lateral femoral circumflex artery courses above the vastus intermedius to supply the rectus femoris, the vastus lateralis, and the extended TFL. Musculocutaneous perforators from the TFL supply the skin of the lateral thigh.[33] The lateral femoral circumflex artery enters the TFL approximately 10 cm below the anterior superior iliac spine.[32] This flap remains particularly useful in that a large portion of the lateral thigh, up to 15 x 40 cm, can be elevated safely based on the small TFL and its perforators (Figure 25-4).[33]

RECTUS ABDOMINUS FLAP

The rectus abdominus flap can be used as both a pedicled or free tissue transfer for soft tissue coverage. We have used the pedicled rectus flap for coverage of open proximal femur fractures in combat-wounded patients.[9] This technique has previously been used in civilian trauma with good success.[34] The rectus abdominus muscle has blood supply from both the deep superior and the inferior epigastric arteries. When providing coverage to the extremity, the flap is usually designed based upon the blood flow from the inferior epigastric artery. The viability of the inferior epigas-

tric artery should be verified prior to proceeding with this flap as the artery may be damaged by previous abdominal surgeries that use transverse incisions, such as a hernia repair or an appendectomy.[35] This flap is advantageous because it provides good tissue volume with an abundant reliable blood supply that originates outside of the zone of injury. The pedicled flap can be performed in a bipolar fashion with the vascular pedicle as the only tether point, allowing for significant transposition.[34] The rectus abdominus is a relatively expendable muscle and does not further compromise extremity function in the often multiple extremity-injured combat casualty. This donor site is frequently available as it is usually spared from the effects of blast injuries by the body armor.

The rectus abdominis is also reliable as a free tissue transfer for small- to moderate-sized defects (see Figure 25-4).[12,36-40] The free flap can be used as a muscle or a musculocutaneous flap. The vascular leash is usually the deep inferior epigastric artery, although the deep superior epigastric artery can also be used. When the rectus flap is used for extremity reconstruction, it is usually taken as a muscle flap alone.[38] The deep inferior epigastric artery is routinely 2.5 to 3 mm in diameter, and usually a pedicle of 5 to 7 cm can be harvested with the muscle.[38] Disadvantages to the pedicled or free rectus transfer include the possibility of abdominal hernia as well as aesthetic concerns for young military servicemembers.[12,34] Despite these concerns, donor site morbidity has proven minimal.[38]

GASTROCNEMIUS FLAP

The gastrocnemius flap has been a commonly used flap in the civilian world. It has also been extensively used in flap coverage about the knee in combat wounded.[9] The medial or lateral head of the gastrocnemius can be used to cover defects overlying the distal femur, quadriceps tendon, patella, patellar tendon, and the proximal one-third of the tibia. The gastrocnemius is the most superficial muscle in the posterior compartment of the leg. The respective heads of the gastrocnemius arise from the medial and lateral condyles of the femur and continue distally where they converge below the knee. At the junction of the middle and distal one-third of the leg, the muscle becomes tendinous and joins with the tendon of the soleus to form the Achilles tendon. The medial head of the gastrocnemius is larger and closer to the anterior leg and thus is harvested more frequently for coverage. The lateral head of the gastrocnemius is 3 to 4 cm shorter and must traverse around the fibula and the common peroneal nerve to reach the anterior leg. This decreases its coverage range and increases the potential morbidity due to the proximity of the peroneal nerve (Figure 25-5).

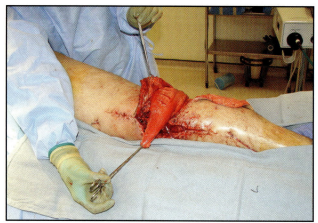

Figure 25-5. The left gastrocnemius flap transposed into the anterior knee soft tissue defect.

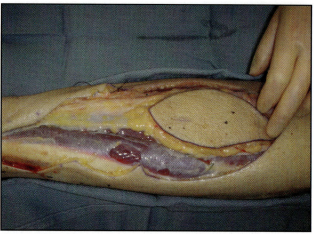

Figure 25-6. The sural artery flap in island configuration prior to inset. Note the broad lower pedicle incorporating the sural nerve and lesser saphenous vein.

The few major contraindications to the performance of a gastrocnemius muscle flap include active infection and damage to the gastrocnemius muscle or the sural arteries supplying the muscle. The medial and lateral sural arteries arise from the popliteal artery and supply the medial and the lateral heads of the gastrocnemius. The presence of any damage to the popliteal artery or sural artery that would compromise the success of the flap is a contraindication to this flap coverage. In the preoperative planning for this flap, close examination for any vascular insufficiency to the leg as well as routine angiography or computed tomographic angiography is frequently performed in the combat casualty due to frequent occult injuries to the popliteal artery.

In our experience, the use of the gastrocnemius flap and in some instances bilateral gastrocnemius flaps has led to the avoidance of free tissue transfer around the knee. While free tissue transfer around the knee is possible and good outcomes have been reported, it is often complicated by the inability to find suitable recipient vessels.[41,42] Additionally, the length of the pedicle that is needed is often longer than the available donor pedicle in trauma cases, especially in the combat wounded. Vein grafts are then frequently needed, increasing both the complexity of the surgery and the failure rates.[41]

Despite these downsides to free tissue transfer around the knee, there are some instances in which a large free muscle flap such as a latissimus dorsi is needed to fill a large void of bone and soft tissue. However, we have found very few instances to perform free tissue transfers around the knee. This is due to both the utility of the gastrocnemius flap and what we feel is a critical selection bias. In situations where large free tissue transfers around the knee have been necessary, the injuries have usually been so severe that a multidisciplinary team of orthopedic and plastic surgeons have recommended early amputation.

SURAL ARTERY FLAP

The distally based sural artery flap has grown in popularity in recent years.[12,43,44] Its clinical utility has been demonstrated in civilian as well as in combat-wounded populations.[44] We have found the sural artery flap useful, and we have considered its use when coverage of the distal tibia, ankle, or hindfoot were required and free tissue transfer was not indicated or possible.

The distally based sural artery flap is a fasciocutaneous flap that is supplied via retrograde blood flow through the superficial sural artery via the anastamoses of the lateral malleolar arteries from the peroneal artery. The superficial sural artery accompanies the sural nerve and lesser saphenous vein on the posterior aspect of the leg. The flap is used for coverage of small- to medium-sized defects around the ankle and hindfoot. The pivot point of the flap is approximately 5 cm proximal to the lateral malleolus. It is recommended that the harvested flap not exceed 9 x 12 cm, although dimensions as large as 9 x 22 cm have been reported without flap necrosis (Figure 25-6).[12,35]

The benefits of the sural artery flap include its consistent anatomy as well as the ability to perform the flap quickly without the sacrifice of one of the major arteries to the foot. It is also a fasciocutaneous flap, which facilitates improved underlying tendon excursion and provides ideal defect contouring. Despite relatively minimal postoperative discomfort and morbidity, the donor site defect usually requires skin grafting for closure, which remains an aesthetic concern.[12,35,43] Potential complications of the flap include the hyposensitivity that results on the lateral border of the foot as a result of transection of the sural nerve as well as the potential for a symptomatic sural neuroma.[35] Additionally, as is the case with most retrograde flaps, the flap is prone to venous congestion.

Prerequisite to performing this flap, the vascular supply to the peroneal artery must be ensured. Venous drainage, specifically the patency of the lesser saphenous vein, must also be verified.[35] In the postoperative setting, the most important considerations are the avoidance of compression of the vascular pedicle and elevation of the leg to facilitate venous return. In the majority of instances, these combat-wounded servicemembers already have external fixators on the lower extremity, and it is relatively easy to construct a "kickstand" to facilitate reliable protected elevation and decompression of the vascular pedicle.[45-47]

One final but exquisitely important consideration in the performance of this flap in the lower extremity combat casualty is that the performance of this flap will definitely compromise a standard Burgess below-the-knee amputation using a long posterior myofasciocutaneous flap. If limb salvage is questionable, then consideration of another flap may be indicated.[12,48]

FREE ANTEROLATERAL THIGH FLAP

The anterolateral thigh flap is a versatile free flap capable of being harvested as a cutaneous, fasciocutaneous, or a musculocutaneous flap with the vastus lateralis. Most commonly, the anterolateral thigh flap is harvested as a fasciocutaneous flap based upon the perforator originating from the descending branch or transverse branch of the lateral femoral circumflex artery.[49] The variability of perforator anatomy can make this flap more challenging but also contributes to its versatility with custom design. The advantages of the anterolateral thigh flap include the potential large size of the flap (up to 35 x 25 cm),[50,51] the ability to use a 2-team approach for harvest, the ability to obtain a long vascular pedicle up to 20 cm with the flap allowing for anastamosis outside the zone of injury, and relatively little donor site morbidity persists if minimal muscle harvest is performed.[35,50-52] These advantages coupled with the improved sensation and gliding surface make the anterolateral thigh flap an ideal flap for free tissue transfer and make it our free flap of choice for reconstruction (Figure 25-7).

In the preoperative planning for this flap, it is imperative that the inflow vessels be identified. In the combat casualty, this usually means that angiography of the lower extremity to receive the flap should be performed. In the postoperative setting, flap monitoring is imperative. To facilitate close monitoring, we recommend 24 hours in an intensive care or step-down unit where adequate time and attention can be devoted to the flap.

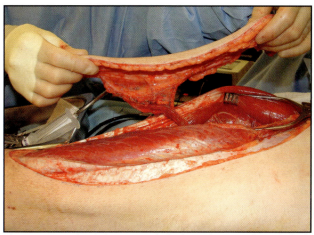

Figure 25-7. The left proximal thigh with anterolateral thigh flap elevated prior to division and inset.

CRITICAL POINTS FOR OPTIMAL SUCCESS WITH FREE TISSUE TRANSFER

A frank objective analysis of the wound and overall patient factors by a team of orthopedic and plastic surgeons is critical to the success of a free tissue transfer. Free tissue transfers should not be performed when the limb is a better candidate for early amputation. In our experience, we performed only 3 free muscle transfers to the lower extremity for soft tissue reconstruction. It was not common that a patient presented with a lower extremity that necessitated bulk muscle free tissue transfer for coverage of a wound and was deemed a good candidate for limb salvage. Similarly, we did not frequently use vein grafts in free tissue transfer, as the wounds that would have required them were frequently better candidates for amputation. In the majority of our free tissue transfers to the lower extremity, we used fasciocutaneous flaps with long vascular pedicles in an effort to maximize vascular anastamoses outside the zone of injury. In addition, it is imperative that patients can safely be placed on anticoagulation therapy following flap reconstruction. We liberally anticoagulated our free flap reconstructions with regional and systemic heparin prior to flap harvest and continued until post-surgical day 4 due to the wide zone of jury associated with blast trauma and multiple concurrent upstream injuries. In appropriately selected patients, we experienced minimal post-surgical hemorrhagic complications.

SOFT TISSUE EXPANSION

In addition to the multiple soft tissue coverage procedures previously discussed, we have found the use of soft tissue expanders useful in the treatment of our patients. In these devastating lower extremity injuries, multiple reconstructive surgeries are frequently necessary. Following early coverage of soft tissue defects, the use of soft tissue expanders in preparation for continued reconstructive surgeries has been used in combat-wounded servicemembers. Soft tissue expanders about the lower extremity have been most commonly used in preparation for total knee arthroplasty or revision arthroplasty in patients who are at high risk of having soft tissue coverage complications.[53] The use of soft tissue expansion has also been reported for preserving amputation length.[54]

The soft tissue expander is a silicone pouch that is inserted in a deflated fashion under the skin. It has a port that is remote from the cavity and is tunneled under the subcutaneous tissue. The cavity is slowly filled with saline via the port over many weeks as the skin stretches. Following maximum necessary expansion, continued reconstruction proceeds. The use of expanders has facilitated the excision of skin grafts and wound closure with newly expanded and more durable, healthy skin flaps. Soft tissue expansion not only increases the skin available for closure, but also improves the quality of the soft tissue obtained. Cherry and colleagues[55] explained that the use of the expanders leads to an increase in the vascularity of the expanded tissue. They hypothesized that the physical forces on the overlying tissue led to increased local angiogenesis. Reported complications of expansion are infection, hematoma, seroma, pain, necrosis of overlying skin, neuropraxia, bone resorption, and flap failure.[56] In our experience with soft tissue expansion, we have seen hematoma formation and infection.

Outcomes/Complications

We reported our flap experience over a 30-month period during Operation Iraqi Freedom and Operation Enduring Freedom entailing 46 lower extremity wounds requiring flap reconstructions.[9] Ten fasciocutaneous, 34 musculocutaneous, and 2 adipofascial flaps were performed on 43 patients. The time to reconstruction was 7 to 82 days (average: 21 days). Total flap loss occurred in only 1 patient and partial flap loss in 2 patients. Our success rate was 98%, defined as eventual wound healing without the need for amputation (see Tables 25-1 through 25-3).

Our flap complication rate was very low with this severely injured cohort of lower extremity combat casualties. We strongly believe that the complication rates in these patients can be minimized with the combination of discriminating and precise patient selection as well as adherence to classic flap and microsurgical principles. In addition to the one early total flap failure, we also had 2 patients with small partial flap losses that were treated successfully with debridements, negative pressure wound therapy, and

flap readvancement for wound closure. Three total amputations were eventually performed on our lower extremity reconstruction cohort. One patient underwent early limb amputation after early total flap failure. In this patient, attempted aggressive limb salvage with a massive zone of injury and damage to deep and superficial venous drainage resulted in loss of an anterolateral thigh free flap. Two additional patients (free latissimus flap, local adipofascial flap) who had flap success and went on to heal their tibia fractures underwent delayed below-knee amputation due to poor function of the salvaged limb (Table 25-4).

In our experience, free and pedicled flaps have been used with equal success for lower extremity reconstruction.[9] Despite this success, we must acknowledge that pedicled tissue transfer occurred 3.7 times more often than free tissue transfer in our lower extremity combat casualty cohort. While we have had good success with free tissue transfer in carefully selected patients, it is of paramount importance in the management of these complicated patients that the ladder of soft tissue reconstruction be followed. In this combat casualty population with multiple extremity injuries, the simplest and least morbid solution to coverage is selected to ensure that the optimal overall outcome is achieved. Recently, in the civilian reconstruction of extremity injuries, there is a trend toward early and more common free tissue transfer over pedicled transfer due to the improved technical skills and surgical abilities of microvascular surgeons. Despite the potential benefits that have been noted with this management, we are less likely to advance up the soft tissue ladder of reconstruction without adequate reason when a very reliable pedicled flap will provide a successful outcome.[57,58] The risks of a prolonged microsurgery flap procedure in a critically injured combat patient are significant. In our experience, joint contractures and stiffness have not been a significant complication when pedicled distant flaps have been used to reconstruct extremity wounds.

Conclusion

Providing wound coverage to a combat-injured limb that would otherwise be amputated is a very rewarding yet humbling experience. It is imperative to recognize the unique nature of combat wounds and the differences in management of these wounds from civilian trauma. An early frank evaluation of the limb should be performed by a multidisciplinary team of orthopedic and plastic surgeons to determine the optimal treatment plan in order to maximize both patient and surgeon expectations. In the majority of instances in the lower extremity, pedicled flaps will provide reliable and durable soft tissue coverage when free tissue

Table 25-4

Tibia Fracture Subgroup Analysis

Patient	Associated Fracture	Flap Type	Time to Flap (Days)	Late Infection	Additional Surgeries	Flap Result	Orthopedic Treatment	Time to Union
1	Open IIIB tibia	Free rectus abdominus flap	20			Flap survived	Taylor Spatial Frame	286
2	Open IIIB tibia	Local pedicled adipofascial flap	16		Amputation	Flap survived, pt desired amputation	Ilizarov	259
3	Open IIIB tibia	Soleus flap, STSG	21			Flap survived	Ilizarov	217
4	Open IIIB tibia	Soleus flap, STSG	16			Flap survived	Taylor Spatial Frame	180
5	Open IIIB tibia	Soleus flap, STSG	8			Flap survived	Taylor Spatial Frame	69
6	Open IIIB tibia	Free rectus abdominus flap, STSG	11	Yes	9	Flap survived	Taylor Spatial Frame	196
7	Open IIIB tibia	Lateral gastrocnemius flap, STSG	20			Flap survived	Taylor Spatial Frame	268
8	Open IIIB tibia	Peroneus brevis flap, STSG	12			Flap survived	Taylor Spatial Frame then IM nail	249
9	Open IIIB tibia	Medial gastrocnemius flap, STSG	12	Yes after delayed bone grafting	5	Flap survived	Taylor Spatial Frame	205
10	Open IIIB tibia	Soleus flap, STSG	22			Flap survived	Taylor Spatial Frame	215
11	Open IIIC tibia	Soleus flap, STSG	41			Flap survived	Taylor Spatial Frame	170
12	Open IIIB tibia	Free latissimus flap, STSG	11	Yes	Amputation	Flap survived, pt desired amputation	Taylor Spatial Frame	
13	Open IIIB tibia	Medial gastrocnemius flap, STSG	26			Flap survived	Taylor Spatial Frame	300
14	Open IIIB tibia	Soleus flap	17			Total flap failure	IM nail	165
14	Open IIIB tibia	Free rectus abdominus flap after failed soleus flap	29			Flap survived	IM nail	165
15	Open IIIB tibia plateau and shaft	Gastrocnemius flap, STSG	21			Flap survived	Taylor Spatial Frame	135
16	Open IIIB tibia plateau	Medial gastrocnemius flap, STSG	17			Flap survived	Spanning knee ex fix	292
17	Open IIIC tibia plateau, open femur	Medial gastrocnemius flap, STSG	27			Flap survived	Taylor Spatial Frame	233
18	Open IIIB prox tibia, open femur	Lateral gastrocnemius flap, STSG	15			Flap survived	ORIF with extensor mechanism allograft	96
19	Open IIIB pilon	Local ankle bipedicled flap x 2 with STSG	13			Flap survived	ORIF then Taylor Spatial Frame	280

IM = intramedullary, ORIF = open reduction and internal fixation, STSG = split-thickness skin graft.

donor sites or patient characteristics prohibit free tissue transfer. When free tissue transfer is indicated, it can be performed successfully with stringent patient selection. With these principles in mind, success in the face of the demanding and unique challenges presented by modern battlefield injuries can be obtained.

References

1. Helling TS, McNabney WK. The role of amputation in the management of battlefield casualties: a history of two millennia. *J Trauma*. 2000;49(5):930-939.
2. Mabry RL, Holcomb JB, Baker AM, et al. United States Army Rangers in Somalia: an analysis of combat casualties on an urban battlefield. *J Trauma*. 2000;49(3):515-528; discussion 528-529.
3. Geiger S, McCormick F, Chou R, Wandel AG. War wounds: lessons learned from Operation Iraqi Freedom. *Plast Reconstr Surg*. 2008;122(1):146-153.
4. Nikolic D, Jovanovic Z, Popovic Z, Vulovic R, Mladenovic M. Primary surgical treatment of war injuries of major joints of the limbs. *Injury*. 1999;30(2):129-134.
5. Owens BD, Kragh JF Jr, Macaitis J, Svoboda SJ, Wenke JC. Characterization of extremity wounds in Operation Iraqi Freedom and Operation Enduring Freedom. *J Orthop Trauma*. 2007;21(4):254-257.
6. Potter BK, Scoville CR. Amputation is not isolated: an overview of the US Army Amputee Patient Care Program and associated amputee injuries. *J Am Acad Orthop Surg*. 2006;14(10 Spec No.):S188-S190.
7. Stansbury LG, Lalliss SJ, Branstetter JG, Bagg MR, Holcomb JB. Amputations in U.S. military personnel in the current conflicts in Afghanistan and Iraq. *J Orthop Trauma*. 2008;22(1):43-46.
8. Kumar AR. Standard wound coverage techniques for extremity war injury. *J Am Acad Orthop Surg*. 2006;14(10 Spec No.):S62-S65.
9. Kumar AR, Grewal NS, Chung TL, Bradley JP. Lessons from operation Iraqi freedom: successful subacute reconstruction of complex lower extremity battle injuries. *Plast Reconstr Surg*. 2009;123(1):218-229.
10. Kumar AR, Grewal NS, Chung TL, Bradley JP. Lessons from the modern battlefield: successful upper extremity injury reconstruction in the subacute period. *J Trauma*. 2009;67(4):752-757.
11. Chattar-Cora D, Perez-Nieves R, McKinlay A, Kunasz M, Delaney R, Lyons R. Operation Iraqi freedom: a report on a series of soldiers treated with free tissue transfer by a plastic surgery service. *Ann Plast Surg*. 2007;58(2):200-206.
12. Baechler MF, Groth AT, Nesti LJ, Martin BD. Soft tissue management of war wounds to the foot and ankle. *Foot Ankle Clin*. 2010;15(1):113-138.
13. Helgeson MD, Potter BK, Evans KN, Shawen SB. Bioartificial dermal substitute: a preliminary report on its use for the management of complex combat-related soft tissue wounds. *J Orthop Trauma*. 2007;21(6):394-399.
14. Godina M. Early microsurgical reconstruction of complex trauma of the extremities. *Plast Reconstr Surg*. 1986;78(3):285-292.
15. Byrd HS, Spicer TE, Cierney G Jr. Management of open tibial fractures. *Plast Reconstr Surg*. 1985;76(5):719-730.
16. Hallock GG. Utility of both muscle and fascia flaps in severe lower extremity trauma. *J Trauma*. 2000;48(5):913-917.
17. Hertel R, Lambert SM, Muller S, Ballmer FT, Ganz R. On the timing of soft-tissue reconstruction for open fractures of the lower leg. *Arch Orthop Trauma Surg*. 1999;119(1-2):7-12.

18. Francel TJ, Vander Kolk CA, Hoopes JE, Manson PN, Yaremchuk MJ. Microvascular soft-tissue transplantation for reconstruction of acute open tibial fractures: timing of coverage and long-term functional results. *Plast Reconstr Surg*. 1992;89(3):478-487; discussion 488-489.
19. Khouri RK, Shaw WW. Reconstruction of the lower extremity with microvascular free flaps: a 10-year experience with 304 consecutive cases. *J Trauma*. 1989;29(8):1086-1094.
20. Yazar S, Lin CH, Lin YT, Ulusal AE, Wei FC. Outcome comparison between free muscle and free fasciocutaneous flaps for reconstruction of distal third and ankle traumatic open tibial fractures. *Plast Reconstr Surg*. 2006;117(7):2468-2475; discussion 2476-2477.
21. Stalekar H, Fuckar Z, Ekl D, Sustic A, Loncarek K, Ledic D. Primary vs secondary wound reconstruction in Gustilo type III open tibial shaft fractures: follow-up study of 35 cases. *Croat Med J*. 2003;44(6):746-755.
22. Le B. *Microsurgery in war wounds*. Scientific Meeting of the American Society of Plastic Surgeons; 2000.
23. Hallock GG. Lower extremity muscle perforator flaps for lower extremity reconstruction. *Plast Reconstr Surg*. 2004;114(5):1123-1130.
24. Yaremchuk MJ, Gan BS. Soft tissue management of open tibia fractures. *Acta Orthop Belg*. 1996;62(Suppl):1188-1192.
25. Steiert AE, Gohritz A, Schreiber TC, Krettek C, Vogt PM. Delayed flap coverage of open extremity fractures after previous vacuum-assisted closure (VAC) therapy—worse or worth? *J Plast Reconstr Aesthet Surg*. 2009;62(5):675-683.
26. Bhattacharyya T, Mehta P, Smith M, Pomahac B. Routine use of wound vacuum-assisted closure does not allow coverage delay for open tibia fractures. *Plast Reconstr Surg*. 2008;121(4):1263-1266.
27. Levin LS. The reconstructive ladder. An orthoplastic approach. *Orthop Clin North Am*. 1993;24(3):393-409.
28. Levin LS, Condit DP. Combined injuries—soft tissue management. *Clin Orthop Relat Res*. 1996;327:172-181.
29. Wolf JM, Athwal GS, Shin AY, Dennison DG. Acute trauma to the upper extremity: what to do and when to do it. *J Bone Joint Surg Am*. 2009;91(5):1240-1252.
30. Lister G, Scheker L. Emergency free flaps to the upper extremity. *J Hand Surg Am*. 1988;13(1):22-28.
31. Nahai F, Silverton JS, Hill HL, Vasconez LO. The tensor fascia lata musculocutaneous flap. *Ann Plast Surg*. 1978;1(4):372-379.
32. Paletta CE, Freedman B, Shehadi SI. The VY tensor fasciae latae musculocutaneous flap. *Plast Reconstr Surg*. 1989;83(5):852-857; discussion 858.
33. Gosain AK, Yan JG, Aydin MA, Das DK, Sanger JR. The vascular supply of the extended tensor fasciae latae flap: how far can the skin paddle extend? *Plast Reconstr Surg*. 2002;110(7):1655-1661; discussion 1662-1663.
34. Windle BH, Stroup RT Jr, Beckenstein MS. The inferiorly based rectus abdominis island flap for the treatment of complex hip wounds. *Plast Reconstr Surg*. 1996;98(1):99-102.
35. Moran SL, Cooney WP. *Master Techniques in Orthopaedic Surgery: Soft Tissue Surgery*. Philadelphia, PA: Lippincott Williams & Wilkins; 2008.
36. Reath DB, Taylor JW. The segmental rectus abdominis free flap for ankle and foot reconstruction. *Plast Reconstr Surg*. 1991;88(5):824-828; discussion 829-830.
37. Musharafieh R, Macari G, Hayek S, Elhassan B, Atiyeh B. Rectus abdominis free-tissue transfer in lower extremity reconstruction: review of 40 cases. *J Reconstr Microsurg*. 2000;16(5):341-345.
38. Meland NB, Fisher J, Irons GB, Wood MB, Cooney WP. Experience with 80 rectus abdominis free-tissue transfers. *Plast Reconstr Surg*. 1989;83(3):481-487.

39. Taylor GI, Corlett R, Boyd JB. The extended deep inferior epigastric flap: a clinical technique. *Plast Reconstr Surg.* 1983;72(6):751-765.

40. Taylor GI, Corlett RJ, Boyd JB. The versatile deep inferior epigastric (inferior rectus abdominis) flap. *Br J Plast Surg.* 1984;37(3):330-350.

41. Liau JE, Pu LL. Reconstruction of a large upper tibial wound extending to the knee with a free latissimus dorsi flap: Optimizing the outcomes. *Microsurgery.* 2007;27(6):548-552.

42. Hong JP, Lee HB, Chung YK, Kim SW, Tark KC. Coverage of difficult wounds around the knee joint with prefabricated, distally based sartorius muscle flaps. *Ann Plast Surg.* 2003;50(5):484-490.

43. Fraccalvieri M, Bogetti P, Verna G, Carlucci S, Fava R, Bruschi S. Distally based fasciocutaneous sural flap for foot reconstruction: a retrospective review of 10 years experience. *Foot Ankle Int.* 2008;29(2):191-198.

44. Orr J, Kirk KL, Antunez V, Ficke J. Reverse sural artery flap for reconstruction of blast injuries of the foot and ankle. *Foot Ankle Int.* 2010;31(1):59-64.

45. Castro-Aragon OE, Rapley JH, Trevino SG. The use of a kickstand modification for the prevention of heel decubitus ulcers in trauma patients with lower extremity external fixation. *J Orthop Trauma.* 2009;23(2):145-147.

46. Berkowitz MJ, Kim DH. Using an external fixation "kickstand" to prevent soft-tissue complications and facilitate wound management in traumatized extremities. *Am J Orthop.* 2008;37(3):162-164.

47. Roukis TS, Landsman AS, Weinberg SA, Leone E. Use of a hybrid "kickstand" external fixator for pressure relief after soft-tissue reconstruction of heel defects. *J Foot Ankle Surg.* 2003;42(4):240-243.

48. Assal M, Blanck R, Smith DG. Extended posterior flap for transtibial amputation. *Orthopedics.* 2005;28(6):542-546.

49. Song YG, Chen GZ, Song YL. The free thigh flap: a new free flap concept based on the septocutaneous artery. *Br J Plast Surg.* 1984;37(2):149-159.

50. Hsu CC, Lin YT, Lin CH, Lin CH, Wei FC. Immediate emergency free anterolateral thigh flap transfer for the mutilated upper extremity. *Plast Reconstr Surg.* 2009;123(6):1739-1747.

51. Koshima I. Free anterolateral thigh flap for reconstruction of head and neck defects following cancer ablation. *Plast Reconstr Surg.* 2000;105(7):2358-2360.

52. Park JE, Rodriguez ED, Bluebond-Langer R, et al. The anterolateral thigh flap is highly effective for reconstruction of complex lower extremity trauma. *J Trauma.* 2007;62(1):162-165.

53. Manifold SG, Cushner FD, Craig-Scott S, Scott WN. Long-term results of total knee arthroplasty after the use of soft tissue expanders. *Clin Orthop Relat Res.* 2000;380:133-139.

54. Wieslander JB, Wendeberg B, Linge G, Buttazzoni G, Buttazzoni AM. Tissue expansion: a method to preserve bone length and joints following traumatic amputations of the leg—a follow-up of five legs amputated at different levels. *Plast Reconstr Surg.* 1996;97(5):1065-1071.

55. Pasyk KA, Austad ED, McClatchey KD, Cherry GW. Electron microscopic evaluation of guinea pig skin and soft tissues "expanded" with a self-inflating silicone implant. *Plast Reconstr Surg.* 1982;70(1):37-45.

56. Gold DA, Scott SC, Scott WN. Soft tissue expansion prior to arthroplasty in the multiply-operated knee. A new method of preventing catastrophic skin problems. *J Arthroplasty.* 1996;11(5):512-521.

57. Hanumadass M, Kagan R, Matsuda T. Early coverage of deep hand burns with groin flaps. *J Trauma.* 1987;27(2):109-114.

58. Lohman RF, Nabawi AS, Reece GP, Pollock RE, Evans GR. Soft tissue sarcoma of the upper extremity: a 5-year experience at two institutions emphasizing the role of soft tissue flap reconstruction. *Cancer.* 2002;94(8):2256-2264.

Chapter 26

COMPLEX FOOT AND ANKLE INJURIES

LTC Scott B. Shawen, MD; CPT Jonathan F. Dickens, MD;
CPT Kelly G. Kilcoyne, MD; and MAJ Benjamin K. Potter, MD

Ground-based blasts have proven common in the current conflicts in Iraq and Afghanistan, producing frequent injuries to the foot and ankle. Both the magnitude and severity of foot and ankle blast injuries are profound. Unlike civilian trauma correlates, battlefield foot and ankle injuries are characterized by an extremely high degree of kinetic energy, producing wide zones of bone and soft tissue injury. Irregularly shaped projectiles create atypical and severely comminuted fractures, often with segmental bone loss. Volumetric muscle and skin loss with damage to critical neurovascular structures further complicate wound management. Additionally, the "outside-in" mechanism of some combat wounds imparts considerable contamination from the projectiles, footwear, and surrounding environment. In addition, blunt force injury secondary to an explosion results as the floor of the vehicle impacts the foot and can cause severe open fracture/dislocation injuries of the forefoot, midfoot, and hindfoot. For these reasons, battlefield foot and ankle trauma is unique and highly variable. Although adherence to the principles outlined in this chapter may serve as a guide to patient management, the orthopedic treatment of foot and ankle blast injuries must proceed in an individually tailored and methodical manner to optimize outcomes.

Epidemiology

Since the onset of Operations Iraqi and Enduring Freedom (OIF/OEF), more than 34,000 US military personnel have sustained musculoskeletal injuries, and more than 16,000 casualties have been unable to return to duty. Of these, 53% of the combat injured have sustained a lower extremity injury. Reports on the characteristics of the combat injured indicate that a blast mechanism accounts for more than 71% of all extremity injuries, and 82% of these injuries are open fractures.[1-3]

Management in Theater

The initial assessment and management of lower extremity blast wounds begins at the forward echelons of care by orthopedic and trauma surgeons. The austere environment, limited resources, and rapidity of the evacuation process require intervention that is focused, methodical, and efficient. The cornerstones for management of severely combat-wounded extremities include early, aggressive wound debridement; hemorrhage control; provisional fracture stabilization; and compartment release, when appropriate.

Early intervention and surgical debridement is critical to preventing infection and stabilizing the combat casualty to prevent loss of life or limb(s). In the current conflicts, the evacuation time from the point of injury to initial surgical care is less than 1 hour in many cases. Unfortunately, this is not always the case, and evacuation may be substantially delayed because of environmental or combat conditions. In the civilian literature, it has traditionally been recommended that open fractures undergo operative assessment and debridement within 6 hours of injury.[4-6] More recent civilian studies have failed to find a significant difference in infection rates with open fractures treated within 6 hours and those treated after 6 hours of

Owens BD, Belmont PJ Jr, eds. *Combat Orthopedic Surgery:
Lessons Learned in Iraq and Afghanistan* (pp 269-282)
© 2011 SLACK Incorporated

injury, placing relatively greater emphasis on the early administration of systemic antibiotics.[7] There have been no studies to date assessing the outcomes of early versus delayed surgical intervention in the grossly contaminated combat casualty; however, we advocate surgical intervention at the earliest feasible time.

Blast injuries require an aggressive treatment approach particularly when the individual is in close proximity to the blast. Meticulous removal of all foreign material and devitalized tissue is integral in the effort to minimize the complications of severe open extremity trauma. Dysvascular, nonarticular bone should be removed. Viable fracture fragments and joints should be reduced and possibly pinned. Nonviable soft tissue should be sharply debrided to a healthy, clean, and bleeding base. Pulsatile lavage, when available, may be useful in the initial debridement procedures to remove large particulate debris and gross foreign material. However, we do not advocate repetitive use of pulsatile lavage during subsequent debridements or at higher echelons of care due to the proven detrimental effects of this irrigation modality on both local bacteria counts and host tissues.[8,9] There is no accepted irrigation volume that definitively decontaminates open wounds, although a large volume of at least 6 to 9 L of normal saline appears to generally provide acceptable dilution of wound contaminants.

Serial wound evaluation with repeat debridement and irrigation should continue every 24 to 72 hours to establish a clean and stable wound bed and prepare the local tissue for definitive management. Unlike lower energy civilian trauma, which requires fewer debridements to obtain a clean wound that is ready for definitive reconstruction, high-energy blast wounds are characterized by projectile penetration across tissue planes often extending beyond the surgeon's initial impression of the zone of injury. Consequently, serial debridements frequently demonstrate progressive soft tissue and bone devitalization with a dynamic wound evolution over a prolonged period. In our experience at Walter Reed Army Medical Center, we have found that even at late debridements beyond 120 hours from the injury, large foreign bodies or significant areas of wound necrosis may be discovered.

Negative pressure wound therapy (NPWT) with reticulated open cell foam (ROCF) has improved the management of severe open wounds, fasciotomies, and surgical incisions that are not amenable to primary closure. The reticulated foam dressing is applied directly to the wound and sealed from the outside environment. The advantages of NPWT include increased local blood flow, accelerated granulation tissue formation, decreased wound volume, and improved bacterial clearance.[10-14] Perhaps the greatest benefit of NPWT has been the decreased resources needed to care for the severe, open wound. Painful and labor intensive dressing changes are minimized, decreasing the workload of caretakers and improving patient comfort and satisfaction.

NPWT has thus been used as a frequent adjunctive treatment for the management of infected or contaminated open blast-related foot and ankle wounds. Controversy remains over the effectiveness of serial NPWT/ROCF in decreasing quantitative bacterial cell counts. Morykwas and colleagues[12] reported that in an animal model infected with *Staphylococcus aureus* and *Staphylococcus epidermidis*, bacterial levels remained below 10^5 organisms per gram of tissue.[11] The authors concluded that NPWT/ROCF created a conducive environment for wound healing. In contrast, Weed and colleagues,[15] in a retrospective review of 25 patients with acute and chronic wounds, found that NPWT/ROCF resulted in no change or an increase in bacterial bioburden with no effect on overall wound healing.[15] Regardless of the discrepency in bacterial bioburden in open wounds treated with NPWT/ROCF, this treatment appears to function as an effective bridge until definite wound closure can safely be obtained.

NPWT/ROCF is also useful in decreasing the wound size following a fasciotomy or blast-related soft tissue wound. The "shoelace" vessel loop technique is commonly performed by interlacing the elastic loops over the ROCF with staples placed at the skin margins (Figure 26-1). This quick and easy technique minimizes skin retraction, although frequently the vessel loops lack adequate tensile strength, and equal force distribution across the wound edges is not ensured.[16]

Despite the numerous advantages of NPWT, its benefits should not be overestimated. There is no substitute for an adequate surgical debridement of the wound. NPWT will not clean or debride the wound. Additionally, care must be taken to avoid application of the foam dressing directly over exposed neurovascular structures. Whenever possible, these vital structures should be covered directly with local soft tissue prior to the application of the foam dressing. Concurrently, deep wounds must be packed with foam to prevent the collapse of the wound and the creation of a dead space with negative pressure. After application, the system must be continuously monitored for failure. Loss of suction creates a closed system conducive to bacterial growth and potential local infection or systemic sepsis.

EARLY STABILIZATION

Expeditious stabilization of the blast-injured foot is integral in the treatment and evacuation of the forward-deployed combat casualty. Isolated injuries to the ankle and hindfoot may be provisionally stabilized with a well-padded splint while more involved

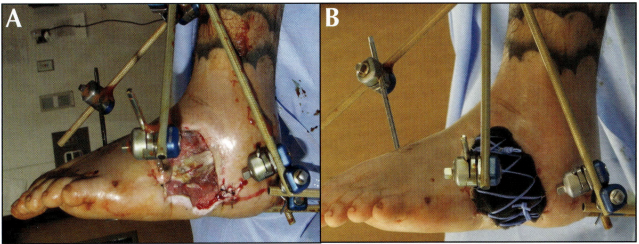

Figure 26-1. Left foot after blunt trauma and open hindfoot fracture dislocation. Fractures have been reduced and the extremity placed into a spanning external fixator (A). After irrigation and debridement of the open wound, the "shoelace" vessel loop technique is utilized over ROCF to minimize skin retraction (B).

injuries are best managed with temporizing external fixation and/or percutaneously placed pins. When the fracture pattern is amenable and circumstance permits, external fixation is the preferred method of provisional stabilization. Monoplanar external fixation provides secure fracture fixation and improved pain control and allows for continuous wound surveillance throughout the evacuation chain. Bridging external fixation for open, comminuted ankle and hindfoot fractures is well described while nonbridging external fixators may be used in cases of isolated midfoot and forefoot trauma. Additionally, external fixation allows for more predictable soft tissue salvage and reduces the risks associated with deep tissue and implant-related infections.

Several principles should be considered when the combat surgeon is applying an external fixator. First, consideration should be given to the injury and future surgical approaches that the definitive reconstructive team might use. The external fixator and pins should be placed away from future surgical approaches. Additionally, the pin sites and frame should be constructed in a manner that allows for continuous wound surveillance and intervention, patient transport, fracture stabilization, and assessment of fracture reduction. In short, provisional external fixation should be placed with the goals of maintaining limb mechanical alignment, joint reduction, and length with a neutral ankle and pins placed as far remote from subsequent fixation sites as practicable.

Injuries to the talus require special consideration and are particularly common secondary to the tremendous force imparted to the plantar foot, causing the talus to dislocate at the talonavicular joint and/or fracture at the neck and potentially dislocate through the calcaneus, plantarmedial skin, and soft

tissue. Reduction should be performed through the wound and fixed with K-wires. If the talonavicular joint is unstable, this should be pinned first with 1 or 2 K-wires, followed by reduction of the calcaneal tuberosity using threaded large-diameter 4- or 5-mm Steinman pins. Fixation of the talonavicular joint first controls the talus and provides a lever to assist with reduction of the calcaneus. Talar neck fractures should be pinned urgently to minimize avascular sequelae and assist with reduction of the talar body. Pinning of the subtalar joint with 2 or 3 K-wires through the posterior calcaneus helps to maintain the reduction. Other fractures and dislocations of the midfoot should be reduced and pinned with attention to minimizing soft tissue injury and violation during the reduction and fixation, maximizing the reconstructive options and operative approaches available during subsequent procedures.

Any patient with lower extremity trauma is at risk for developing heel pressure ulcers. Compromised tissue perfusion, traumatic or iatrogenic sensory deficits (traumatic nerve injury, regional or neuraxial anesthetic blocks), prolonged immobility, and lack of vigilance along the evacuation chain all contribute to the development of heel decubiti. Ultimately, these unnecessary wounds may cause serious dilemmas in the definitive treatment strategy. The early and liberal application of a "kickstand" is an effective means of unloading the heel and may be constructed in a timely and efficient manner (Figure 26-2).[17,18]

COMPARTMENT SYNDROME

The incidence of overt compartment syndrome in "at risk" limbs in evacuated combat casualties is estimated

Figure 26-2. Foot in spanning external fixator demonstrating a "kickstand" extended posteriorly to avoid any heel pressure and possible skin breakdown over the heel.

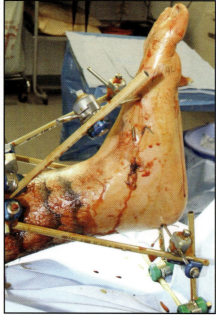

to be 15%.[19] Blast injuries, high-velocity gunshot wounds, blunt trauma, and any extremity with a field tourniquet in place are at risk for compartment syndrome. When left untreated, the complications of compartment syndrome are severe, and myoneural fibrosis, contractures, infection, amputation, and systemic complications may result. In the combat casualty, there should be a low threshold for performing fasciotomies when the clinical exam is suggestive of this diagnosis. Compartmental pressure measurements infrequently aid the treating surgeon and may not be available for use. Additionally, when evaluating an "at risk" limb, the possibility of injury progression during transport must be considered. Further evacuation in which surgical treatment options are limited should lead the surgeon toward performing prophylactic fasciotomies, even in the absence of abundant clinical signs.

Multiple approaches have been used to decompress the compartments of the foot including plantar, medial plantar, medial only, lateral, and dorsal approaches.[20] The choice of fasciotomy is governed by surgeon preference, other planned procedures, and pre-existing soft tissue injuries. We recommend release through either a 2-dorsal incision or single medial incision technique. The 2-incision dorsal approach centered above the second and fourth metatarsals is technically easier and may be more familiar to the combat orthopedic surgeon. When using this approach, the medial incision should be made medial to the second metatarsal and the lateral incision lateral to the fourth metatarsal in order to minimize skin-bridge necrosis and facilitate access to the interossei. The medial-only fasciotomy begins at the origin of the abductor

hallucis, 3 cm above the plantar surface and 4 cm from the posterior aspect of the heel, and is extended parallel to the plantar surface for approximately 6 cm.[21] Myerson and colleagues[22] in a cadaveric model reported that the 2-incision dorsal and medial-only approaches adequately decompressed the compartments, although the pressures more quickly normalized with the medial approach. Consideration should be made to perform a medial-only fasciotomy as this approach can adequately decompress all compartments while preserving the soft tissues of the foot for future calcaneus, midfoot, and forefoot reconstructive procedures.

Fasciotomy-related complications secondary to exposure of susceptible muscle and deep tissues commonly include infection, iatrogenic nerve injury, and soft tissue compromise. Additionally, fasciotomies may significantly jeopardize the already limited soft tissue envelope in the blast-injured foot, making definitive reconstruction difficult. When considering foot fasciotomies, the potential limb-saving benefit of fasciotomy must outweigh the potential infectious or soft tissue coverage complications. Combat surgeons, however, should not withhold fasciotomy when clinically indicated for fear that this procedure will adversely affect limb salvage. It has been the author's experience that even though fasciotomy wounds are frequently colonized, overt clinical signs of wound infection generally do not occur. Colonization, even when resulting in minor infection, can be managed successfully with local measures without adverse effects on the eventual outcome.

LIMB SALVAGE VERSUS AMPUTATION

The decision to proceed with limb salvage or amputation begins in the combat zone soon after the blast injury. Despite extensive research, there are no scoring systems that reliably and reproducibly predict the need for amputation. The most accepted indications for amputation include an overtly mangled extremity in a patient in extremis, completion of a blunt or grossly contaminated traumatic amputation, and a vascular injury that is either irreparable or for which the warm ischemia time has exceeded 6 hours.[23] Overt transection of the tibial nerve and ipsilateral severe open hindfoot and distal tibia trauma are relative indications. However, advancements in combat casualty care have made salvage of even the most severely mutilated extremities possible in many instances. Similar to civilian open extremity trauma, the military experience of blast-related lower extremity trauma has demonstrated that the ability to salvage the limb is primarily related to the extent of soft issue compromise as opposed to the extent of osseous injury.[24]

In the early post-blast period, the combat surgeon should pursue limb salvage as long as the patient's overall health is not compromised. Early limb salvage allows a multidisciplinary team of plastic, vascular, and trauma surgeons to evaluate the extent of injury at the definitive treatment facility. After serial wound evaluations, the reconstructive team is able to better characterize the wound and make well-informed treatment recommendations.[24] Additionally, forgoing amputation at the initial presentation affords the patient and family the opportunity to learn about the injury, treatments, and risks and benefits of limb salvage versus amputation. Patients will benefit in this period from peer counseling and support groups that may aid in increasing patient satisfaction while decreasing anxiety. Finally, if amputation is later elected or necessitated, initial preservation of the traumatized limb retains maximal soft tissue and bone for definitive treatment by the reconstructive team, thus potentially minimizing morbidity and salvaging residual limb length.[25]

Particular attention should be paid to the casualty with combined ipsilateral tibia and foot fractures as well as multilevel segmental fractures of the foot and ankle, as these patients have a higher risk of subsequent amputation due to failed limb salvage.[26-28] Patients with these ipsilateral and multilevel open fractures should be given special consideration for early amputation at the definitive treatment facility.[29]

Definitive Management

FOREFOOT INJURIES

Blast-related trauma to the forefoot includes injury to one or multiple toes, metatarsal fractures, and associated bone and/or distal soft tissue loss. If a fracture is not associated with a large soft tissue deficit or partial or complete amputation, it can often be treated with percutaneous retrograde pinning or internal fixation. Unfortunately, closed fractures without amputations are not as common in these high-energy injuries as partial or complete amputation and large bone deficits.

Amputations of the third and fourth toes are the most straightforward amputations to complete and may be easily treated with toe spacers and shoe fillers. These amputations are tolerated without the painful functional deficits that can complicate amputation of the first, second, and fifth toes. Amputation of the fifth toe requires removal of the lateral metatarsal condyle to appropriately taper the foot and prevent a painful lateral prominence. When amputating the second toe, the amputation should extend to the level of the proximal metaphysis (ray resection). Otherwise, a hallux valgus deformity can occur as a result of the loss of the lateral support of the great toe. The resulting gap that initially results between the first and third toes usually reapproximates on its own, and a hallux valgus deformity is avoided.[29]

Injury to the great toe may represent the most challenging of the forefoot injuries. The importance of the great toe is emphasized by its role in the push-off phase of the gait cycle. Strategies from the civilian literature to preserve the great toe include replacement of the associated bone loss with vascularized and nonvascularized bone grafts and fusion of the first metatarsophalangeal (MTP) joint.[30,31] Vascularized bone grafting from the supracondylar ridge of the distal femur may provide protection from infection due to the vascular nature of the graft while effectively incorporating into the local bone bed. Bone grafting following blast-related injuries is usually delayed approximately 6 weeks from the time of definitive soft tissue closure with interval placement of an antibiotic-impregnated polymethylmethacrylate (PMMA) spacer or antibiotic beads to decrease incidence of infection.[32] Fusion of the first MTP joint with concomitant structural bone loss has been successfully accomplished in civilian trauma centers with autograft bone block arthrodesis.[33] Myerson and colleagues reported 100% satisfactory outcomes in patients undergoing first MTP fusion with structural allograft bone block, although 3 of 24 required repeat arthrodesis.[30,34]

Metatarsal fractures without large soft tissue loss or severe comminution can be treated with percutaneous pin fixation or internal fixation. In situations of multiple metatarsal fractures, comminution, segmental fractures, or any combination thereof, external fixation is often the best treatment option. Metatarsal bone loss also presents challenges, with the column of involvement generally dictating the treatment. The lateral column is the more mobile column and can often be treated with a partial amputation and shoe filler. A partial amputation of the lateral column may allow soft tissue coverage elsewhere on the dorsum of the foot. The medial column is critical for ambulation and should be restored to length with autograft or allograft (Figure 26-3). Bone grafting may be structural or cancellous, but defects larger than 1 cm often necessitate structural grafting.[35] Vascularized grafts incorporate quickly and have a high remodeling potential; however, they are associated with significant donor site morbidity, prolonged operative times, and increased technical demands. Structural allografts have an unlimited supply and reduced donor site morbidity, but may be at risk for incomplete or slow incorporation.

Figure 26-3. Fragment injury to the left foot with open first metatarsal segmental fracture (A). After external fixation and bone grafting (B). After healing and external fixator removal (C).

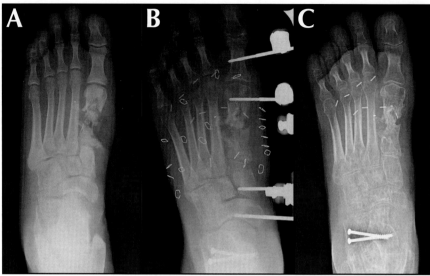

MIDFOOT INJURIES

The approach to midfoot reconstruction in the civilian setting hinges on the identification of the complete injury and obtaining an open reduction to restore normal anatomy. Residual metatarsal angulation and diastasis between the base of the first and second metatarsals of greater than 2 mm are factors associated with treatment failure.[36,37] Included in the critical concepts for the diagnosis and treatment of midfoot injuries are subsequent reconstructive options for the treatment of missed or chronic injuries. If a dislocation is not associated with a fracture, it can successfully be treated. Additionally, in the more acute injury, closed reduction and percutaneous screw fixation is often possible.[33] These options for delayed and/or percutaneous fixation are important to consider when dealing with an open or otherwise contaminated midfoot injury, as the soft tissue envelope may not permit early intervention.

The associated soft tissue injury and wound contamination associated with these war wounds and the need for staged management is outlined previously in the chapter. An additional challenge specific to the midfoot is fasciotomy incisions that are often present and must be accounted for when planning definitive soft tissue coverage and/or closure.

The use of ringed external fixators as the definitive fixation specifically for midfoot injuries has evolved with the experience of military orthopedic surgeons and offers several advantages over open reduction and internal fixation techniques.[32,38] The need for further insult to the often compromised soft tissues is minimized, and the need for internal hardware in contaminated wounds is obviated. Moreover, the extensive energy imparted by the blast frequently results in unreconstructable osseous comminution

of the articular surfaces. Additionally, patients can often bear weight and perform ankle range of motion during the consolidation phase of the ringed fixation (Figure 26-4).[38-40]

The ringed external fixator is created using multiple olive wires to initially realign the first ray with the medial column and subsequently sequentially building the midfoot reduction. The reconstruction aims to effect a near-anatomic alignment of the midfoot, restore the plantar weight-bearing forefoot cascade, and avoid further bone or soft tissue manipulation in the zone of injury. The fractures are then allowed to consolidate, and, if needed, selective bone grafting may be performed in a delayed fashion for painful nonunions.[32]

Significant shortening of the medial or, more commonly, the lateral column must be prevented. Ring external fixators or monolateral external fixators can also be used to restore length to the medial or lateral column if shortening is encountered in more proximal midfoot injuries (Figure 26-5). As seen with injuries to the great toe, antibiotic-impregnated PMMA spacers can be used in conjunction with delayed bone grafting to restore column length.

HINDFOOT INJURIES

Blast-related injuries to the calcaneus and talus are often accompanied by significant soft tissue loss as well as intra- and extra-articular bone loss. These are devastating injuries because the calcaneus and talus are critical for stance, gait, and hindfoot alignment. Calcaneus and talus fractures secondary to blasts are often associated with injury at a more proximal level in one or both extremities and frequently occur with associated nerve and vascular injury, making it difficult for the treating surgeon to decide if limb salvage

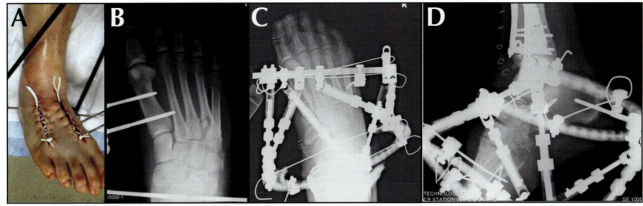

Figure 26-4. Blunt trauma causing tibial pilon fracture and midfoot fracture dislocation. (A) Foot fasciotomies performed in theater. (B) Radiograph demonstrating the midfoot fractures with lateral dislocation of the talar head through the fractured lateral navicular. (C) Placement of a mitre-type ringed external fixator, allowing reduction of the talar head utilizing an olive wire and re-establishing the length of the lateral column. (D) The external fixator does not cross the ankle joint, allowing immediate range of motion across the ankle.

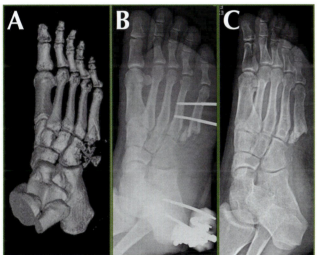

Figure 26-5. High-velocity gunshot wound to the lateral foot. (A) 3-D computed tomography reconstruction of the foot demonstrating loss of the 5th metatarsal base and a portion of the cuboid. (B) External fixation to maintain the length of the lateral column of the foot. (C) Final follow-up demonstrating maintenance of the lateral column length after healing.

or amputation is the best option for the patient. Severe open injuries of the hindfoot are also associated with high rates of late infection and subsequent amputation despite ostensibly successful initial limb salvage.

Calcaneal alignment, as one part of the foot tripod, is critical to maintain appropriate length, width, and height to allow for near-normal shoe wear and gait. Bone loss in the calcaneus and subtalar joint destruction as a result of high-energy open trauma are often accompanied by critical soft tissue loss. Soft tissue reconstructions for the lateral and posterior aspects of the calcaneus have been described with moderate success, but there are no reliable reconstruction options for wounds of the plantar fat pad.[41-43] Plantar soft tis-

sue wounds are known predictors of poor outcomes with associated open calcaneus fractures.[44,45] It is unclear whether soft tissue transfers in the presence of open calcaneus fractures may reproduce the function of the plantar fat pad, and amputation should be considered in these cases.

Closed calcaneus fractures do occur and may be treated in the standard fashion, although following combat-related trauma, these tend to fall on the severe end of the spectrum. A recent biomechanical study comparing percutaneous screw fixation versus lateral plating of Sanders type IIB fractures in cadavers demonstrated similar mean-to-load failure and construct stiffness.[46,47] More research is needed, but percutaneous screws for definitive fixation may be an attractive alternative to plating with the traditional lateral exposure, possibly leading to decreased infection rates. Similarly, techniques combining limited incision and percutaneous screw fixation for closed type II and III fractures have been described with decreased rates of infection and equivalent accuracy and maintenance of reduction.[47] Unfortunately, percutaneous screw fixation is often not an option for definitive fixation in the war-related calcaneus fracture as most of these fractures are open and severely comminuted.

The treatment of open calcaneus fractures is burdened with increased rates of infection and complications compared with closed fractures. Sanders reviewed 43 open calcaneus fractures with medial wounds and concluded that Gustilo type I and II fractures can be treated with open reduction and internal fixation with closure of the medial wounds. Based on their review, type II and III calcaneus fractures with wounds in different locations (other than medial) were associated with high rates of infection when treated acutely. The authors concluded that open type II and III fractures with lateral, dorsal, or plantar soft

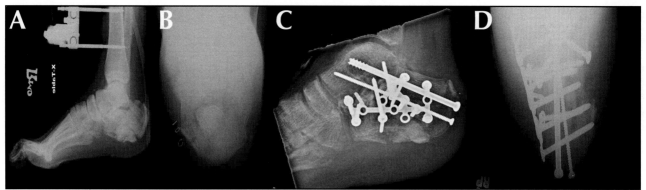

Figure 26-6. Blunt trauma resulting in open right calcaneus fracture. Injury films demonstrate a widely displaced fracture (A,B). Open reduction and primary subtalar arthrodesis with restoration of calcaneal pitch and alignment (C,D).

tissue injury should not be treated acutely as these are associated with unacceptably high rates of osteomyelitis and delayed amputation. The rate of infection of type III fractures in this study was 50%, with osteomyelitis occurring in 27%. The mainstay of initial treatment of all open calcaneus fractures, regardless of the grade, should consist of intravenous administration of antibiotics, serial irrigation and debridement, NPWT or other wound coverage, and initial temporary stabilization of the limb.[44] For blast-related calcaneus fractures, the aforementioned war-time treatment protocol is followed. Ring fixation alone or in conjunction with limited internal or percutaneous fixation is often the most effective temporizing treatment until delayed internal fixation, if elected, can be safely performed. A primary subtalar arthrodesis is performed if the amount of comminution or articular bone loss precludes a near-anatomic reconstruction of the subtalar joint (Figure 26-6).

Management of intra- and extra-articular bone loss in the calcaneus is determined by the extent of injury, presence of infection, and available soft tissue envelope. The use of bone graft substitutes, autograft and allograft, with or without the addition of local antibiotics may be combined with internal fixation to manage bone loss in the calcaneus.[34,35,43,48-50] Intra-articular bone loss of the calcaneus presents a more challenging treatment dilemma and frequently requires subtalar fusion. Augmenting the fusion with autograft or allograft may be necessary depending on the amount of bone loss and need to reconstruct the calcaneal height.[35,49] If autograft is chosen, the patient's ipsilateral proximal tibia is a safe and reliable source and offers decreased morbidity compared to the iliac crest.[51]

The talus plays a critical role in gait and stance and serves as the junction between the vertical and horizontal components of the lower extremity. Treatment of talar fractures is challenging largely as a result of its unique anatomy, including the large percentage of its surface area being covered in articular cartilage,

4 articulations, and retrograde blood flow. As seen in other areas with retrograde blood flow, avascular necrosis can complicate both open and closed injuries. Treatment of talus fractures is most often dictated by the location of fracture within the talus. Talar neck fractures without significant bone loss can be treated with staged internal fixation. These fractures tend to collapse into varus, which ultimately leads to a change in subtalar contact stresses, complicating outcomes.[52] Talar body fractures can be treated with internal fixation if the soft tissues are amenable. External fixation and percutaneous screws or pins can be used acutely or, if soft tissues allow, internal fixation can be performed (Figure 26-7).

The extruded talus presents a unique problem, and, regardless of mechanism, the appropriate treatment is difficult and controversial. There is no published literature on management of the extruded talus as a result of combat-related injury; however, a review of 27 patients with an extruded talus from a civilian trauma center touts the safety and versatility of reimplantation. Smith et al report no cases of late infection and only one case of acute infection that occurred after a tibiocalcaneal arthrodesis. They argued that reimplantation is not only safe, but it also restores the most normal joint mechanics, hindfoot height, and bone stock for future function and reconstructive procedures.[53] In contrast, Marsh's review of 12 complete and partial talar extrusions reported an infection rate of 38%.[54] Among the additional risks of implantation, the development of collapse and avascular necrosis may also be encountered. Following blast-related combat injury, talar extrusions often present in the setting of grossly contaminated wounds and only in the rare circumstance of a pristine-appearing wound should reimplantation be attempted. An alternative management strategy includes tibiocalcaneal fusion, although this frequently leaves a patient with a leg length discrepancy unless large bone grafts or delayed tibial bone transport are used.[55]

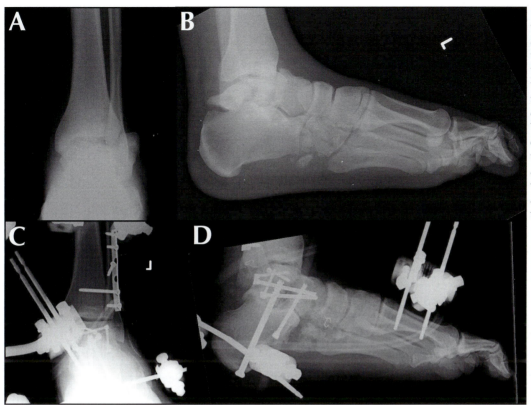

Figure 26-7. Blunt trauma resulting in a comminuted left talar body and neck fractures. (A,B) Injury films demonstrate the displaced nature of the fracture. (C,D) Through a fibular osteotomy, open reduction of the talar body and neck fractures with primary subtalar arthrodesis were performed.

ANKLE INJURIES

Rotational ankle injuries occur in the battlefield setting and may or may not be associated with a blast mechanism. Heavy loads carried by soldiers and frequent battlefield operations make rotational ankle injuries a common occurrence. Depending on the severity, this may necessitate splinting, external fixation if grossly unstable, and evacuation for further care. The majority of these injuries are closed and can be treated with open reduction and internal fixation as per standard, non-combat trauma.

Ankle injuries associated with a blast are more likely to be accompanied by soft tissue loss. These open injuries often require initial placement of a monoplanar external fixator for stability and soft tissue control. As seen with blast injuries in the foot, the extent of soft tissue destruction usually dictates the timing for definitive fixation. If soft tissue coverage can be readily accomplished with a flap or skin substitute, fractures are treated with delayed internal fixation. More commonly in the setting of delayed soft tissue coverage, the use of limited internal or percutaneous fixation, with or without spanning external fixation, is recommended for definitive treatment (Figure 26-8).

Treatment of high-energy tibial plafond, or pilon, fractures remains a challenge for the civilian and military orthopedic surgeon alike. High-energy pilon fractures are often accompanied by soft tissue disruption and fracture comminution as a result of axial load and shear forces. To combat the historically high infection rates associated with internal fixation of both closed and open pilon fractures, a staged treatment protocol was developed. In a retrospective review of 56 pilon fractures, 34 closed and 22 open, in a civilian trauma setting, Sanders and colleagues[52] concluded that when a staged protocol of initial restoration of fibular length with plating and tibial external fixation is followed, soft tissue stabilization is possible, decreasing infection rates. In their review, they found a 3.4% deep infection rate with closed pilon fractures and 10.5% with open pilon fractures.[56] The final stage of the protocol was anatomic reduction and internal fixation after soft tissue swelling decreased, which was performed an average of 14 days from external fixation. Similar to staging used in civilian trauma, a staged approach for treatment of blast-related pilon fractures is generally recommended. While the extent of soft tissue injury often precludes plate fixation of the fibula, limited internal fixation used in conjunction with circular external fixators and fine wires allows maintenance of subtalar motion and limits the need for further soft tissue disruption associated with early open reduction and internal fixation. Concurrent percutaneous or delayed minimal open reduction and internal fixation of the articular surface can then be performed as soft tissue status permits. At the time of this chapter, there are no published data on infection rates of pilon fractures from a blast mechanism.

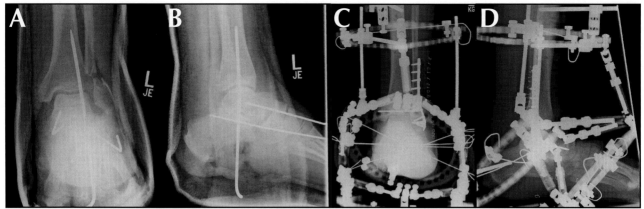

Figure 26-8. Left ankle fracture and dislocation from blunt trauma. Percutaneous fixation of the ankle maintaining the reduction (A,B). After open reduction of the fibula, external fixation was used to maintain reduction of the ankle. Hinges were used to allow motion across the joint while holding the reduction (C,D).

SOFT TISSUE COVERAGE AND WOUND MANAGEMENT

Even in areas with significant soft tissue coverage as part of the normal anatomy, coverage of bone, tendon, and neurovascular structures can be a challenge. These vital structures are particularly vulnerable in the foot and ankle with tenuous skin and only a thin layer of subcutaneous fat. Options for local coverage include flap coverage and skin substitutes.

Civilian literature assessing time to flap coverage found increased risk of infection and flap failure after 7 days from time of injury.[57,58] The unusual bacteria associated with blast injuries in the desert environment, time delays for evacuation and definitive care, and the extensive soft tissue loss associated with high-energy blasts have forced military surgeons to extend the time to soft tissue coverage. A review of 43 patients with lower extremity open fractures from blast injuries requiring flap coverage demonstrated good success despite increasing time to coverage. In his review, Kumar and colleagues show a 98% success rate, with 22% of flaps covering foot and ankle injuries, with a time to flap coverage from 7 to 82 days.[59] The most commonly used flap to the foot and ankle in this series was a free anterolateral thigh fasciocutaneous flap.[59]

Military surgeons have also successfully used skin substitutes for wound coverage in many areas including the foot and ankle. One series showed successful results, defined by achieving soft tissue coverage over exposed tendon and bone, in 83% of patients using Integra bilayer dermal regeneration dressing (Integra LifeSciences, Plainsboro, NJ).[60] The successful use of these skin substitutes obviates the need for more complex and invasive flap coverage. Split-thickness skin grafting is then performed 1 to 3 weeks later, after successful incorporation of the dermal analog.

BONE DEFECT MANAGEMENT

High-energy combat trauma imparts a significant force to the foot and ankle, frequently producing segmental bone defects that require carefully tailored treatment strategies. Bone defect management may commence after wound closure has been achieved and infection avoided. The surgeon must frequently span large unsupported bone defects while minimizing the risks of infection, thus making internal fixation implants less attractive initially.

Fixation may include traditional internal fixation, monoplanar external fixation, ring external fixation, or a combination thereof. As a general rule, more severe wounds with higher degrees of bone and articular cartilage damage are treated with spanning external fixation. Internal fixation is reserved for fracture fixation with a relatively uninjured soft tissue envelope that is healthy and able to be closed primarily. Limited internal fixation with bridging external fixation may add improved structural support and articular reconstruction while limiting soft tissue disruption and infection.

Bone defects are typically managed in a staged approach to avoid chronic infection and/or autograft loss. Initially, the defect may be filled with antibiotic-impregnated PMMA beads, typically consisting of heat-stable vancomycin and tobramycin mixed with cement.[61] Following initial wound healing without clinical, laboratory, or radiologic evidence of infection, bone grafting may commence. Autogenous bone grafting may be vascularized or nonvascularized. Vascularized autograft is more quickly and reliably incorporated with presumed decreased rates of infection; however, this comes at the expense of increased donor site morbidity in the already debilitated patient. Structural allograft bone is frequently used to fill defects owing to relatively abundant supply and lack of donor site morbidity. Bone graft substitutes such as rhBMP-2 (recombinant human bone morphogenetic protein, INFUSE; Medtronic Sofamor Danek, Memphis, TN) may be used in combination with allograft or autograft and supplemented with local antibiotic(s) to aid in bone regeneration. Metal cages with cancellous bone grafting[62] and the use of tantalum[63] have also been described for bone defect management, but the risk of deep infection in open, contaminated blast-related foot trauma is generally considered unacceptably high.

Complications

Functional impairment in the foot and ankle following a blast injury is determined by the degree of nerve, bone, and articular surface loss, as well as the magnitude of the soft tissue injury and subsequent sequelae. Importantly, the degree of soft tissue loss and residual function of the intrinsic and extrinsic foot and leg compartments contributes significantly to the patient's outcome.[64-66] Nonoperative modalities are employed first in an attempt to obtain and preserve joint mobility, increase strength, and provide a stable foot with corrective bracing and accommodative shoe wear. Persistent deformity and functional impairment may benefit from surgical intervention with the specific goals to relieve nerve compression, release contractures, stabilize joints, and provide a functional weight-bearing terminal extremity.

NERVE DEFICIT AND NEUROPATHIC PAIN

The evolution of military medical care to manage polytrauma combat casualties has been accompanied by advances in the diagnosis, management, and modulation of acute and chronic trauma-related pain. Pain management is initiated at the point of injury and aggressively managed throughout the continuum of care using a multimodal approach encompassing a wide range of procedures and medications. These include regional and neuraxial anesthesia with continuous epidural or peripheral nerve block infusions, judicious opioids, acetaminophen, anti-inflammatory agents, anticonvulsants, ketamine, clonidine, and antidepressants as options to treat pain at various sites of action. Ultimately, skilled pain management is integral in the prevention of neurogenic pain, which, if untreated, may evolve to a complex regional pain syndrome and may also contribute to the spectrum of post-traumatic stress disorder or lead to late amputation.[67]

The nerves of the foot and ankle function primarily to provide proprioception and protective sensation. In addition to providing sensation, the tibial nerve provides motor innervations to the majority of the intrinsic muscles of the foot, and the deep peroneal nerve innervates the extensor digitorum brevis and extensor hallucis brevis. Injury to the nerves of the foot and ankle are highly variable in the blast injury and are dependent on the type, location, and extent of injury as well as the function of the injured nerve. Isolated lacerations to the nerves of the foot and ankle are rare in typical blast injuries. The long-term morbidity of nerve injuries of the foot is generally related to damage to the sensory nerves. Injury to sensory nerves results in numbness, loss of protective sensation, neuroma formation, and in some cases complex regional pain syndrome type I (reflex sympathetic dystrophy) or type II (pain of neurogenic origin or causalgia). Damage to the motor branches of these nerves frequently results in an imbalance between the extrinsic and intrinsic musculature of the foot and the development of claw toes.

Nerve injuries to the foot should be treated with acute epineurial repair and primary wound closure when possible. In cases where surgical debridement is required, nerve repair adds little morbidity while decreasing the occurrence of painful neuromas and claw toes. Generally, lesions distal to the arch are not repaired due to their small size and minimal contribution to the sensation of the foot. In more proximal lesions, if the transected nerve ends cannot be identified or a tension-free repair is not possible, the proximal nerve stump is sharply transected and buried within the muscle to prevent symptoms from the resulting neuroma or delayed nerve grafting approximately 6 to 8 weeks after wound closure is performed. The treatment of painful neuromas begins with nonsurgical therapies including mechanical desensitization, transcutaneous electrical nerve stimulation (TENS), local corticosteroids, medications, and custom shoe wear to offload the neuroma. Diagnostic nerve blocks may be used to isolate the neuroma. If nonsurgical treatment fails, surgery to resect the neuroma and bury the proximal nerve within the muscle should be performed.[68,69]

Injury to the tibial nerve at the ankle may produce a sensory deficit to the entire plantar aspect of the foot and has been considered to be an indication for amputation in the civilian literature. In the setting of blast trauma with severe soft tissue injury, identification of the transected nerve may not be possible, and many patients will have a reversible defect due to neuropraxia or axonotmesis from the blast itself or surgical debridements. Improvement in protective sensation may be noted up to 2 years after injury, and some patients develop enough protective sensation to allow for a good functional outcome.[70] A period of watchful waiting may be especially important for patients with a presumed tibial nerve injury and a contralateral lower extremity amputation to prevent bilateral lower extremity amputations.

Transection of a tibial nerve that is not amenable to direct repair may be considered for cable grafting when the soft tissue envelope allows. Because the transected nerve in this setting lies within the primary zone of injury, nerve grafting in the acute period should be avoided as the injury to the truncated nerve ends is frequently underestimated. Over time, the initially apparent fascicular architecture of the nerve will be replaced by dense scar. At the time of delayed nerve grafting, the truncated nerve may be trimmed up to 1 cm to expose healthy nerve ends with normal-appearing fascicles. Several authors have reported favorable results with delayed nerve grafting with return of protective superficial sensation and resolution of neurogenic pain, but ultimate recovery may require up to 4 years.[71]

CHRONIC INFECTION

Deep wound infection and osteomyelitis are well-recognized complications in the treatment of combat-related extremity injuries. A recent review of infections in combat casualties demonstrated a rate of osteomyelitis between 2% and 15%, with lower extremity injuries twice as likely to develop infections as upper extremity trauma. *Acinetobacter baumanni-calcoaceticus* complex, *Klebsiella pneumoniae,* and *Pseudomonas aeruginosa* were more likely to be isolated at the initial presentation; however, gram-positive cocci such as *Staphylococcus aureus* are the most common isolate at the time of overt infection or late recurrence.[61,72] All open, blast-related fractures are considered colonized, and consequently routine collection of pre- or post-debridement cultures is not recommended. Differentiating between colonization and clinically significant infection should be based on the clinical scenario. Only cultures obtained because of concern for ongoing symptoms or wound infection, appearance of the wound, elevated inflammatory markers, or concerning radiographic findings (radiographs, computed tomography, magnetic resonance imaging, indium-111 labeled leukocyte scans, and positron emission tomography) should be used to make clinical decisions.

The management of the delayed deep wound infection begins with identification of the offending organism, followed by surgical debridement and parenteral antibiotics. Adjuvants such as antibiotic-impregnated cement beads or spacers may be used to increase the local delivery of antibiotic to the wound. Once the local infection has been successfully controlled via a combination of debridement and local and systemic antimicrobial therapy, reconstructive efforts may recommence.

POST-TRAUMATIC ARTHRITIS AND STIFFNESS

Loss of motion about the foot and ankle leads to increased contact stresses and altered kinematics of the foot and ankle, knee, and hip, thus predisposing the patient to post-traumatic arthritis at both local and remote joints. The patient should be counseled on the importance of preserving articular motion, and occupational therapy and physical therapy should be initiated as soon as feasible. In particular, equinus contractures, which may develop from prolonged external fixation and complicated lower extremity injuries, must be avoided. The foot is especially prone to edema, and this may also limit motion. The use of compression stockings following soft tissue stabilization may minimize the magnitude of this edema.

Despite appropriate early treatment, many of the severe foot and ankle injuries will result in post-traumatic arthritis or dysfunction secondary to loss of bone stock or articular cartilage. Arthrodesis remains the mainstay of treatment of end-stage arthritis by providing a stable, plantigrade, pain-free foot. Late osteotomies or joint fusions are accomplished in the standard manner; however, consideration should be given to the increased risks of latent infection, limitations of an impaired soft tissue envelope, and the problems inherent with significant bone loss. Compression fixation, when possible, is the treatment of choice. When significant bone defects are present, however, neutralization fixation may be necessary to prevent a secondary deformity that could result from impaction into a bone defect. Although the loss of a major motion segment in the ankle or hindfoot often leads to arthritis in surrounding joints, most patients have improvement in pain relief and function and are satisfied with their outcomes decades after fusion procedures.[73]

Conclusion

Combat-related trauma to the foot and ankle encompasses a large spectrum of injuries. Despite the variation in injury type and severity, the treating orthopedic surgeon should always approach each injury in a stepwise fashion. One should not become overwhelmed with the complexity of injuries in the combat wounded. Initial treatment of every open injury begins with aggressive wound irrigation and debridement, temporizing stabilization of fractures, and serial debridements and surveillance of soft tissues. Definitive fixation most often occurs in a delayed fashion after appropriate soft tissue healing or coverage at higher echelons of care. The treating orthopedic surgeon at every echelon of care must consider him- or herself a member of a larger team and consider the short- and long-term implications of each treatment decision. Although complications are frequent, remarkably good results can be achieved in many patients through diligent effort, careful attention to osseous reconstruction, and respect for the often compromised soft tissue envelope.

References

1. Covey DC. Blast and fragment injuries of the musculoskeletal system. *J Bone Joint Surg Am*. 2002;84-A(7):1221-1234.

2. Owens BD, Kragh JF Jr, Macaitis J, Svoboda SJ, Wenke JC. Characterization of extremity wounds in Operation Iraqi Freedom and Operation Enduring Freedom. [Report]. *J Orthop Trauma*. 2007;21(4):254-257.

3. Ritenour AE, Dorlac WC, Fang R, et al. Complications after fasciotomy revision and delayed compartment release in combat patients. *J Trauma*. 2008;64(2 Suppl):S153-S161.

4. Crowley DJ, Kanakaris NK, Giannoudis PV. Debridement and wound closure of open fractures: the impact of the time factor on infection rates. *Injury*. 2007;38(8):879-889.

5. Khatod M, Botte MJ, Hoyt DB, Meyer RS, Smith JM, Akeson WH. Outcomes in open tibia fractures: relationship between delay in treatment and infection. *J Trauma*. 2003;55(5):949-954.

6. Pollak AN, Jones AL, Castillo RC, Bosse MJ, MacKenzie EJ; LEAP Study Group. The relationship between time to surgical debridement and incidence of infection after open high-energy lower extremity trauma. *J Bone Joint Surg Am*. 2010;92(1):7-15.

7. Charalambous CP, Siddique I, Zenios M, et al. Early versus delayed surgical treatment of open tibial fractures: effect on the rates of infection and need of secondary surgical procedures to promote bone union. *Injury*. 2005;36(5):656-661.

8. Hassinger SM, Harding G, Wongworawat MD. High-pressure pulsatile lavage propagates bacteria into soft tissue. *Clin Orthop Relat Res*. 2005;439:27-31.

9. Owens BD, White DW, Wenke JC. Comparison of irrigation solutions and devices in a contaminated musculoskeletal wound survival model. *J Bone Joint Surg Am*. 2009;91(1):92-98.

10. Herscovici D Jr, Sanders RW, Scaduto JM, Infante A, DiPasquale T. Vacuum-assisted wound closure (VAC therapy) for the management of patients with high-energy soft tissue injuries. *J Orthop Trauma*. 2003;17(10):683-688.

11. Morykwas MJ, Argenta LC, Shelton-Brown EI, McGuirt W. Vacuum-assisted closure: a new method for wound control and treatment: animal studies and basic foundation. *Ann Plast Surg*. 1997;38(6):553-562.

12. Morykwas MJ, Simpson J, Punger K, Argenta A, Kremers L, Argenta J. Vacuum-assisted closure: state of basic research and physiologic foundation. *Plast Reconstr Surg*. 2006;117(7 Suppl):121S-126S.

13. Pollak AN. Use of negative pressure wound therapy with reticulated open cell foam for lower extremity trauma. *J Orthop Trauma*. 2008;22(10 Suppl):S142-S145.

14. Skagen K, Henriksen O. Changes in subcutaneous blood flow during locally applied negative pressure to the skin. *Acta Physiologica Scandinavica*. 1983;117(3):411-414.

15. Weed T, Ratliff C, Drake DB. Quantifying bacterial bioburden during negative pressure wound therapy: does the wound VAC enhance bacterial clearance? *Ann Plast Surg*. 2004;52(3):276-279.

16. Berman SS, Schilling JD, McIntyre KE, Hunter GC, Bernhard VM. Shoelace technique for delayed primary closure of fasciotomies. *Am J Surg*. 1994;167(4):435-436.

17. Berkowitz MJ, Kim DH. Using an external fixation "kickstand" to prevent soft-tissue complications and facilitate wound management in traumatized extremities. *Am J Orthop*. 2008;37(3):162-164.

18. Castro-Aragon OE, Rapley JH, Trevino SG. The use of a kickstand modification for the prevention of heel decubitus ulcers in trauma patients with lower extremity external fixation. *J Orthop Trauma*. 2009;23(2):145-147.

19. Bumbasirevic M, Lesic A, Mitkovic M, Bumbasirevic V. Treatment of blast injuries of the extremity. *J Am Acad Orthop Surg*. 2006;14(10 Spec No.):S77-S81.

20. Frink M, Zeckey C, Haasper C, Krettek C, Hildebrand F. [Injury severity and pattern at the scene: what is the influence of the mechanism of injury?]. *Unfallchirurg*. 2010;113(5):360-365.

21. Manoli A 2nd, Weber TG. Fasciotomy of the foot: an anatomical study with special reference to release of the calcaneal compartment. *Foot Ankle*. 1990;10(5):267-275.

22. Myerson MS. Experimental decompression of the fascial compartments of the foot—the basis for fasciotomy in acute compartment syndromes. *Foot Ankle*. 1988;8(6):308-314.

23. Dougherty PJ. Open tibia fracture: amputation versus limb salvage. Opinion: below-the-knee amputation. *J Orthop Trauma*. 2007;21(1):67-68.

24. Tintle SM, Keeling JJ, Shawen SB. Combat foot and ankle trauma. *J Surg Orthop Adv*. 2010;19(1):70-76.

25. Shawen SB, Keeling JJ, Branstetter J, Kirk KL, Ficke JR. The mangled foot and leg: salvage versus amputation. *Foot Ankle Clin*. 2010;15(1):63-75.

26. Lantry JM, Perumal V, Roberts CS. Can patterns of segmental injuries of the foot and ankle predict amputation and disability? *J Surg Orthop Adv*. 2009;18(3):134-138.

27. MacKenzie EJ, Bosse MJ. Factors influencing outcome following limb-threatening lower limb trauma: lessons learned from the Lower Extremity Assessment Project (LEAP). *J Am Acad Orthop Surg*. 2006;14(10 Spec No.):S205-S210.

28. MacKenzie EJ, Bosse MJ, Kellam JF, et al. Factors influencing the decision to amputate or reconstruct after high-energy lower extremity trauma. *J Trauma*. 2002;52(4):641-649.

29. Smith DG, Michael JW, Bowker JH, eds. *Atlas of Amputations and Limb Deficiencies: Surgical, Prosthetic, and Rehabilitation Principles*. 3rd ed. Rosemont, IL: American Academy of Orthopaedic Surgeons; 2004:xvii, 965.

30. Myerson MS, Schon LC, McGuigan FX, Oznur A. Result of arthrodesis of the hallux metatarsophalangeal joint using bone graft for restoration of length. *Foot Ankle Int*. 2000;21(4):297-306.

31. Nakamura K, Yokoyama K, Wakita R, Itoman M. Segmental bony defect of the proximal phalanx of the great toe reconstructed by free vascularized bone graft from the supracondylar region of the femur: a case report. *J Orthop Trauma*. 2007;21(7):499-502.

32. Keeling JJ, Beer R, Forsberg JA, Andersen RC, Mazurek MT, Shawen SB. Open midfoot blast trauma treated with ring external fixation: case report. *Foot Ankle Int*. 2009;30(3):262-267.

33. Brodsky JW, Baum BS, Pollo FE, Mehta H. Prospective gait analysis in patients with first metatarsophalangeal joint arthrodesis for hallux rigidus. *Foot Ankle Int*. 2007;28(2):162-165.

34. Myerson MS, Neufeld SK, Uribe J. Fresh-frozen structural allografts in the foot and ankle. *J Bone Joint Surg Am*. 2005;87(1):113-20.

35. Neufeld SK, Uribe J, Myerson MS. Use of structural allograft to compensate for bone loss in arthrodesis of the foot and ankle. *Foot Ankle Clin*. 2002;7(1):1-17.

36. Myerson MS. The diagnosis and treatment of injury to the tarso-metatarsal joint complex. *J Bone Joint Surg Br.* 1999;81(5):756-763.

37. Myerson MS, Fisher RT, Burgess AR, Kenzora JE. Fracture dislocations of the tarsometatarsal joints: end results correlated with pathology and treatment. *Foot Ankle.* 1986;6(5):225-242.

38. Keeling JJ, Gwinn DE, Tintle SM, Andersen RC, McGuigan FX. Short-term outcomes of severe open wartime tibial fractures treated with ring external fixation. *J Bone Joint Surg Am.* 2008;90(12):2643-2651.

39. Lerner A, Fodor L, Soudry M. Is staged external fixation a valuable strategy for war injuries to the limbs? *Clin Orthop Relat Res.* 2006;448:217-224.

40. McGuigan FX, Forsberg JA, Andersen RC. Foot and ankle reconstruction after blast injuries. *Foot Ankle Clin.* 2006;11(1):165-182.

41. Peek A, Giessler GA. Functional total and subtotal heel reconstruction with free composite osteofasciocutaneous groin flaps of the deep circumflex iliac vessels. *Ann Plast Surg.* 2006;56(6):628-634.

42. Wei FC, Chen HC, Chuang CC, Noordhoff MS. Reconstruction of Achilles tendon and calcaneus defects with skin-aponeurosis-bone composite free tissue from the groin region. *Plast Reconstr Surg.* 1988;81(4):579-589.

43. Yazar S, Lin CH, Wei FC. One-stage reconstruction of composite bone and soft-tissue defects in traumatic lower extremities. *Plast Reconstr Surg.* 2004;114(6):1457-1466.

44. Heier KA, Infante AF, Walling AK, Sanders RW. Open fractures of the calcaneus: soft-tissue injury determines outcome. *J Bone Joint Surg Am.* 2003;85-A(12):2276-2282.

45. Ikuta Y, Murakami T, Yoshioka K, Tsuge K. Reconstruction of the heel pad by flexor digitorum brevis musculocutaneous flap transfer. *Plast Reconstr Surg.* 1984;74(1):86-96.

46. Smerek JP, Kadakia A, Belkoff SM, Knight TA, Myerson MS, Jeng CL. Percutaneous screw configuration versus perimeter plating of calcaneus fractures: a cadaver study. *Foot Ankle Int.* 2008;29(9):931-935.

47. Weber M, Lehmann O, Sagesser D, Krause F. Limited open reduction and internal fixation of displaced intra-articular fractures of the calcaneum. *J Bone Joint Surg Br.* 2008;90(12):1608-1616.

48. Kelly CM, Wilkins RM, Gitelis S, Hartjen C, Watson JT, Kim PT. The use of a surgical grade calcium sulfate as a bone graft substitute: results of a multicenter trial. *Clin Orthop Relat Res.* 2001;382:42-50.

49. Scranton PE Jr. Use of bone graft substitutes in lower extremity reconstructive surgery. *Foot Ankle Int.* 2002;23(8):689-692.

50. Thornton SJ, Cheleuitte D, Ptaszek AJ, Early JS. Treatment of open intra-articular calcaneal fractures: evaluation of a treatment protocol based on wound location and size. *Foot Ankle Int.* 2006;27(5):317-323.

51. Geideman W, Early JS, Brodsky J. Clinical results of harvesting autogenous cancellous graft from the ipsilateral proximal tibia for use in foot and ankle surgery. *Foot Ankle Int.* 2004;25(7):451-455.

52. Sanders DW, Busam M, Hattwick E, Edwards JR, McAndrew MP, Johnson KD. Functional outcomes following displaced talar neck fractures. *J Orthop Trauma.* 2004;18(5):265-270.

53. Smith CS, Nork SE, Sangeorzan BJ. The extruded talus: results of reimplantation. *J Bone Joint Surg Am.* 2006;88(11):2418-2424.

54. Marsh JL, Saltzman CL, Iverson M, Shapiro DS. Major open injuries of the talus. *J Orthop Trauma.* 1995;9(5):371-376.

55. Dennison MG, Pool RD, Simonis RB, Singh BS. Tibiocalcaneal fusion for avascular necrosis of the talus. *J Bone Joint Surg Br.* 2001;83(2):199-203.

56. Sirkin M, Sanders R, DiPasquale T, Hersovici D Jr. A staged protocol for soft tissue management in the treatment of complex pilon fractures. *J Orthop Trauma.* 2004;18(8 Suppl):S32-S38.

57. Byrd HS, Spicer TE, Cierney G 3rd. Management of open tibial fractures. *Plast Reconstr Surg.* 1985;76(5):719-730.

58. Godina M. Early microsurgical reconstruction of complex trauma of the extremities. *Plast Reconstr Surg.* 1986;78(3):285-292.

59. Kumar AR, Grewal NS, Chung TL, Bradley JP. Lessons from operation Iraqi freedom: successful subacute reconstruction of complex lower extremity battle injuries. *Plast Reconstr Surg.* 2009;123(1):218-229.

60. Helgeson MD, Potter BK, Evans KN, Shawen SB. Bioartificial dermal substitute: a preliminary report on its use for the management of complex combat-related soft tissue wounds. *J Orthop Trauma.* 2007;21(6):394-399.

61. Murray CK, Hsu JR, Solomkin JS, et al. Prevention and management of infections associated with combat-related extremity injuries. *J Trauma.* 2008;64(3 Suppl):S239-S251.

62. Clements JR, Carpenter BB, Pourciau JK. Treating segmental bone defects: a new technique. *J Foot Ankle Surg.* 2008;47(4):350-356.

63. Bouchard M, Barker LG, Claridge RJ. Technique tip: tantalum: a structural bone graft option for foot and ankle surgery. *Foot Ankle Int.* 2004;25(1):39-42.

64. Botte MJ, Santi MD, Prestianni CA, Abrams RA. Ischemic contracture of the foot and ankle: principles of management and prevention. *Orthopedics.* 1996;19(3):235-244.

65. Brey JM, Castro MD. Salvage of compartment syndrome of the leg and foot. *Foot Ankle Clin.* 2008;13(4):767-772.

66. Perry MD, Manoli A 2nd. Reconstruction of the foot after leg or foot compartment syndrome. *Foot Ankle Clin.* 2006;11(1):191-201.

67. Malchow RJ, Black IH. The evolution of pain management in the critically ill trauma patient: emerging concepts from the global war on terrorism. *Crit Care Med.* 2008;36(7 Suppl):S346-S357.

68. Glazebrook MA, Paletz JL. Treatment of posttraumatic injuries to the nerves in the foot and ankle. *Foot Ankle Clin.* 2006;11(1):183-190.

69. Thordarson DB, Shean CJ. Nerve and tendon lacerations about the foot and ankle. *J Am Acad Orthop Surg.* 2005;13(3):186-196.

70. McGuigan FX, Forsberg JA, Andersen RC. Foot and ankle reconstruction after blast injuries. *Foot Ankle Clin.* 2006;11(1):165-182.

71. Nunley JA, Gabel GT. Tibial nerve grafting for restoration of plantar sensation. *Foot Ankle.* 1993;14(9):489-492.

72. Valenziano CP, Chattar-Cora D, O'Neill A, Hubli EH, Cudjoe EA. Efficacy of primary wound cultures in long bone open extremity fractures: are they of any value? *Arch Orthop Trauma Surg.* 2002;122(5):259-261.

73. Thordarson DB. Fusion in posttraumatic foot and ankle reconstruction. *J Am Acad Orthop Surg.* 2004;12(5):322-333.

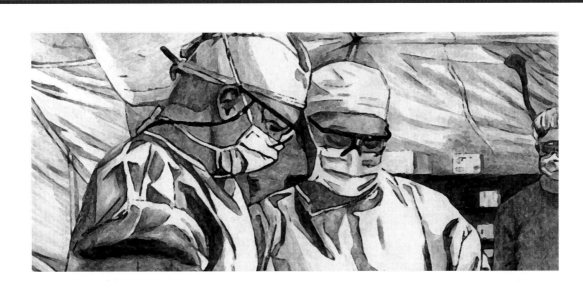

SECTION V
SPINE/PELVIS

COMBAT INJURIES TO THE PELVIS AND ACETABULUM

LtCol Wade Gordon, MD; CPT Matthew Kluk, MD; CDR Joseph E. Strauss, DO; and LTC(P) Romney C. Andersen, MD

The Global War on Terrorism has resulted in severe, high-energy injuries in military servicemembers not routinely seen in civilian practice.[1] Because of improved body armor and an efficient medical evacuation system, many servicemembers are surviving with severe musculoskeletal injuries that would have proven fatal in prior conflicts.[2] Many of these injuries involve the lumbar spine and pelvic girdle.

When a blunt mechanism of injury is responsible, these combat-related pelvic injuries are generally similar to those seen in civilian trauma. There are, however, a significant number of open blast injuries to the pelvic girdle, which are unique to combat. Both blast injuries and high-velocity military gunshots impart significantly more contamination compared to open pelvic fractures typically seen in a civilian setting, and this contamination often penetrates deep into the tissues of the pelvis. Similar to civilian pelvic and acetabular fractures, combat injuries to the pelvis typically occur in the setting of polytrauma, with other associated injuries.[3,4] Additionally, with blast mechanisms of injury, the complexity of these injuries is increased by a high incidence of concomitant open abdominal and vascular injuries, as well as extensive osseous destruction and soft tissue wounds.

In the combat environment, medical care is provided in increasingly capable echelons of care. This starts with the medics providing first aid at the point of injury, and the patient is then stepwise transferred through the medical evacuation system, culminating in definitive management in the United States.[5]

Epidemiology

The Joint Theater Trauma Registry provides us with the best estimates of pelvic and acetabular fractures sustained in casualties of Operation Iraqi Freedom and Operation Enduring Freedom. The exact incidence is difficult to determine, as some percentage of battlefield deaths certainly include fractures to the pelvis as part of the fatal injury pattern. As of May 2009, there have been 271 pelvic ring fractures, and 146 of these were open fractures (54%). There have also been 108 acetabular fractures, of which 34 (31%) were open injuries.[6] This percentage of open fractures is not seen in civilian trauma, where the rate of open pelvis fractures has been documented as 4%.[7,8]

Management in Theater

The initial evaluation and management of the patient is subject to the limitations of the fluid and relatively austere combat environment, but the same Advanced Trauma Life Support (ATLS) principles apply as in civilian practice.[9] Patients are stabilized and resuscitated to the extent possible in the field, where a sheet may be applied.[10,11] They are then evacuated to forward surgical teams (Echelon II) or combat support hospitals (Echelon III) where the first surgical capability is provided to the patient. Pelvic binders will typically not be available until arrival at an Echelon III facility, where external fixation also becomes available. For this reason, their use is often

Owens BD, Belmont PJ Jr, eds. *Combat Orthopedic Surgery:*
Lessons Learned in Iraq and Afghanistan (pp 285-296)
© 2011 SLACK Incorporated

limited to temporizing in situations within those facilities when a surgical delay is inevitable.

Once patients reach the combat support hospital, injuries are systematically evaluated. Wounds are inspected, a musculoskeletal physical examination is conducted to assess for neurovascular status, radiographs are taken to assess for fractures, and tourniquets are taken down if possible. Trauma resuscitation protocols are continued, and external fixation may be applied to the unstable pelvis; open wounds are addressed, and damage control intervention for vascular, abdominal, or concomitant musculoskeletal injuries can be performed. This includes diverting colostomy in the case of pelvic fractures with associated hollow visceral injuries.[12,13]

Unstable injuries to the pelvic ring are typically treated with some form of pelvic binder prior to arrival at an echelon of care where surgical management of the fracture is possible.[7,8] At that point, an external fixator will be placed, using either supra-acetabular or iliac wing half-pins for fixation. In the austere combat environment, there are often significant limitations of equipment (absence of power drills), operative time, and fluoroscopy, as well as surgeon comfort level with pelvis external fixator placement.

It is therefore advisable, in this setting, to insert iliac wing pins for initial placement of the resuscitation frame. When necessary, this can be done via open technique, under direct visualization without fluoroscopy, and is much less technically demanding than placement of supra-acetabular pins. Two or 3 pins are placed, depending on the perceived quality of purchase in the bone. The pins are then connected to the external fixator bar construct, either by individual pin-to-bar clamps or with multiple pin clamps, subsequently attached to the construct with outriggers. Stacked bars brought in a V-shape distally over the symphysis are typically placed, all clamps are tightened after a reduction maneuver has been performed, and reduction is verified by fluoroscopy when available.

This construct allows for safe transport of the patient to higher echelons of care[14] and allows access to the abdomen for potential laparotomy. It does, however, make it difficult for the patient to sit up in bed. In the obese patient, or the patient with a distended abdomen, a third transverse bar may be added to clear the abdomen. If external fixation becomes the patient's definitive fixation, it should be revised to a "sport frame," with supra-acetabular pins, a construct that facilitates sitting and mobilization. Sport frames consist of a single Schantz pin placed in each hemipelvis. Each pin is placed at the anterior inferior iliac spine and directed toward the subchondral bone at the greater sciatic notch.

The most severely injured patients will arrive in the United States within 4 to 5 days after injury, and

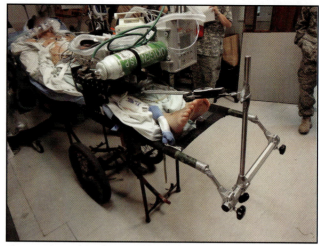

Figure 27-1. This photograph depicts a typical distal femoral traction set up for aeromedical evacuation. The weight is set with a pulley system that does not require free weights to assist in ease of transport.

definitive management is normally delayed until this point. Unstable acetabular fractures in which the femoral head is in contact with the acetabulum should be placed into skeletal traction initially with approximately 15% of the patient's body weight. This will minimize the amount of cartilage damage incurred by the contact pressure between the femoral head and acetabulum. While possible, maintaining skeletal traction throughout the medical evacuation system is difficult (Figure 27-1). Alternatively, closed reduction and external fixation spanning the hip joint can be performed. Routine broad-spectrum prophylactic antibiotics are administered,[15] and serial irrigation and debridement procedures are performed as the patient moves through the medical evacuation system. Once sufficiently stable to tolerate a prolonged flight, the patient is evacuated through Landstuhl Medical Center in Germany (Echelon IV) to an Echelon V facility at one of the major US military hospitals. Definitive management, including internal fixation of pelvic and acetabular fractures, is delayed until arrival at one of these medical centers, where polytraumatized patients can be cared for by a multidisciplinary team of general, orthopedic, vascular, and urologic surgeons, as well as intensive care providers.[1,5]

Definitive Management

INDICATIONS AND CONTRAINDICATIONS

The indications for surgical fracture management are similar to that seen in the civilian setting, with added consideration given to the nature of any soft tissue injuries. The bulk of these combat pelvis and acetabular fractures are the result of blast injuries or other penetrating trauma. Even blunt injuries to the pelvic girdle are frequently associated with open abdominal or extremity wounds of variable degrees of severity and contamination with foreign material. With a clean soft tissue envelope, standard fixation techniques of plating and screw fixation can be used.[16]

Contraindications include deep infection, which is a severe clinical problem in the management of combat pelvic and acetabular fractures. In many cases, the pelvis is contaminated with foreign material and bowel contents. Otherwise, operative pelvis and acetabular fractures may be definitively managed with external fixation or nonoperatively if the wound is not amenable despite appropriate management.[17,18]

Soft Tissue Management

Up to 54% percent of combat injuries to the pelvis and acetabulum are open injuries, compared to 4% in the setting of civilian trauma.[7,8] It is the nature of these wounds that dictates the management of the osseous injury in many cases. Even in combat-related fractures of the pelvis and acetabulum that are closed, there are often associated severe, open extremity and abdominal wounds. There is frequently a large burden of foreign body contamination, bowel contamination, volumetric muscle loss, bone loss, and neurovascular injury.

Open wounds are serially debrided throughout the medical evacuation process and are routinely debrided every 48 to 72 hours until the wounds are clean. In cases of severe contamination, the wounds may be debrided daily until stable. Open soft tissue wounds, as well as open abdominal injuries, are usually covered with a negative pressure wound therapy dressing. The use of the vacuum-assisted closure dressing was shown to be safe and effective for use in open pelvic fractures in the civilian setting,[19] as well as for transport of combat casualties. Negative pressure wound therapy dressings afford protection of the wound from environmental factors as well as assist with nursing care as the patient proceeds through the evacuation system.[20,21] Antibiotic-impregnated cement beads can also be used for both dead-space management and local delivery of broad-spectrum antibiotics.[9]

In many cases of combat pelvic and acetabular trauma, the location and severity of open wounds about the pelvic girdle dictate the surgical approach to the fracture. In these cases, the most appropriate surgical approach for management of the fracture may be prohibited. Alternate, less desirable surgical approaches may then be used, external fixation can be used as definitive management, or surgical management may be deferred altogether.

Surgical Technique

Combat Injuries to the Pelvic Ring

The principles for management of combat-related injuries to the pelvic ring are not significantly different from those of civilian injuries. The primary differences are related to the timing of definitive fixation, strategies to manage associated soft tissue wounds, the risk for deep infection, and certain specific technical considerations.

As in civilian pelvis fractures, the strategy for definitive management is based on fracture stability.[22] Traditionally, open pelvic fractures have been treated entirely with external fixation.[13,14] However, Leenen and colleagues reported on the successful treatment of open pelvic fractures with internal fixation after appropriate soft tissue management.[23]

Rotationally unstable fractures (Tile B) are treated with reduction of the symphysis pubis and anterior plating, provided the soft tissues are amenable. If open pelvic or abdominal wounds preclude the ability to safely place implants, anterior external fixation should be used to provide definitive fixation. In these cases, the patient is routinely transitioned to a sport frame to facilitate sitting and rehabilitation over a long course of external fixation. Open combat pelvic fractures that are rotationally and vertically unstable (Tile C) and associated with gluteal or buttock open wounds are particularly challenging. In these patients, the need for posterior stabilization exists despite the suboptimal soft tissue envelope, and the posterior injury is often treated with sacroiliac screws. In cases of severe wound contamination, the posterior pelvic ring is treated nonoperatively after it is reduced and alignment maintained as sufficiently as possible with an anterior external fixator.

In select cases where anterior pelvic fixation is required but the patient's wounds are not amenable to internal fixation, the use of a "subcutaneous external fixator" is appropriate. This technique is particularly helpful when anterior soft tissues preclude definitive internal fixation and there are significant buttock or posterior thigh wounds that require multiple episodes of prone positioning for surgery.

In this technique, top-loading spinal instrumentation is employed, and 2 long pedicle screws are placed percutaneously in the supra-acetabular bone, in the same position as in a sport frame. A curved bar is then tunneled subcutaneously, and top-loading set screws are then used to stabilize the construct after reduction of the pelvic ring has been achieved.

The surgical management of displaced and unstable pelvic ring injuries can also be challenging in patients with lower extremity amputations. In these patients, the reduction of the posteriorly displaced hemi-pelvis

Figure 27-2. (A) Inlet view showing 2 cm of diastasis at the right sacroiliac (SI) joint as well as a comminuted right superior and inferior pubic rami fracture and SI diastasis. There is no gross displacement of the SI joint in the anteroposterior plane. (B) Outlet view showing 2 cm of diastasis at the right SI joint with 1 cm of vertical displacement of the right sacral ala and a comminuted superior and inferior pubic rami fracture. (C) Computed tomography (CT) showing pubic diastasis and a right superior pubic rami fracture. (D) CT cut showing right SI diastasis with a left-sided zone II sacral fracture.

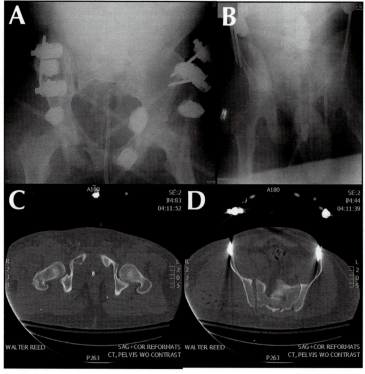

can be very difficult with a very short residual limb through which to impart a reduction force via skeletal or manual traction. Additionally, volumetric muscle loss as well as segmental nerve injuries and vascular injuries represent unique problems in the management of blast injuries to the pelvic ring. Often, split-thickness skin grafting is required, and in rare instances, free tissue transfer can be effective in achieving soft tissue coverage.[24,25]

CASE 1

The patient is a 23-year-old male servicemember who sustained a blast injury and was partially ejected from his vehicle. The patient was initially evaluated at an Echelon III facility and was found to be hemodynamically unstable. He was resuscitated, had an external fixator placed for an unstable pelvic ring injury, and underwent exploratory laparotomy for abdominal compartment syndrome. He was transferred to Landstuhl Regional Medical Center, where his right gluteal open wounds were debrided and a diverting colostomy was performed.

The patient arrived at Walter Reed Army Medical Center (WRAMC) 4 days after his injury. Initial radiographs revealed a left zone III sacral fracture, right sacroiliac joint diastasis, and a comminuted fracture of the right pubic rami (Figure 27-2). He underwent serial irrigation and debridement procedures for both his open abdominal and gluteal wounds. Wound cultures from the irrigation and debridement procedures were positive for *Escherichia coli* as well as methicillin-resistant *Staphylococcus aureus* (MRSA).

Seven days after injury, bilateral sacroiliac screws were placed, and an external fixator was used to definitively treat his open combat pelvic ring injury (Figure 27-3). The external fixator was removed 3 months after injury, and the open gluteal wound was ultimately covered with split-thickness skin grafting. His postoperative course was complicated by a deep wound infection, which was treated with irrigation, debridement, and systemic antibiotics. Sacroiliac screw removal was delayed and was performed after fracture union was achieved. The patient also developed significant, painful heterotopic ossification limiting motion in his right hip, which was excised 7 months after injury. One year after injury, the patient subsequently fell out of his wheelchair, sustaining a minimally displaced right femoral neck fracture. This was treated by internal fixation with cannulated screws. The patient did well postoperatively, but developed a recurrence of the heterotopic ossification about his right hip (Figure 27-4).

CASE 2

The patient is a 28-year-old male servicemember who sustained a blast injury while on foot, and had multiple other injuries. His injuries included a splenic rupture, a proximal left transfemoral amputation, and right transfemoral amputation. He also sustained an APC II pelvis injury with a pubic diastasis of 38 mm

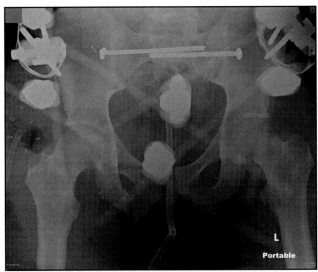

Figure 27-3. Postoperative films showing near anatomic reduction of the right sacroiliac joint using a partially threaded cannulated screw and fixation of the left-sided sacral fracture using a fully threaded cannulated screw. The patient was maintained in his original external fixator.

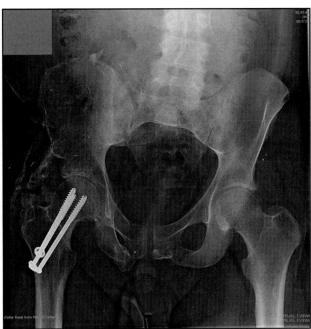

Figure 27-4. Postoperative films after the patient sustained a right femoral neck fracture treated with 3 cannulated screws. The patient had recurrence of significant heterotopic ossification about his right hip.

and severe soft tissue injuries to the buttocks, which extended to the sacrum and were confluent with a rectal injury. At an Echelon III facility, he was treated with irrigation and debridement of his multiple open wounds, as well as laparotomy, with fecal diversion, and splenectomy.

The patient arrived at WRAMC 5 days after injury and underwent serial debridement of his wounds and ultimate delayed primary closure of his bilateral lower extremity amputations. Secondary to the severity of his open wounds and the high risk of infection, definitive internal fixation was determined not to be safe. The patient's posterior soft tissue injuries also required serial debridements in the prone position, making external fixation less desirable as definitive management.

A subcutaneous external fixator was placed percutaneously using top-loading spinal instrumentation, maintaining the reduction of the pelvic ring and simplifying positioning for multiple procedures in the prone position (Figure 27-5). The external fixator was removed 3 months postoperatively.

Combat Injuries to the Acetabulum

Acetabular fractures caused by blast injuries or other penetrating combat trauma are quite different from those seen in civilian practice. Combat acetabular fractures tend to be difficult to classify and often have unusual fracture morphology. Combat acetabular frac-

tures may be associated with large soft tissue wounds, vascular injuries, and a high degree of foreign contamination. There are limited data in the literature on the management of open acetabular fractures. Overall, recently published infection rates with internal fixation of all acetabular fractures is 5% to 12%.[26,27] In open, combat-related acetabular fractures, the soft tissues are managed in a similar fashion to that discussed earlier for open pelvic ring injuries.

The condition of the soft tissues, particularly the presence of large soft tissue defects, often dictates fracture management. This is true with respect to timing of surgery, surgical approach, and in some cases can prohibit the surgical stabilization of the osseous injury altogether. Time and multiple debridement procedures are often necessary to achieve a clean and stable soft tissue envelope prior to the placement of internal fixation implants.[9] Otherwise, the standard principles of fracture exposure coupled with reduction and fixation using meticulous soft tissue handling are employed.

CASE 3

The patient is a 23-year-old male servicemember who sustained an open, comminuted both column acetabular fracture from small arms fire. He was hemodynamically unstable at initial presentation in theater and required a large volume of blood products during resuscitation. His internal iliac artery

Figure 27-5. (A) Preoperative anteroposterior pelvis film with 3 cm of diastasis of the pubic symphasis and a widened right SI joint. (B) Clinical photograph of the subcutaneous external fixator being placed. The 2 posts are pedicle screws, which were placed superior to the patient's acetabulum bilaterally in the same fashion that SPORT frame pins are placed. The rod was passed subcutaneously. (C) Postoperative inlet showing 2 cm of residual diastasis at the pubic symphasis and a reduced pelvic ring. (D) Postoperative outlet showing 2 cm of residual diastasis and no vertical displacement of the bony pelvis.

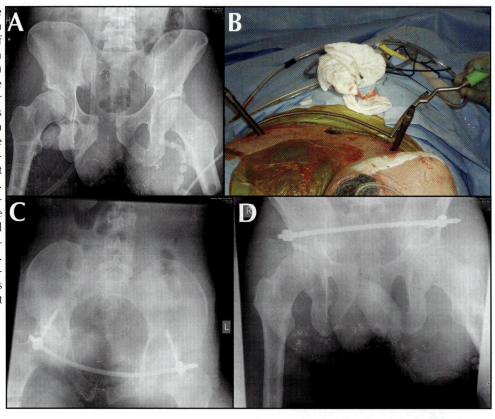

at the time was ligated as a life-saving measure. The patient arrived at WRAMC 4 days after injury. His initial films revealed a comminuted iliac wing and both column acetabular fracture (Figure 27-6). The patient underwent serial irrigation and debridement procedures until his wounds were amenable to definitive fixation 2 weeks after injury. At that time, he underwent internal fixation using a Stoppa approach, as well as the lateral window of the ilioinguinal approach (Figure 27-7). The Stoppa approach accesses the intrapelvic surfaces of the anterior pelvis via a single extraperitoneal window through the rectus abdominus muscle by lifting the neurovascular structures and retracting the contents of the peritoneal sac away from the fracture.[28,29] Nine months postoperatively, the patient was ambulating without significant pain, although he continues to use a cane secondary to abductor muscle weakness. As no further surgical insult was imparted on the abductor muscle mass, it is likely that this loss of abductor strength is secondary to internal iliac ligation and subsequent ischemic injury.

CASE 4

The patient is a 26-year-old male servicemember who was injured by an improvised explosive device while in a vehicle. He sustained a suprafoveal (Pipkin II) femoral head fracture, along with an acetabular roof fracture from a penetrating fragment (Figure 27-8). He also sustained a traumatic right above-elbow

amputation. He presented to an Echelon III facility and was treated with irrigation and debridement of his wounds, as well as exploratory laparotomy. He arrived at WRAMC 6 days after injury.

The patient underwent serial irrigation and debridement procedures until his wounds were amenable to internal fixation on post-injury day 13. A Kocher-Langenbeck approach was performed, along with a trochanteric osteotomy to gain access to the acetabular roof fracture. An anterior surgical dislocation of the hip was performed to access the femoral head fracture. This fracture was stabilized with headless compression screws, and he was treated with plate fixation of his acetabular fracture (Figure 27-9).

Despite postoperative irradiation for heterotopic ossification prophylaxis (700 cGy delivered on postoperative day 1), his postoperative course was complicated by extensive heterotopic ossification that bridged and ankylosed the patient's right hip (Figure 27-10).

He subsequently underwent excision of the heterotopic bone, which was noted to have completely encased the sciatic nerve as it exited the greater sciatic notch (Figure 27-11).

At his 6-month follow-up, the patient is full weight bearing on his right lower extremity and ambulating without assistive devices with minimal pain and good range of motion of the right hip to 110 degrees flexion, 10 degrees extension, 45 degrees external rotation, and 60 degrees internal rotation.

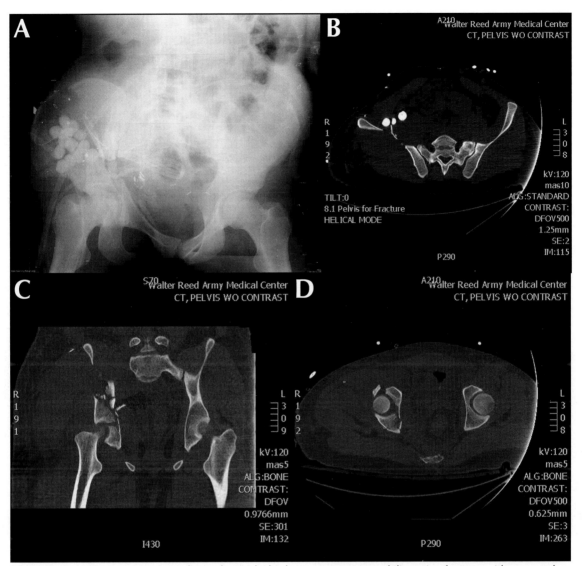

Figure 27-6. (A) Anteroposterior pelvis radiograph displaying a comminuted iliac wing fracture with an acetabular fracture involving both columns. (B) Axial CT cut displaying dead space management with antibiotic impregnated beads as well as the patient's comminuted iliac wing fracture. (C) Coronal CT cut showing comminution within the patient's posterior column. (D) Axial CT cut showing comminution within the patient's quadrilateral plate, the fracture extending into the posterior column, and an anterior wall fragment.

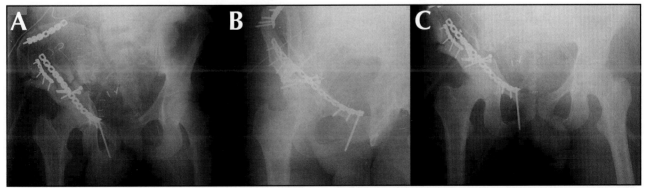

Figure 27-7. (A) Postoperative anteroposterior pelvis radiograph displaying reduction of the patient's iliac wing with multiple pelvic recon plates as well as interfragmentary screws. (B) Obturator oblique showing reduction of the anterior column. (C) Iliac oblique showing reduction of the posterior column.

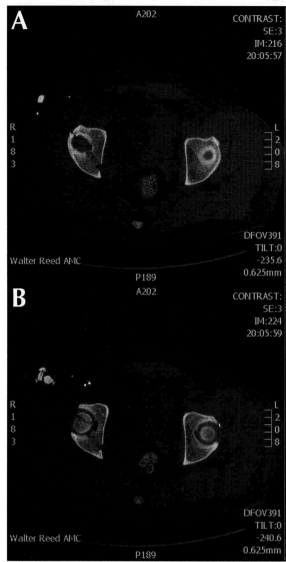

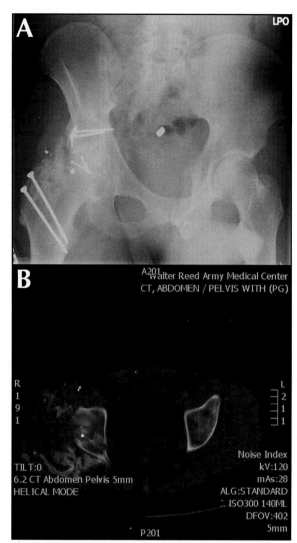

Figure 27-8. (A) Comminuted fracture of the acetabulum in the posterior column. (B) Comminuted suprafoveal fracture of the femoral head.

Figure 27-10. (A) Anteroposterior pelvis with significant heterotopic ossification of the patient's abductors causing ankylosis of the hip. (B) Axial CT cut with significant heterotopic ossification within the patient's abductors.

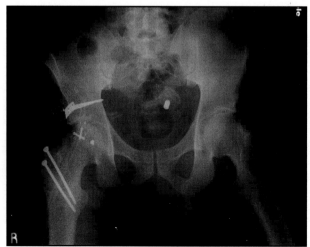

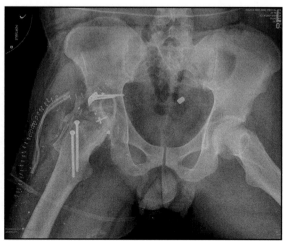

Figure 27-9. Postoperative radiographs displaying reduction of the femoral head with headless compression screws as well as a plate for fixation of the patient's acetabular fracture.

Figure 27-11. Postoperative radiograph after removal of heterotopic ossification from the patient's abductors, showing residual heterotopic ossification within the patient's short external rotators.

Complications

Complications are frequent when dealing with combat-related pelvic trauma. Infection is the primary early complication, whereas heterotopic ossification is the most concerning late complication. Post-traumatic arthritis, neurovascular injuries, femoral head osteonecrosis, and deep vein thrombosis occur[23] and are not significantly different than in civilian injuries.

INFECTION

Infectious complications are common in combat pelvic and acetabular fractures, particularly in conjunction with open injuries. Broad-spectrum antibiotics are recommended in the setting of open pelvic fractures, switching to bacteria-specific antibiotics as cultures dictate.[11] Adequate debridement of necrotic and nonviable soft tissue, as well as removal of foreign body and bowel contamination, is paramount in decreasing infection rates.[9,30] Antibiotic-impregnated beads are also used in large open wounds for local delivery of antibiotics and dead space management. Finally, the judicious use of internal fixation is advisable secondary to the severity and difficulty in managing infectious complications of pelvic and acetabular fractures. Avoiding the placement of permanent implants in patients with contaminated pelvic wounds is recommended, despite the likelihood that this will result in a suboptimal radiographic and clinical outcome.

Despite optimal management, late infections still occur. Fluid collections can be diagnosed on physical and laboratory exams as well as radiologic studies including computed tomography (CT) and ultrasound. Soft tissue and bone infections should be treated with incision and debridement along with proper antibiotics and antibiotic beads. Removal of hardware and replacement with external fixators should be considered when feasible.

HETEROTOPIC OSSIFICATION

Heterotopic ossification is a significant problem in the management of all combat-related musculoskeletal injuries, particularly those resulting from blasts, where the rate has been reported as 65%.[31,32] Heterotopic ossification is also increased in the setting of head injuries and spinal cord injuries, and this risk is multiplied by the presence of musculoskeletal injury. In Garland and O'Hollaren's study of patients with closed head injuries, heterotopic ossification developed in only 4% of those with isolated traumatic brain injury, but in 89% of those with concurrent musculoskeletal injury.[33] Combat pelvic and acetabular fractures are no different in this regard, and heterotopic ossification can be especially severe in patients

with significant associated injury to the gluteal musculature. Trochanteric osteotomy also increases risk of heterotopic ossification formation after surgical management of acetabular fractures.[23] Irradiation and indomethacin are typically employed for prophylaxis when indicated, though due to concerns regarding inhibition of healing in large open wounds in the pelvic girdle, these modalities are not always used in pelvic and acetabular fractures caused by blast mechanisms. The standard dose of radiation is 700 to 800 cGy administered within 48 hours of surgery. When indomethacin is employed, 25 mg is given 3 times a day for 3 to 6 months.

At WRAMC, postoperative irradiation (700 cGy in a single dose) is administered postoperatively on the day after surgery, except in the cases of severe open wounds, where the risk of wound complications are greater than the potential risk of heterotopic ossification formation. The importance of aggressive debridement of all damaged muscle in preventing heterotopic bone formation cannot be understated. Whether the result of surgical trauma or blast injury, all injured musculature must be debrided adequately.

Heterotopic bone around the pelvic girdle can result in loss of hip motion or muscle weakness from functional muscle loss. If problematic, heterotopic ossification can be excised once mature. Care must be taken during excision to protect neurovascular structures, which are commonly encased in the ectopic bone. CT can be very helpful in the preoperative planning of these procedures. Excision can also result in the creation of dead spaces, formation of large hematomas, and difficulty in obtaining closure of friable soft tissue envelopes. Drains and negative pressure dressings are used in an attempt to avoid complications, and irradiation or indomethacin is normally employed to prevent recurrence.

Possible Concerns, Future of the Technique

The greatest potential future advances in the treatment of combat pelvic and acetabular fractures may be found in the areas of modulation of heterotopic bone formation, developing anti-infective implants, and regenerative medicine. Ongoing research on each of these topics is promising.

Current work on the etiology of heterotopic bone is related to the identification and modulation of the cytokine and other cell-signaling factors responsible for bone formation. This may ultimately be extremely helpful in the management of future acetabular fractures, both in preventing heterotopic ossification[25] and promoting fracture union.

The osseous components of combat injuries to the pelvic girdle are often secondary in their functional impact when compared to the related soft tissue injuries. Nerve, muscle, blood vessel, and connective tissue deficits are frequently the most devastating and the most difficult to treat. As a result, there has been increased interest in, as well as Department of Defense funding for, research in regenerative medicine. These efforts include the induction of pluripotent cells to regenerate injured nerves, muscle tissue, and bone in the setting of fracture healing. While in its very early stages, the potential clinical value of this research is promising.

Along similar lines, the high rate of deep infection in combat injuries has led to research into the development of anti-infective fracture fixation implants, by various mechanisms. These include nanotechnology incorporation of antibiotics directly into the metal implants and coating implants with infection-resistant bio-active ceramics.

In summary, as a result of the high-energy fracture patterns and devastating open associated soft tissue injuries, combat pelvic and acetabular fractures present a challenging clinical problem. They are typically only a single component of a severely multiply injured patient, carry a high complication rate, and often require modifications of standard techniques in their management. With increasing experience and refined techniques, high complication rates can be diminished, resulting in better clinical outcomes for combat veterans.

References

1. Andersen RC, Frisch HM, Farber GL, Hayda RA. Definitive treatment of combat casualties at military medical centers. *J Am Acad Orthop Surg.* 2006;14:S24-S31.
2. Nessen SC, Lounsbury DE, Hetz SP, eds. *War Surgery in Afghanistan and Iraq: A Series of Cases, 2003-2007.* Washington, DC: Borden Institute; 2008.
3. Rothenberger DA, Fischer RP, Strate RG, Velasco R, Perry JF Jr. The mortality associated with pelvic fractures. *Surgery.* 1978;84:356-361.
4. Poole GV, Ward EF, Muakkassa FF, Hsu HS, Griswold JA, Rhodes RS. Pelvic fracture from major blunt trauma: outcome is determined by associated injuries. *Ann Surg.* 1991;213:532-539.
5. Bagg MR, Covey DC, Powell ET 4th. Levels of medical care in the global war on terrorism. *J Am Acad Orthop Surg.* 2006;14:S7-S9.
6. Hsu JR. *Joint Theater Trauma Registry Data.* Personal communication: July 2010.
7. Perry JF. Pelvic open fractures. *Clin Orthop Relat Res.* 1980;151:41-45.
8. Brenneman FD, Katyal D, Boulanger BR, Tile M, Riedelmeier DA. Long-term outcomes in open pelvic fractures. *J Trauma.* 1997;42:773-777.
9. American College of Surgeons. *Advanced Trauma Life Support for Doctors Student Course Manual.* 8th ed. Chicago, IL: Author; 2008.
10. Krieg JC, Mohr M, Ellis TJ, Simpson TS, Madey SM, Bottlang M. Emergent stabilization of pelvic ring injuries by controlled circumferential compression: a clinical trial. *J Trauma.* 2005;59:659-664.
11. Routt ML Jr, Falicov A, Woodhouse E, Schildhauer TA. Circumferential pelvic antishock sheeting: a temporary resuscitation aid. *J Orthop Trauma.* 2002;16:45-48.
12. Grotz MR, Allami MK, Harwood P, Pape HC, Krettek C, Giannoudis PV. Open pelvic fractures: epidemiology, current concepts of management and outcome. *Injury.* 2005;36(1):1-13.
13. Jones AL, Powell JN, Kellam JF, McCormack RG, Dust W, Wimmer P. Open pelvic fractures. A multicenter retrospective analysis. *Orthop Clin North Am.* 1997;28(3):345-350.
14. Riemer BL, Butterfield SL, Diamond DL, et al. Acute mortality associated with injuries to the pelvic ring: the role of early patient mobilization and external fixation. *J Trauma.* 1993;35:671-677.
15. Gosselin R, Roberts I, Gillespie W. Antibiotics for preventing infection in open limb fractures. *Cochrane Database Syst Rev.* 2004;1:CD003764.
16. Tile M. Acute pelvic fractures: II. Principles of management. *J Am Acad Orthop Surg.* 1996;4:152-161.
17. Tang P, Meredick R, Prayson MJ, Gruen GS. External fixation of the pelvis. *Tech Orthop.* 2002;17:228-238.
18. Tile M. Fractures of the pelvis. In: Schatzker J, Tile M, eds. *The Rationale of Operative Fracture Care.* Berlin, Germany: Springer; 1987:256-269.
19. Labler L, Trentz O. The use of vacuum assisted closure (VAC) in soft tissue injuries after high energy pelvic trauma. *Langenbecks Arch Surg.* 2007;392(5):601-609.
20. Pollak AN. The use of negative pressure wound therapy with reticulated open cell foam for lower extremity trauma. *J Orthop Trauma.* 2008;22(10 Suppl):S142-S145.
21. Powell ET 4th. The role of negative pressure wound therapy with reticulated open cell foam in the treatment of war wounds. *J Orthop Trauma.* 2008;22(10 Suppl):S138-S141.
22. Pennal GF, Tile M, Waddell JP, Garside H. Pelvic disruption: assessment and classification. *Clin Orthop Relat Res.* 1980;151:12-21.
23. Leenen LP, van der Werken C, Schoots F, Goris RJ. Internal fixation of open pelvic fractures. *J Trauma.* 1993;35:220-225.
24. Kottmeier SA, Wilson SC, Born CT, Hanks GA, Iannacone WM, DeLong WG. Surgical management of soft tissue lesions associated with pelvic ring injury. *Clin Orthop.* 1996;329:46-53.
25. Gwinn DE, Morgan RA, Kumar AR. Gluteus maximus avulsion and closed degloving lesion associated with a thoracolumbar burst fracture: a case report. *J Bone Joint Surg Am.* 2007;89:408-412.
26. Suzuki T, Morgan SJ, Smith WR, Stahel PF, Gillani SA, Hak DJ. Postoperative surgical site infection following acetabular fracture fixation. *Injury.* 2010;41(4):396-399.
27. Kaempffe FA, Bone LB, Border JR. Open reduction and internal fixation of acetabular fractures: heterotopic ossification and other complications of treatment. *J Orthop Trauma.* 1991;5(4):439-445.
28. Hirvensalo E, Lindahl J, Bostman O. A new approach to the internal fixation of unstable pelvic fractures. *Clin Orthop Relat Res.* 1993;297:28-32.
29. Cole JD, Bolhofner BR. Acetabular fracture fixation via a modified Stoppa limited intrapelvic approach. Description of operative technique and preliminary treatment results. *Clin Orthop.* 1994;305:112-123.
30. Birolini D, Steinman E, Utiyama EM, Arroyo AA. Open pelviperineal trauma. *J Trauma.* 1990;30:492-495.
31. Forsberg JA, Pepek JM, Wagner S, et al. Heterotopic ossification in high-energy wartime extremity injuries: prevalence and risk factors. *J Bone Joint Surg Am.* 2009;91(5):1084-1091.

32. Potter BK, Burns TC, Lacap AP, Granville RR, Gajewski DA. Heterotopic ossification following traumatic and combat-related amputations. Prevalence, risk factors, and preliminary results of excision. *J Bone Joint Surg Am.* 2007;89(3):476-486.

33. Garland DE, O'Hollaren RM. Fractures and dislocations about the elbow in the head-injured adult. *Clin Orthop Relat Res.* 1982;168: 38-41.

Chapter 28

SPINE FRACTURES

CPT Daniel G. Kang, MD and LTC Ronald A. Lehman Jr, MD

The current conflicts in Iraq and Afghanistan have brought unique challenges in the treatment of spinal column injuries, due to young, healthy combatants subjected to high-energy blast trauma. In contrast to previous US military conflicts, orthopedic surgeons have taken an increasing role in the treatment of spine fractures sustained during the wars in Iraq and Afghanistan.

Epidemiology

Spine injuries are commonly encountered in civilian trauma, with approximately 75% to 90% of spinal fractures occurring in the thoracic and lumbar spine.[1] In a multicenter review of more than 1000 patients with thoracolumbar fractures from civilian institutions, 16% of injuries occurred between T1 and T10, 52% between T11 and L1 (thoracolumbar junction), and 32% between L1 and L5.[1-4] Significant three-column injuries, including fracture-dislocations, make up approximately 50% of thoracolumbar fractures, with approximately 75% of these injuries resulting in a complete neurologic deficit.[1,5] There is also a high association between spinal injuries and sacral and pelvic fractures, with 26% of sacral fractures and 8% of pelvic fractures having an associated spinal fracture.[6,7] In the Iraq and Afghanistan conflicts, the use of improvised explosive devices (IEDs) by insurgent forces has created a high incidence of less common injury patterns to the spinal column, in particular low lumbar burst fractures and lumbosacral dissociation injuries.[8,9]

Combat casualty care of spine fractures is significantly different than civilian trauma practice because injuries are often open, contaminated, and associated with injuries to other organ systems.[10] Spinal column injuries rarely occur in isolation, and high-energy blast or high-velocity ballistic weapons often result in polytrauma combat casualties with associated traumatic brain injury, thoracic and visceral injuries, and extremity injuries. Thus, the resuscitation and comprehensive care of the multiply injured combat casualty takes precedence, with initial management of a suspected spine injury focusing on immobilization and prevention of further neurologic injury and deterioration.

ANATOMY

The spinal column consists of 7 cervical, 12 thoracic, and 5 lumbar vertebrae, as well as the sacrum and coccyx. The cervical spine is vulnerable to injury because of its mobility and exposure. The spinal cord is particularly prone to damage in this region because of the coupling of a large mass (the head) to the lever arm of great flexibility (the cervical spine).[11] The cervical canal is relatively wide in the upper cervical region from the foramen magnum to the lower part of C2. Thus, the majority of patients with injuries above C2 who survive are often neurologically intact. However, approximately one-third of patients with upper cervical spine injures die at the scene of the injury from apnea caused by loss of phrenic nerve function.[11] Below C3, the diameter of the cervical spinal canal is much smaller relative to the diameter of the spinal cord, and vertebral column injuries are at higher risk of causing spinal cord injuries.[11,12]

Owens BD, Belmont PJ Jr, eds. *Combat Orthopedic Surgery:*
Lessons Learned in Iraq and Afghanistan (pp 297-310)
© 2011 SLACK Incorporated

The thoracic spine requires significant force to disrupt the protective enclosure of the thoracic spinal cord. The sternum and rib cage significantly limit motion and offer rotatory stability in the thoracic spine,[13] while the surrounding paraspinal musculature offers additional protection.[12,14,15] As a result, the incidence of thoracic fractures is much lower than in other areas of the spine. Compression fractures are the most prevalent in this region and are rarely associated with spinal cord injuries. However, due to the narrow thoracic canal, when a fracture-dislocation in the thoracic spine does occur, there is a high incidence of spinal cord injury, with a 6-to-1 ratio of complete to incomplete cord injury.[12] The T2 to T10 area has the smallest ratio of canal size to cord diameter in the spine, and is a circulatory watershed with the artery of Adamkiewicz providing blood supply at approximately T8-T12 levels.[14,15]

The thoracolumbar junction from T11 to L1 acts as a fulcrum between the immobile, inflexible thoracic region and the stronger, flexible lumbar levels, making this transition area more vulnerable to injury. This is the most common location of burst-type fractures, and 52% of spine fractures occur in this region.[1,12,14]

The lumbar spine is more mobile compared to the thoracic spine, particularly in flexion and extension with 12 degrees at T12-L1 versus 25 degrees at L5-S1 vertebral motion segments.[15] Fractures occurring about the lumbar spine generally have a better prognosis due to the increased ratio of the canal area to the neural elements. The lumbar spine also marks the termination of the spinal cord at the L1 level, with the cauda equina being less susceptible to permanent damage. Injury to the nerve roots may carry a better prognosis due to regenerative properties not normally seen in the cord or conus. There is often difficulty in determining the extent of injury and prognosis with an injury at the L1-L2 levels due to the variable anatomy and commingling of cord, conus, and cauda equina.[14,16] Another unique anatomic and biomechanical characteristic of the lower lumbar spine (L3-L5) is that vertebral bodies are caudal to the apex of lordosis, resulting in the center of gravity running posterior to the vertebral axis and in evenly distributed flexion and axial forces along the vertebral body.[17] The lower lumbar spine is also stabilized by the iliolumbar ligaments and further protected by its location below the pelvic brim.[17]

Evaluation and Management in Theater

The principles of pre-hospital care are similar in the care of combat casualties compared to civilian trauma systems, with a focus on adhering to the standards of Advanced Trauma Life Support (ATLS) protocols.[18] Effective treatment of the combat casualty with spine and spinal cord injury begins with recognition of the injury. In 1985, Bohlman found 100 of 300 cervical spine injuries presenting in a civilian emergency department setting were initially missed.[5,19] While the current incidence of missed spine injures is likely less than 1-in-3 as reported in Bohlman's review from the 1980s, the primary reasons for failure to identify spine injuries are likely unchanged: the presence of multiple injuries, medical instability, and altered level of consciousness.[5,19] Thus, the general or orthopedic surgeon should always suspect and rule out spine injury in the polytrauma patient.

Modes of extrication and evacuation during combat differ from the civilian emergency medical trauma transport system because care is delivered in an austere and dangerous combat environment. Also, the first responder on the battlefield is another servicemember, often with minimal medical training. The first responder's focus is to expeditiously remove the wounded comrade from danger rather than to maintain spinal stability. On the battlefield, preservation of life of the combat casualty and of the combat medic takes precedence over spine immobilization. The training of combat medics has emphasized the importance of spine immobilization during extrication and evacuation when conditions and equipment permit. Thus, effective care of a combat casualty with suspected spine injury begins with a clear and comprehensive field protocol to ensure rapid and safe removal from the combat zone while working in tandem with a well-organized battalion aid station where resuscitation is initiated.[20] A forward surgical team, Echelon II facility, is often staffed with 3 general surgeons and an orthopedic surgeon, where the initial evaluation and management of spine fractures is usually performed.[18]

Discussion of the initial management of the polytrauma combat casualty is beyond the scope of this chapter. However, when a combat casualty presents with clinical instability and when complex wounds involving the head, thorax, abdomen, or extremities co-exist with spinal column injury, life-saving measures take precedence over the definitive diagnosis and management of spinal column and cord injury. During resuscitation, initial management of suspected spine injury should focus on appropriate immobilization and preventing neurologic deterioration. Upon arrival at an Echelon II facility, initial evaluation in the trauma bay should include primary survey with focus on the stepwise ATLS protocol. The neck should never be hyperextended, and if endotracheal intubation is necessary, in-line neck stabilization should be performed.[10]

Once the airway is secure and the primary survey is complete, a cervical collar should be placed on the patient if not already present. During the secondary survey of the patient, the physical examination should concentrate on the spine. In suspected thoracic and lumbar spine injuries, transfers and movement of the patient should be performed using a log-roll technique with the most experienced provider performing in-line neck stabilization, and the entire spine must be inspected and palpated. Physical exam findings suggesting injury to the spinal column include ecchymoses, tenderness, or a palpable step-off between the spinous processes. Patients with persistent, localized tenderness to the thoracolumbar spine and no other injury on initial radiographs still have a 30% incidence of occult spinal fracture.[15] Neurologic examination must be documented and repeated at regular intervals to note any change that may occur during the treatment process. A detailed and systematic neurologic exam, often performed in accordance with determination of an American Spinal Injury Association grade, should include motor testing, dermatomal sensory testing, lumbar and sacral root evaluation, and rectal examination.[15,16] During early assessment, it is critical to determine whether the patient sustained transient paresis following the trauma.[20] Vaccaro emphasizes that, although some patients experiencing transient paralysis may appear to have a normal neurologic status on arrival at the emergency department, they require immediate and careful assessment for a possible unstable cervical spine fracture or dislocation.[20]

IMAGING

Combat casualty care of any trauma patient with a suspected spine fracture should include appropriate radiographic imaging with supplemental studies such as computed tomographic (CT) scanning or magnetic resonance imaging (MRI) as indicated and when first available through the echelons of care. Spine injury/instability should be assumed and suspected in any patient complaining of cervical instability pain along the vertebral column, tenderness to palpation along the midline over the spinous processes, neurologic deficit, or altered mental status.[10]

Initial radiographic assessment can be first obtained at an Echelon II facility and begins with a lateral cervical spine radiograph. A quality lateral view should include the entire cervical spine down to the endplate of T1. A swimmer's view (lateral view with maximally abducted arm) can be obtained if unable to obtain adequate visualization of the most caudal cervical vertebra on a standard lateral image. A combat casualty who is awake, alert, and cooperative with no neck pain or tenderness and is neurologically intact does not require further radiographic evaluation if the lateral view is negative and is cleared from cervical spine precautions.[20,21] Upon arrival at an Echelon III

facility, a spiral CT traumagram is performed for the multiply injured combat casualty. The use of spiral CT traumagram is indicated in a blunt trauma patient who is unconscious or unable to provide a reliable clinical exam due to altered mental status or distracting injuries. Spiral CT of the spine has been found to identify 99% of all fractures of the cervical, thoracic, and lumbar spine and provides more accurate assessment of bone injury and spinal canal compromise when compared to plain radiographs.[22-24] Antevil and colleagues reported use of CT to evaluate cervical spine injury and found 100% sensitivity versus 70% using plain radiographs. They also noted significantly shorter mean time for initial radiologic evaluation for CT (1.0 hours) versus plain films (1.9 hours).[25] CT of the chest, abdomen, and pelvis has also been highly effective in recognizing thoracic and lumbar spine trauma, with reported 100% sensitivity and 97% specificity compared to plain radiographs with 73% sensitivity and 100% specificity.[23] If a spine fracture is identified with routine spiral CT traumagram or on plain radiographs, a CT scan of the entire spine should be carefully reviewed due to the high incidence of additional, noncontiguous spinal column fractures, which has been reported to be from 10% to 20% and may be even higher because of the high-energy blast injuries sustained by combat casualties.[6,26,27]

MRI is more accurate in assessing soft tissue injury, is the definitive diagnostic modality in the evaluation of spinal cord injury, and can be obtained at an Echelon IV facility. MRI is indicated in a combat casualty with a neurologic deficit, a deteriorating neurologic exam, or if the injured individual is obtunded or otherwise unable to participate in an exam. MRI is also useful in detecting compressive lesions such as spinal epidural hematoma or traumatic herniated disk after subluxation or dislocation, as well as spinal cord contusions or disruption.[12] However, MRI is frequently not available in a combat support hospital (CSH) in theater and often is not feasible in an acutely injured combat casualty with hemodynamic instability. In addition, MRI should not be performed in a combat casualty with retained metallic foreign bodies or with non-MRI compatible implants. Once at an Echelon IV or V facility, dynamic lateral plain radiographs of the spine may be performed to demonstrate instability without associated fracture due to purely ligamentous spine injury. Dynamic flexion/extension lateral radiographs of the spine are delayed until 2 weeks after injury when pain and spasm have sufficiently subsided and are indicated in a combat casualty with persistent mild neck or back pain and tenderness, who is cooperative and neurologically normal.[28] Cervical instability is defined on lateral radiographs as either more than 3.5 mm of sagittal displacement/translation, angulation more than 11 degrees between motion segments, or more than

1 mm of occipito-atlantal translation.[29,30] Thoracic and lumbar spine instability is defined by more than 5 mm of sagittal translation or sagittal angulation more than 20 to 30 degrees between motion segments, or more than 50% loss of vertebral body height.[15]

As previously stated, effective treatment of the combat casualty with spine or spinal cord injury begins with recognition of the injury. Thus, the general or orthopedic surgeon entrusted with the care of combat casualties should maintain heightened vigilance and obtain adequate and appropriate images of the spine when injury is suspected.

In-Theater Treatment

The goal of in-theater care is to maximize the potential for neurologic recovery from the moment of injury to the time of arrival at a CSH where advanced medical and surgical resources are available.[20] Once a patient arrives at the CSH, the ultimate goal is to ensure the patient has a stable, painless spine and an optimal neurologic evaluation. For the combat casualty with spinal column injury without a neurologic deficit, the goal is to do no further harm.

Initial resuscitation efforts should prevent secondary spinal cord injury from hypoxia, hypotension, hyperthermia, and edema. The optimal target of opportunity for mitigating the effects of further neurologic deterioration is prevention of the secondary injury cascade that often accompanies spinal cord injury. Any pharmacologic treatment of spinal cord injury must take into account the significant controversy regarding the use of high-dose methylprednisolone and its influence on neurologic recovery.[31-34] The spine surgeon should be apprised of all of the information pertaining to the patient before considering the initiation of the corticosteroid protocol. Additionally, the corticosteroid protocol is not recommended in spinal cord injury resulting from penetrating trauma.[35,36] The role of halo immobilization in the combat setting is limited and often is not feasible due to lack of equipment in theater. Immobilization with a rigid cervical collar or sand bags for nonpenetrating trauma to the cervical spine is preferable until arrival at a definitive treatment site. In cervical spine trauma with facet joint dislocation or burst fractures with worsening neurologic status, the patient should be placed in Gardner-Wells tongs traction, with extreme care exercised by surgeons not experienced with this procedure. Appropriate initial traction is estimated at 5 pounds of weight per level of injury, with 5 to 15 pounds of traction released once radiographs demonstrate appropriate reduction. It is important to ensure the absence of an occipitocervical dissociation prior to the application of in-line weight to the skull. Contraindications to Gardner-Wells tong traction include depressed skull

fractures near the insertion site of the pins or injury to the occipitocervical articulation, which could cause severe neurologic injury and/or death. Post-traction radiographs (at 10- to 15-pound increments) should always be obtained to verify appropriate reduction and to ensure cervical spine ligamentous injury has not been missed or exacerbated by overdistraction.[10]

Spinal column fractures associated with penetrating abdominal injury should undergo surgical abdominal exploration, with evaluation for visceral injury and with repair or intestinal diverting procedures as indicated. It is critical to recognize a bullet or ballistic fragment that may have caused colonic perforation before passing through the spine because of the high rate of spine infection if not treated with an appropriate antibiotic regimen.[28] Broad-spectrum intravenous antibiotics should be initiated as soon as possible, with 72 hours of prophylaxis appropriate for the combat casualty with a low-velocity gunshot wound or ballistic fragment injury to the spine not complicated by visceral injury. For penetrating spine injury with colonic perforation, the lowest infection rates have been documented with antibiotics continued for 10 to 14 days after injury.[28,37-42] Surgical debridement of low-energy penetrating spine injuries, with or without visceral perforation, does not provide substantial clinical benefit and is not routinely performed for our combat casualties in theater.[28] High-velocity ballistic injuries, which are more common in combat casualties compared to civilian trauma patients, are associated with significantly more soft tissue destruction and a larger zone of injury. There are few reported case series of combat casualties treated for high-velocity ballistic injury to the spinal column.[43,44] In the current conflicts, they are treated with 14 days of broad-spectrum intravenous antibiotics with aggressive surgical debridement in theater to remove devitalized tissue, followed by decompressive laminectomy with instrumentation once at an Echelon IV or V treatment facility.

Fractures of the spine caused by low-velocity bullet wound or ballistic fragmentation are usually stable, and surgical intervention is rarely necessary. The majority of cases of spine instability and late deformity after penetrating injury have been associated with overly aggressive laminectomy.[28,45] There are few indications for urgent decompression in a neurologically intact patient, including new-onset progressive neurologic deficit associated with an intracanal bullet or ballistic fragment, bone fragment, or expanding epidural hematoma.[28] Regardless of the level of spine injury, a combat casualty previously neurologically intact or with incomplete spinal cord injury with progressive neurologic deficit should have urgent decompression by the first available orthopedic spine surgeon or neurosurgeon in theater, usually at an Echelon III treatment facility, or if unavailable in theater, the combat casualty should be urgently transported to an Echelon IV treatment facility.

A prospective study by Waters and Adkins reported statistically significant motor improvement after surgical decompression for retained intracanal bullets from T12 to L4 levels compared with patients treated nonoperatively.[42,46] In the current conflict, combat casualties with an intracanal bullet or ballistic fragment below T12 undergo removal and decompression to improve the rate of motor recovery in the lumbar and sacral nerve roots. In this select patient population, decompression and bullet fragment removal occurs within 5 to 7 days from injury at an Echelon IV or V treatment facility by an orthopedic spine surgeon or neurosurgeon. There is no literature to support early decompression, and timing of surgical intervention was evaluated in a retrospective study by Cybulski and colleagues, who reported similar rates of neurologic recovery in patients undergoing decompression after gunshot injury below the conus level within 72 hours (47.5%) versus after 72 hours (48.1%) from injury.[47] However, higher rates of infection and arachnoiditis have been reported when surgery was performed more than 2 weeks from injury.[47]

The role of removal and decompression of an intracanal bullet or ballistic fragment at the cervical and thoracic levels with incomplete neural injury remains unclear in the literature.[45,46,48] In combat casualties with an incomplete spinal cord injury and a thoracic spine intracanal bullet or ballistic fragment, removal and decompression is not performed. However, removal and decompression is considered at the cervical level with incomplete spinal cord injury due to the potential of improved functional neurologic recovery.[28] Cervical spine intracanal bullet or fragment removal can be performed through a posterior laminectomy for the lower cervical spine when the bullet or fragment can be removed without extensive dural dissection, and for the upper cervical spine (C1-C2), decompression can be performed through a transoral approach.[28,49]

For complete neural deficits at the cervical and thoracic levels, early or late operative decompression is not indicated, and it has not shown improvement in neurologic recovery, while causing higher complication rates compared to nonsurgical management.[28,42] Also, the use of corticosteroids for penetrating spinal cord injury is not recommended and is associated with pancreatitis and gastrointestinal complications.[28,35,36,50]

Emergent surgical decompression and instrumentation is indicated only in rare instances of blunt spinal column injuries, including progressive neurologic deterioration and irreducible canal compromise. In our institutional experience at Walter Reed Army Medical Center (WRAMC) regarding combat casual-

ties with blunt spinal column injury and complete neurologic injury, the likelihood of neurologic recovery is minimal and is not influenced by emergent surgical intervention.[51,52] Patients with evidence of incomplete neurologic injury at the resolution of spinal shock, progressive neurologic deterioration, and an unstable fracture pattern with significant spinal cord compression may benefit from acute surgical decompression and instrumentation.[10] The optimal timing of surgical intervention is unclear, and a critical window of opportunity may exist in which the decompression of the spinal canal and spinal stabilization may enhance functional neurologic outcome. However, the literature has shown no difference in long-term neurologic recovery with early versus late decompression. Vaccaro and colleagues reported the only controlled, prospective, randomized study on the timing of surgical intervention in cervical spinal cord injury.[52] The authors found no difference in functional neural recovery when patients were operated on either early (<3 days) or late (5 days). In contrast, a multi-center study found neurologic deterioration in 4 of 26 patients who had surgery within 5 days after spinal cord injury, but in none of 108 patients who had an operation after 5 days.[51,53,54]

In the combat casualty with spinal canal compromise and no neurologic deficit, there has been no report of substantial benefit achieved by acute surgical intervention to offset the risk of causing neurologic deficit in a previously neurologically intact patient. One possible argument for surgical intervention is that significant spinal canal compromise may develop stenotic symptoms in the future. However, there are only rare reports of spinal stenosis symptoms developing in long-term outcome studies.[6,55-57] Sandor and colleagues found patients with as much as 93% canal compromise resorbed fracture fragments over time with nonsurgical management.[58] In another series of 41 neurologically intact patients, two-thirds of retropulsed bone resorbed at long-term follow-up.[59]

Definitive Management

The definitive management of a combat casualty with spine injury should be performed following evacuation to an Echelon V facility with an available orthopedic spine surgeon or neurosurgeon. Severely injured combat casualties often arrive at such a facility within 72 to 96 hours from the time of injury and upon admission should have a thorough and complete re-evaluation. Radiographs and other imaging studies should be repeated if previous studies are unavailable or there is any concern about change regarding clinical status or neurologic exam. Medical records should be obtained, and previous neurologic exams should be reviewed for evidence of resolution of spinal shock during the transport process. Patients should have a repeat detailed neurologic exam, performed in accordance with the American Spinal Injury Association classification, and bulbocavernosus reflex and rectal exam should be performed to document resolution of spinal shock. Emphasis is placed on repeat evaluation and examination of the combat casualty from head to toe to ensure there have been no missed injuries and there has not been a change in the neurologic status of the patient during the transport process. A tertiary medical treatment facility offers the advantage of a well-trained surgical team, advanced medical and surgical resources, the availability of multiple consulting surgical services, and a fully capable intensive care unit to assist in management of other injuries or medical problems.

Most spinal column fractures in the absence of neurologic deficit are stable and can be treated successfully nonoperatively. Nonoperative management is also favorable in the combat casualty with multiple noncontiguous spine fractures as surgical stabilization requires instrumenting large portions of the patient's spinal column. Open injuries require aggressive and repeated irrigation and debridement procedures prior to consideration of definitive fixation with placement of implants. The presence of an open injury, particularly if highly contaminated, may sway the surgeon toward nonoperative management to reduce the significant morbidity of an infection. Patients with injury of the posterior osteoligamentous complex (supraspinous ligament, interspinous ligament, ligamentum flavum, and facet joint capsules) are not candidates for nonoperative management because there is a low likelihood the ligamentous injury will heal.[6] A new thoracolumbar injury classification and severity score (TLICS/TLISS) has categorized posterior ligamentous injury as one of 3 major injury characteristics. The 2 other major injury characteristics include injury morphology and neurologic status, and a scoring system based on summation of points from all 3 major injury characteristics (if greater than 4 points) guides the surgeon toward operative management.[3,60] A patient with a distraction injury (+4 points), intact neurologic status (0 points), and disrupted posterior ligamentous (+3 points) would have a summed TLISS of more than 4, which would indicate the need for operative management.[3] Advances in nonoperative management protocols and the development of spine injury rehabilitation centers have minimized the problems associated with prolonged immobilization. Rechtine and colleagues have advocated the use of an aggressive treatment plan in patients treated nonoperatively, with emphasis on chemical and mechanical deep venous thrombosis prophylaxis, early active physical therapy programs with exercise and strengthening initiated

as soon as possible to decrease muscle atrophy and deconditioning, and specialized beds and turning protocols to reduce decubitus ulcer formation.[6]

Despite advancements in spinal instrumentation and radiographic imaging techniques, controversy continues regarding the indications for surgical intervention, the timing of intervention, and the approach with which to decompress and stabilize traumatic spinal deformity. In a literature review concerning management of traumatic fractures of the thoracic and lumbar spine, the authors found insufficient evidence in the literature showing significant advantage in patient outcome when comparing various surgical techniques for the reduction and fixation of spinal fractures.[61] Regardless of surgical technique, the ultimate goals in managing the combat casualty with a spinal column injury are to maximize neurologic recovery and to stabilize the spine expeditiously for early rehabilitation and an early return to military service and a productive lifestyle.[15]

Definitive surgical treatment of spinal column fracture remains necessary if the biomechanical stability of the spine is severely compromised or if a neurologic deficit is imminent or worsening.[61] Discussion of the definitive surgical management of all injury and fracture patterns of the spinal column is beyond the scope of this chapter. We will discuss injuries unique to the combat-related injuries experienced at our military treatment facility during the Iraq and Afghanistan conflicts, in particular low lumbar burst fractures and lumbosacral dissociation.

Low Lumbar Spine Burst Fracture

Low lumbar spine (L3 to L5) burst fractures are relatively uncommon and account for only 1% of all spinal injuries in the civilian trauma population. During the Iraq and Afghanistan conflicts, combat casualties have experienced an increased incidence of low lumbar spine burst fractures due to high-energy blast injuries from IEDs.

The low lumbar spine has unique anatomic and biomechanical characteristics, which provide increased stability.[17] Most notable is the location of the low lumbar spine caudal to the apex of lordosis. This characteristic allows the body's center of gravity to fall posterior to the vertebral axis at the L3 level, thus a flexion and axial compression force results in relative neutral sagittal alignment, and forces are distributed uniformly across the 3 columns of the spine. This is compared to the L1-L2 level, cephalad to the apex of lordosis, in which flexion and axial compression forces are directed through the anterior column, subsequently producing injury with less significant force than in the low lumbar spine and creating kyphotic deformity.

Also of note is that the low lumbar spine has the widest spinal canal, with termination of the spinal cord at L2 with continuation as the cauda equina. This anatomic characteristic of the low lumbar spine results in rare neurologic deficit, and as much as 90% canal compromise has been reported without neurologic injury.[62,63]

The indications and outcomes of operative management for low lumbar spine burst fractures have not been fully determined in the literature. However, in the combat casualty with low lumbar spine burst fracture and no neurologic deficit, the literature is consistent in recommending nonoperative management with bracing and early ambulation.[64-66] There has been evidence to support both nonoperative and operative management of a patient with low lumbar spine burst fracture with neurologic deficit. There has been no correlation between neurologic deficit and canal compromise, no difference in neurologic sequelae, no evidence of lumbar stenosis development or progression of kyphosis as a long-term complication of nonoperative management, no significant difference in pain relief or patient satisfaction, and similar radiologic outcomes.[6,17,57,62,67-71]

Lumbosacral Dissociation

Lumbosacral dissociation injuries are rare injuries in the civilian trauma population. During the Iraq and Afghanistan conflicts, combat casualties have experienced an increased incidence of lumbosacral dissociation, with a total of 23 lumbosacral dissociation injuries treated between 2001 and 2008. The increased incidence of this rare injury is likely due to high-energy blast injuries from IEDs and increased survival from the protection offered by advances in body and vehicular armor.

Lumbosacral dissociation injuries are characterized by an anatomic separation of the pelvis from the spinal column and are the result of high-energy trauma. In civilian trauma practice, these injuries are most often associated with high-speed motor vehicle collisions or falls from a height. Other terms used to describe the relatively rare injury pattern of lumbosacral dissociation are *spondylopelvic dissociation*, *spinopelvic dissociation*, and *lumbosacral fracture-dislocation*.[72-76] Different patterns of lumbosacral injury can result in anatomic separation and instability of the spine and pelvis, and often present as an H-type sacral fracture, traumatic high-grade spondylolisthesis, disruption of iliolumbar and sacroiliac ligaments from sacroiliac dislocation, or multiple lumbar transverse process fractures.[73,76-78] However, we believe lumbosacral dissociation injuries represent a specific injury pattern causing mechanical separation and instability of the spine and pelvis, which is characterized by a sacral fracture with both vertical and horizontal components resulting in the lack of contiguity of the cephalad endplate of S1 with the ilium.[79-81] A combat casualty with an L4 or L5 transverse process fracture should be evaluated with advanced imaging as sacral and pelvic fractures are frequently associated and may represent a disruption of the iliolumbar ligamentous complex.[79,81-85] A lumbosacral dissociation injury also results in kyphotic deformity due to deforming forces of the iliopsoas muscle and the pull of gravity. Even when the patient is non-ambulatory, the cephalad portion of the spine or sacrum tends to rotate into flexion relative to the pelvis. The long-term sequelae of lumbosacral dissociation injury and post-traumatic kyphosis include increased local degenerative changes, lumbago and lumbar muscle weakness, and difficulty with seating and gait efficiency.

The indications and outcomes of operative management for lumbosacral dissociation injuries have not been fully determined in the literature. Nork and colleagues, in a review of U-shaped sacral fractures, recommended operative treatment with percutaneous sacroiliac screw fixation without decompression and found improvement in the majority of patients with sacral nerve root symptoms.[79] These authors also noted that percutaneous sacroiliac screw fixation should not be used for cases in which deformity restricted screw placement. Based on our experience with lumbosacral dissociation injuries, there is no evidence of improved patient outcomes with early stabilization. Factors influencing operative versus nonoperative treatment include the presence and degree of neurologic compromise, co-morbidities, condition of soft tissue envelope, extent of the deformity, bony versus ligamentous instability, and the experience of the surgical team. Table 28-1 summarizes the indications for nonoperative management of lumbosacral dissociation.

Combat casualties with lumbosacral dissociation often have other multiple severe injuries, along with large open wounds and compromised soft tissue envelope about the pre-sacral and gluteal area, which often forces the surgeon toward nonoperative management, especially with expected immobility of more than 3 months because of the necessity for fracture consolidation. Operative management for lumbosacral dissociation injuries include stabilization with or without sagittal plane reduction using instrumented posterior spinal fusion with sacral nerve root decompression, percutaneous sacroiliac screw, or sacral plate. Percutaneous sacroiliac screw fixation alone is considered in the patient expected to be only immobilized for 6 weeks with an amenable injury pattern.

Table 28-1

Lumbosacral Dissociation Injury Treatment

Indications for nonoperative treatment:
• Severely compromised soft tissue envelope
• Multiple severe injuries with expected immobility >3 months
Operative treatment:
• Closed lumbosacral dissociation injury
• No other significant injury preventing mobility
• Posterior spinal fusion with instrumentation and decompression with evidence of sacral nerve root deficit
• Percutaneous sacroiliac screw fixation if expected immobility 6 weeks and appropriate injury pattern

Table 28-2

Summary of Institutional Review of Low Lumbar Spine Burst Fractures From September 2001 to May 2008

Inclusion criteria:
• Burst fracture from T12-L5
• At least 1-year clinical follow-up
• Damage to at least 1 vertebral endplate or body
• Loss of vertebral body height with retropulsion into the spinal canal
Patients:
• 32 patients with 39 thoracolumbar burst fractures (7 patients with multiple fractures)
• 20/32 patients with low lumbar burst fracture
• 14/39 (35.9%) thoracolumbar junction fractures
• 25/39 (64.1%) low lumbar spine fractures
• 14/25 (56%) low lumbar spine burst fractures with major neurologic injury
Outcomes:
• 12/20 (60%) patients with L3-L5 burst fracture operative management
• 10/12 (83.3%) patients T12-L2 burst fracture operative management
• 10/32 patients treated with nonoperative management
• 4/22 (18.2%) infection rate operative management
• 1/14 low lumbar burst fractures with initial neurologic injury with persistent neurologic deficit at 1-year follow-up
• 1.6/10 mean VAS L3-L5 operative management
• 2.0/10 mean VAS T12-L2 operative management

INSTITUTIONAL REVIEW OUTCOMES AND COMPLICATIONS

WRAMC performed a retrospective review of medical records and imaging studies of all combat casualties with thoracolumbar fractures treated during the Iraq and Afghanistan conflicts between September 2001 and May 2008, and with at least 1-year clinical follow-up.[8] WRAMC treated 32 patients with thoracolumbar spine burst fractures in a 7-year time period (Table 28-2). There were a total of 39 thoracolumbar burst fractures, with 25 of 39 (64.1%) at the L3 to L5 level, and there was an infection rate of 18.2% in all thoracolumbar spine fractures treated with operative management. The combat casualties with low lumbar spine burst fracture experienced major neurologic injury in 14 of 25 fractures (56%). However, after 1 year of follow-up, only 1 patient with initial neurologic injury had a continued neurologic deficit.

Table 28-3

Summary of Institutional Review of Lumbosacral Dissociation Injuries From September 2001 to May 2008

Inclusion criteria:
• Evidence of zone 3 sacral fracture with associated lumbar fractures indicating loss of iliolumbar ligamentous complex integrity
• At least 1-year clinical follow-up
Patients:
• 23 lumbosacral dissociation injuries
• 6/23 (26.1%) open sacral fracture
• 15/23 (65.2%) H or U type zone 3 sacral fracture
• 8/23 (34.8%) severely comminuted sacral fracture
• 20/23 with neurologic injury at presentation (10 with sacral nerve root deficit and 7/10 having severely comminuted sacral fractures)
Outcomes:
• 9/23 (39.1%) nonoperative management
• 8/23 (34.8%) sacroiliac screw fixation
• 5/23 (21.7%) posterior spinal fusion with instrumentation and decompression
• 1/23 (4.4%) sacral plate
• 11/23 (48%) with residual pain and mean VAS 1.7, no difference between treatment groups
• 3/23 (13%) infection rate (2/3 open injury treated nonoperatively and 1/3 posterior spinal fusion requiring removal of instrumentation)
• 11/15 H or U type zone 3 sacral fractures presented with kyphosis, mean increase at follow-up 12 degrees
• 2/15 H or U type zone 3 sacral fractures treated nonoperatively, both with initial kyphosis >20 degrees had progression (1/2 required sacral nerve root decompression for progressive deficit)

WRAMC also performed a retrospective review of medical records and imaging studies of all combat casualties with lumbosacral dissociation injuries, defined by evidence of a zone III sacral fracture with associated lumbar fractures indicating loss of iliolumbar ligamentous complex integrity, treated during the Iraq and Afghanistan conflicts between September 2001 and May 2008, and with at least 1 year of clinical follow-up.[9] WRAMC has treated 23 such combat casualties with lumbosacral dissociation (Table 28-3). The criteria outlined by Denis and Roy-Camille were used to classify all sacral fractures.[80,86] Sacral kyphosis was determined using sagittal reconstructions of CT scans, with measurements taken from the cephalad endplate of S1 to the caudal aspect of S2 based on the CT sagittal reconstructions. WRAMC had an overall 13% infection rate, with a 33% rate in open lumbosacral dissociation injuries. Nonoperative management should be considered in patients with multiple severe injuries or large, open wounds, with expected immobility of more than 3 months. We found that most combat casualties with sacral nerve root injury

have gradual improvement within 1 year, and we recommend exploration and decompression of sacral nerve roots be individualized based on the patient's associated injuries and whether there is progressive neurologic deficit. Patients with operative management often complained of prominent instrumentation with associated skin ulceration, and therefore in these instances minimizing the prominence of iliac screws and posterior instrumentation should be a routine part of lumbopelvic fixation.

TREATMENT RECOMMENDATIONS: LOW LUMBAR SPINE BURST FRACTURE

Compared to the civilian trauma population, our combat casualty population has experienced an increased incidence of low lumbar spine burst factures sustained during the Iraq and Afghanistan conflicts, which is most likely secondary to the use of high-energy blast trauma from IEDs. These spine combat casualties have also demonstrated more significant neurologic injury. The high-energy blast experienced

Figure 28-1. Low lumbar burst fracture in a 26-year-old active duty soldier who sustained trauma from an air cargo resupply pallet that struck him on the right side of his body during an uncontrolled descent due to a parachute malfunction. He suffered a closed right distal humerus and distal fibula fracture, T8 compression fracture, and a low lumbar burst fracture at L5. He was wearing his protective body armor at the time of injury. On presentation, the patient had weakness in his L5 distribution with 4-/5 extensor hallusis longus strength and numbness within his first dorsal web space. (A-D) Preoperative reconstructed computed tomography axial and sagittal views at L5 demonstrate a burst fracture extending into the right pedicle and left lamina/facet, with an approximately 5-mm retropulsed fragment eccentric to the right, congenitally narrow canal with approximately 8.5-mm residual available canal diameter, and right L5 transverse process fracture.

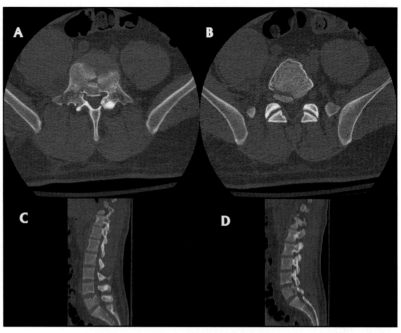

at the time of injury may also explain the persistence of neurologic deficit in one of our combat casualties with low lumbar spine burst fracture. This is compared to previous literature from civilian trauma institutions, which found resolution of neurologic deficit in all studied patients.[66,67,69-71] The increased incidence of low lumbar spine burst fractures is complex and multifactorial; however, another etiology is likely the recent advances, design, and rigidity of body armor, effectively lowering the transition zone that normally occurs at the thoracolumbar junction to the low lumbar spine. Based on our experience, we recommend surgical decompression and stabilization with interbody fusion and pedicle screw instrumentation in the presence of neurologic deficit or multiple injuries requiring early rehabilitation and mobilization in the combat casualty with a low lumbar spine fracture (Figures 28-1 through 28-3).

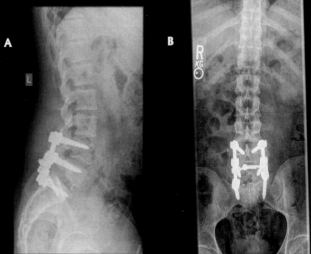

Figure 28-2. (A,B) Postoperative plain radiographs anterior-posterior and lateral views demonstrate posterior interbody fusion at L5-S1 with bilateral L4-S1 pedicle screw instrumentation.

TREATMENT RECOMMENDATIONS: LUMBOSACRAL DISSOCIATION

Lumbosacral dissociation injuries are rare in the civilian trauma population; however, there has been an increased incidence during the Iraq and Afghanistan conflicts, which is most likely secondary to exposure to high-energy blast trauma. Operative stabilization promotes healing and earlier mobilization, but is not without significant perioperative risk. We recommend operative fixation in patients with H or U type zone III sacral injury with initial kyphosis more than 20 degrees, as they may be more likely to have progression of kyphosis and subsequent sacral nerve root

impingement regardless of potential mobility status (Figures 28-4 through 28-7).

References

1. Gertzbein SD. Scoliosis Research Society. Multicenter spine fracture study. *Spine (Phila Pa 1976)*. 1992;17(5):528-540.
2. Wood K, Buttermann G, Mehbod A, et al. Operative compared with nonoperative treatment of a thoracolumbar burst fracture without neurological deficit. A prospective, randomized study. *J Bone Joint Surg Am*. 2003;85-A(5):773-781.
3. Patel AA, Vaccaro AR. Thoracolumbar spine trauma classification. *J Am Acad Orthop Surg*. 2010;18(2):63-71.

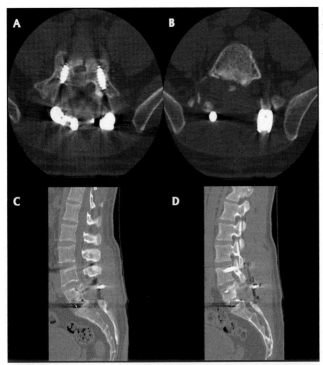

Figure 28-3. (A-D) Postoperative reconstructed computed tomography axial and sagittal views at L5, demonstrate L5 laminectomy and foraminal decompression, reduction of retropulsed fragments, with posterior interbody fusion with pedicle screw instrumentation.

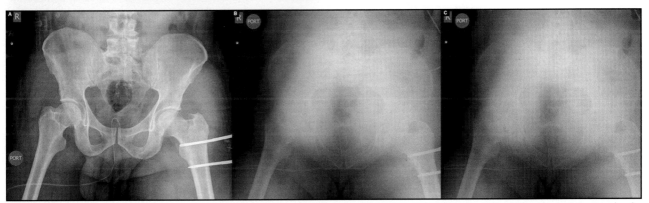

Figure 28-4. Lumbosacral dissociation in a 39-year-old active duty Marine who sustained trauma after his mine-resistant ambush-protected vehicle struck an IED. He sustained a left closed femur fracture, left closed comminuted calcaneus fracture, left minimally displaced metatarsal fracture, C1 lateral mass fracture, bilateral L5 transverse process fractures, T4/5 compression fractures, intraventricular/subarachnoid hemorrhages, and a complex H-type sacral fracture with lumbosacral dissociation. On presentation, the patient had no ability to move his left lower extremity. (A-C) Preoperative plain radiographs anteroposterior/inlet/outlet views demonstrate complex bilateral sacral fractures with minimal displacement and proximal pins of femur external fixator.

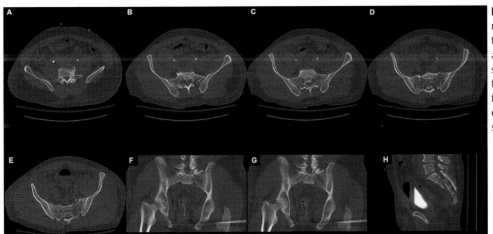

Figure 28-5. Preoperative reconstructed computed tomography axial, coronal, and sagittal views demonstrate complex H-type transforaminal through S1/2 sacral fracture with kyphosis and dorsal displacement of distal sacral segment S2/3.

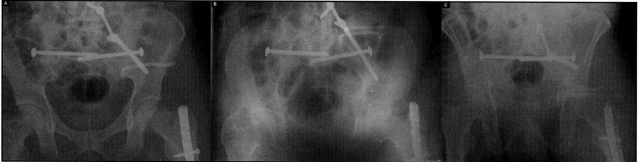

Figure 28-6. (A-D) Postoperative plain radiographs AP/inlet/outlet views demonstrate bilateral sacroiliac screw placement, with unilateral L4 to ilium pedicle screw instrumentation.

Figure 28-7. Postoperative reconstructed computed tomography axial, coronal, and sagittal views demonstrate bilateral sacroiliac screw placement, with unilateral L4 to ilium pedicle screw instrumentation.

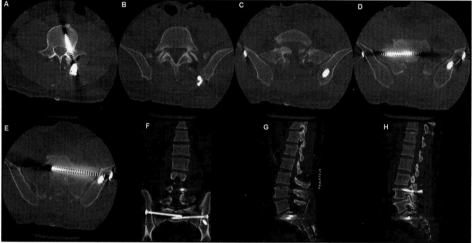

4. Hu R, Mustard CA, Burns C. Epidemiology of incident spinal fracture in a complete population. *Spine (Phila Pa 1976)*. 1996;21(4):492-499.

5. Bohlman HH. Treatment of fractures and dislocations of the thoracic and lumbar spine. *J Bone Joint Surg Am*. 1985;67(1):165-169.

6. Rechtine GR. Nonsurgical treatment of thoracic and lumbar fractures. *Instr Course Lect*. 1999;48:413-416.

7. Albert TJ, Levine MJ, An HS, Cotler JM, Balderston RA. Concomitant noncontiguous thoracolumbar and sacral fractures. *Spine (Phila Pa 1976)*. 1993;18(10):1285-1291.

8. Eckel TT, Lehman RA, Helgeson MD, Cooper, PB, Bellabarba C. Low lumbar burst fractures: a unique fracture mechanism sustained in our current overseas conflicts. In: 2nd Annual Lumbar Spine Research Society Meeting; April 2-3, 2009; Chicago, IL.

9. Helgeson MD, Lehman RA, Moore FM, Andersen RC, Frisch M. Retrospective review of lumbosacral dissociations in blast injuries. In: Society of Military Orthopedic Surgeons Annual Meeting; Dec 8-13, 2008; Las Vegas, NV.

10. Szul AC, Davis LB, Walter Reed Army Medical Center Borden Institute, eds. *Emergency War Surgery*. 3rd US rev. Washington, DC: Walter Reed Army Medical Center Borden Institute; 2004.

11. Slucky AV, Eismont FJ. Treatment of acute injury of the cervical spine. *Instr Course Lect*. 1995;44:67-80.

12. American College of Surgeons. *Advanced Trauma Life Support for Doctors Student Course Manual*. 8th ed. Chicago, IL: Author; 2008:157-186.

13. Berg EE. The sternal-rib complex. A possible fourth column in thoracic spine fractures. *Spine (Phila Pa 1976)*. 1993;18(13):1916-1919.

14. Cotler JM. Introduction to thoracolumbar fractures. *Instr Course Lect*. 1999;48:427-428.

15. Singh K, Vaccaro AR. Thoracic and lumbar trauma. In: Bono CM, Garfin SR, eds. *Spine*. Philadelphia, PA: Lippincott Williams & Wilkins; 2004:45-57.

16. Wiesel SW, Lauerman WC. The spine. In: Wiesel SW, Delahay JN, eds. *Principles of Orthopedic Medicine and Surgery*. Philadelphia, PA: WB Saunders; 2001:439-511.

17. Seybold EA, Sweeney CA, Fredrickson BE, Warhold LG, Bernini PM. Functional outcome of low lumbar burst fractures. A multicenter review of operative and nonoperative treatment of L3-L5. *Spine (Phila Pa 1976)*. 1999;24(20):2154-2161.

18. Hetz SP. Introduction to military medicine: a brief overview. *Surg Clin North Am*. 2006;86(3):675-688.

19. Bohlman HH, Kirkpatrick JS, Delamarter RB, Leventhal M. Anterior decompression for late pain and paralysis after fractures of the thoracolumbar spine. *Clin Orthop Relat Res*. 1994;300:24-29.

20. Vaccaro AR, An HS, Betz RR, Cotler JM, Balderston RA. The management of acute spinal trauma: prehospital and in-hospital emergency care. *Instr Course Lect*. 1997;46:113-125.

21. Sears W, Fazl M. Prediction of stability of cervical spine fracture managed in the halo vest and indications for surgical intervention. *J Neurosurg*. 1990;72(3):426-432.

22. Brown CV, Antevil JL, Sise MJ, Sack DI. Spiral computed tomography for the diagnosis of cervical, thoracic, and lumbar spine fractures: its time has come. *J Trauma*. 2005;58(5):890-895; discussion 895-896.

23. Berry GE, Adams S, Harris MB, et al. Are plain radiographs of the spine necessary during evaluation after blunt trauma? Accuracy of screening torso computed tomography in thoracic/lumbar spine fracture diagnosis. *J Trauma*. 2005;59(6):1410-1413; discussion 1413.

24. Sanchez B, Waxman K, Jones T, Conner S, Chung R, Becerra S. Cervical spine clearance in blunt trauma: evaluation of a computed tomography-based protocol. *J Trauma*. 2005;59(1):179-183.

25. Antevil JL, Sise MJ, Sack DI, Kidder B, Hopper A, Brown CV. Spiral computed tomography for the initial evaluation of spine trauma: a new standard of care? *J Trauma*. 2006;61(2):382-387.

26. Vaccaro AR, An HS, Lin S, Sun S, Balderston RA, Cotler JM. Noncontiguous injuries of the spine. *J Spinal Disord*. 1992;5(3):320-329.

27. Henderson RL, Reid DC, Saboe LA. Multiple noncontiguous spine fractures. *Spine (Phila Pa 1976)*. 1991;16(2):128-131.

28. Bono CM, Heary RF. Gunshot wounds to the spine. *Spine J*. 2004;4(2):230-240.

29. Bono CM, Vaccaro AR, Fehlings M, et al. Measurement techniques for lower cervical spine injuries: consensus statement of the Spine Trauma Study Group. *Spine (Phila Pa 1976)*. 2006;31(5):603-609.

30. Moore TA, Vaccaro AR, Anderson PA. Classification of lower cervical spine injuries. *Spine (Phila Pa 1976)*. 2006;31(11 Suppl):S37-S43; discussion S61.

31. Bracken MB, Shepard MJ, Collins WF Jr, et al. Methylprednisolone or naloxone treatment after acute spinal cord injury: 1-year follow-up data. Results of the second National Acute Spinal Cord Injury Study. *J Neurosurg*. 1992;76(1):23-31.

32. Bracken MB, Shepard MJ, Collins WF, et al. A randomized, controlled trial of methylprednisolone or naloxone in the treatment of acute spinal-cord injury. Results of the Second National Acute Spinal Cord Injury Study. *N Engl J Med*. 1990;322(20):1405-1411.

33. Bracken MB, Shepard MJ, Holford TR, et al. Methylprednisolone or tirilazad mesylate administration after acute spinal cord injury: 1-year follow up. Results of the third National Acute Spinal Cord Injury randomized controlled trial. *J Neurosurg*. 1998;89(5):699-706.

34. Coleman WP, Benzel D, Cahill DW, et al. A critical appraisal of the reporting of the National Acute Spinal Cord Injury Studies (II and III) of methylprednisolone in acute spinal cord injury. *J Spinal Disord*. 2000;13(3):185-199.

35. Levy ML, Gans W, Wijesinghe HS, SooHoo WE, Adkins RH, Stillerman CB. Use of methylprednisolone as an adjunct in the management of patients with penetrating spinal cord injury: outcome analysis. *Neurosurgery*. 1996;39(6):1141-1148; discussion 1148-1149.

36. Heary RF, Vaccaro AR, Mesa JJ, et al. Steroids and gunshot wounds to the spine. *Neurosurgery*. 1997;41(3):576-583; discussion 583-574.

37. Kumar A, Wood GW 2nd, Whittle AP. Low-velocity gunshot injuries of the spine with abdominal viscus trauma. *J Orthop Trauma*. 1998;12(7):514-517.

38. Kihtir T, Ivatury RR, Simon R, Stahl WM. Management of transperitoneal gunshot wounds of the spine. *J Trauma*. 1991;31(12):1579-1583.

39. Kitchel SH. Current treatment of gunshot wounds to the spine. *Clin Orthop Relat Res*. 2003;408:115-119.

40. Roffi RP, Waters RL, Adkins RH. Gunshot wounds to the spine associated with a perforated viscus. *Spine (Phila Pa 1976)*. 1989;14(8):808-811.

41. Romanick PC, Smith TK, Kopaniky DR, Oldfield D. Infection about the spine associated with low-velocity-missile injury to the abdomen. *J Bone Joint Surg Am*. 1985;67(8):1195-1201.

42. Waters RL, Sie IH. Spinal cord injuries from gunshot wounds to the spine. *Clin Orthop Relat Res*. 2003;408:120-125.

43. Parsons TW 3rd, Lauerman WC, Ethier DB, et al. Spine injuries in combat troops—Panama, 1989. *Mil Med*. 1993;158(7):501-502.

44. Splavski B, Vrankovic D, Saric G, Blagus G, Mursic B, Rukovanjski M. Early management of war missile spine and spinal cord injuries: experience with 21 cases. *Injury*. 1996;27(10):699-702.

45. Stauffer ES, Wood RW, Kelly EG. Gunshot wounds of the spine: the effects of laminectomy. *J Bone Joint Surg Am*. 1979;61(3):389-392.

46. Waters RL, Adkins RH. The effects of removal of bullet fragments retained in the spinal canal. A collaborative study by the National Spinal Cord Injury Model Systems. *Spine (Phila Pa 1976)*. 1991;16(8):934-939.

47. Cybulski GR, Stone JL, Kant R. Outcome of laminectomy for civilian gunshot injuries of the terminal spinal cord and cauda equina: review of 88 cases. *Neurosurgery*. 1989;24(3):392-397.

48. Robertson DP, Simpson RK, Narayan RK. Lumbar disc herniation from a gunshot wound to the spine. A report of two cases. *Spine (Phila Pa 1976)*. 1991;16(8):994-995.

49. Maniker AH, Gropper MR, Hunt CD. Transoral gunshot wounds to the atlanto-axial complex: report of five cases. *J Trauma*. 1994;37(5):858-861.

50. Fehlings MG. Editorial: recommendations regarding the use of methylprednisolone in acute spinal cord injury: making sense out of the controversy. *Spine (Phila Pa 1976)*. 2001;26(24 Suppl):S56-S57.

51. Marshall LF, Knowlton S, Garfin SR, et al. Deterioration following spinal cord injury. A multicenter study. *J Neurosurg*. 1987;66(3):400-404.

52. Vaccaro AR, Daugherty RJ, Sheehan TP, et al. Neurologic outcome of early versus late surgery for cervical spinal cord injury. *Spine (Phila Pa 1976)*. 1997;22(22):2609-2613.

53. Ducker TB, Bellegarrigue R, Salcman M, Walleck C. Timing of operative care in cervical spinal cord injury. *Spine (Phila Pa 1976)*. 1984;9(5):525-531.

54. Wagner FC Jr, Chehrazi B. Early decompression and neurological outcome in acute cervical spinal cord injuries. *J Neurosurg*. 1982;56(5):699-705.

55. Yazici M, Atilla B, Tepe S, Calisir A. Spinal canal remodeling in burst fractures of the thoracolumbar spine: a computerized tomographic comparison between operative and nonoperative treatment. *J Spinal Disord*. 1996;9(5):409-413.

56. Chakera TM, Bedbrook G, Bradley CM. Spontaneous resolution of spinal canal deformity after burst-dispersion fracture. *AJNR Am J Neuroradiol*. 1988;9(4):779-785.

57. de Klerk LW, Fontijne WP, Stijnen T, Braakman R, Tanghe HL, van Linge B. Spontaneous remodeling of the spinal canal after conservative management of thoracolumbar burst fractures. *Spine (Phila Pa 1976)*. 1998;23(9):1057-1060.

58. Sandor L, Barabas D. [Spontaneous "regeneration" of the spinal canal in traumatic bone fragments after fractures of the thoraco-lumbar transition and the lumbar spine]. *Unfallchirurg*. 1994;97(2):89-91.

59. Mumford J, Weinstein JN, Spratt KF, Goel VK. Thoracolumbar burst fractures. The clinical efficacy and outcome of nonoperative management. *Spine (Phila Pa 1976)*. 1993;18(8):955-970.

60. Vaccaro AR, Lehman RA Jr, Hurlbert RJ, et al. A new classification of thoracolumbar injuries: the importance of injury morphology, the integrity of the posterior ligamentous complex, and neurologic status. *Spine (Phila Pa 1976)*. 2005;30(20):2325-2333.

61. Verlaan JJ, Diekerhof CH, Buskens E, et al. Surgical treatment of traumatic fractures of the thoracic and lumbar spine: a systematic review of the literature on techniques, complications, and outcome. *Spine (Phila Pa 1976)*. 2004;29(7):803-814.

62. Dai LD. Low lumbar spinal fractures: management options. *Injury.* 2002;33(7):579-582.

63. Blanco JF, De Pedro JA, Hernandez PJ, Paniagua JC, Framinan A. Conservative management of burst fractures of the fifth lumbar vertebra. *J Spinal Disord Tech.* 2005;18(3):229-231.

64. Gertzbein SD. Neurologic deterioration in patients with thoracic and lumbar fractures after admission to the hospital. *Spine (Phila Pa 1976).* 1994;19(15):1723-1725.

65. Kraemer WJ, Schemitsch EH, Lever J, McBroom RJ, McKee MD, Waddell JP. Functional outcome of thoracolumbar burst fractures without neurological deficit. *J Orthop Trauma.* 1996;10(8):541-544.

66. Levine AM, Edwards CC. Low lumbar burst fractures. Reduction and stabilization using the modular spine fixation system. *Orthopedics.* 1988;11(10):1427-1432.

67. Andreychik DA, Alander DH, Senica KM, Stauffer ES. Burst fractures of the second through fifth lumbar vertebrae. Clinical and radiographic results. *J Bone Joint Surg Am.* 1996;78(8):1156-1166.

68. Korovessis P, Baikousis A, Zacharatos S, Petsinis G, Koureas G, Iliopoulos P. Combined anterior plus posterior stabilization versus posterior short-segment instrumentation and fusion for mid-lumbar (L2-L4) burst fractures. *Spine (Phila Pa 1976).* 2006;31(8):859-868.

69. Mick CA, Carl A, Sachs B, Hresko MT, Pfeifer BA. Burst fractures of the fifth lumbar vertebra. *Spine (Phila Pa 1976).* 1993;18(13):1878-1884.

70. Butler JS, Fitzpatrick P, Ni Mhaolain AM, Synnott K, O'Byrne JM. The management and functional outcome of isolated burst fractures of the fifth lumbar vertebra. *Spine (Phila Pa 1976).* 2007;32(4):443-447.

71. Finn CA, Stauffer ES. Burst fracture of the fifth lumbar vertebra. *J Bone Joint Surg Am.* 1992;74(3):398-403.

72. Schildhauer TA, Bellabarba C, Nork SE, Barei DP, Routt ML Jr, Chapman JR. Decompression and lumbopelvic fixation for sacral fracture-dislocations with spino-pelvic dissociation. *J Orthop Trauma.* 2006;20(7):447-457.

73. Vresilovic EJ, Mehta S, Placide R, Milam RA. Traumatic spondylopelvic dissociation. A report of two cases. *J Bone Joint Surg Am.* 2005;87(5):1098-1103.

74. Bellabarba C, Schildhauer TA, Vaccaro AR, Chapman JR. Complications associated with surgical stabilization of high-grade sacral fracture dislocations with spino-pelvic instability. *Spine (Phila Pa 1976).* 2006;31(11 Suppl):S80-S88; discussion S104.

75. Bents RT, France JC, Glover JM, Kaylor KL. Traumatic spondylopelvic dissociation. A case report and literature review. *Spine (Phila Pa 1976).* 1996;21(15):1814-1819.

76. Van Savage JG, Dahners LE, Renner JB, Baker CC. Fracture-dislocation of the lumbosacral spine: case report and review of the literature. *J Trauma.* 1992;33(5):779-784.

77. Marcus RE, Hansen ST Jr. Bilateral fracture-dislocation of the sacrum. A case report. *J Bone Joint Surg Am.* 1984;66(8):1297-1299.

78. Singh AK, Fleetcroft JP. Bilateral fracture-dislocation of the sacrum. *Injury.* 1989;20(5):301-303.

79. Nork SE, Jones CB, Harding SP, Mirza SK, Routt ML Jr. Percutaneous stabilization of U-shaped sacral fractures using iliosacral screws: technique and early results. *J Orthop Trauma.* 2001;15(4):238-246.

80. Roy-Camille R, Saillant G, Gagna G, Mazel C. Transverse fracture of the upper sacrum. Suicidal jumper's fracture. *Spine (Phila Pa 1976).* 1985;10(9):838-845.

81. Sabiston CP, Wing PC. Sacral fractures: classification and neurologic implications. *J Trauma.* 1986;26(12):1113-1115.

82. Strange-Vognsen HH, Lebech A. An unusual type of fracture in the upper sacrum. *J Orthop Trauma.* 1991;5(2):200-203.

83. Fountain SS, Hamilton RD, Jameson RM. Transverse fractures of the sacrum. A report of six cases. *J Bone Joint Surg.* 1977;59(4):486-489.

84. Bucknill TM, Blackburne JS. Fracture-dislocations of the sacrum. Report of three cases. *J Bone Joint Surg Br.* 1976;58-B(4):467-470.

85. Ebraheim NA, Biyani A, Salpietro B. Zone III fractures of the sacrum. A case report. *Spine.* 1996;21(20):2390-2396.

86. Denis F, Davis S, Comfort T. Sacral fractures: an important problem. Retrospective analysis of 236 cases. *Clin Orthop Relat Res.* 1988;227:67-81.

Chapter 29

SPINE NEUROLOGIC INJURY

CDR David E. Gwinn, MD and LTC Michael K. Rosner, MD

Spinal cord and spinal nerve injury can cause significant functional limitations to the injured patient. These injuries often result from a high degree of trauma with possible spinal column instability, head injury, and hollow organ injury. Open, contaminated wounds may accompany combat-related neurologic injuries if the etiology is a penetrating mechanism of high-velocity projectiles and blast fragments. The purpose of this chapter is to provide a detailed overview of spine neurologic injury resulting from combat and the management of these injuries at the different echelons of care.

Epidemiology

The characteristics of spine neurologic injury differ significantly between the civilian and combat-injured populations. The vast majority of civilian spine neurologic injuries are secondary to blunt force trauma sustained in motor vehicle accidents, falls, and recreational sport activities. In combat, approximately 40% of spine neurologic injuries are due to penetrating trauma.[1] The high-velocity nature of the bullet and blast wounds causing these injuries may lead to a degree of wound contamination and spinal column instability not seen in civilian penetrating injuries. Although the percentage of penetrating injuries is higher in combat casualties in Operation Iraqi Freedom/Operation Enduring Freedom (OIF/OEF), the percentage of thoracic wounds that could potentially cause a spine neurologic injury is significantly less than historical data from World War II and the Vietnam War due to the efficacy of modern body armor.[2]

Whereas the civilian-injured patient usually has near immediate care at Level I trauma centers providing both resuscitation and definitive spinal management, the combat casualty requires evacuation through echelons of care before definitive treatment can be administered. These evacuations may cause a time delay in definitive treatment. Potter and colleagues reported that definitive treatment of spine combat casualties averaged 8.3 days during the beginning of the Iraq and Afghanistan Wars.[1] Despite the lengthy evacuation chain required in a combat environment, treatment of spinal column and spinal cord injury has yielded comparable results, in regard to neurologic outcomes, to the civilian population.

Management in Theater

Tenets of initial management of the patient with suspected spine neurologic injury are similar between the combat casualty and civilians, with the exception of available resources and physical safety. Aspects of management will be specifically discussed according to the echelon of care and available resources. The echelon of care is the classic definition for care often used in warfare manuals regarding medical management. Current conflicts have often merged the echelons of care as combat support hospitals have moved closer to the front lines of the battlefields and are equipped with resources similar to a Level I trauma center.

Owens BD, Belmont PJ Jr, eds. *Combat Orthopedic Surgery: Lessons Learned in Iraq and Afghanistan (pp 311-318)*
© 2011 SLACK Incorporated

ECHELON I

Resources for the combat medic in the battlefield may be limited to dressings, cervical collars, stretchers for evacuation, and intravenous fluids. Specific skills and knowledge required at this level of care include Advanced Trauma Life Support (ATLS), recognition of the patient with potential spinal column or cord injury, and immobilization and transportation techniques. The combat medic prioritizes the need for evacuation to a more secure area over all other aspects. Evacuation to a more secure area takes precedence over spine immobilization in order to provide safety to both the combat casualty and provider, and immediate life-preserving measures (ATLS) take precedence over spine evaluation and immobilization.

The primary survey to identify and manage airway, breathing, and circulatory dysfunction according to ATLS guidelines should begin as soon as possible. A rapid neurologic assessment, part of the secondary survey, should be done to unmask the presence of spinal cord or column injury. On the battlefield, this may be as basic as observing for, or eliciting, purposeful lower extremity movement or testing sacral sensation.

Patients suspected of sustaining spinal injury should be immobilized for transportation as quickly as possible. Specifically, the criteria most predictive of the need for immobilization of a potential spinal column injury include focal neurologic deficits, altered mental status, spinal pain or tenderness, and evidence of an extremity fracture in cases of blunt trauma.[3] Patients resisting trunk movement, holding their head in their hands, or with palpable spinal step-off should also be suspected of having an unstable injury. Immobilization includes application of a rigid cervical collar, placement on a firm backboard using the 2-man log-roll technique, and in-line immobilization of the head in an eyes-forward posture using tape or sandbags. This principle of early prehospital recognition and immobilization, although not directly supported by Level I evidence, has accompanied a dramatic decrease in complete spinal cord injuries during the past 30 years.[4] Patients who cannot be immobilized due to an austere environment can be manually transported to a safe place using a 2-man carry; however, the cervical spine is not stabilized during this maneuver. Evidence from the current conflict shows that rigid cervical immobilization is rarely required in cases of penetrating neck trauma.[5]

All patients with a suspected spinal cord injury should be given supplemental oxygen, if available, to limit further neurologic injury due to hypoxemia. Obtunded patients should have early placement of an endotracheal or nasotracheal tube, which can be safely accomplished with limited neck extension. Intravenous isotonic saline solution infusion should be initiated.

Transportation to higher echelons of care should be achieved as soon as possible. Efforts at continued hemodynamic resuscitation and immobilization should occur in route but cannot delay transportation.[6] Air and ground transportation has been shown to be equally safe depending on the combat location, and the transport decisions should be based on availability, terrain environment, and speed.[7]

ECHELON II (FORWARD SURGICAL TEAMS) AND ECHELON III (COMBAT SUPPORT HOSPITALS)

Resources at these levels of care include medical and surgical capabilities allowing for emergency room-type triage, wound debridement, hemorrhage control, vascular repair, basic imaging (advanced at some current locations to include computed tomography [CT]), and advanced medical stabilization capabilities. In addition to managing airway and hemodynamic problems, providers must be able to conduct a detailed neurologic exam, classify the level and extent of neurologic injury, and conduct emergent surgical decompression. Surgical spine specialists may be located at the Combat Support Hospital locations and can assist with all management of spinal column instability.

The primary survey is repeated at initial entry to this level of care, and ATLS principles continue to be followed regarding the airway, breathing, and circulation. This may be the first place that frequent hemodynamic monitoring is available, and mean arterial pressure should be kept above 85 mm Hg to limit the effect of hypotension on an already injured spinal cord.[8] Neurogenic shock, which can result from high thoracic and cervical spinal cord injury, needs to be identified early when hypotension is accompanied by bradycardia. Advanced cardiac monitoring and the use of vasopressors are required to control hypotension in these patients when it is available at these echelons of care and no contraindications exist.

Hypoxemia should be addressed with supplemental oxygen. Patients with decreased respiratory drive due to unconsciousness or with poor mechanical ventilation due to a cervical spinal cord injury above the C5 level should be intubated. PaO_2 should be kept above 100 mm Hg in these individuals.[9]

Providers should recognize and document spinal shock, characterized by areflexic, anesthetic, flaccid paralysis and an absent bulbocavernosus reflex. Spinal shock, when it subsides, following the return of the bulbocavernosus reflex, allows complete classification of the neurologic deficit. It should be noted, however, that in the case of injuries to the conus medullaris, the bulbocavernosus reflex may not return.

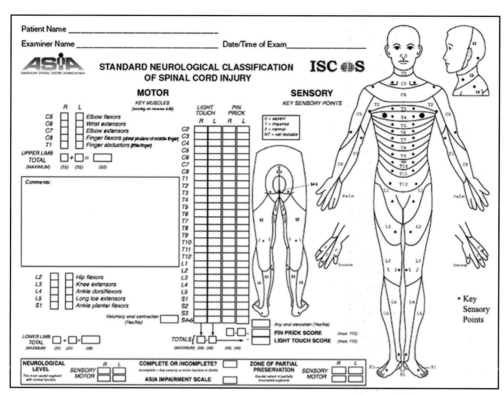

Figure 29-1. American Spinal Injury Association Standard Neurological Classification of Spinal Cord Injury. (Reprinted with permission from American Spinal Injury Association: International Standards for Neurological Classification of Spinal Cord Injury, revised 2000; Atlanta, GA. Reprinted 2008.)

A detailed neurologic exam, according to the American Spinal Injury Association (ASIA), should be conducted as early as possible to establish the level and extent of injury (Figure 29-1). Determination of an initial ASIA grade is necessary in order to monitor for new or progressive neurologic injury throughout the evacuation chain, to communicate to the next echelon when transferring care, and to determine prognosis.

Noncontiguous spine fractures may occur in up to 16.7% of cases when blunt trauma causes a spinal column injury regardless of neurologic status.[10] For this reason, orthogonal radiographs should be obtained for the entire spine at this level of care when spinal column injury is suspected or detected.

New or worsening neurologic deficits should be detected with periodic exams. Emergent decompression, when facilities and expertise allow, should be accomplished as quickly as possible in these cases to maximize neurologic outcomes. Although instrumentation for definitive spinal column stabilization is not always available at these levels of care, in our experience, decompression can be safely performed and patients transported with external immobilization.

Cervical dislocation with spinal cord injury should be reduced with manual or controlled weighted traction and externally immobilized. There is significant debate in regard to the protocol for evaluating and treating patients with cervical facet dislocations in the civilian sector.[11,12] This debate revolves around the use of magnetic resonance imaging (MRI) to detect herniated disks, which are present in up to 50% of

these injuries, that may cause neurologic worsening in obtunded or incoherent patients who cannot participate in neurologic exams during attempted closed reductions.[13] At this level of care, without access to MRI and with potential for delay in transfer, it is reasonable to reduce these dislocations as soon as possible and to apply external immobilization.

Based on timing within the evacuation chain, it is at this level that neuroprotective medical interventions, such as administration of high-dose methylprednisolone during the first 8 hours after injury, would be applied in the civilian community. The National Acute Spinal Cord Injury Study (NASCIS) II and III trials showed beneficial effects of these high-dose steroids in improving motor function of spinal cord-injured patients.[14,15] However, these studies are considered controversial based on scrutiny of their methods (functional outcomes were not assessed) and post-hoc statistical analysis. Furthermore, due to the significant side effects including increased risk of infection, this intervention is not recommended for use in the battlefield where open contaminated wounds and penetrating spinal cord injury are commonplace.[16]

It is important for the provider at this level of care to recognize when unnecessary spinal immobilization has been applied. Immobilized patients have an increased risk of aspiration, respiratory limitations, and increased intracranial pressures.[17,18] Some patients suspected of spinal column injuries may have been immobilized on the battlefield but upon further evaluation do not have a neurologic deficit or spinal column instability. The alert patient with neck pain and a normal neurologic exam can be cleared of cervical spine bracing with patient-controlled dynamic flexion extension radiographic examination if CT imaging is not available. Those patients without neck pain or a history of distracting injuries can be cleared without x-rays.[19] In those cases with mental status changes, advanced imaging such as CT scan or MRI is required. These imaging modalities may not be available at lower echelons of care and management may be at the discretion of the treating physician.

ECHELON IV AND ECHELON V

Resources at these levels include advanced imaging, intensive care units, spine surgeons, spinal implants, and operative capabilities for definitive care. Transfer of patients with stable neurologic deficits from Echelon III to Echelons IV and V can usually be accomplished in 24 to 72 hours.

Definitive Management

Definitive management involves decompression, restoring spinal column stability, and initiating functional rehabilitation in the neurologically injured patient. This section will focus on the principles, timing, and techniques of decompression.

The decision to decompress the spinal canal depends on multiple factors, including the mechanism of injury (penetrating or blunt) and the location (anterior or posterior) of ongoing compressive pathology.

PENETRATING TRAUMA

All spine combat casualties with penetrating spinal column trauma should receive tetanus prophylaxis and broad-spectrum antibiotic coverage as quickly as possible. Antibiotic coverage should be continued for a minimum of 48 to 72 hours. If associated abdominal viscous injury has occurred, particularly injury to the colon, intravenous antibiotics should be continued for 7 to 14 days.[20-22] In the typical scenario, antibiotics will be continued for 14 days. Wound cultures have limited utility in this setting, and antibiotics should not be delayed in order to obtain them. This protocol has resulted in an extremely low rate of spinal infection and meningitis.[21-23] The use of diverting colostomy or wound debridement has not appeared to influence the rate of spinal infection.[24]

Surgical intervention is rarely indicated in patients with penetrating spinal column trauma. Decompressive surgery has not been shown to improve neurologic outcomes in patients with complete or stable incomplete spinal cord injuries when compared to observation.[25] Surgically treated patients may be at risk for a

higher rate of complications, including spinal instability, wound infection, and spinal fistulae. The only absolute surgical indication, other than spinal column instability, is a progressive or new neurologic deficit with a radiologically identifiable cause. Preferably, serial neurologic exams by a single experienced observer would be used to detect these changes. This is not possible within the evacuation chain required in combat casualty care and highlights the importance of a detailed documented neurologic exam at a lower level of care and the communication (verbal and written) that is essential upon transfer to higher echelons of care. Plain radiography, available at lower echelons of care, may be able to identify patients with metallic or bony fragments causing neural compression. CT myelogram may additionally detect compressive epidural hematoma. This technology will likely be available at an Echelon IV treatment facility and would be preferable to use diagnostically if accessible in a timely manner. MRI for patients with penetrating spinal trauma remains controversial over concerns that metallic fragment migration may worsen neurologic insult. It is advisable to avoid MRI early in the care of these patients.

The patient with a new or progressive neurologic deficit should receive decompression, generally with a laminectomy via a posterior approach, with removal of the compressive pathology. Principles for providing concurrent spinal stability with instrumentation should be followed as outlined in the previous chapter. If spinal instrumentation or technical expertise in using the instrumentation is not available at the lower echelons of care, decompression should still be accomplished by a qualified provider with spinal precautions maintained postoperatively. Traditionally, penetrating spinal column trauma does not induce instability requiring operative stabilization. However, the high-velocity nature of modern weaponry has increased the incidence of spinal instability as evidenced by a study from Potter and colleagues in which 36% of penetrating spinal wounds were found to require stabilization.[1]

Cerebrospinal fluid (CSF) leak, CSF fistula, and prevention of metal toxicity have been identified by some surgeons as relative indications for surgery. In most cases, these situations can be managed safely with nonoperative treatment including subarachnoid drains and wound packing for CSF leaks and observation for symptoms in those with retained intradural metallic fragments. Although intradural lead and copper fragments have induced toxicity in laboratory animals, relatively few clinical cases of fragment migration or elution toxicity have been reported.[26-28] In these cases, surgery can be delayed in favor of conservative treatment and can be performed on an elective basis.

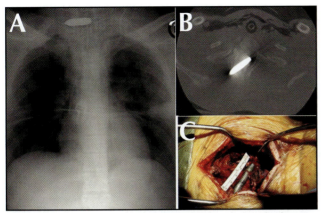

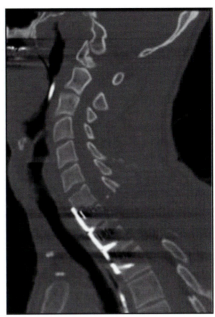

Figure 29-4. Postoperative mid-canal sagittal CT scan showing anterior plate and interbody grafts following C7-T2 anterior discectomy and fusion.

Figure 29-2. (A) Anterior-posterior chest radiograph showing metallic foreign body lodged in the midline at the T2 level. (B) Axial CT scan showing the the metallic foreign body lodged within the spinal canal and through the right T2 lamina. (C) Intraoperative photograph showing the foreign body following laminectomy and removal.

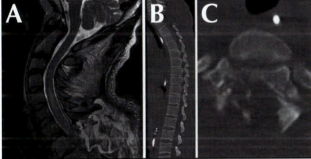

Figure 29-3. Post-decompression imaging obtained upon transfer to tertiary care facility. (A) Sagittal T2-weighted MRI demonstrating posterior cerebrospinal fluid leak. (B) Sagittal CT scan demonstrating laminectomy and anterolisthesis of T1 on T2. (C) Axial CT image at the level of the T2 costovertebral joint showing destruction of the pedicles.

Case 1

A 22-year-old male servicemember sustained a high-velocity gunshot wound to the neck with complete spinal cord injury, ASIA A classification, below the level of injury. A cervical collar was applied, and broad-spectrum antibiotics were initiated. Within 24 hours, he was transferred to an Echelon IV facility in Germany. Initial radiographs and CT scans demonstrated a large metallic fragment that traversed the left T2 pedicle and shattered the posterior elements while remaining incarcerated in the spinal canal (Figure 29-2). Because of the size and location of the foreign body, and the potential for persistent CSF fistula or leak, a posterior T1 and T2 decompression with foreign body removal was performed. Upon arrival at Walter Reed Army Medical Center (WRAMC), an MRI and CT scan were obtained (Figure 29-3). The studies revealed a transection of the spinal cord at T1-2, partial destruc-

tion of the T1 posterior inferior vertebral body with anterolisthesis of T1 on T2, and complete destruction of the left T2 pedicle and costovertebral joints. CSF leaks were appreciated both anterior and posterior to the spinal canal. Because of the spinal instability, C7-T2 anterior discectomy and instrumented fusion were performed (Figure 29-4). The patient was transferred to a rehabilitation center 1 week following surgery.

CLOSED/BLUNT TRAUMA

Patients with a neurologic injury associated with a closed spinal column injury almost universally have some degree of instability requiring surgical intervention, including decompression and possibly instrumented stabilization. Decompression of compressive spinal cord lesions should be performed as soon as the patient is medically stable. Immediate decompression compared to nonoperative treatment has been found to result in substantial improvements in neurologic recovery and patient outcomes.[29] Although no prospective randomized series has shown a benefit of early (less than 72 hours) versus late decompression, animal studies have shown significant benefits for decompression performed within 24 hours.[30-32] Most clinicians consider incomplete spinal cord injuries to be more urgent than complete injuries because of the potential for ongoing compression to contribute to worsening neurologic injury. In spine combat casualties with contaminated open wounds, an increased concern for infection exists when considering spinal instrumentation. This concern should not delay early decompression in instances where external spinal immobilization can provisionally stabilize until the spine instrumentation can occur.

Spinal cord decompression should be performed from the direction of the compressive insult except in some instances where a thoracolumbar burst fracture may be reduced and neural elements decompressed via a posterior approach.[33] Dislocated and deformed segments should be reduced and stabilized with instrumented fusion to maximize canal diameter and prevent the deleterious effects of persistent deformity.

Case 2

A 24-year-old male servicemember sustained an axial load injury to the head while unloading a helicopter. He was completely neurologically intact upon initial evaluation (ASIA E), was placed in a cervical collar, and was transported to the nearest combat support hospital. Upon arrival, radiographs showed a cervical compression-extension injury (Figure 29-5). A neurosurgeon at the combat support hospital recognized progressive quadraparesis by serial exam and performed an urgent posterior decompression via laminectomy at C5. The patient was placed in a cervical collar and was transferred to WRAMC. Upon arrival, he had regained full strength and sensory function. The patient underwent a posterior instrumented spinal fusion from C4 to C6 (see Figure 29-5). This case highlights the benefits of early decompression, the importance of serial neurologic exams along the evacuation chain, and the safety of transportation in external immobilization prior to definitive fixation.

Outcomes

In the most recent review of combat-related spinal injuries evacuated to WRAMC during the current conflict, 112 of 5000 patients sustained spinal column injuries.[1] Of these patients, 78 (70%) were treated surgically, 61 had multilevel injuries (11 noncontiguous), and 31 had complete or incomplete spinal cord injuries. By anatomic region, 36% were cervical, 33% lumbar, 22% thoracic, and 9% were sacral. Fifty-two (67%) of the 78 patients treated surgically received stabilization procedures, including 36% of penetrating and 54% of blunt injuries. Nine of the 20 spinal cord-injured patients who received stabilizing surgery had neurologic improvement of at least one Frankel grade. It should be noted that the patients included in this study were all evacuated through the echelons of care as previously described. Fewer than 1% of these patients experience neurologic deterioration during evacuation.[1]

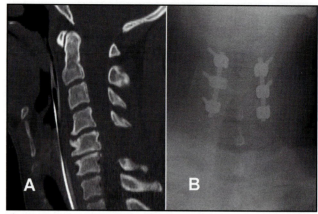

Figure 29-5. (A) Initial post-decompression mid-canal sagittal CT scan showing laminectomy defect at C5. (B) Anterior-posterior cervical radiograph following posterior instrumented fusion from C4 to C6.

Complications

After decompression and stabilization, the most important aspect of managing the neurologically injured patient is prevention and management of complications related to the injury itself as well as surgical intervention. This section will highlight some of the complications directly managed by the spine surgeon, including early and late perioperative complications. This section does not discuss long-term concerns such as diet, bladder management, and functional rehabilitation.

DEEP VEIN THROMBOSIS/ PULMONARY EMBOLISM

Deep vein thrombosis (DVT) and pulmonary embolism (PE) have a frequency between 67% and 100% in the spinal cord-injured patient in the absence of thromboprophylaxis.[34,35] PE is the third most common cause of death in this population.[36] Hypercoagulability begins within hours of injury and persists for 2 to 3 weeks. The risk of DVT and PE is the greatest within the first 12 weeks after injury.[37]

Thromboprophylaxis should be used in all patients and should be initiated as soon as possible. Prophylaxis should last at least 3 months or until the conclusion of inpatient rehabilitation.[38] Mechanical prophylaxis should be used in all patients as soon as possible. Patients with intracranial bleeding, active hemorrhage, hemothorax, or intra-abdominal bleeding should have pharmacologic prophylaxis delayed until neurologically and hemodynamically stable.[34] Heparin and oral anticoagulants are effective for the prevention of DVT and PE in spinal cord-injured patients. Low-molecular weight heparin is more effective for preventing DVT and causes less bleeding complications when compared with unfractionated heparin.[38] Pharmacologic treatment should be used for an additional 6 to 12 months in patients who develop DVT or PE. Placement of a temporary IVC filter should be considered in patients with contraindications to pharmacoprophylaxis, long-bone fractures, pending surgery, or DVT/PE despite mechanical or pharmacologic prophylaxis.[39]

GASTROINTESTINAL STRESS ULCERATION

Gastrointestinal ulcers are a common finding in spine-injured patients and may lead to significant morbidity and mortality. Spinal cord injury has been identified as an independent risk factor for stress ulceration and can be difficult to diagnose and treat in this population due to neurologic dysfunction. Prevention with acid-neutralizing pharmacoprophylaxis should be instituted in all patients for at least 3 weeks following the injury and continued further until normal diet routines are established.[40]

RESPIRATORY COMPLICATIONS

Due to decreased respiratory drive and vital capacity, respiratory complications occur with high frequency in spinal cord injury patients and are the most common cause of acute morbidity and mortality in this population.[41] After the first 3 weeks, there are generally improvements in respiratory function with decreasing edema and spasticity of the costal musculature. Early respiratory physiotherapy to clear secretions and maintain lung volumes consists of breathing exercises, postural drainage, chest percussion, and assisted coughing. Use of these techniques has decreased the incidence of pneumonia, atelectasis, tracheostomy, and prolonged mechanical ventilation and has decreased intensive care unit stays.[42,43]

DECUBITI

Pressure ulcers also increase morbidity and mortality in the patient with a spinal cord injury. Pressure ulceration may occur within 2 hours of backboard immobilization and as early as 30 minutes in a hypotensive patient. Infections due to pressure ulcers may result in amputations, prolonged hospitalizations, additional surgical procedures, and death. Prevention with frequent turning, specialty beds, padding of bony surfaces, and skin examinations twice per day should be initiated as soon as possible.

POST-TRAUMATIC SYRINGOMYELIA

Intramedullary cysts can form when CSF flow is disrupted at the site of spinal cord injury. When these cysts form cephalad to the injury site, patients can experience ascending paralysis or sensory loss. Post-traumatic syringomyelia has a reported incidence between 3% and 28% and can appear from days to years after initial injury.[44,45] Risk factors for development of post-traumatic syringomyelia include residual canal stenosis or deformity, highlighting the importance of surgical planning and technique in the acute phase.[45,46] Treatment involves surgery to address residual canal stenosis and/or deformity, subarachnoid adhesions, and shunting of CSF to the peritoneum.[46,47] Treatment with these techniques has generally been successful in stabilizing or reversing neurologic deficits secondary to syringomyelia, making prompt recognition and patient education on this process extremely important.

References

1. Potter BK, Groth AT, Javernick MA, et al. Evacuation and management of patients with combat-related spinal injuries. *Contemporary Spine Surgery.* 2005;6(8):53-60.
2. Belmont PJ, Goodman GP, Zacchelli M, et al. Incidence and epidemiology of combat injuries sustained during "the surge" portion of Operation Iraqi Freedom by a U.S. Army Brigade Combat Team. *J Trauma.* 2010;68(1):204-210.
3. Domeier RM, Swor RM, Evans RW, et al. Multicenter prospective validation of prehospital clinical spinal clearance criteria. *J Trauma.* 2002;53(4):744-750.
4. Garfin SR, Shackford SR, Marshall LF, et al. Care of the multiply injured patient with cervical spine injury. *Clin Orthop.* 1989;239:19-29.
5. Ramasamy A, Midwinter M, Mahoney P, et al. Learning the lessons from conflict: pre-hospital cervical spine stabilization following ballistic neck trauma. *Injury.* 2009;40(12):1342-1345.
6. American College of Surgeons. *Advanced Trauma Life Support Program for Doctors Instructor Course Manual.* 6th ed. Chicago, IL: Author; 1997:263-300.
7. Burney RE, Waggoner R, Maynard FM. Stabilization of spinal injury for early transfer. *J Trauma.* 1989;29:1497-1499.
8. Vale FL, Burns J, Jackson AB, et al. Combine medical and surgical treatment after acute spinal cord injury: results of a prospective pilot study to assess the merits of aggressive medical resuscitation and blood pressure management. *J Neurosurg.* 1997;87:239-246.
9. Dyson-Hudson TA, Stein AB. Acute management of traumatic cervical spinal cord injuries. *Mt Sinai J Med.* 1999;66:170-178.
10. Tearse DS, Keene JS, Drummond DS. Management of non-contiguous vertebral fractures. *Paraplegia.* 1987;25(2):100-105.
11. Arnold PM, Brodke DS, Rampersaud YR, et al. Differences between neurosurgeons and orthopedic surgeons in classifying cervical dislocation injuries and making assessment and treatment decisions: a multicenter reliability study. *Am J Orthop.* 2009;38(10):E156-E161.
12. Grauer JN, Vaccaro AR, Lee JY, et al. The timing and influence of MRI on the management of patients with cervical facet dislocations remains highly variable: a survey of members of the Spine Trauma Study Group. *J Spinal Disord Tech.* 2009;22(2):96-99.
13. Vaccaro AR, Madigan L, Schweitzer ME, et al. Magnetic resonance imaging analysis of soft tissue disruption after flexion distraction injuries of the cervical spine. *Spine.* 2001;26(17):1866-1872.
14. Bracken MB, Shepard MJ, Collins WF, et al. A randomized, controlled trial of methylprednisolone or naloxone in the treatment of acute spinal-cord injury: results of the Second National Acute Spinal-Cord Injury Study. *N Engl J Med.* 1990;322:1405-1411.

15. Bracken MB, Shepard MJ, Holford TR, et al. Administration of methylprednisolone for 24 or 48 hours or tirilizad mesylate for 48 hours in the treatment of acute spinal cord injury. Result of the Third National Acute Spinal Cord Injury Randomized Controlled Trial. National Acute Spinal Cord Injury Study. *JAMA.* 1997;277(20):1597-1604.

16. Matsumoto T, Tamaki T, Kawakami M, et al. Early complications of high-dose methylprednisolone sodium succinate treatment in the follow-up of acute spinal-cord injury. *Spine.* 2001;26:426-430.

17. Davies G, Deakin C, Wilson A. The effect of a rigid collar on intracranial pressure. *Injury.* 1996;27(9):647-649.

18. Tintinalli JE, Claffey J. Complications of nasotracheal intubation. *Ann Emerg Med.* 1981;10:142-144.

19. Anderson PA, Muchow RD, Munoz A, et al. Clearance of the asymptomatic cervical spine: a meta-analysis. *J Orthop Trauma.* 2010;24(2):100-106.

20. Kumar A, Wood GW 2nd, Whittle AP. Low-velocity gunshot injuries of the spine with abdominal viscous trauma. *J Orthop Trauma.* 1998;12:514-517.

21. Roffi RP, Waters RL, Adkins RH. Gunshot wounds to the spine associated with a perforated viscous. *Spine.* 1989;14(8):808-811.

22. Romanick PC, Smith TK, Kopaniky DR, et al. Infection about the spine associated with low-velocity-missile injury to the abdomen. *J Bone Joint Surg Am.* 1985;67(8):1195-1201.

23. Heary RF, Vaccaro AR, Mesa JJ, et al. Thoracolumbar infections in penetrating injuries to the spine. *Orthop Clin North Am.* 1996;27:69-81.

24. Bono CM, Heary RF. Gunshot wounds to the spine. *Spine J.* 2004;4(2):230-240.

25. Stauffer ES, Wood RW, Kelly EG. Gunshot wounds of the spine: the effects of laminectomy. *J Bone Joint Surg Am.* 1979;61:389-392.

26. Tindel NL, Marcillo AE, Tay BK, et al. The effect of surgically implanted bullet fragments on the spinal cord in a rabbit model. *J Bone Joint Surg Am.* 2001;83:884-890.

27. Kuijlen JM, Herpers MJ, Beuls EA. Neurogenic claudication, a delayed complication of retained bullet. *Spine.* 1997;22:910-914.

28. Scuderi GJ, Vaccaro AR, Fitzhenry LN, et al. Long-term clinical manifestations of retained bullet fragments within the intervertebral disk space. *J Spinal Disord Tech.* 2004;17:108-111.

29. Papadopoulos SM, Selden NR, Quint DJ, et al. Immediate spinal cord decompression for cervical spinal cord injury: feasibility and outcome. *J Trauma.* 2002;52:323-332.

30. Vaccaro AR, Daugherty RJ, Sheehan TP, et al. Neurologic outcome of early versus late surgery for cervical spinal cord injury. *Spine.* 1997;22(22):2609-2613.

31. Dimar JR, Glassman SD, Raque GH, et al. The influence of spinal canal narrowing and timing of decompression on neurologic recovery after spinal cord contusion in a rat model. *Spine.* 1999;24:1623-1633.

32. Fehlings MG, Sekhon LH, Tator C. The role and timing of decompression in acute spinal cord injury: what do we know? What should we do? *Spine.* 2001;26(24 Suppl):S101-S110.

33. Haiyun Y, Rui G, Shucai D, et al. Three-column reconstruction through single posterior approach for the treatment of unstable thoracolumbar fracture. *Spine.* 2010;35(8):295-302.

34. Geerts WH, Code KI, Jay RM, et al. A prospective study of venous thromboembolism after major trauma. *N Engl J Med.* 1994;331(24):1601-1606.

35. Myllynen P, Kammonen M, Rokkanen P, et al. Deep venous thrombosis and pulmonary embolism in patients with acute spinal cord injury: a comparison with nonparalyzed patients immobilized due to spinal fractures. *J Trauma.* 1985;25(6):541-543.

36. Devivo MJ, Kartus PL, Stover SL, et al. Cause of death for patients with spinal cord injuries. *Arch Intern Med.* 1989;149(8):1761-1766.

37. Jones T, Ugalde V, Franks P, et al. Venous thromboembolism after spinal cord injury: incidence, time course, and associated risk factors in 16,240 adults and children. *Arch Phys Med Rehabil.* 2005;86(12):2240-2247.

38. Ploumis A, Ponnappan RK, Maltenfort MG, et al. Thromboprophylaxis in patients with acute spinal cord injuries: an evidence-based analysis. *J Bone Joint Surg Am.* 2009;91(11):2568-2576.

39. Rosner MK, Kuklo TR, Tawk R, et al. Prophylactic placement of an inferior vena cava filter in high-risk patients undergoing spinal reconstruction. *Neurosurg Focus.* 2004;17:E6.

40. Simons RK, Hoyt DB, Winchell RJ, et al. A risk analysis of stress ulceration after trauma. *J Trauma.* 1995;39:289-293.

41. Lemons VR, Wagner FC Jr. Respiratory complications after cervical spinal cord injury. *Spine.* 1994;19:2315-2320.

42. McMichan JC, Michel L, Westbrook PR. Pulmonary dysfunction following traumatic quadriplegia; recognition, prevention, and treatment. *JAMA.* 1980;243:528-531.

43. Berney S, Stockton K, Berlowitz D, et al. Can early extubation and intensive physiotherapy decrease length of stay of acute quadriplegic patients in intensive care? A retrospective case control study. *Physiother Res Int.* 2002;7:14-22.

44. Masry WS, Biyani A. Incidence, management, and outcome of posttraumatic synringomyelia. *J Neurol Neurosurg Psychiatry.* 1996;60:141-146.

45. Perrouin-Verbe B, Lenne-Aurier K, Auffray-Calvier E, et al. Posttraumatic syringomyelia and posttraumatic spinal canal stenosis: a direct relationship: review of 75 patients with a spinal cord injury. *Spinal Cord.* 1998;36:137-143.

46. Schurch B, Wichmann W, Rossier AB. Posttraumatic syringomyelia: a prospective study of 449 patients with spinal cord injury. *J Neurol Neurosurg Psychiatry.* 1996;60:61-67.

47. Williams B, Terry AF, Francis-Jones HW, et al. Syringomyelia as a sequel to traumatic paraplegia. *Paraplegia.* 1981;19:67-80.

FINANCIAL DISCLOSURES

Dr, Romney C. Andersen has received research support from the MARP and PRORP and travel support from the TRUE.

Dr. Martin F. Baechler has no financial or proprietary interest in the materials presented herein.

Dr. Philip J. Belmont Jr has no financial or proprietary interest in the materials presented herein.

Dr. Michael J. Beltran has no financial or proprietary interest in the materials presented herein.

Dr. James P. Bradley has not disclosed any relevant financial relationships.

Dr. Trevor S. Brown has no financial or proprietary interest in the materials presented herein.

Dr. Chester C. Buckenmaier III has no financial or proprietary interest in the materials presented herein.

Dr. Travis C. Burns has no financial or proprietary interest in the materials presented herein.

Dr. Joseph Carney has no financial or proprietary interest in the materials presented herein.

Dr. D.C. Covey has not disclosed any relevant financial relationships.

Dr. Jonathan F. Dickens has no financial or proprietary interest in the materials presented herein.

Dr. Matthew L. Drake has no financial or proprietary interest in the materials presented herein.

Dr. Gerald L. Farber has no financial or proprietary interest in the materials presented herein.

Dr. James R. Ficke has no financial or proprietary interest in the materials presented herein.

Dr. Mark E. Fleming has no financial or proprietary interest in the materials presented herein.

Dr. Jonathan Agner Forsberg has no financial or proprietary interest in the materials presented herein.

Dr. Brett A. Freedman has no financial or proprietary interest in the materials presented herein.

Dr. Tad Gerlinger has no financial or proprietary interest in the materials presented herein.

Dr. Gens P. Goodman has no financial or proprietary interest in the materials presented herein.

Dr. Wade Gordon has received research funding from the Congressionally Directed Peer-Reviewed Orthopaedic Research Program.

Dr. David E. Gwinn has no financial or proprietary interest in the materials presented herein.

Dr. Kathryn H. Hanna has no financial or proprietary interest in the materials presented herein.

Mr. Zach Harvey has no financial or proprietary interest in the materials presented herein.

Dr. Roman Hayda has no financial or proprietary interest in the materials presented herein.

Dr. Eric P. Hofmeister has no financial or proprietary interest in the materials presented herein.

Dr. Joseph R. Hsu has received institutional research support from the Geneva Foundation and the Henry Jackson Foundation.

Dr. Wesley Jackson has no financial or proprietary interest in the materials presented herein.

Dr. Daniel G. Kang has no financial or proprietary interest in the materials presented herein.

Dr. Kelly G. Kilcoyne has no financial or proprietary interest in the materials presented herein.

Dr. Matthew Kluk has no financial or proprietary interest in the materials presented herein.

Dr. John F. Kragh Jr is an employee of the US Government and has consulted at no cost with Tiger Tourniquet LLC, Tactical Medical Solutions LLC, Combat Medical Solutions Inc, Composite Resources Inc, Delfi Medical Innovations Inc, North American Rescue Products LLC, H & H Associates Inc, Creative & Effective Technologies Inc, TEMS Solutions LLC, Blackhawk Products Group, and Hemaclear. He has received honoraria for work for the Food and Drug Administration for device panel consultation. He has received honoraria for trustee work for the nonprofit Musculoskeletal Transplant Foundation.

Dr. Leo T. Kroonen has no financial or proprietary interest in the materials presented herein.

Dr. Anand R. Kumar has no financial or proprietary interest in the materials presented herein.

Dr. Ronald A. Lehman Jr has no financial or proprietary interest in the materials presented herein.

Dr. Alan A. Lim has no financial or proprietary interest in the materials presented herein.

Dr. Robert McGill has no financial or proprietary interest in the materials presented herein.

Dr. Clinton K. Murray has no financial or proprietary interest in the materials presented herein.

Dr. Leon J. Nesti has not disclosed any relevant financial relationships.

Dr. Brett D. Owens has no financial or proprietary interest in the materials presented herein.

Dr. Mark Pallis has no financial or proprietary interest in the materials presented herein.

Dr. Benjamin K. Potter has no financial or proprietary interest in the materials presented herein.

Dr. Damian Rispoli has no financial or proprietary interest in the materials presented herein.

Dr. Michael K. Rosner has no financial or proprietary interest in the materials presented herein.

Dr. Andrew J. Schoenfeld has no financial or proprietary interest in the materials presented herein.

Dr. Scott B. Shawen has no financial or proprietary interest in the materials presented herein.

Dr. Dirk L. Slade has no financial or proprietary interest in the materials presented herein.

Dr. Daniel J. Stinner has no financial or proprietary interest in the materials presented herein.

Dr. Joseph E. Strauss has no financial or proprietary interest in the materials presented herein.

Dr. Kenneth F. Taylor has no financial or proprietary interest in the materials presented herein.

Dr. Joachim Jude Tenuta has no financial or proprietary interest in the materials presented herein.

Dr. Scott Tintle has no financial or proprietary interest in the materials presented herein.

Dr. Jared A. Vogler has not disclosed any relevant financial relationships.

Dr. Scott Waterman has not disclosed any relevant financial relationships.

INDEX